Bladder Exstrophy and Epispadias

Aseem R. Shukla • Rakesh S. Joshi
Editors-in-Chief

Joao Luiz Pippi Salle • Pramod P. Reddy
Dana A. Weiss • Paul A. Merguerian
Jaishri Ramji
Associate Editors

Bladder Exstrophy and Epispadias

A Compendium

Springer

Editors-in-Chief
Aseem R. Shukla, MD, MHCI
Division of Urology
Children's Hospital of Philadelphia
Philadelphia, PA, USA

Perelman School of Medicine
University of Pennsylvania
Philadelphia, PA, USA

Rakesh S. Joshi, MCh, DNB
Department of Paediatric Surgery
B. J. Medical College and Civil Hospital
Ahmedabad, Gujarat, India

Associate Editors
Joao Luiz Pippi Salle, MD
Division of Urology
SickKids Hospital and Co-Director of the
Center for Pelvic Reconstruction
Toronto, Canada

Dana A. Weiss, MD
Division of Urology
Childrens Hospital of Philadelphia
Philadelphia, PA, USA

Jaishri Ramji, MCh
Department of Paediatric Surgery
Ahmedabad Civil Hospital
Ahmedabad, India

Pramod P. Reddy, MD
Burnet Campus
Cincinnati Children's
Cincinnati, OH, USA

Paul A. Merguerian, MD
Division of Urology
Seattle Children's Hospital
Seattle, WA, USA

ISBN 978-3-031-91237-5 ISBN 978-3-031-91238-2 (eBook)
https://doi.org/10.1007/978-3-031-91238-2

This Springer imprint is published by the registered company Springer Nature Switzerland AG
The registered company address is: Gewerbestrasse 11, 6330 Cham, Switzerland

To the courageous children affected by bladder exstrophy and epispadias, whose indefatigable spirit, determination, and hope compel us to do better by them each day.

To Douglas Canning, Richard Grady, and Atul Thakre, our mentors lost too soon, whose exemplary lives of selflessness, grit, and love inspire us every day to be better.

Foreword

My fascination with congenital anomalies dates back to my time as a bright-eyed medical student and the correlation of how a seemingly small embryological miscue could lead to a major anatomical defect. The excitement of restoring form and function as I rotated on the surgical services propelled me to a career in urology and perhaps no clearer example between embryological maldevelopment and eventual anatomic anomaly exists than with the exstrophy-epispadias complex.

Driven to pursue reconstructive pediatric urology, I was fortunate to learn from Sir Herbert Johnston, one-half of the duo that founded the specialty of pediatric urology in the United Kingdom, at Alder Hey Children's Hospital in Liverpool, England, the first center to successfully close a child with cloacal exstrophy, and have him survive, in 1965. After completing additional training in pediatric surgical techniques, I truly believed I would return to Georgia and begin practice in pediatric urology; however, as fate—or a serendipitous plan by Robert Jeffs and Patrick C. Walsh—my plan and subsequent career was rerouted to Baltimore, MD.

I arrived at Johns Hopkins on February 1, 1985, and was fortunate to benefit from the knowledge and mentorship Bob (a pioneering surgeon and a founding father of pediatric urology in North America) offered in complex congenital genitourinary disorders. Though care for exstrophy at Johns Hopkins dated back to the 1920s with Hugh Hampton Young, Bob was the first to really establish a dedicated unit of excellence at Johns Hopkins specifically, and only, designated for children with exstrophy or epispadias. While he had established his multi-staged approach in the 1970s, with this now high-volume center, we worked to refine it and always sought to improve it. In 1996, I was fortunate, and humbled, to succeed him as Director of Pediatric Urology.

This second addition of *The Exstrophy-Epispadias Complex*, a book I originally edited with Dr. Ranjiv Mathews back in 1999, is more than a collection of authors and articles; it is the representation of many individuals' tireless work. Though my life's work has been the treatment and correction of the anatomical insult in exstrophy, I very much view the congenital spectrum with the same bright-eyed awe as I did during medical school each time I assuage a young couple's anxiety regarding a prenatal diagnosis. We have collectively gained much ground, but the work remains.

John P. Gearhart, MD, FAAP, FACS (Ed) (Hon)
Professor and Chief,
Jeffs Division of Pediatric Urology
The Brady Urological Institute,
Johns Hopkins Hospital
Baltimore, MD, USA

Foreword

I had the good fortune to be Dr. Hendren's second Fellow in Pediatric Urology. It was the period when Dr. Hendren was Chief of Pediatric Surgery at the MGH (later he was to become Chief at Boston Children's). He was a master surgeon and his teachings focused on the complex reconstruction of urologic malformations and form the basics of complete primary repair of exstrophy. Dr. W. Leadbetter (of ureteral reimplant) appreciated the surgical talent of Dr. Hendren and supported his active involvement in the training of pediatric urologic residents which included training Pediatric Urology Fellows. As Chief, of Pediatric Surgery, Dr. Hendren did it all, megaureter repairs, hypospadias, ureteral reimplants, and exstrophy closures (many as one stage procedures). Dr. Hendren trained only three Pediatric Urology Fellows at the MGH, but many after returning to Boston Children's.

I was fortunate to be one of those fellows and lifelong interest in bladder exstrophy was ignited. My observation of this anomaly has confirmed for me that bladder exstrophy presents on a spectrum, and whether a baby presents with cloacal exstrophy, bladder exstrophy, or penopubic epispadias depends on the timing of the premature rupture of the infra-umbilical membrane in relation to the descent of the urorectal septum.

While my preference developed for the complete primary repair of exstrophy, as surgeons we can only try to establish "normal anatomy" and anticipate that "normal" physiology will follow. We must recognize that likelihood of "normal" function depends in large part on where the exstrophy anomaly sits on the spectrum between cloacal exstrophy and epispadias.

I am pleased that this book dedicated to bladder exstrophy is bringing together today's surgeons that are committed to taking the baton and continuing to make strides in understanding, caring for, and advocating for children affected by exstrophy. I do hope that it is informative for the reader, and ideally, will ignite a passion in caregivers as Dr. Hendren did in me in those early days of my career in Boston.

Children's Hospital of Wisconsin
Medical College of Wisconsin
Milwaukee, WI, USA

Michael E. Mitchell, MD

Preface

Every book has an origin story, and this book's antecedents beg the reader's indulgence in sharing some recollections.

Nearly two decades ago, we met for the first time in an office that sat astride a small patient holding area, directly across the entrance to a solitary operating room that held two operating tables arrayed in parallel. We stood in a ward among the labyrinthine corridors of one of the largest hospitals in Asia, the Civil Hospital-Ahmedabad, a safety-net and tertiary hospital serving the 60 million inhabitants of India's state of Gujarat. Aseem, visiting from Minneapolis, was accompanied by the already well-known bladder exstrophy expert surgeon from Seattle, Richard Grady. Across the table sat Rakesh, a pediatric surgeon at Civil Hospital, and a partner to the host that day, Atul Thakre, who had recently completed a pediatric urology fellowship and was embarking on a practice at Civil Hospital.

That patient holding area across from the office reverberated with the giggles and cries of a dozen children with bladder exstrophy at various stages—primary, failed, and complex variants—in the laps of their bewildered parents, looking expectantly for a solution to an anomaly they could not understand, but would bear out of their love for their child.

Beholding that gaggle of children that day in 2009—more than we might see at an American children's hospital in an entire year—Richard and Aseem, joined in ensuing years by pediatric anesthesiologist Anjana Kundu, Cincinnati's Pramod P. Reddy, Civil Hospital's own Jaishri Ramji, Toronto's Joao Luiz Pippi Salle, Seattle's Paul A. Merguerian, and Philadelphia's Douglas Canning and Dana Weiss, each a co-editor of this compendium, committed to returning every year to work together at Civil Hospital to surgically repair, research, and teach bladder exstrophy and epispadias surgery. The care for these children is possible only because of the expert faculty, residents, administration, nurses, and entire tireless staff of Civil Hospital for welcoming, nurturing, and hosting the annual gathering. Our growing cohort of surgeons, anesthesiologists, nurses, advocates, and affected families soon took on an appellation: the International Bladder Exstrophy Collaborative (IBEC).

As IBEC grew—the cohort now includes close to 300 children with bladder exstrophy and epispadias—and our research endeavors began grappling with fundamental questions about technique and outcomes with dozens of pediatric urologists from around the world descending on Ahmedabad to immerse in the annual IBEC workshop, the contours of this book were contemplated.

The venerable authority on bladder exstrophy, Dr. John Gearhart last edited a book dedicated to bladder exstrophy in 1999, which he published with Springer Nature. We are honored that this successor book to Dr. Gearhart's pioneering effort is also hosted by the same Springer Nature in making this present effort a reality. We sincerely hope that this book conveys the advances in bladder exstrophy embryology, radiological diagnosis, and genetics and comprehensively shares—with vivid videos—the nuances of the modern staged repair, complete primary repair, and radical soft tissue mobilization (Kelly repair) approach to repairing bladder exstrophy and penopubic epispadias. We also explore long-term concerns of exstrophy such as incontinence, cosmesis, sexual function, and most importantly, how our efforts, as physicians, impact a patient's sense of self and satisfaction. This book also offers the perspective on the critical role of nursing and also that of caregivers and advocates.

A book comes to fruition only with a legion of support. We are indebted firstly to the courageous children and caregivers affected by the rare and devastating anomaly of bladder exstrophy and epispadias. It is their hopes, aspirations, and indefatigable smiles in the face of immense adversity that inspire us as every day as practitioners, and whose wellness is the North Star to this effort.

We are grateful to Dr. Michael Mitchell and Dr. John Gearhart, living legends who have transformed the lives of children with bladder exstrophy not only as surgeons but as dogged perfectionists and students of their discipline, spending careers articulating their chosen approaches to exstrophy surgery while setting the highest bar in elucidating outcomes with honesty and transparency. We are honored to have their reflections as a preface to this book. We are profoundly thankful to our co-editors—each of whom is a surgical leader of IBEC—for sharing in this undertaking, and every chapter author and co-author without whose exhaustive effort and willingness to share their precious time and expertise, this book would not exist. Our deep appreciation to the efforts of our editors with Springer Nature, Priyanka Dey, and Paige Ripperger, whose daily nudges became a fixture of our inbox to ensure completion of this undertaking.

To Suhag, Parth, and Nimai: thank you for your love. And thank you for your encouragement, patience, and endurance in the face of another weekend of, "Can't help around the house, have this book to finish!"

To Rima, Vidhi, and Dev: thank you for your unconditional love and everlasting support despite extended working hours balancing the responsibilities of a pediatric surgery department and Medical Superintendent duties at Civil Hospital.

Atul Thakre, Richard Grady, and Doug Canning wrote the first chapters of the IBEC story, but fate determined that they would not write the epilogue. Their joyful spirit animates and suffuses the totality of this book—every written word, each chapter and video—and they continue to gently guide our hands whenever we embark on the care of an affected child. Doug's dictum—start with the child and go out from there, is our IBEC motto. This book is dedicated to their eternal spirit. Om Sadgati.

With appreciation,

Philadelphia, PA, USA — Aseem R. Shukla
Ahmedabad, Gujarat, India — Rakesh S. Joshi

Contents

Contributors

Rita Agarwal Department of Anesthesiology, Lucille Packard Children's Hospital, Stanford University, Palo Alto, CA, USA

Pamela Artigas Association for the Bladder Exstrophy Community (A-BE-C), Vero Beach, FL, USA

Pavai Arunachalam Department of Pediatric Surgery, PSG IMS&R, Coimbatore, Tamil Nadu, India

Susan J. Back Department of Radiology, Children's Hospital of Philadelphia, Philadelphia, PA, USA

Perelman School of Medicine, University of Pennsylvania, Philadelphia, PA, USA

Soroush Baghdadi Department of Orthopedic Surgery, UCLA, Los Angeles, CA, USA

Darius Bagli Division of Urology, Department of Surgery, Sickkids Hospital, University of Toronto, Toronto, ON, Canada

Ravi Kishore Barla Department of Pediatric Surgery, CMC Hospital, Vellore, Tamil Nadu, India

Caroline Bergh Department of Physical Therapy, Children's Hospital of Philadelphia, Philadelphia, PA, USA

Joseph Borer Department of Surgery, Harvard Medical School, Boston, MA, USA

Lesley Breech University of Cincinnati School of Medicine, Department of Obstetrics and Gynecology, Cincinnati, OH, USA

Cincinnati Children's Hospital Medical Center, Cincinnati, OH, USA

Stefano Cardin Division of Pediatric Orthopaedics, Orlando Health – Arnold Palmer Hospital for Children, Orlando, FL, USA

Michael Chua Division of Pediatric Urology, Hospital for Sick Children, University of Toronto, Toronto, ON, Canada

Stephanie Cizek Stanford University School of Medicine, Department of Obstetrics and Gynecology, Division of Pediatric and Adolescent Gynecology, Palo Alto, CA, USA

Lucille Packard Children's Hospital, Palo Alto, CA, USA

Sarah Cooper Department of Physical Therapy, Children's Hospital of Philadelphia, Philadelphia, PA, USA

Chad B. Crigger Jeffs Division of Pediatric Urology, The Brady Urological Institute, Johns Hopkins Hospital, Baltimore, MD, USA

Carolyn Fazzini Children's Hospital of Philadelphia, Philadelphia, PA, USA

Nicolas Fernandez Division of Pediatric Urology, Seattle Children's Hospital, Seattle, WA, USA

University of Washington, Seattle, WA, USA

Vinod Gautam Department of Orthopedics, Government Medical Collage, Gujarat, India

John P. Gearhart Jeffs Division of Pediatric Urology, The Brady Urological Institute, Johns Hopkins Hospital, Baltimore, MD, USA

Juliana Gebb Richard D. Wood Jr. Center for Fetal Diagnosis and Treatment, Children's Hospital of Philadelphia, Philadelphia, PA, USA

Perelman School of Medicine at University of Pennsylvania, Philadelphia, PA, USA

Karl F. Godlewski Children's Hospital of Philadelphia, Philadelphia, PA, USA

Travis Groth Pediatric Urology, Children's Wisconsin, Medical College of Wisconsin, Milwaukee, WI, USA

Archika Gupta Department of Pediatric Surgery, King Geroge's Medical University, Lucknow, India

Emily Haddad Association for the Bladder Exstrophy Community (A-BE-C), Vero Beach, FL, USA

Amber Heberling Seattle Children's Hospital, Seattle, WA, USA

Sangeeta Hingorani University of Washington School of Medicine, Department of Pediatrics, Division of Nephrology, Seattle Children's Hospital, Seattle, WA, USA

B. David Horn Department of Orthopedic Surgery, The Children's Hospital of Philadelphia, Philadelphia, PA, USA

V. Rama Jayanthi Department of Pediatric Urology, Nationwide Children's Hospital, Columbus, OH, USA

Navroop S. Johal Department of Paediatric Urology, Great Ormond Street Hospital for Children NHS Foundation Trust, London, UK

Rakesh S. Joshi Department of Pediatric Surgery, B. J. Medical College and Civil Hospital, Ahmedabad, Gujarat, India

Department of Paediatric Surgery, Ahmedabad Civil Hospital, Ahmedabad, Gujarat, India

John Kryger Pediatric Urology, Children's Wisconsin, Medical College of Wisconsin, Milwaukee, WI, USA

Anjana Kundu Department of Anesthesiology and Perioperative Medicine, Golisano Children's Hospital and University of Rochester, Rochester, NY, USA

S. N. Kureel Department of Pediatric Surgery, King Geroge's Medical University, Lucknow, India

Ted Lee Department of Urology, Boston Children's Hospital, Boston, MA, USA

Paul A. Merguerian Seattle Children's Hospital, University of Washington, Seattle, WA, USA

Michael E. Mitchell Children's Hospital of Philadelphia, Philadelphia, PA, USA

Children's Hospital of Wisconsin, Medical College of Wisconsin, Milwaukee, WI, USA

Piyush Sudamalal Mittal Department of Orthopaedic, Civil Hospital, B.J. Medical College & Government Spine Institute, Ahmedabad, Gujarat, India

Julie S. Moldenhauer Richard D. Wood Jr. Center for Fetal Diagnosis and Treatment, Children's Hospital of Philadelphia, Philadelphia, PA, USA

Perelman School of Medicine at University of Pennsylvania, Philadelphia, PA, USA

Camila Moreno Division of Urology, Department of Surgery, Sickkids Hospital, University of Toronto, Toronto, ON, Canada

Jacqueline P. Morin Department of Pediatric Urology, Nationwide Children's Hospital, Columbus, OH, USA

Imran Mushtaq Department of Paediatric Urology, Great Ormond Street Hospital for Children NHS Foundation Trust, London, UK

Edward R. Oliver Department of Radiology and Richard D. Wood Jr. Center for Fetal Diagnosis and Treatment, Children's Hospital of Philadelphia, Philadelphia, PA, USA

Perelman School of Medicine, University of Pennsylvania, Philadelphia, PA, USA

Lisa Pilchman Children's Hospital Los Angeles, Los Angeles, CA, USA

Jaishri Ramji Department of Pediatric Surgery, B. J. Medical College and Civil Hospital, Ahmedabad, Gujarat, India

Pramod P. Reddy Division of Pediatric Urology, Cincinnati Children's, Cincinnati, OH, USA

Rodrigo L. P. Romao Division of Pediatric Urology, Division of Pediatric General and Thoracic Surgery, Hospital for Sick Children, University of Toronto, Toronto, ON, Canada

Elizabeth Roth Pediatric Urology, Children's Wisconsin, Medical College of Wisconsin, Milwaukee, WI, USA

Christina M. Rouse Division of Urology, Children's Hospital of Philadelphia, Philadelphia, PA, USA

Joao Luiz Pippi Salle Division of Urology, SickKids Hospital and Co-Director of the Center for Pelvic Reconstruction, Toronto, Canada

Mehak Sehgal Department of Paediatric Urology, Great Ormond Street Hospital for Children NHS Foundation Trust, London, UK

Sudipta Sen Department of Pediatric Surgery, PSG IMS&R, Coimbatore, Tamil Nadu, India

Department of Pediatric Surgery, CMC Hospital, Vellore, Tamil Nadu, India

Margarett Shnorhavorian University of Washington, Department of Urology, Seattle, WA, USA

Seattle Children's Hospital, Division of Pediatric Urology, Seattle, WA, USA

Aseem R. Shukla Children's Hospital of Philadelphia, Philadelphia, PA, USA

Perelman School of Medicine, University of Pennsylvania, Philadelphia, PA, USA

Katelyn A. Spencer Children's Hospital of Philadelphia, Philadelphia, PA, USA

Perelman School of Medicine, University of Pennsylvania, Philadelphia, PA, USA

Raimund Stein Center for Pediatric, Adolescent and Reconstructive Urology, University Medical Center Mannheim, Medical Faculty Mannheim Heidelberg University, Mannheim, Germany

Kanoujia Sunil Chandan Institute of Pediatric and Neonatology, Lucknow, India

Brian A. VanderBrink Division of Pediatric Urology, Cincinnati Children's Hospital Medical Center, Cincinnati, OH, USA

John K. Weaver Cleveland Clinic Lerner College of Medicine at Case Western Reserve University School of Medicine, Cleveland, OH, USA

Dana A. Weiss Children's Hospital of Philadelphia, Philadelphia, PA, USA

Perelman School of Medicine at the University of Pennsylvania, Philadelphia, PA, USA

Chen-Han Wilfred Wu Case Western Reserve University School of Medicine, Cleveland, OH, USA

Lissa Yu University of Washington School of Medicine, Department of Obstetrics and Gynecology, Division of Pediatric and Adolescent Gynecology, Seattle, WA, USA

Seattle Children's Hospital, Seattle, WA, USA

Arvid Yung Department of Anesthesiology and Perioperative Medicine, Golisano Children's Hospital and University of Rochester, Rochester, NY, USA

Epidemiology and Embryology of the Bladder Exstrophy: Epispadias Complex

1

Nicolas Fernandez, Camila Moreno, and Darius Bagli

Introduction

Bladder exstrophy and epispadias complex is a spectrum of anomalies that affect genital and bladder development.

The embryology and developmental pathology are complex and involve interaction between multiple tissue and cell types. Currently, most of the mechanistic details regarding the precise etiology of bladder exstrophy remain unknown. Our understanding remains limited to several published theories given the inability to follow early human embryological events to the final development of exstrophy in the late fetus.

The purpose of this chapter is to present the available epidemiology and review the present embryological, physiopathological, and molecular understanding of this complex condition.

Epidemiology

Bladder exstrophy is a rare and complex birth defect. It is considered a spectrum that includes epispadias, classic bladder exstrophy, and omphalocele-exstrophy imperforated anus spinal anomaly (OEIS) [1]. The global reported prevalence is 2–8

N. Fernandez
Division of Pediatric Urology, Seattle Children's Hospital, Seattle, WA, USA

University of Washington, Seattle, WA, USA
e-mail: Nicolas.fernandez@seattlechildrens.org

C. Moreno · D. Bagli (✉)
Division of Urology, Department of Surgery, Sickkids Hospital, University of Toronto, Toronto, ON, Canada
e-mail: darius.bagli@sickkids.ca

A. R. Shukla, R. S. Joshi (eds.), *Bladder Exstrophy and Epispadias*, https://doi.org/10.1007/978-3-031-91238-2_1

cases per 100,000 newborns [2, 3]. Depending on the type of defect, different prevalence rates have been reported. For epispadias, the reported prevalence is 2.4 per 100,000 newborns, with 2–4 per 100,000 newborns for bladder exstrophy and 0.5–1 per 100,000 newborns for OEIS [4]. One of the largest epidemiological analyses on bladder exstrophy reported 546 cases per 24,355,094 newborns, which results in a prevalence of 2 per 100,000 newborns. Reports of prevalence changes over time and high/low prevalence geographical clusters have been described in the past [3]. An initial report from the International Clearinghouse for Birth Defects Monitoring Systems (ICBDSR) between 1980 and 2006 reported a prevalence of 2.07 per 100,000 newborns (95% CI = 1.90–2.25) [2]. Another multinational study reported a prevalence of 3.3 per 100.000 newborns during the period between 1967 and 1985 [5] (Fig. 1.1).

Stillbirth prevalence has been reported to be 11 per 1000 stillborn fetuses [3]. Recent publications have reported a reduction in live birth prevalence over time, probably related to pregnancy terminations [3]. Interestingly, areas with prevalence below the worldwide average have been reported in China and South America [2]. The lack of epidemiological data from large, densely populated countries like India, where there are no national surveillance systems, limits the ability to conclude prevalence trends in this region [6]. Variations can be attributed to differences in case detection or variations in inclusion criteria used in different surveillance systems and whether epispadias cases alone are included in the spectrum or not. Specifically, case definition is reported to be different within surveillance systems, as seen in the EUROCAT [3].

Prenatal detection of bladder exstrophy was reported for the first time in 1995 by Gearhart et al. Diagnostic criteria include: (1) absence of a distended bladder, (2)

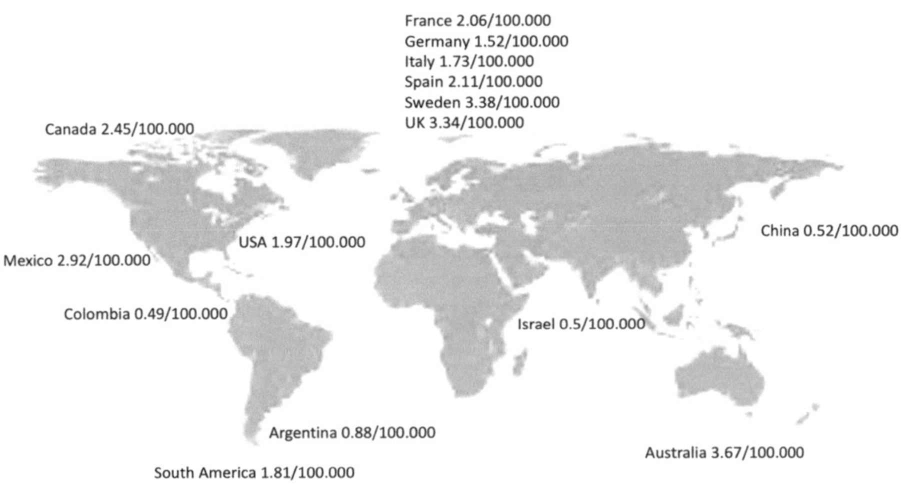

Fig. 1.1 Reported prevalence rates in literature for different regions in the world. Data from each region do not fall withing the same time periods [2, 3]

low insertion of the umbilical cord, (3) wide ramus pubis, (4) small genitalia, and (5) abdominal mass [7]. An accurate report of prenatal prevalence diagnosis is difficult to interpret given the technical difficulties in its detection, the timing of ultrasounds during pregnancy, and the regulations about pregnancy terminations in different regions of the world. A longitudinal cohort of prenatally screened patients reported that only one-quarter of the babies born with bladder exstrophy were detected with prenatal ultrasounds [8].

Bladder exstrophy presents 1.5–2.3 times more frequently in male patients than in females [9]. It is important to remember that in severe OEIS cases, initial gender designation itself may be challenging, requiring multidisciplinary management. For this reason, initial case identification by gender may not always be prospectively known [10].

The most common risk factors associated with bladder exstrophy are low birth weight and Caucasian ethnicity [2, 11, 12]. Smoking during pregnancy and prior family/siblings history of bladder exstrophy have been reported to be highly associated. Maternal age has also been identified as a risk factor, with older mothers having a higher risk. Exposure to endocrine disruptors and in vitro fertilization have also been described to support a 7.5-fold increased risk [13]. A large multinational study has reported a mortality of 6% in the first day of life and 3.5% in the first 6 days of life [3].

About one-third of patients born with bladder exstrophy have associated anomalies. Upper urinary tract anomalies are the most frequent, present in about 40% of the cases. Omphalocele is present in 34% of the cases, followed by anorectal malformations in 21%, neural tube defects in 18%, and cardiac anomalies in 15% [2, 12]. The risk of another child being born with bladder exstrophy in a given family is 1 in 100 cases [14]. Moreover, for pregnant women with bladder exstrophy, the reported risk of carrying a fetus with bladder exstrophy is 500 times greater than in the general pregnant population and is reported to be 1 in 70 newborns [9]. A higher risk of bladder exstrophy has also been reported within families with other members harboring midline congenital anomalies [15].

Embryology and Pathophysiology

Etymology

The term "exstrophy" in the medical context is used primarily to refer to conditions related to the abnormal development and exposure of internal organs. As is often the case, the term originates from the Greek. The word "ek" translates as "out," and "strophe" translates to "a turning." Thus, the term literally means a "turning inside out," capturing the medical conditions where internal organs are exposed or externalized. This accurately describes the nature of bladder exstrophy and, where present, penile epispadias, whose internal structures are presented outside the body cavity. Indeed, exstrophy of the bladder often co-presents with spinal, abdominal wall, and colorectal anomalies.

Normal Development

In normal development at the beginning of the third week of gestation, the future cloacal plate is discernible and composed of ectoderm and endoderm [16]. At the beginning of the fourth week of gestation, the paired genital tubercle forms along the upper part of the cloacal membrane. Fusion of the tubercles into a single genital structure occurs at the fifth week. Critical medial migration of mesenchymal cells will give origin to the muscular and skeletal structures of the pelvis and abdominal wall (Fig. 1.2).

Once the urorectal septum has grown sufficiently in the caudal direction, cloacal division into the bladder anlage and urogenital sinus ventrally and the rectum and hindgut dorsally is complete by the seventh week. This normally occurs after the aforementioned medial mesenchymal cell migration has been completed. The most distal aspect of the septum then defines the origin of the urogenital and rectal openings (formerly the single cloacal opening), both of which are covered by the urogenital and anal membranes, respectively (formerly the single cloacal membrane) (Fig. 1.3).

Whether an extension of these migration processes also enables the later medial closure or tubularization and ventralization of the urethra and spongiosal tissues and their final placement underneath the future corporal bodies is unknown. However, it must be remembered that the even rarer occurrence of isolated penile epispadias (without exstrophy) suggests that epispadias formation can be uncoupled from bladder exstrophy development, suggesting this may be governed by a separate mechanism (Figs. 1.4 and 1.5).

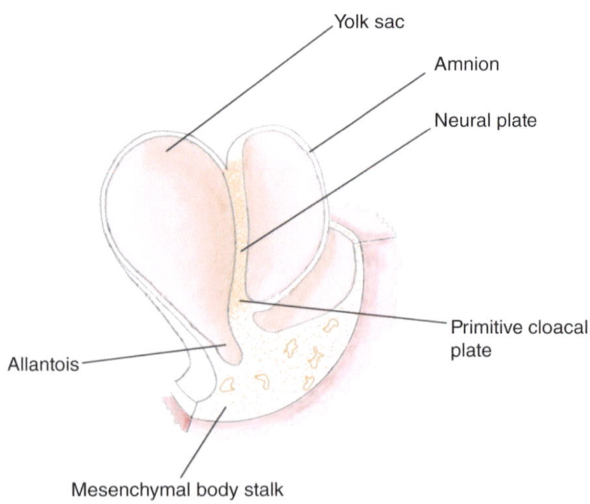

Fig. 1.2 Early embryological appearance of the cloacal plate at 2 weeks of gestation. Sagittal image of embryo

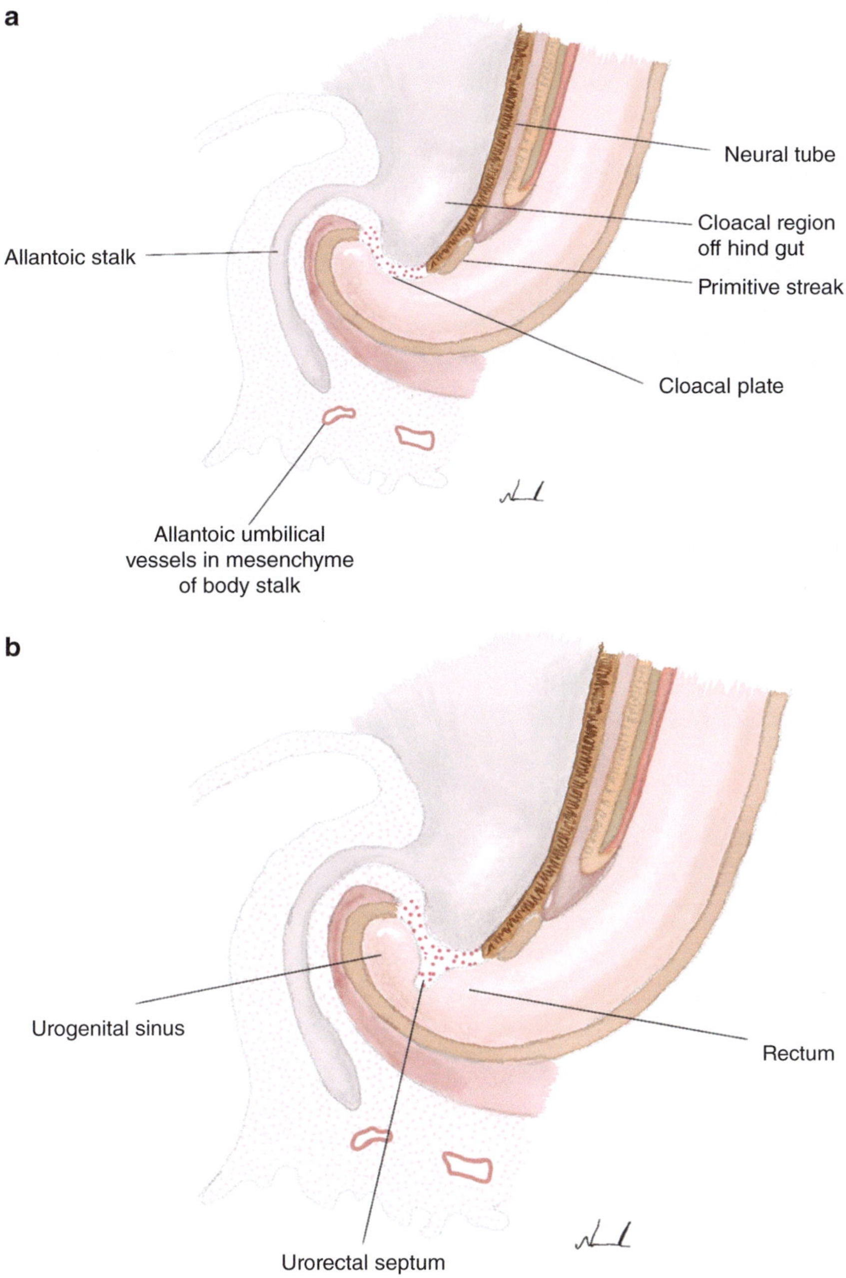

Fig. 1.3 (**a**) Cloacal plate begins the process of developing into the urorectal septum. (**b**) At 3 weeks of gestation, the septum will separate the urogenital sinus ventrally and the rectum dorsally

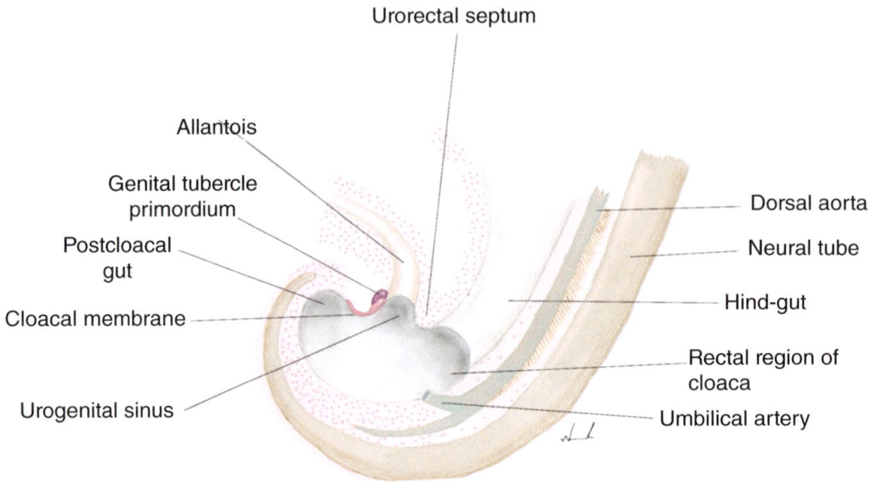

Fig. 1.4 Early formation of the genital tubercle and its relation to the cloacal membrane at 4 weeks of gestation

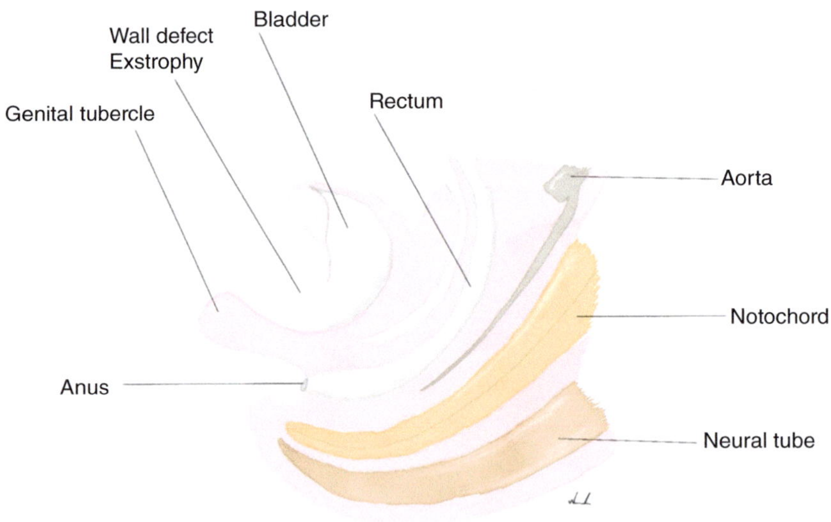

Fig. 1.5 Five weeks of gestation depicting the embryo with exstrophy and abdominal wall defect

It is important to point out that most of the embryologic etiologies for bladder exstrophy remain largely conjecture or hypothesis. No animal studies of bladder exstrophy to date have followed early embryonic development through to the late embryo and fetus to confirm the typically described events leading to bladder exstrophy. Nevertheless, some of the structural and molecular factors discussed below have been found to be associated with bladder exstrophy in mammalian models and in patients with bladder exstrophy. Bladder exstrophy development has essentially been centered around the caudal migration of the urorectal septum, where most embryologic theories are based around physical descriptions of disordered medial migration of mesenchymal tissues destined to become muscle and body wall and attempt to provide a rationale for this migration failure.

Historical Perspective and Proposed Theories

The earliest events in bladder development are concerned with increasing cellular differentiation into discrete mesenchymal (outer serosa, smooth muscle, and subepithelial lamina propria) and epithelial (uroepithelium) tissues. Additional cell types also invest the bladder wall, ultimately comprising its vascular and neural components, including resident cells such as macrophages with immunological or other functions. Whether and how these components are rendered abnormal at the cellular level during or after the earliest events leading to exstrophy and epispadias are not completely understood. Some of the prevailing cellular theories are discussed later below.

The first proposed hypothesis for bladder exstrophy was published by Patten and Barry in 1952 [17]. They proposed that a low insertion of the genital tubercle in relation to the cloacal membrane prevents normal mesodermal migration. This then causes an abnormal or premature rupture of the cloacal membrane. One cited problem with this theory is that if the genital tubercle is forming more caudally, bladder exstrophy should present regularly with penile structures in the perineal region, which is not seen in most cases of bladder exstrophy-epispadias [16].

The most accepted embryologic theory proposes a "wedge effect" and was initially described in 1962 by Marshall and Muecke [18, 19]. In 1988, Mildenberger elaborated on this idea, proposing that a caudal insertion of the embryo body stalk prevents the interposition of the mesenchymal tissue in the midline [20]. In this case, the most cephalad portion of the cloacal membrane remains in contact with the lower portion of the body stalk, causing a wedge effect. This hypothesis is thought to support the origin of severe OEIS cases.

Malrotation of pelvic ring primordia is another hypothesis proposed in 1997 by Beaudoin et al. [21]. This theory involving skeletal maldevelopment was later supported by Kumar et al. hypothesizing that the well-known pubic diastasis of bladder exstrophy is the inciting mechanism for bladder exstrophy formation as the principal disruptive phenomenon that occurs after organ formation [16]. They suggest that the levator muscles, rather than encircling the bladder neck/anal sphincter complex, form a hammock configuration due to the diastasis. The hammock becomes a pushing force moving the hindgut anteriorly (hence anterior displacement of the anus in exstrophy). The resulting progressive stretch on the remaining anterior bladder/developing penis structures leads to thinning (covered bladder exstrophy?) or outright rupture (exposed bladder exstrophy) [16]. While this hypothesis remains to be supported by any scientific evidence, it does add new consideration of the role of muscular and skeletal structures in the etiology of bladder exstrophy.

Around the same time, Stec et al. published a hypothesis involving three steps or opportunities for cellular dysfunction. Initially, premature rupture of the cloacal membrane occurs, followed by a mechanical obstruction or failure in mesodermal cell migration. This then results in cellular dysfunction leading to the anomaly [22], although how these events are orchestrated is unknown.

Bladder Exstrophy Pathophysiology

The failure of medial mesenchymal cell migration between the ectoderm of the abdomen and the cloaca is the most currently accepted pathophysiologic basis for bladder exstrophy [4]. Marshall and Muecke reported that the center of the anomaly originates at the area where the future bladder neck should form [19, 21]. This phenomenon occurs in the first 4 weeks of gestation, where an overdeveloped cloacal membrane then physically prevents mesenchymal cell migration, resulting in premature cloacal membrane rupture [4]. Conversely, it is unclear if normal mesenchymal migration is then preventing premature rupture of the cloacal membrane. Moreover, since the anus is often intact, normally developed, and patent, though somewhat anteriorly displaced in simple bladder (non-cloacal) exstrophy, this presumes the premature membrane rupture is limited to the urogenital membrane, sparing the anal membrane to open at the correct time. The timing of this crucial step of membrane rupture is thought to generate the different subtypes of the anomaly: isolated epispadias, bladder exstrophy, or—if the anal membrane or early single cloacal membrane ruptures prematurely—OEIS. Nevertheless, it remains paradoxical and unknown how a premature rupture of the anal membrane still results in imperforate anus. Presumably, premature lesser ruptures of the cloacal membrane before the urorectal septum has completely reached the cloacal membrane will result in an enterovesical fistula. Regarding isolated epispadias and membrane rupture, if only very distal/caudal membrane rupture occurs later when mesenchymal migration has completed abdominal wall formation covering the embryonic bladder but not yet contributed to tubularization/ventralization of the urethra and spongiosum, this could underlie the formation of isolated epispadias.

A rare subtype is the occult or so-called "covered" bladder exstrophy where a musculoskeletal defect exists without visceral exstrophy. The exact prevalence of this subtype has not been reported, and only isolated case reports have been published [23]. It is believed to be due to a sufficient mesodermal invasion into the infraumbilical cloacal membrane to thinly close the body wall, but insufficient deeper medial mesodermal migration to result in bladder closure itself [24].

Other theories of exstrophy development include an abnormal coordination of spatial-temporal formation of the pelvic bones and bladder [4].

It bears repeating that the observed uncoupling of events such as body wall closure, bladder closure, and penile closure raises the possibility that distinct mechanisms are involved and/or that temporal or spatial processing of a more unified process can be interrupted at various stages of development. Indeed, some authors have challenged the concept of grouping epispadias, bladder exstrophy, and OEIS together as a spectrum of a single condition. This is supported by the fact that the original experiments were performed using chicken embryos, which possess a normal persistent cloaca postnatally and have no pubic symphysis [21]. Also, as mentioned earlier, there is no stage in embryonal development where cloacal membrane rupture could physically result in displacement of the open urethral plate dorsally [21].

Newer Cellular Theories Underlying the Bladder Exstrophy-Epispadias Formation

While the above discussion has centered around anatomical and embryological theories, it is even more important to consider candidates at the cell and molecular level that may mediate the formation of bladder exstrophy-epispadias.

Sonic Hedgehog One of the key molecular steps in the normal development of the bladder involves epithelial-mesenchymal interplay or interaction between the urothelium and the underlying undifferentiated mesenchyme, destined to form bladder muscle (detrusor) [25, 26]. During normal bladder development, a group of signaling molecules becomes orchestrated by a protein known as sonic hedgehog (SHH). The secretion of SHH by the urothelium activates a cascade or pathway of additional proteins (SHH → Ptc1 → Gli2 → Bmp4) [27–29]. Acting together, this pathway results in the mesenchyme differentiating into bladder smooth muscle cells. Given the importance of these cellular events to bladder development, it is reasonable to hypothesize that spatial disruption of this pathway, particularly in the ventral aspect of the bladder, may be involved in the genesis of bladder exstrophy [27, 29, 30].

P63 A master regulator of epithelial development is the tumor suppressor protein TP63, transcribed from the p63 gene and a member of the P53 tumor suppressor family. The basal and intermediate layers of the urothelium express p63 during organogenesis [31–33]. Since p63 is responsible for normal urothelial development and function, and the urothelium is responsible for mesenchymal induction (see above), this presents two opportunities for potential disruption of bladder development in exstrophy. Indeed, p63 mice engineered to lack p63 expression ($p63^{-/-}$ knockout mice) show apoptosis and decreased proliferation in the urothelium with loss of urothelial smooth muscle development, *particularly in the ventral bladder wall* [30, 34, 35] (Fig. 1.6).

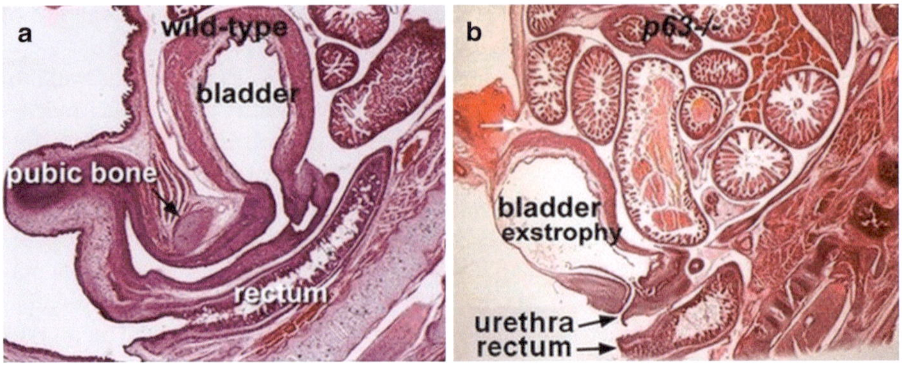

Fig. 1.6 (**a**) Histology of E18 wild-type mouse fetus. (**b**) $p63^{-/-}$ mouse fetus with thin ventral bladder wall. (Used with permission. Permission Pending)

Indeed, a study comparing 163 patients (98% with classic bladder exstrophy) and 285 ethnically matched controls revealed 7 single nucleotide polymorphisms (SNPs) and 4 insertion/deletion (in/del) polymorphisms in a region of the p63 gene promoter named ΔNP63. Importantly, ΔNP63 is a key regulator of anti-apoptosis in the urothelium. While none of the SNPs were significantly associated with bladder exstrophy incidence, a statistically significant increased risk of bladder exstrophy-epispadias was associated with three out of four in/del ΔNP63 polymorphisms [36].

PERP and Desmosomes PERP (p53 apoptosis effector related to PMP-22) is a plasma membrane protein. In humans, it is encoded by the PERP gene. PERP emerged as a possible effector in bladder exstrophy from a gene expression profiling study by Qi et al. of human exstrophy and human and murine embryonic bladder tissues [37]. The significance of this finding is that the PERP promoter is bound not only by p53 but also by p63 (see above), suggesting that PERP is regulated by p63 signaling [38, 39] P63-PERP regulation indeed has a clinical correlate in at least one human syndrome [40].

Knockout studies reveal PERP is an essential component of the desmosome, a cell complex critical for cells to adhere to each other in maintaining tissue integrity. Without PERP, tissue integrity is compromised [41]. Furthermore, of the 162 differentially expressed genes identified in Qi's gene profiling study, 30% are associated with the desmosome. Three key components of the desmosome, desmoplakin (DSP), desmin (DES) and desmulin (DMN) were the sixth most overexpressed (DSP) and two most underexpressed (DES & DMN) genes, respectively, in the bladder exstrophy samples [37]. Furthermore, multiple studies confirm that PERP and desmosomal components work tightly together at the physical molecular level to maintain the integrity of all epithelia [38, 41, 42].

Based on the above interactions drawn from human and knockout animal data, Mahfuz et al. have proposed a unifying hypothesis that p63 → PERP ↔ desmosomes may be a pathway of molecular epithelial and mesenchymal signaling disruption leading to bladder exstrophy formation [30].

Additional Molecular Candidates The WNT5A gene has been found up-regulated 14-fold in bladder exstrophy patient samples. In murine cloacal mesoderm, mouse Gli2 overexpression induced the expression of Wnt5A, and in cloacal ectoderm, Gli2 also up-regulated p63 expression. Together this allows speculation that there is a common upstream pathway regulating both p63 and Wnt5A [43].

A review by Hall et al. discusses additional candidate genes linked to bladder exstrophy, including human chromosomal duplication in the region of 22q11.21 [44–46], which includes a novel heterozygous missense variant in the LZRT1 gene [47]. A genome-wide association study on 110 bladder exstrophy patients vs. 1177 controls identified that changes in a locus involving a variant of ISL-1 (encoding the insulin gene enhancer protein) on chromosome 5q11.1 were associated with increased risk for bladder exstrophy [48].

Given the importance of the cloacal membrane discussed above, progenitor cells adjacent to the cloacal mesenchyme are regulated by transcription factors Six1 and Six2 and signaling by Dkk1. These factors are required for normal growth and development of the perineum and could also be target molecular candidates in bladder exstrophy development [49, 50].

Kasprenski et al. (2020) reported reduced uroplakin-II (UPII) and p63 expression in specimens from the entire bladder exstrophy spectrum (CBE, CE, and epispadias) when compared to controls. Uroplakins are key molecules involved in urothelial differentiation and permeability barrier development [51]. After surgical closure, bladder exstrophy is also associated with a persistent increase in the expression of protein markers including CK13, CK29, UPIIIa, claudin 4, UPII, and p63 [52]. Whether or not these gene changes are solely related to bladder exposure to the external environment or also regulate the genesis of the anomaly itself, they serve as potential targets for developmental study.

Conclusion

The etiology of the bladder exstrophy and epispadias complex involves multiple systems, including the urogenital, colorectal, and musculoskeletal tissues. Several theories try to explain the physiopathology and embryology, but no consensus currently exists. The most critical embryological structures and events include the cloacal membrane, the timing of its rupture, the presence or absence of a urorectal septum, and an abnormal migration of mesenchymal cells. Moreover, the molecular aspects of this condition have also been studied with suspected involvement of the SHH cascade and P63 master regulator influence on mesenchymal induction. Despite this considerable data, it is clear a great deal remains to be elucidated to better understand the physiopathological, embryological, or molecular mechanisms of bladder exstrophy development. Such insight may one day pave the way for improved management of this challenging condition, or even its prevention altogether.

References

1. Lowentritt BH, Sean Van Zijl P, Frimberger D, Baird A, Lakshmanan Y, Gearhart JP. Variants of the exstrophy complex: a single institution experience. J Urol. 2005;173:1732–7.
2. Siffel C, Correa A, Amar E, Bakker MK, Bermejo-Sánchez E, Bianca S, et al. Bladder exstrophy: an epidemiologic study from the International Clearinghouse for Birth Defects Surveillance and Research, and an overview of the literature. Am J Med Genet C Semin Med Genet. 2011;157(4):321–32.
3. Kancherla V, Tandaki L, Sundar M, Lux A, Bakker MK, Bergman JE, et al. A multicountry analysis of prevalence and mortality among neonates and children with bladder exstrophy. Am J Perinatol. 2022;41:1143.
4. Lee T, Borer J. Exstrophy-epispadias complex. Urol Clin North Am. 2023;50:403–14. W.B. Saunders.
5. International Clearinghouse for Birth Defects Monitoring Systems (ICBDMS). Epidemiology of bladder exstrophy and epispadias: a communication from the International Clearinghouse for Birth Defects Monitoring Systems. Teratology. 1987;36(2):221–7.
6. Joshi RS, Shrivastava D, Grady R, Kundu A, Ramji J, Reddy PP, et al. A model for sustained collaboration to address the unmet global burden of bladder exstrophy-epispadias complex and penopubic epispadias the international bladder exstrophy consortium. JAMA Surg. 2018;153(7):618–24.
7. Gearhart J, Ben-Chaim J, Jeffs R, Sanders R. Criteria for the prenatal diagnosis of classic bladder exstrophy. Obstet Gynecol. 1995;85:961–4.
8. Goyal A, Fishwick J, Hurrell R, Cervellione RM, Dickson AP. Antenatal diagnosis of bladder/cloacal exstrophy: challenges and possible solutions. J Pediatr Urol. 2012;8(2):140–4. Available from: https://doi.org/10.1016/j.jpurol.2011.05.003.
9. Shapiro E, Lepor H, Jeffs R. The inheritance of the exstrophy-epispadias complex. J Urol. 1984;132:308–10.
10. Gordetsky J, Joseph DB. Cloacal exstrophy: a history of gender reassignment. Urology. 2015;86(6):1087–9. Available from: https://doi.org/10.1016/j.urology.2015.06.056.
11. Ebert AK, Zwink N, Jenetzky E, Stein R, Boemers TM, Lacher M, et al. Association between exstrophy-epispadias complex and congenital anomalies: a German multicenter study. Urology. 2019;123:210–20.
12. Gearhart JP, Benson J, Silver RI, Caddedu J, Lakshmanan Y, Jeffs RD. Spinal anomalies in classic bladder exstrophy. Br J Urol. 1997;79(Suppl. 4):16.
13. Wood H, Trock B, Gearhart J. In vitro fertilization and the cloacal-bladder exstrophy-epispadias complex: is there an association? J Urol. 2003;2003:1512–5.
14. Ives E, Coffey R, Carter C. A family study of bladder exstrophy. J Med Genet. 1980;17(2):139–41.
15. Boyadijiev S, Dodson J, Radford C. Clinical and molecular characterization of the bladder exstrophy-epispadias complex: analysis of 232 families. BJU Int. 2004;94:1337.
16. Kumar S, Mammen A, Varma K. Pathogenesis of bladder exstrophy a new hypothesis. J Pediatr Urol. 2015;11(314):318.
17. Patten J, Barry A. The genesis of exstrophy of the bladder and epispadias. Am J Anat. 1952;90(1):35–57.
18. Muecke EC. The role of the cloacal membrane in exstrophy: the first successful experimental study. J Urol. 1964;92:659–67. Available from: http://www.ncbi.nlm.nih.gov/pubmed/14241195.
19. Marshall V, Muecke E. Variations in exstrophy of the bladder. J Urol. 1962;88:766–96.
20. Mildenberger H, Kluth D, Dzuiba M. Embryology of bladder exstrophy. J Pediatr Surg. 1988;23(2):166–70.
21. Beaudoin S, Simon L, Bargy F. Anatomical basis of a common embryological origin for epispadias and bladder or cloacal exstrophies. Surg Radiol Anat. 1997;19:11–6.

22. Stec A. Embryology and bony and pelvic floor anatomy in the bladder exstrophy-epispadias complex. Semin Pediatr Surg. 2011;20:66–70.
23. Borwankar SS, Kasat LS, Naregal A, Jain M, Bajaj R. Covered exstrophy: a rare variant. Pediatr Surg Int. 1998;14:129.
24. Chadha R, Sharma A, Bagga D, Mahajan JK. Covered exstrophy with incomplete duplication of the bladder. Pediatr Surg Int. 1999;15:422.
25. Baskin L, Hayward S, Young P, Cunha G. Role of mesenchymal epithelial interactions in normal bladder development. J Urol. 1996;156:1820e–7e.
26. Baskin LS, Hayward SW, Sutherland RA, DiSandro MJ, Thomson AA, Goodman J, et al. Mesenchymal-epithelial interactions in the bladder. World J Urol. 1996;14(5):301.
27. Cheng W, Yeung CK, Ng YK, Zhang JR, Hui CC, Kim PCW. Sonic hedgehog mediator Gli2 regulates bladder mesenchymal patterning. J Urol. 2008;180(4):1543–50.
28. Shiroyanagi Y, Liu B, Cao M, Agras K, Li J, Hsieh MH, et al. Urothelial sonic hedgehog signaling plays an important role in bladder smooth muscle formation. Differentiation. 2007;75(10):968–77.
29. Haraguchi R, Motoyama J, Sasaki H, Satoh Y, Miyagawa S, Nakagata N, et al. Molecular analysis of coordinated bladder and urogenital organ formation by Hedgehog signaling. Development. 2007;134(3):525–33.
30. Mahfuz I, Darling T, Wilkins S, White S, Cheng W. New insights into the pathogenesis of bladder exstrophy–epispadias complex. J Pediatr Urol. 2013;9(6):996–1005.
31. Castillo-Martin M, Domingo-Domenech J, Karni-Schmidt O, Matos T, Cordon-Cardo C. Molecular pathways of urothelial development and bladder tumorigenesis. Urol Oncol. 2010;28(4):401–8.
32. Karni-Schmidt O, Castillo-Martin M, HuaiShen T, Gladoun N, Domingo-Domenech J, Sanchez-Carbayo M, et al. Distinct expression profiles of p63 variants during urothelial development and bladder cancer progression. Am J Pathol. 2011;178(3):1350–60.
33. Yang A, Schweitzer R, Sun D, Kaghad M, Walker N, Bronson RT, et al. p63 is essential for regenerative proliferation in limb, craniofacial and epithelial development. Nature. 1999;398(6729):714–8.
34. Cheng W, Jacobs WB, Zhang JJR, Moro A, Park JH, Kushida M, et al. ΔNp63 plays an anti-apoptotic role in ventral bladder development. Development. 2006;133(23):4783–92.
35. Tourchi A, Inouye BM, Di Carlo HN, Young E, Ko J, Gearhart JP. New advances in the pathophysiologic and radiologic basis of the exstrophy spectrum. J Pediatr Urol. 2014;10(2):212–8.
36. Wilkins S, Zhang KW, Mahfuz I, Quantin R, D'Cruz N, Hutson J, et al. Insertion/deletion polymorphisms in the ΔNp63 promoter are a risk factor for bladder exstrophy epispadias complex. PLoS Genet. 2012;8(12):e1003070.
37. Qi L, Chen K, Hur DJ, Yagnik G, Lakshmanan Y, Kotch LE, et al. Genome-wide expression profiling of urinary bladder implicates desmosomal and cytoskeletal dysregulation in the bladder exstrophy-epispadias complex. Int J Mol Med. 2011;27(6):755–65.
38. Ihrie RA, Reczek E, Horner JS, Khachatrian L, Sage J, Jacks T, et al. Perp is a mediator of p53-dependent apoptosis in diverse cell types. Curr Biol. 2003;13(22):1985–90.
39. Flores ER, Tsai KY, Crowley D, Sengupta S, Yang A, McKeon F, et al. p63 and p73 are required for p53-dependent apoptosis in response to DNA damage. Nature. 2002;416(6880):560–4.
40. Beaudry VG, Pathak N, Koster MI, Attardi LD. Differential PERP regulation by TP63 mutants provides insight into AEC pathogenesis. Am J Med Genet A. 2009;149A(9):1952–7.
41. Ihrie RA, Marques MR, Nguyen BT, Horner JS, Papazoglu C, Bronson RT, et al. Perp is a p63-regulated gene essential for epithelial integrity. Cell. 2005;120(6):843–56.
42. Ihrie RA, Attardi LD. A new Perp in the lineup: linking p63 and desmosomal adhesion. Cell Cycle. 2005;4(7):873–6.
43. Liu G, Moro A, Zhang JJR, Cheng W, Qiu W, Kim PCW. The role of Shh transcription activator Gli2 in chick cloacal development. Dev Biol. 2007;303(2):448–60.
44. Hall SA, Manyevitch R, Mistry PK, Wu W, Gearhart JP. New insights on the basic science of bladder exstrophy-epispadias complex. Urology. 2021;147:256–63.

45. Draaken M, Reutter H, Schramm C, Bartels E, Boemers TM, Ebert AK, et al. Microduplications at 22q11.21 are associated with non-syndromic classic bladder exstrophy. Eur J Med Genet. 2010;53(2):55–60.
46. Lundin J, Söderhäll C, Lundén L, Hammarsjö A, White I, Schoumans J, et al. 22q11.2 microduplication in two patients with bladder exstrophy and hearing impairment. Eur J Med Genet. 2010;53(2):61–5.
47. Lundin J, Markljung E, Baranowska Körberg I, Hofmeister W, Cao J, Nilsson D, et al. Further support linking the 22q11.2 microduplication to an increased risk of bladder exstrophy and highlighting *LZTR1* as a candidate gene. Mol Genet Genomic Med. 2019;7(6):e666.
48. Draaken M, Knapp M, Pennimpede T, Schmidt JM, Ebert AK, Rösch W, et al. Genome-wide association study and meta-analysis identify ISL1 as genome-wide significant susceptibility gene for bladder exstrophy. PLoS Genet. 2015;11(3):e1005024.
49. Guo C, Sun Y, Guo C, MacDonald BT, Borer JG, Li X. Dkk1 in the peri-cloaca mesenchyme regulates formation of anorectal and genitourinary tracts. Dev Biol. 2014;385(1):41–51.
50. Wang C, Wang J, Borer JG, Li X. Embryonic origin and remodeling of the urinary and digestive outlets. PLoS One. 2013;8(2):e55587.
51. Kasprenski M, Michaud J, Yang Z, Maruf M, Benz K, Jayman J, et al. Urothelial differences in the exstrophy-epispadias complex: potential implications for management. J Urol. 2021;205(5):1460–5.
52. Rubenwolf PC, Eder F, Ebert AK, Hofstaedter F, Woodhouse CRJ, Roesch WH. Persistent histological changes in the exstrophic bladder after primary closure—a cause for concern? J Urol. 2013;189(2):671–7.

Bladder Exstrophy-Epispadias Complex: Prenatal Diagnosis and Counseling

2

Juliana Gebb, Lisa Pilchman, and Julie S. Moldenhauer

Introduction

The bladder exstrophy-epispadias complex (BEEC) describes a spectrum of rare congenital genitourinary malformations that includes epispadias, classic bladder exstrophy (CBE), and cloacal exstrophy (CE) in order of increasing severity. Optimal care of affected infants and children requires a large multidisciplinary team providing coordinated management, typically in specialized centers. Identification of fetuses affected with BEEC helps to optimize prenatal counseling, maternal care, and delivery planning such that neonates can be born in centers with the appropriate subspecialists available for immediate evaluation and complex management.

Prenatal diagnosis of BEEC presents a challenge due to the rarity of the complex, but also because nuanced findings can be missed or inappropriately characterized. In older studies, prenatal identification of BEEC through routine ultrasound was reported to be very low at 10% [1]; however, more recent single- and multi-institutional studies have demonstrated an approximately 46–47% prenatal diagnosis rate of classic bladder exstrophy [2, 3]. When looking at diagnosis over time, however, the rate has increased, from around 30% in the early 2000s to 61% from 2015 to 2020 [2]. The prenatal diagnosis of CE has been more common, ranging from 78% to 82%, likely due to the more extreme anomalies [2, 4].

J. Gebb (✉) · J. S. Moldenhauer
Richard D. Wood Jr. Center for Fetal Diagnosis and Treatment, Children's Hospital of Philadelphia, Philadelphia, PA, USA

Perelman School of Medicine at University of Pennsylvania, Philadelphia, PA, USA
e-mail: gebbj@chop.edu; moldenhauerj@chop.edu

L. Pilchman
Children's Hospital Los Angeles, Los Angeles, CA, USA

A. R. Shukla, R. S. Joshi (eds.), *Bladder Exstrophy and Epispadias*,
https://doi.org/10.1007/978-3-031-91238-2_2

A prenatal diagnosis of BEEC is not considered to be life-limiting, with 1-year survival rates reported to be 90–100% [1]. However, surgical intervention is required in all cases, and many patients require multiple surgeries. There are currently no in utero interventions available for the treatment of BEEC. Accuracy of the prenatal diagnosis of BEEC helps to provide improved parental counseling and delivery venue optimization, timely referral to pediatric subspecialists, and assistance to families in preparation for a neonate that will require complex care and often prolonged hospitalization.

Prenatal Imaging

Ultrasound is the most utilized fetal imaging modality for anatomic assessment as it is safe, cost-effective, and accessible even in remote settings. With improving technology, fetal malformations can now be diagnosed at earlier gestational ages. Genitourinary malformations can be suspected in the first trimester at the time of a standard nuchal translucency screening ultrasound between 12 and 14 weeks gestation [5–7]. At this early gestational age, fetal gender is determined based on the direction that the genital tubercle points. More detailed anatomic evaluation of the fetus typically occurs at 18–22 weeks of gestation with well-established standard guidelines and reporting requirements [8–10]. Additionally, in cases with omphalocele and/or open spina bifida, elevation of the maternal serum alpha-fetoprotein at 16 weeks may be present prior to the mid-trimester scan [11, 12]. The gestational timing of prenatal screening and imaging techniques employed in the prenatal diagnosis of BEEC are presented in the Table 2.1.

Assessment of the external fetal genitalia that occurs in the mid-trimester can better evaluate the appearance of the penis/scrotum and the labia, allowing for fetal phenotypic sex determination. An abnormal appearance of the genitalia, ambiguous genitalia, or discrepancy between phenotypic sex and genetic sex falls under disorders of sex development and requires further evaluation. Parental counseling regarding fetal sex determination should include options for invasive and non-invasive methods. Cell-free fetal DNA screening is a non-invasive method that involves a maternal blood draw to evaluate fetal DNA circulating in the maternal plasma that originates from the trophoblast and is available beginning at 9–10 weeks gestation [13]. It is considered diagnostic with regard to fetal sex determination [14]. The ability to further diagnose specific disorders of sex development is limited with cffDNA and requires additional testing. Amniocentesis is an invasive testing option available for sex determination in the mid-trimester and is associated with a procedure-related pregnancy loss rate of approximately 0.1–0.3% [15, 16]. Third trimester amniocentesis can also be performed for those receiving a late diagnosis and is not associated with a risk for pregnancy loss, but complications such as preterm premature rupture of membranes and placental abruption can lead to preterm delivery [17]. A more complete genetic assessment, including the use of genome sequencing, could also be performed on the amniotic fluid specimen.

Table 2.1 Prenatal imaging and screening pertinent to diagnosing BEEC

	First trimester	Second trimester	Third trimester
Imaging	Ultrasound Estimate of gestational age Nuchal translucency measurement (10–14 weeks) Detailed first trimester anatomy (12 weeks 0 days–13 weeks 6 days)	Ultrasound 18–22 weeks detailed anatomic evaluation	Ultrasound Anatomic evaluation Evaluation of growth and amniotic fluid
		Fetal echocardiogram	Fetal echocardiogram
		MRI	MRI
Screening	Cell-free fetal DNA Available from 9 to 10 weeks	Cell-free fetal DNA	Cell-free fetal DNA
		Maternal serum alpha-fetoprotein (15–20 weeks) Levels elevated ≥2.5 MoM associated with open neural tube defects with a detection rate of 65–80%	
Definitive genetic testing	Chorionic villus sampling (10–13 weeks) Pregnancy loss rate ~ 0.1–0.3%	Amniocentesis (15–23 weeks) Pregnancy loss rate ~ 0.1–0.3%	Amniocentesis (≥24 weeks) Complication rate 1.2–7.2%

As described in more detail in the section on prenatal imaging (Chap. 4), findings of classic bladder exstrophy include: (1) non-visualization of the fetal bladder over 30–60 min with normal appearance of the kidneys and amniotic fluid; (2) low-set umbilical cord with abdominal bulge below; (3) splayed pubic bones; (4) anteriorly displaced "target" sign (anal dimple); (5) genital abnormalities; and (6) umbilical cord insertion-to-genital tubercle length below the fifth centile [18–21]. Findings in cloacal exstrophy include the findings of classic bladder exstrophy as well as: (1) sub-umbilical omphalocele; (2) "elephant trunk-like" appearance of the prolapsed ileum between the two hemi-bladders; (3) absence of "target" sign implicating anal atresia; and (4) spinal defects that can range from vertebral anomalies to tethered cord to various forms of open and closed spina bifida [22, 23]. Additional findings may include renal anomalies in one-third of cases as well as lower limb and brain anomalies associated with spina bifida [24].

Detailed anatomic survey should therefore focus not only on the fetal pelvis, bladder, genitalia, and anus/rectum but should also fully evaluate other structures such as the spine, brain, limbs, kidneys, and abdominal wall. In cases of CE, the thoracic circumference is also an important consideration given the risk of pulmonary hypoplasia in the presence of large omphaloceles and/or significant scoliosis. Ultrafast fetal MRI can aid ultrasound in differentiating complex anatomical differences and can provide lung volumes [4, 25]. Although the association with congenital heart disease is typically low, fetal echocardiography is generally recommended, as there are reports of cardiac disease in conjunction with BEEC.

Prenatal Counseling

As with any prenatally diagnosed congenital anomaly, disclosure of findings, discussion regarding the diagnosis and long-term outcomes, and presentation of pregnancy management options are included in prenatal counseling. Long-term outcomes in BEEC vary widely, depending on the specific diagnosis, as below. In general, pregnancy management options include continuation with a plan for multidisciplinary maternal and neonatal care or termination. Gestational age limitations and methods of termination are dictated by state laws and local practice patterns. After a prenatal diagnosis of BEEC, the rates of termination of pregnancy vary widely based on geographic location and may be as low as 8% or as high as 100% [26, 27].

Parents should be offered the opportunity to consult with pediatric subspecialists, including urology, surgery, neurosurgery, and neonatology, in the prenatal period. Delivery venue will largely be dictated by the availability of pediatric subspecialists to care for the neonate. Therefore, parents should be referred to specialty centers to optimize delivery and neonatal care planning. Additionally, expectant parents may benefit from participation in a parent support group or psychosocial support resources, as high rates of caregiver mental health disorders and stress have been reported [28, 29].

Epispadias

Epispadias has traditionally been prenatally diagnosed as one of the findings in fetal classic bladder exstrophy. Cases of isolated epispadias are rarer and may be missed on prenatal ultrasound. Kidneys and amniotic fluid typically appear normal and remain as such throughout the pregnancy. The appearance of the external fetal genitalia in isolated epispadias most commonly will be deemed ambiguous, prompting additional evaluation, as it implies an underlying disorder of sex development. At a minimum, a prenatal diagnosis of ambiguous genitalia warrants determination of fetal genotypic sex. Fetal imaging might suggest a shortened phallus in males or a bifid clitoris in females, which could be easily missed if a clear image of the perineum is not obtained in utero. The anogenital distance (AGD), visualization of the fetal vagina, and identification of the fetal uterus have also been proposed as additional sonographic markers to determine phenotypic sex [30–33]. Incorrect determination of fetal sex can have a negative impact on maternal well-being and infant care [34].

In cases of isolated epispadias, the goal is to optimize cosmetic and functional outcomes, including reproductive outcomes and continence. For male infants, we counsel that parents will have to refrain from attempting circumcision after birth to avoid injury to the penis and urethra and so that the foreskin can be used during the surgical repair. Maternal prenatal care follows a typical course, and the mode of delivery is anticipated to be vaginal, with cesarean delivery reserved for routine obstetric indications. Delivery venue should be optimized to allow availability of the appropriate pediatric subspecialists to evaluate the neonate; however, the treatment of epispadias is not urgent, and surgery will not usually be undertaken until at least 6 months of age, allowing for postnatal consultation well after discharge from the hospital.

Classic Bladder Exstrophy

Outcomes in cases of classic bladder exstrophy have improved greatly but continue to require complex multidisciplinary care that is best undertaken at a center with a high volume of cases. Prenatally, the kidneys appear normal, and the amniotic fluid is generally normal throughout pregnancy. Urinary reflux tends to develop after bladder reconstruction occurs, but prior to bladder closure, there is no reflux and there is a low risk of urinary tract infections. At birth, the exposed bladder mucosa is protected from abrasion from a diaper by covering it with a smooth covering such as clear double-backed transparent dressing such as Tegaderm™, plastic wrap, or hydrogel sheets that can retain moisture. The anus is anteriorly displaced, but this does not cause functional concerns in most situations. Anal atresia or rectal stenosis/prolapse has been reported in 1.8% of patients with classic bladder exstrophy, and these may require intervention; however, rectal prolapse often resolves after the bladder closure [35]. Inguinal hernias are common and are addressed surgically if present. Genital reconstruction may be performed at the time of bladder closure, as in the complete primary repair of exstrophy, or later in a staged repair. Females often have normal sexual function and reproductive outcomes but may have vaginal stenosis. Males often have difficulties with reproduction due to low sperm count and ejaculation volume.

In the setting of fetal bladder exstrophy, maternal prenatal care follows a typical course, and mode of delivery is anticipated to be vaginal, with cesarean delivery reserved for routine obstetric indications. Delivery venue should be optimized to allow availability of the appropriate pediatric subspecialists to evaluate the neonate.

Cloacal Exstrophy

The prognosis in cloacal exstrophy cases is poorer due to the involvement not only of the bladder but also of the intestines and the spine. The combination of structural differences associated with cloacal exstrophy is often referred to as the OEIS (Omphalocele—Exstrophy of the Cloaca—Imperforate Anus—Spinal Defects) Complex. Surgical management involves multiple procedures over many years. Initial surgeries include repair of the omphalocele with colostomy creation and reapproximation of the posterior bladder plates. Closure of open spinal dysraphism may occur before this or at 3 months of age for closed defects. These infants often have long-term nutritional challenges due to short gut physiology. Only once the infant has grown and is thriving, often at 1–2 years of age, is there an attempt to close the bladder plate with osteotomies of the iliac bones to internally rotate the pelvis. Due to the combination of minimal hindgut, as well as spinal dysraphism, pull-through procedures are rare and have a very poor success rate for becoming clean (7%) or achieving continence (1%) [36].

After these initial procedures, other major urologic reconstruction procedures may be necessary, and genital reconstruction surgery is also undertaken. Because of the complicated condition and need for staged surgical repair, consultation with the parents includes the discussion of the possibility of long-term urologic complications and bowel incontinence.

Additionally, if there is a presence of spina bifida, counseling includes a discussion of the associated neuromuscular weakness that can lead to talipes and difficulty with ambulation, as well as compromise to the nerves that innervate the bladder, bowel, and external genitalia. In cases of open spina bifida, Arnold-Chiari II malformation is often present and can lead to the need for treatment of hydrocephalus after birth. When hydrocephalus is severe, or if there are complications from ventriculoperitoneal shunting, neurocognitive outcome may be affected.

Maternal prenatal care should follow a typical course. Prior reports have suggested an increased association with fetal growth restriction and in utero fetal death [37, 38]. Therefore, serial ultrasounds to monitor fetal growth throughout the pregnancy are recommended. Antenatal surveillance to monitor fetal well-being should also be considered. Oligohydramnios can also develop over the course of the pregnancy given the association with inherent renal abnormalities, requiring close monitoring of amniotic fluid throughout the pregnancy. There is an increased risk for prematurity associated with CE, with median gestational age at delivery reported to be 36 weeks [4, 39]. The most optimal mode of delivery is unknown. However, in the setting of liver-containing omphalocele and/or open neural tube defect, cesarean delivery should be considered. Delivery should occur in a center with experience caring for these complex neonates.

BEEC Variants

Approximately 10% of fetuses with BEEC will have anatomic variations from the classic forms [40–43]. It is therefore critical to tailor counseling to the individual findings for each fetus. Reported variants include epispadias with bladder prolapse, pseudoexstrophy, superior vesical fissure, duplicate exstrophy/duplicate bladder, covered exstrophy, and covered cloacal exstrophy [40].

In all cases of BEEC and variants, pediatric urology and surgery (as appropriate) consultations should be obtained to discuss in detail the planned postnatal evaluation, surgical interventions, and reported outcomes, including quality of life assessments. Psychosocial support of expectant parents of fetuses with congenital anomalies is an integral part of many fetal centers and greatly benefits this population.

Prenatal Management

Prenatal diagnosis of BEEC does not typically alter obstetric management or delivery timing in cases of epispadias and CBE. However, preterm delivery occurs commonly in CE. Serial growth scans are recommended for prenatally diagnosed BEEC. Evaluation of the amniotic fluid and fetal kidneys is warranted, although they remain normal in the vast majority of fetuses with epispadias and CBE. Renal differences and oligohydramnios are more commonly seen with CE, requiring serial monitoring throughout pregnancy. Additionally, antenatal surveillance should be considered in cases of CE, as fetal death in utero has been reported. Delivery at term in a specialty center is recommended to facilitate postnatal evaluation and management. Vaginal delivery is offered, with cesarean reserved for normal obstetric indications except in cases with a concomitant open spina bifida or large omphalocele, for whom cesarean is recommended.

Genetic Counseling

In approximately 98.5% of cases with BEEC, the finding is isolated with neurodevelopmental outcomes similar to the general population [24, 44]. Although karyotype and microarray are generally normal, duplication of 22q11.21 has been associated with classic bladder exstrophy, and invasive prenatal genetic testing is offered [45]. Even when genetic testing is normal, prenatal diagnosis can determine fetal sex, which can aid in counseling and postnatal management in cases with ambiguous genitalia. Moreover, the systematic application of modern genetic testing with microarray and next-generation sequencing techniques in large BEEC cohorts has begun to identify putative disease-causing genes and regions in the human genome for both Mendelian and multifactorial phenotypes [24]. Two recent studies of BEEC/CBE using whole exome sequencing of trios revealed numerous de novo variants and inherited variants that require further study [46–48].

The recurrence risk for future pregnancies is 1.4% [44]. Because the BEEC spectrum is rarely associated with an underlying genetic diagnosis, genetic evaluations in subsequent pregnancies, such as chorionic villus sampling or amniocentesis, are not informative. The application of IVF with preimplantation genetic diagnosis also has limited utility for couples planning future pregnancies after an affected child. Diagnosis of BEEC in subsequent pregnancies is largely limited to imaging studies in the late first trimester and second trimester.

Conclusion

The prenatal diagnosis of BEEC spectrum continues to be challenging and is largely limited to imaging techniques. Counseling, education, and support can assist expectant parents to prepare to care for a surgically complex neonate. Optimization of long-term childhood outcomes remains the goal of prenatal diagnosis.

References

1. Jayachandran D, Bythell M, Platt MW, Rankin J. Register based study of bladder exstrophy-epispadias complex: prevalence, associated anomalies, prenatal diagnosis and survival. J Urol. 2011;186(5):2056–60.
2. Lee T, Weiss D, Roth E, Bortnick E, Jarosz S, Eftekharzadeh S, et al. Prenatal diagnosis of bladder exstrophy and OEIS over 20 years. Urology. 2023;172:174–7.
3. Hirsch AM, Morrill CC, Haffar A, Harris TGW, Crigger C, Jelin AC, et al. Optimizing prenatal diagnosis and referral of classic bladder exstrophy: lessons from a single-institution experience. J Pediatr Urol. 2024;20:630.
4. Morrill CC, Haffar A, Crigger C, Black M, Jelin A, Nasr I, et al. A single-institutional experience with prenatal diagnosis of cloacal exstrophy: room for improvement. J Pediatr Surg. 2023;58(10):1949–53.
5. Rossi AC, Prefumo F. Accuracy of ultrasonography at 11-14 weeks of gestation for detection of fetal structural anomalies: a systematic review. Obstet Gynecol. 2013;122(6):1160–7.
6. Syngelaki A, Hammami A, Bower S, Zidere V, Akolekar R, Nicolaides KH. Diagnosis of fetal non-chromosomal abnormalities on routine ultrasound examination at 11-13 weeks' gestation. Ultrasound Obstet Gynecol. 2019;54(4):468–76.
7. American Institute of Ultrasound in Medicine. AIUM practice parameter for the performance of detailed diagnostic obstetric ultrasound examinations between 12 weeks 0 days and 13 weeks 6 days. J Ultrasound Med. 2021;40(5):E1–E16.
8. American Institute of Ultrasound in Medicine. AIUM-ACR-ACOG-SMFM-SRU practice parameter for the performance of standard diagnostic obstetric ultrasound examinations. J Ultrasound Med. 2018;37(11):E13–24.
9. American Institute of Ultrasound in Medicine. AIUM practice parameter for the performance of detailed second- and third-trimester diagnostic obstetric ultrasound examinations. J Ultrasound Med. 2019;38(12):3093–100.
10. Salomon LJ, Alfirevic Z, Berghella V, Bilardo CM, Chalouhi GE, Da Silva Costa F, et al. ISUOG Practice Guidelines (updated): performance of the routine mid-trimester fetal ultrasound scan. Ultrasound Obstet Gynecol. 2022;59(6):840–56.
11. Practice Bulletin No. 187: neural tube defects. Obstet Gynecol. 2017;130(6):e279–e90.
12. Glowska-Ciemny J, Szmyt K, Kuszerska A, Rzepka R, von Kaisenberg C, Kocylowski R. Fetal and placental causes of elevated serum alpha-fetoprotein levels in pregnant women. J Clin Med. 2024;13(2):466.
13. American College of Obstetricians and Gynecologists' Committee on Practice Bulletins—Obstetrics; Committee on Genetics; Society for Maternal-Fetal Medicine. Screening for fetal chromosomal abnormalities: ACOG practice bulletin summary, number 226. Obstet Gynecol. 2020;136(4):859–67.
14. Mackie FL, Hemming K, Allen S, Morris RK, Kilby MD. The accuracy of cell-free fetal DNA-based non-invasive prenatal testing in singleton pregnancies: a systematic review and bivariate meta-analysis. BJOG. 2017;124(1):32–46.
15. Practice Bulletin No. 162: prenatal diagnostic testing for genetic disorders. Obstet Gynecol. 2016;127(5):e108–e22.
16. Salomon LJ, Sotiriadis A, Wulff CB, Odibo A, Akolekar R. Risk of miscarriage following amniocentesis or chorionic villus sampling: systematic review of literature and updated meta-analysis. Ultrasound Obstet Gynecol. 2019;54(4):442–51.
17. Zemet R, Ali Maktabi M, Tinfow A, Giordano JL, Heisler TM, Yan Q, et al. Amniocentesis in pregnancies at or beyond 24 weeks: an international multicenter study. Am J Obstet Gynecol. 2024;80:3.
18. Jaffe R, Schoenfeld A, Ovadia J. Sonographic findings in the prenatal diagnosis of bladder exstrophy. Am J Obstet Gynecol. 1990;162(3):675–8.
19. Gearhart JP, Ben-Chaim J, Jeffs RD, Sanders RC. Criteria for the prenatal diagnosis of classic bladder exstrophy. Obstet Gynecol. 1995;85(6):961–4.

20. Fishel-Bartal M, Perlman S, Messing B, Bardin R, Kivilevitch Z, Achiron R, et al. Early diagnosis of bladder exstrophy: quantitative assessment of a low-inserted umbilical cord. J Ultrasound Med. 2017;36(9):1801–5.
21. Antomarchi J, Moeglin D, Laurichesse H, Combourieu D, Bigi N, Maisonneuve E, et al. The pubic diastasis measurement, a key element for the diagnosis, management, and prognosis of the bladder exstrophy. Fetal Diagn Ther. 2019;45(6):435–40.
22. Meizner I, Levy A, Barnhard Y. Cloacal exstrophy sequence: an exceptional ultrasound diagnosis. Obstet Gynecol. 1995;86(3):446–50.
23. Della Monica M, Nazzaro A, Lonardo F, Ferrara G, Di Blasi A, Scarano G. Prenatal ultrasound diagnosis of cloacal exstrophy associated with myelocystocele complex by the "elephant trunk-like" image and review of the literature. Prenat Diagn. 2005;25(5):394–7.
24. Reutter H, Keppler-Noreuil K, Keegan CE, Thiele H, Yamada G, Ludwig M. Genetics of bladder-exstrophy-epispadias complex (BEEC): systematic elucidation of Mendelian and multifactorial phenotypes. Curr Genomics. 2016;17(1):4–13.
25. Weiss DA, Oliver ER, Borer JG, Kryger JV, Roth EB, Groth TW, et al. Key anatomic findings on fetal ultrasound and MRI in the prenatal diagnosis of bladder and cloacal exstrophy. J Pediatr Urol. 2020;16(5):665–71.
26. Mallmann MR, Mack-Detlefsen B, Reutter H, Pohle R, Gottschalk I, Geipel A, et al. Isolated bladder exstrophy in prenatal diagnosis. Arch Gynecol Obstet. 2019;300(2):355–63.
27. Xie D, Liang C, Xiang Y, Wang A, Xiong L, Kong F, et al. Prenatal diagnosis of birth defects and termination of pregnancy in Hunan Province, China. Prenat Diagn. 2020;40(8):925–30.
28. Mednick L, Gargollo P, Oliva M, Grant R, Borer J. Stress and coping of parents of young children diagnosed with bladder exstrophy. J Urol. 2009;181(3):1312–6; discussion 17.
29. Spencer KA, Ramji J, Unadkat P, Nadeem I, Lalakia PA, Shah J, et al. Caregiver distress: a mixed methods evaluation of the mental health burden of caring for children with bladder exstrophy. Front Pediatr. 2022;10:948490.
30. Soriano D, Lipitz S, Seidman DS, Maymon R, Mashiach S, Achiron R. Development of the fetal uterus between 19 and 38 weeks of gestation: in-utero ultrasonographic measurements. Hum Reprod. 1999;14(1):215–8.
31. Glanc P, Umranikar S, Koff D, Tomlinson G, Chitayat D. Fetal sex assignment by sonographic evaluation of the pelvic organs in the second and third trimesters of pregnancy. J Ultrasound Med. 2007;26(5):563–9; quiz 70–1.
32. Gilboa Y, Kivilevitch Z, Oren M, Cohen YP, Katorza E, Achiron R. Anogenital distance in male and female fetuses at 20 to 35 weeks of gestation: centile charts and reference ranges. Prenat Diagn. 2014;34(10):946–51.
33. Smet ME, Bethe R, Papworth A, McLennan A, Scott F. Sonographic assessment of fetal sex: more than external genitalia. Fetal Diagn Ther. 2023;50(1):29–36.
34. Chigbu CO, Odugu B, Okezie O. Implications of incorrect determination of fetal sex by ultrasound. Int J Gynaecol Obstet. 2008;100(3):287–90.
35. Stec AA, Baradaran N, Tran C, Gearhart JP. Colorectal anomalies in patients with classic bladder exstrophy. J Pediatr Surg. 2011;46(9):1790–3.
36. Srinivas S, Knaus ME, Avansino JR, Badillo A, Calkins CM, Dickie BH, et al. Outcomes from colonic pull-through for cloacal exstrophy differ by colon length: a multi-institutional study. J Pediatr Surg. 2024;59(2):225–9.
37. Martinez-Frias ML, Bermejo E, Rodriguez-Pinilla E, Frias JL. Exstrophy of the cloaca and exstrophy of the bladder: two different expressions of a primary developmental field defect. Am J Med Genet. 2001;99(4):261–9.
38. Gondo K, Yokomine M, Yoshizato T, Furuta T, Ushijima K. Clues and pitfalls in prenatal diagnosis of classic cloacal exstrophy using ultrasonography and magnetic resonance imaging: a case with sequential observation from 17 to 30 weeks' gestation and literature review. J Obstet Gynaecol Res. 2020;46(8):1443–9.
39. Tiblad E, Wilson RD, Carr M, Flake AW, Hedrick H, Johnson MP, et al. OEIS sequence--a rare congenital anomaly with prenatal evaluation and postnatal outcome in six cases. Prenat Diagn. 2008;28(2):141–7.

40. Lowentritt BH, Van Zijl PS, Frimberger D, Baird A, Lakshmanan Y, Gearhart JP. Variants of the exstrophy complex: a single institution experience. J Urol. 2005;173(5):1732–7.
41. Mallmann MR, Reutter H, Muller A, Boemers TM, Geipel A, Berg C, et al. Prenatal diagnosis of covered cloacal exstrophy. Fetal Diagn Ther. 2014;36(4):333–6.
42. Ozcan T, Woo L, Wien M, Lazebnik N. Prenatal ultrasound findings of covered bladder exstrophy and persistent cloaca. J Clin Ultrasound. 2021;49(8):834–7.
43. Vinit N, Glenisson M, Chalouhi G, Salomon LJ, Millischer-Bellaiche AE, Beaudoin S, et al. Prenatal diagnosis of unusual variant of exstrophy-epispadias complex. Ultrasound Obstet Gynecol. 2023;62(1):155–6.
44. Reutter H, Holmdahl G. Genetic counseling for bladder exstrophy-epispadias complex. Eur J Pediatr Surg. 2021;31(6):468–71.
45. Draaken M, Baudisch F, Timmermann B, Kuhl H, Kerick M, Proske J, et al. Classic bladder exstrophy: frequent 22q11.21 duplications and definition of a 414 kb phenocritical region. Birth Defects Res A Clin Mol Teratol. 2014;100(6):512–7.
46. Pitsava G, Feldkamp ML, Pankratz N, Lane J, Kay DM, Conway KM, et al. Exome sequencing of child-parent trios with bladder exstrophy: findings in 26 children. Am J Med Genet A. 2021;185(10):3028–41.
47. Kollges R, Stegmann J, Schneider S, Waffenschmidt L, Fazaal J, Breuer K, et al. Exome survey and candidate gene re-sequencing identifies novel exstrophy candidate genes and implicates LZTR1 in disease formation. Biomolecules. 2023;13(7):1117.
48. Jelin AC, Wohler E, Martin R, Di Carlo H, Isaacs W, Ko J, et al. De novo variants identified by trio whole exome sequencing of bladder exstrophy epispadias complex. Am J Med Genet A. 2024;194(4):e63501.

Bladder Exstrophy Genetics: Our Current Understanding

3

John K. Weaver and Chen-Han Wilfred Wu

Bladder Exstrophy Genetics

Bladder exstrophy is a devastating congenital abnormality of the urinary tract in which infants are born with the urinary bladder extruded through their abdominal wall, a urethra that is open dorsally, and significant secondary abnormalities of the genitalia. While the etiology of bladder exstrophy is not known, a clear genetic component has been highlighted.

Epidemiologic and Observational Studies

In 1984, using survey data, Shapiro et al. found that bladder exstrophy recurred in 9 of approximately 2500 families (1 in 275) who already had a history of bladder exstrophy or complete epispadias [17]. This is a far higher rate than is seen in the general population (approximately 1 in 10,000–100,000) [9]. Shapiro et al. also found that 3 of 215 offspring from patients with bladder exstrophy or epispadias inherited bladder exstrophy or epispadias, i.e., at an even higher rate of 1 in 70 live births. Finally, they identified 17 sets of twins where at least 1 of the twins was affected by bladder exstrophy. Bladder exstrophy did not occur in both members of any of the five sets of fraternal twins. Both members of identical male twins were affected with exstrophy in five monozygotic pairs, whereas only one member of the three pairs of identical female twins was affected. Information on gender or twin

J. K. Weaver (✉)
Cleveland Clinic Lerner College of Medicine at Case Western Reserve University School of Medicine, Cleveland, OH, USA
e-mail: weaverj3@chop.edu

C.-H. W. Wu
Case Western Reserve University School of Medicine, Cleveland, OH, USA

A. R. Shukla, R. S. Joshi (eds.), *Bladder Exstrophy and Epispadias*,
https://doi.org/10.1007/978-3-031-91238-2_3

type was unavailable in four cases [17]. In a separate study, Lattimer and Smith cited a set of identical twins with bladder exstrophy and another set of twins in whom only one child had exstrophy [18].

In another study using survey data, Ives et al. followed the families of 102 index patients with bladder exstrophy treated at The Hospital for Sick Children, Great Ormond Street. Of the 102 patients, 97 had BE and 5 had cloacal exstrophy. In all they had 162 siblings, none of whom had bladder exstrophy. They concluded that the risk to siblings is low and probably less than 1% [8].

In 2003, Reutter et al., in conjunction with Shapiro, published seven new cases of familial isolated bladder exstrophy and epispadias complex (BEEC). The seven new families were noteworthy for their cumulative patterns of inheritance and the genetic implications. In six pedigrees, two family members were affected: two siblings, two 3rd-degree cousins, and two uncle–nephew pairs. This pattern is more suggestive of a complex inheritance, pointing toward polygenic with an environmental component, as opposed to conventional Mendelian inheritance. There were a total of 13 probands in these families, comprised of 10 males and 3 females, for a male-to-female ratio of 3.3:1. Probands in four families had the identical classical bladder exstrophy phenotype. In two families, one proband had bladder exstrophy and the other epispadias. The family with a single proband had epispadias [16].

In 2004, Boyadjiev et al., from a cohort of 285 families with BEEC, obtained epidemiological information from 151 families [2]. They also performed a detailed clinical genetic examination of 94 probands. In all, 440 DNA samples were collected from 163 families for cytogenetics and molecular analysis. Karyotype analysis on 37 cases detected two chromosomal abnormalities, i.e., 46XY t(8;9)(p11.2;q13) and 47XYY. Molecular analysis of the HLXB9 gene, which causes Currarino syndrome (sacral fusion abnormality), did not detect pathogenic variants in the blood or bladder DNA of ten patients with bladder or cloacal exstrophy. From this analysis, the authors concluded BEEC most commonly occurs as an isolated sporadic birth defect with a recurrence risk of less than 1%. There was no evidence of a single-gene effect or common environmental factor in this study population. However, there was a statistically significant association with advanced parental age.

The following year, Boyadjiev et al. reported on their patient with sporadic bladder exstrophy and de novo apparently balanced chromosomal translocation 46,XY,t(8;9)(p11.2;q13) [2]. This was analyzed by fluorescence in situ hybridization (FISH) and molecular methods, and they were able to map both translocation breakpoints to single genomic clones. The chromosome 8p11.2 breakpoint was mapped to bacterial artificial chromosome (BAC) clone RP4-547J18, predicted to contain several hypothetical genes. Characterization of the chromosome 9q13 breakpoint indicated a disruption in the 5′ region of CNTNAP3 within BAC RP11-292B8. This observation suggested possible involvement of CNTNAP3 in the etiology of bladder exstrophy. Additionally, FISH analysis identified several genomic copies of CNTNAP3 on both sides of the chromosome 9 centromere flanking the polymorphic heterochromatin. Northern blot analysis of lymphoblast and bladder tissue RNA confirmed CNTNAP3 transcripts in these tissues and did not show abnormal CNTNAP3 expression in the proband and two unrelated patients with bladder exstrophy. The authors concluded that CNTNAP3 and/or other genes on chromosome 9q13 or chromosome 8p11.2 may contribute to the etiology of BEEC. They also identified multiple copies of three BAC clones, indicating that segmental duplications of the pericentric region of chromosome 9 and its flanking genes have occurred due to a combination of repeated pericentric inversions and unequal crossing over during evolution.

An increased rate of BEEC in IVF pregnancies has been reported. Wood et al. in 2007 found that under the hypothesis of no association between IVF and BEEC, the expected incidence of IVF in BEEC children ranged between 0.60% and 1.59% [21]. However, the observed incidence of IVF in BEEC children evaluated at Johns Hopkins University ranged between 4.2% and 6.7%. Comparison of the expected and observed incidence using a Pearson-type chi-squared test resulted in a bootstrapped *P* value of 0.0182. The authors concluded that the incidence of IVF in BEEC children appears to be higher than what would be expected if there was no association between IVF and BEEC.

Advanced Genetic Technology and Methods

Strides have been made in recent years with respect to identifying candidate genes. Multiple studies have utilized advanced genetic technology and methods. In 2008, Ludwig et al. sought to identify genetic risk loci using parametric and nonparametric linkage analysis, searching for homozygous segments and more complex inherited loci, respectively [10]. Two pedigrees, Spanish and German, each comprising two members affected with classic bladder exstrophy, were analyzed by genome-wide linkage scan. They identified evidence for possible risk/modifying loci on chromosomes 2p22.1–p21, 2p25.2–p25.1, 4q23–q32.3, 7q21.3–q33, 7q34–q36.1, 14q31.1–q32.2, and 19q13.33–q13.43 (LOD scores >1.50). This study was the first positional approach to identify chromosomal candidate regions causally related to BEEC. Their results suggested the presence of causal genes in the regions identified, but the authors concluded that these regions needed further validation in future studies.

A murine p63+/+ knockout model showed the full picture of classic exstrophy of the bladder and other urogenital defects within the BEEC spectrum. This led Ching et al. to study in depth the role of p63 in urogenital development in mice and the implication of p63 in human BEEC. They performed whole mount in situ analysis in mice to investigate the ventro-caudal expression of the p63 transcript at gestational days (GD) 9.5–12.5, the equivalent of human gestational weeks 4–6, which is the postulated time of BEEC organogenesis in humans [3]. In addition, p63 expression analysis was performed in human blood and bladder tissue of 15 BEEC newborns, accompanied by sequencing analysis of their genomic DNA. They also conducted sequencing analysis of genomic DNA in an additional 22 BEEC patients. In mouse embryos, p63 expression was detected at days 9.5–12.5 in the cloacal membrane and urethral epithelium, supporting its role in the morphogenesis of the external genitalia and the bladder. Tissue-specific expression of a novel and already-known mRNA isoforms was established, and a reproducible dysregulation of variable p63 isoforms was observed in 11 of 15 patients, indicating altered gene expression. However, no obvious p63 gene mutations were identified in any of the patients. The authors concluded that these results strongly suggest that p63 is not only involved in embryonic formation of the urogenital and ventrocaudal anatomy but is also highly dysregulated in human BEEC bladder tissue. They hypothesized that since p63 has been shown to self-regulate its expression through a balance of its isoforms, the dysregulation observed may contribute to the formation of BEEC. In 2013, Qi et al. conducted a candidate gene association study to further investigate the role of p63 in BEEC [15]. They conducted a family-based association study of p63 using 154 Caucasian patients with BEEC and their unaffected parents. High-throughput single nucleotide polymorphism (SNP) genotyping was carried out for 109 selected tagging SNPs localized within p63 with a minor allele frequency > 0.01. Individual and haplotype SNP transmission disequilibrium tests were conducted using Plink and Haploview, respectively. Nominally significant associations were identified between BEEC and six SNPs, and four haplotype blocks include or are near these significant SNPs. They also examined parent-of-origin effects using paternal asymmetry tests. Analysis of parent-of-origin effects showed significant results for seven SNPs. None of these results remained significant after multiple testing corrections. The authors concluded that the altered transmission of p63 variants in BEEC patients may be suggestive of its involvement in the disease etiology.

Copy Number Variant (CNV) Studies

Multiple array-based genome-wide CNV studies for BEEC have been performed. An early study from Draaken et al. identified a de novo 0.9 Mb microduplication on chromosome 19p13.12 in a single BE patient [5]. In another study, Draaken et al. identified duplications in 22q11.21. Two other studies that included a total of 102 BE patients identified a duplication of 22q11.21 in four individuals [4, 11]. An additional case report described an array-based CNV analysis in a single CBE patient with a duplication of 22q11.21 [14].

Following their array-based genome-wide CNV studies, Draaken et al. used a multiplex ligation-dependent probe amplification (MLPA)-based approach to perform a regional screen for 22q11.21 duplications in 244 independent BEEC patients. The authors identified four novel duplications of variable size in four unrelated BE patients [6].

To detect further CNVs, von Lowtzow et al. performed an array analysis on 169 BEEC patients [20]. Following the application of stringent filter criteria, seven rare CNVs were identified. These CNVs ranged from 1 to 6.08 Mb in size. To identify smaller CNVs, relaxed filter criteria used in the detection of previously reported BEEC-associated chromosomal regions were applied. This resulted in the identification of six additional rare CNVs. These CNVs ranged from 0.03 to 0.08 Mb in size. For 10 of these 13 CNVs, confirmation and segregation analyses were performed (5 of maternal origin; 5 of paternal origin). Interestingly, one female with classic bladder exstrophy carried a 1.18 Mb duplication of 22q11.1.

In 2023, Nordenskjold et al., citing that there is a clear genetic background with chromosome aberrations but so far no consistent findings apart from 22q11 duplications detected in about 2–3% of all patients, performed chromosomal microarray analysis on a cohort of 140 persons born with BE to look for submicroscopic chromosomal deletions and duplications [13]. Pathogenic or possibly pathogenic microdeletions or duplications were found in 16 patients (11.4%) and 9 with unknown significance. Two findings were in known syndromic regions (chr16:29645396–30168276 and chrX:154822249–155197455).

Most recently, in 2025, Weaver et al. presented findings of their array-based genome-wide CNV studies [19]. This study was unique in that it was the first genetic analysis of BEEC patients of non-European origin. The cohort included 57 patients of European origin and 93 patients of South Asian origin. The authors identified a total of 38 CNVs of statistical significance following filtering using ParseCNV. This study revealed numerous CNVs that had not been reported previously. Of note, they identified a CNV deletion at chr16:28635133–28636902, which was near one of the CNVs Nordenskjold et al. identified in a known syndromic region (chr16:29645396–30168276).

Gene Expression Studies

In 2011, Qi et al. used genome-wide expression profiling to identify 162 BEEC candidate genes that have twofold or higher expression differences between exstrophic and normal bladder smooth muscles in mouse and human embryologic bladder tissues [15]. They also found 16 candidate genes that are expressed in the infraumbilical endoderm and mesoderm. Most of these genes have functions related to cellular assembly, musculoskeletal system development, and connective tissue morphology. Specifically, 30% of these genes were related to the desmosomal structure and cytoskeleton assembly, of which 69% were under-expressed in exstrophic bladders. In this study, the two most downregulated genes in exstrophic bladders, *DES* (*DESMIN*) and *SYNM* (*DESMUSLIN*), encode muscle-specific proteins that interact with *DSP* (*DESMOPLAKIN*), the sixth most overexpressed gene in exstrophic bladders.

In 2018, Ching et al. reported that deletion of Isl1 from the genital mesenchyme in mice led to hypoplasia of the genital tubercle and prepuce, with an ectopic urethral opening and epispadias-like phenotype [3]. These mice also developed hydroureter and hydronephrosis. Identification of ISL1 transcriptional targets via ChIP-Seq and expression analyses revealed that Isl1 regulates several important signaling pathways during embryonic genital development, including the BMP, WNT, and FGF cascades. An essential function of Isl1 during development of the external genitalia is to induce Bmp4-mediated apoptosis in the genital mesenchyme. Together, these studies demonstrated that Isl1 plays a critical role during development of the external genitalia and potentially formed the basis for a greater understanding of the molecular mechanisms underlying the pathogenesis of BEEC and urinary tract defects in humans.

Genome-wide Association Study (GWAS)

A genome-wide association study (GWAS) meta-analysis combining 568 BE patients and 3241 controls of European origin identified an association with a locus containing the transcriptional enhancer *ISL1* ($p = 2.22 \times 10 - 8$) [7]. Further functional and model organism studies reinforced a possible causal role for *ISL1* in BE. For example, developmental biology models were used to clarify the location of *ISL1* activity in the forming urinary tract, and genetic lineage analysis of *ISL1*-expressing cells by a lineage tracer mouse model showed *ISL1*-expressing cells in the urinary tract of mouse embryos [1, 22].

In a follow-up to their prior GWAS study that identified *ISL1* as a candidate gene, Mingardo et al. published a GWAS meta-analysis of 628 patients with BE and 7352 ethnically matched controls comprising seven independent cohorts [12]. In this study they redemonstrated the significance of their previously identified *ISL1*-containing loci and identified seven novel genome-wide loci of significance. In these regions reside ten coding and four non-coding genes. Among the coding genes was *EFNA1*, which is strongly expressed in mouse embryonic genital tubercle, urethra, and primitive bladder. Re-sequencing of *EFNA1* in the investigated classic bladder exstrophy cohort displayed an enrichment of rare protein-altering mutations at a statistically significant higher rate than the general population. Additionally, they showed that all coding genes were expressed and/or significantly regulated in both mouse and human embryonic developmental bladder stages. Finally, nine of the coding genes residing in the regions of genome-wide significance were differentially expressed in bladder cancers. The authors postulated that differential expression turns these developmental genes on later in life and that these genes may play a role in the known bladder cancer susceptibility of BE patients. Similar to Mingardo et al., Weaver et al. found that a high percentage of our regions of interest include genes with known cancer associations. In our CNV study of a European and South Asian cohort, 10 of the 23 duplication CNVs and 6 of the 18 deletion CNVs contain genes with known cancer associations. However, the genes Weaver et al. identified did not overlap with the genes identified by Mingardo et al. Further investigation will be needed to better define the associations between the genes implicated in bladder exstrophy and cancer, as they could provide insight into methods for cancer prevention in this population.

Future Directions

Overall, the genetic analysis of bladder exstrophy is still in its infancy. Due to the rare nature of this disease, future collaborations across research groups will be needed to make significant strides in gaining a more complete understanding of the genetic underpinnings of bladder exstrophy. Almost all published studies to date, with the exception of one, include only European populations. Studies including non-European populations will be particularly critical to furthering our understanding in the future.

References

1. Arkani S, Cao J, Lundin J, Nilsson D, Källman T, Barker G, Holmdahl G, Clementsson Kockum C, Matsson H, Nordenskjöld A. Evaluation of the ISL1 gene in the pathogenesis of bladder exstrophy in a Swedish cohort. Hum Genome Var. 2018;5:18009. https://doi.org/10.1038/hgv.2018.9.
2. Boyadjiev SA, Dodson JL, Radford CL, Ashrafi GH, Beaty TH, Mathews RI, Broman KW, Gearhart JP. Clinical and molecular characterization of the bladder exstrophy-epispadias complex: analysis of 232 families. BJU Int. 2004;94(9):1337–43. https://doi.org/10.1111/j.1464-410X.2004.05170.x.
3. Ching ST, Infante CR, Du W, Sharir A, Park S, Menke DB, Klein OD. Isl1 mediates mesenchymal expansion in the developing external genitalia via regulation of Bmp4, Fgf10 and Wnt5a. Hum Mol Genet. 2018;27(1):107–19. https://doi.org/10.1093/hmg/ddx388.
4. Draaken M, Reutter H, Schramm C, Bartels E, Boemers TM, Ebert A-K, Rösch W, Schröder A, Stein R, Moebus S, Stienen D, Hoffmann P, Nöthen MM, Ludwig M. Microduplications at 22q11.21 are associated with non-syndromic classic bladder exstrophy. Eur J Med Genet. 2010;53(2):55–60. https://doi.org/10.1016/j.ejmg.2009.12.005.
5. Draaken M, Mughal SS, Pennimpede T, Wolter S, Wittler L, Ebert A-K, Rösch W, Stein R, Bartels E, Schmidt D, Boemers TM, Schmiedeke E, Hoffmann P, Moebus S, Herrmann BG, Nöthen MM, Reutter H, Ludwig M. Isolated bladder exstrophy associated with a de novo 0.9 Mb microduplication on chromosome 19p13.12. Birth Defects Res A Clin Mol Teratol. 2013;97(3):133–9. https://doi.org/10.1002/bdra.23112.
6. Draaken M, Baudisch F, Timmermann B, Kuhl H, Kerick M, Proske J, Wittler L, Pennimpede T, Ebert A-K, Rösch W, Stein R, Bartels E, von Lowtzow C, Boemers TM, Herms S, Gearhart JP, Lakshmanan Y, Kockum CC, Holmdahl G, et al. Classic bladder exstrophy: frequent 22q11.21 duplications and definition of a 414 kb phenocritical region. Birth Defects Res A Clin Mol Teratol. 2014;100(6):512–7. https://doi.org/10.1002/bdra.23249.
7. Draaken M, Knapp M, Pennimpede T, Schmidt JM, Ebert A-K, Rösch W, Stein R, Utsch B, Hirsch K, Boemers TM, Mangold E, Heilmann S, Ludwig KU, Jenetzky E, Zwink N, Moebus S, Herrmann BG, Mattheisen M, Nöthen MM, et al. Genome-wide association study and meta-analysis identify ISL1 as genome-wide significant susceptibility gene for bladder exstrophy. PLoS Genet. 2015;11(3):e1005024. https://doi.org/10.1371/journal.pgen.1005024.
8. Ives E, Coffey R, Carter CO. A family study of bladder exstrophy. J Med Genet. 1980;17(2):139–41. https://doi.org/10.1136/jmg.17.2.139.
9. Ludwig M, Utsch B, Reutter H. Genetic and molecular biological aspects of the bladder exstrophy-epispadias complex (BEEC). Urologe A. 2005;44(9):1037–8, 1040–1044. https://doi.org/10.1007/s00120-005-0863-z.
10. Ludwig M, Rüschendorf F, Saar K, Hübner N, Siekmann L, Boyadjiev SA, Reutter H. Genome-wide linkage scan for bladder exstrophy-epispadias complex. Birth Defects Res A Clin Mol Teratol. 2009;85(2):174–8. https://doi.org/10.1002/bdra.20512.
11. Lundin J, Söderhäll C, Lundén L, Hammarsjö A, White I, Schoumans J, Läckgren G, Kockum CC, Nordenskjöld A. 22q11.2 microduplication in two patients with bladder exstrophy and hearing impairment. Eur J Med Genet. 2010;53(2):61–5. https://doi.org/10.1016/j.ejmg.2009.11.004.

12. Mingardo E, Beaman G, Grote P, Nordenskjöld A, Newman W, Woolf AS, Eckstein M, Hilger AC, Dworschak GC, Rösch W, Ebert A-K, Stein R, Brusco A, Di Grazia M, Tamer A, Torres FM, Hernandez JL, Erben P, Maj C, et al. A genome-wide association study with tissue transcriptomics identifies genetic drivers for classic bladder exstrophy. Commun Biol. 2022;5(1):1203. https://doi.org/10.1038/s42003-022-04092-3.
13. Nordenskjöld A, Arkani S, Pettersson M, Winberg J, Cao J, Fossum M, Anderberg M, Barker G, Holmdahl G, Lundin J. Copy number variants suggest different molecular pathways for the pathogenesis of bladder exstrophy. Am J Med Genet A. 2023;191(2):378–90. https://doi.org/10.1002/ajmg.a.63031.
14. Pierquin G, Uwineza A. 22q11.2 microduplication in a patient with bladder exstrophy and delayed psychomotor development. Eur J Hum Genet. 2012;20(1):89.
15. Qi L, Wang M, Yagnik G, Mattheisen M, Gearhart JP, Lakshmanan Y, Ebert A-K, Rösch W, Ludwig M, Draaken M, Reutter H, Boyadjiev SA. Candidate gene association study implicates p63 in the etiology of nonsyndromic bladder-exstrophy-epispadias complex. Birth Defects Res A Clin Mol Teratol. 2013;97(12):759–63. https://doi.org/10.1002/bdra.23161.
16. Reutter H, Shapiro E, Gruen JR. Seven new cases of familial isolated bladder exstrophy and epispadias complex (BEEC) and review of the literature. Am J Med Genet A. 2003;120A(2):215–21. https://doi.org/10.1002/ajmg.a.20057.
17. Shapiro E, Lepor H, Jeffs RD. The inheritance of the exstrophy-epispadias complex. J Urol. 1984;132(2):308–10. https://doi.org/10.1016/s0022-5347(17)49605-4.
18. Smith MJ, Lattimer JK. The management of bladder exstrophy. Surg Gynecol Obstet. 1966;123(5):1015–8.
19. Weaver JK, Weiss DA, Thompson A, Joshi R, Ramji J, Shukla AR, D'Souza N, Kim E, Lee J, Wu CW, Broms R, Glessner J, Mentch F, Hakonarson H, Pyle LC. Genetic analysis of two bladder exstrophy populations of South Asian and North American origin. J Pediatr Urol. 2025;S1477–5131(25):00234–7. https://doi.org/10.1016/j.jpurol.2025.04.018. Epub ahead of print. PMID: 40340191.
20. von Lowtzow C, Hofmann A, Zhang R, Marsch F, Ebert A-K, Rösch W, Stein R, Boemers TM, Hirsch K, Marcelis C, Feitz WFJ, Brusco A, Migone N, Di Grazia M, Moebus S, Nöthen MM, Reutter H, Ludwig M, Draaken M. CNV analysis in 169 patients with bladder exstrophy-epispadias complex. BMC Med Genet. 2016;17(1):35. https://doi.org/10.1186/s12881-016-0299-x.
21. Wood HM, Babineau D, Gearhart JP. In vitro fertilization and the cloacal/bladder exstrophy-epispadias complex: a continuing association. J Pediatr Urol. 2007;3(4):305–10. https://doi.org/10.1016/j.jpurol.2006.10.007.
22. Zhang R, Knapp M, Suzuki K, Kajioka D, Schmidt JM, Winkler J, Yilmaz Ö, Pleschka M, Cao J, Kockum CC, Barker G, Holmdahl G, Beaman G, Keene D, Woolf AS, Cervellione RM, Cheng W, Wilkins S, Gearhart JP, et al. ISL1 is a major susceptibility gene for classic bladder exstrophy and a regulator of urinary tract development. Sci Rep. 2017;7:42170. https://doi.org/10.1038/srep42170.

4 Prenatal and Postnatal Imaging of the Bladder Epispadias-Exstrophy Complex

Edward R. Oliver and Susan J. Back

Introduction

In many countries, the diagnosis of the epispadias-exstrophy complex (EEC) is frequently made through the second-trimester anatomic screening obstetric ultrasound. Although fetal magnetic resonance imaging (MRI) may not be as readily accessible as ultrasound, it can be a powerful imaging adjunct in assessing cases of suspected EEC. Postnatally, imaging is frequently employed to confirm prenatal findings and assess for complications—either prior to or after surgical correction—such as urinary obstruction. Ultrasound remains the preferred modality for assessing the genitourinary anatomy in the EEC; however, other modalities, such as MRI, fluoroscopy, and CT, may often be employed. In this chapter, we review the prenatal imaging features of isolated bladder exstrophy and cloacal exstrophy and briefly discuss the imaging features of the much less common exstrophy variants. In addition, we review common postnatal imaging findings and share some of our experience and tips for performing and interpreting imaging studies at a tertiary pediatric center that sees a high volume of EEC patients.

E. R. Oliver (✉)
Department of Radiology and Richard D. Wood Jr. Center for Fetal Diagnosis and Treatment, Children's Hospital of Philadelphia, Philadelphia, PA, USA

Perelman School of Medicine, University of Pennsylvania, Philadelphia, PA, USA
e-mail: olivere1@chop.edu

S. J. Back
Department of Radiology, Children's Hospital of Philadelphia, Philadelphia, PA, USA

Perelman School of Medicine, University of Pennsylvania, Philadelphia, PA, USA
e-mail: backs@chop.edu

A. R. Shukla, R. S. Joshi (eds.), *Bladder Exstrophy and Epispadias*,
https://doi.org/10.1007/978-3-031-91238-2_4

Prenatal Imaging Findings

Bladder Exstrophy

Demonstration of a fluid-filled urinary bladder is a required component of all fetal anatomic examinations, regardless of whether the examination is a routine second-trimester screening ultrasound, a detailed fetal anatomic survey performed for a known or suspected anomaly, or a late first-trimester anatomic survey for patients in whom earlier assessment is indicated [1–3]. The normal fetal urinary bladder is located in the midline anterior pelvis, is bordered on both sides by the umbilical arteries (Fig. 4.1), and should fill and empty over the course of an examination. In the case of bladder exstrophy, the anterior abdominal wall and bladder fail to fuse and result in an infraumbilical wall defect with bladder mucosa exposed to the amniotic fluid. Fetal urine is released directly into amniotic space, leading to the pathognomonic finding of bladder exstrophy—a non-visualized, or "absent," urinary bladder (Figs. 4.2 and 4.3) [4, 5].

In addition to an "absent" urinary bladder, several other sonographic findings are typically present that assist in prenatally diagnosing bladder exstrophy. These include a low abdominal cord insertion (Figs. 4.2 and 4.3); genital abnormalities (Fig. 4.4), such as epispadias or bifid penis in males and bifid clitoris and vaginal and/or uterine anomalies in females; and bony pelvic abnormalities, such as pubic diastasis and flattening of the iliac bones (Figs. 4.2 and 4.3) [4–7]. The exstrophied bladder may vary in appearance and range from irregularity of the infraumbilical abdominal wall (Fig. 4.4) to a bulging infraumbilical mass mimicking an omphalocele (Fig. 4.5) [4, 8]. In the former instance, the infraumbilical irregularity is secondary to inflammation of the exposed posterior bladder wall mucosa, whereas in the latter instance, the mass-like appearance is secondary to protrusion and eversion of the bladder plate.

MRI is a powerful imaging adjunct for the assessment of complex fetal anomalies, and, unlike ultrasound, is not subject to some of the limitations that can constrain sonographic evaluation, such as fetal positioning, anterior placenta, and maternal body habitus [9]. In addition, MRI offers excellent tissue contrast, which is particularly helpful in evaluating genitourinary and gastrointestinal abnormalities.

The primary MRI findings of isolated bladder exstrophy are identical to those of ultrasound—non-visualized urinary bladder, infraumbilical abdominal wall defect with a low cord insertion, and pubic diastasis (Figs. 4.6, 4.7, and 4.8)—however, the added value of MRI is in confirming the absence of other anomalies that may confer a more severe diagnosis on the EEC spectrum. The T1-signal characteristics of meconium allow for thorough assessment for hindgut abnormalities, which should be absent in isolated bladder exstrophy. T1-hyperintense meconium should be seen

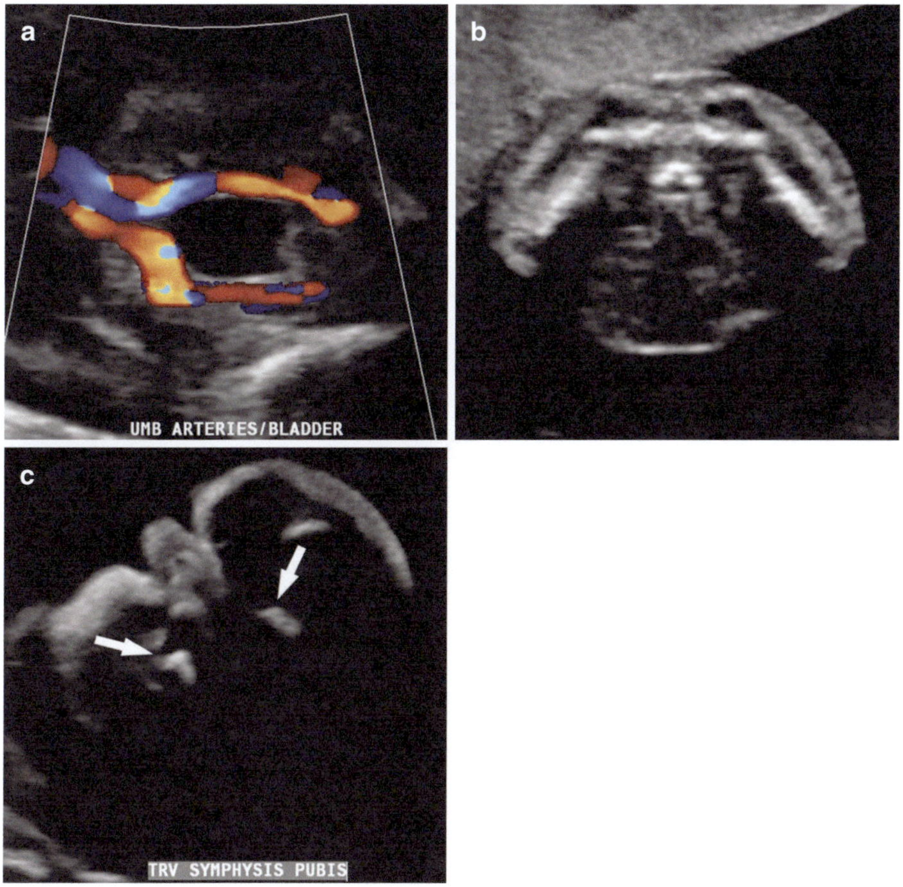

Fig. 4.1 Normal ultrasound findings in a 21-week gestation fetus (**a**) and a 22-week gestation fetus (**b** and **c**). (**a**) Color Doppler image through the pelvis demonstrates a normal anechoic and fluid-filled bladder bordered by both umbilical arteries. (**b**) Transverse grayscale image through the iliac wings demonstrates a normal iliac angle. (**c**) A transverse grayscale image through the lower pelvis shows a normal configuration of the symphysis pubis with the ossification centers (arrows) appropriately angled toward the midline. Distance between the ossified portions of the symphysis pubis measured <1 cm (not shown)

within the rectum after 20 weeks gestational age, and there should be progressive filling of the more proximal colon as the pregnancy advances [10]. If an anteriorly displaced anus is present, the course of the rectum to the perineum may be easier to appreciate on MRI, as the rectal meconium signal should be readily identifiable (Figs. 4.6, 4.7, and 4.8).

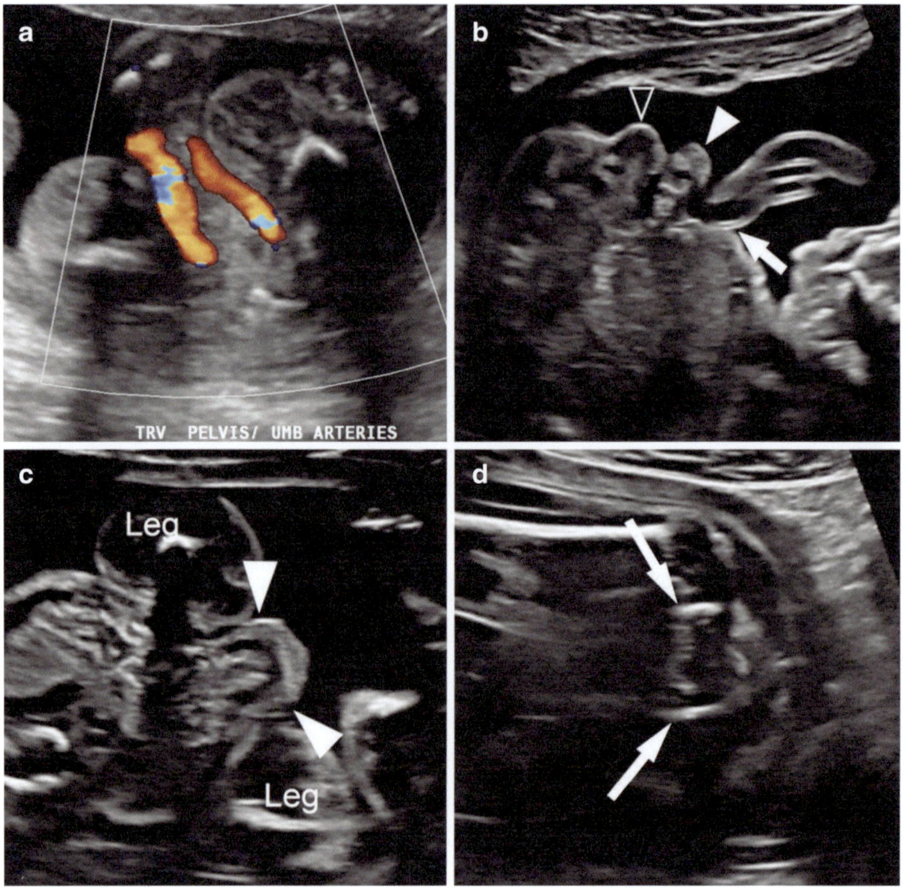

Fig. 4.2 Ultrasound findings of classic bladder exstrophy at 21 weeks gestation. (**a**) Transverse color Doppler image through the pelvis and umbilical arteries demonstrates the absence of an anechoic fluid-filled bladder between the two umbilical arteries, consistent with bladder exstrophy. (**b**) Sagittal grayscale image through the lower abdomen demonstrates an infraumbilical defect (arrowhead) representing the exstrophied bladder immediately below the abdominal cord insertion (arrow) and cephalad to the external genitalia (open arrowhead), which were abnormal in appearance (not shown). (**c**) Transverse grayscale image through the pelvis demonstrates the infraumbilical defect (arrowheads) and bladder plate bulging between the flexed and adducted legs. (**d**) Transverse grayscale image through the anterior bony pelvis reveals separation of the symphysis pubis (arrows) with the ossified portions demonstrating an abnormal parallel configuration. In addition, the distance between the ossified portions of the symphysis is abnormal and >1 cm (1.3 cm, not shown), and the findings are consistent with pubic diastasis. (**e**) Transverse grayscale image through the perineum reveals normal hyperechoic anal mucosa (*) surrounded by a ring of normal hypoechoic anal sphincter muscle (open arrows). (**f**) Sagittal grayscale image through the pelvis and perineum reveals the normal echogenic rectal mucosa (*) extending to the anal orifice (open arrow). (**g**) Postnatal photograph demonstrating the exstrophied bladder (between open arrows) and the abnormal external male genitalia consistent with epispadias (circle)

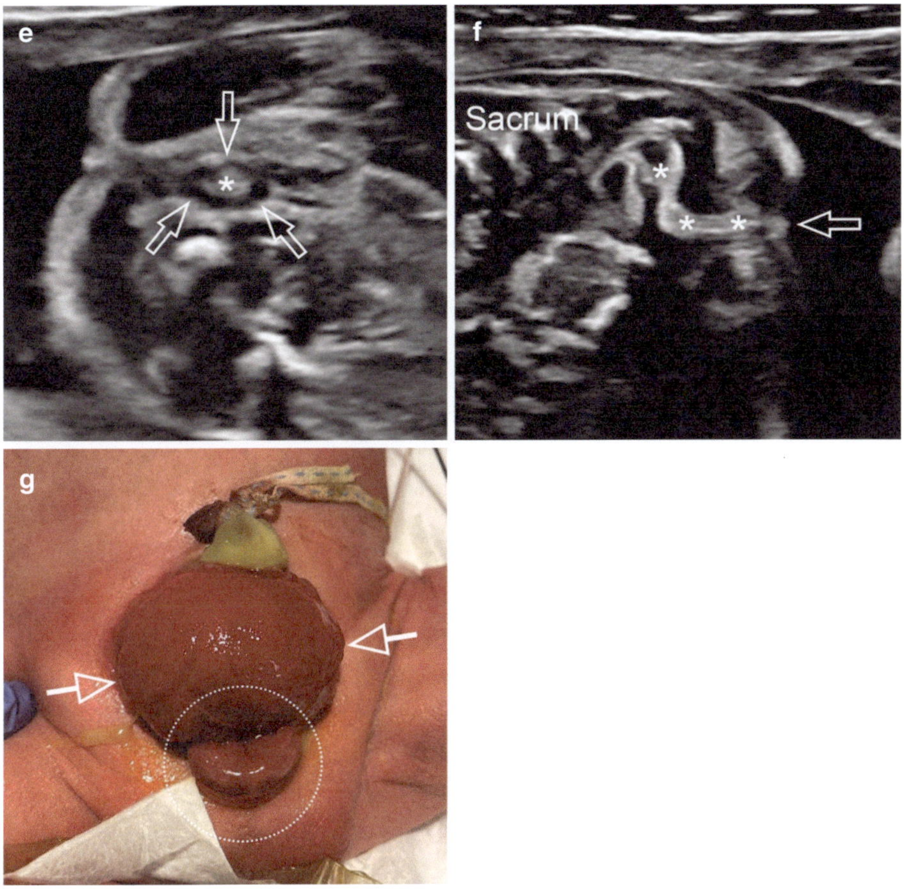

Fig. 4.2 (continued)

Careful assessment of the abdomen and pelvis is crucial in distinguishing isolated bladder exstrophy from bladder exstrophy associated with cloacal exstrophy, which is discussed in greater detail in the following section. In isolated bladder exstrophy, there should be no abnormalities of the spine, such as spinal dysraphisms or anomalous vertebrae. Similarly, abnormalities of the hindgut, such as imperforate anus, should not be present in isolated bladder exstrophy. It is important to note that the anus may be anteriorly displaced in isolated bladder exstrophy and slightly difficult to demonstrate, potentially giving the false impression of an associated imperforate anus. Careful assessment of the perineum can often identify a displaced anus and avoid misdiagnosis. Free-floating intra-amniotic bowel loops also should not be seen in cases of isolated bladder exstrophy, as fusion of the posterior bladder plate halves prevents extrusion of bowel loops into the amniotic fluid; identification of intra-amniotic bowel loops arising through an infraumbilical defect strongly suggests that the bladder halves are separate and unfused, which is a feature of cloacal exstrophy. Lastly, the abdominal wall defect present in isolated bladder exstrophy should be infraumbilical and not involve or extend above the level of the cord insertion, as would be seen with an omphalocele.

Fig. 4.3 Ultrasound findings of classic bladder exstrophy at 24 weeks gestation. (**a**) Transverse color Doppler image through the pelvis and umbilical arteries demonstrates the absence of an anechoic fluid-filled bladder between the two umbilical arteries. (**b**) Sagittal grayscale image through the lower abdomen demonstrates an infraumbilical defect (arrowhead) representing the exstrophied bladder immediately below the abdominal cord insertion (arrow) and cephalad to the external genitalia (open arrow). (**c**) Three-dimensional image of the lower abdominal and pelvic wall shows the abdominal cord insertion (arrow), the bladder plate (arrowhead) bulging between the flexed and adducted legs, and the external genitalia (open arrowhead). (**d**) Transverse grayscale image through the anterior bony pelvis demonstrates pubic diastasis (arrows). Although one ossification center is angled toward the midline, the other is not, and the distance between the ossified portions is abnormal and >1 cm (1.6 cm, not shown). (**e**) Transverse grayscale image through the bony pelvis at the level of the lumbosacral junction reveals posterior rotation of the iliac bones, resulting in an abnormally increased iliac wing angle

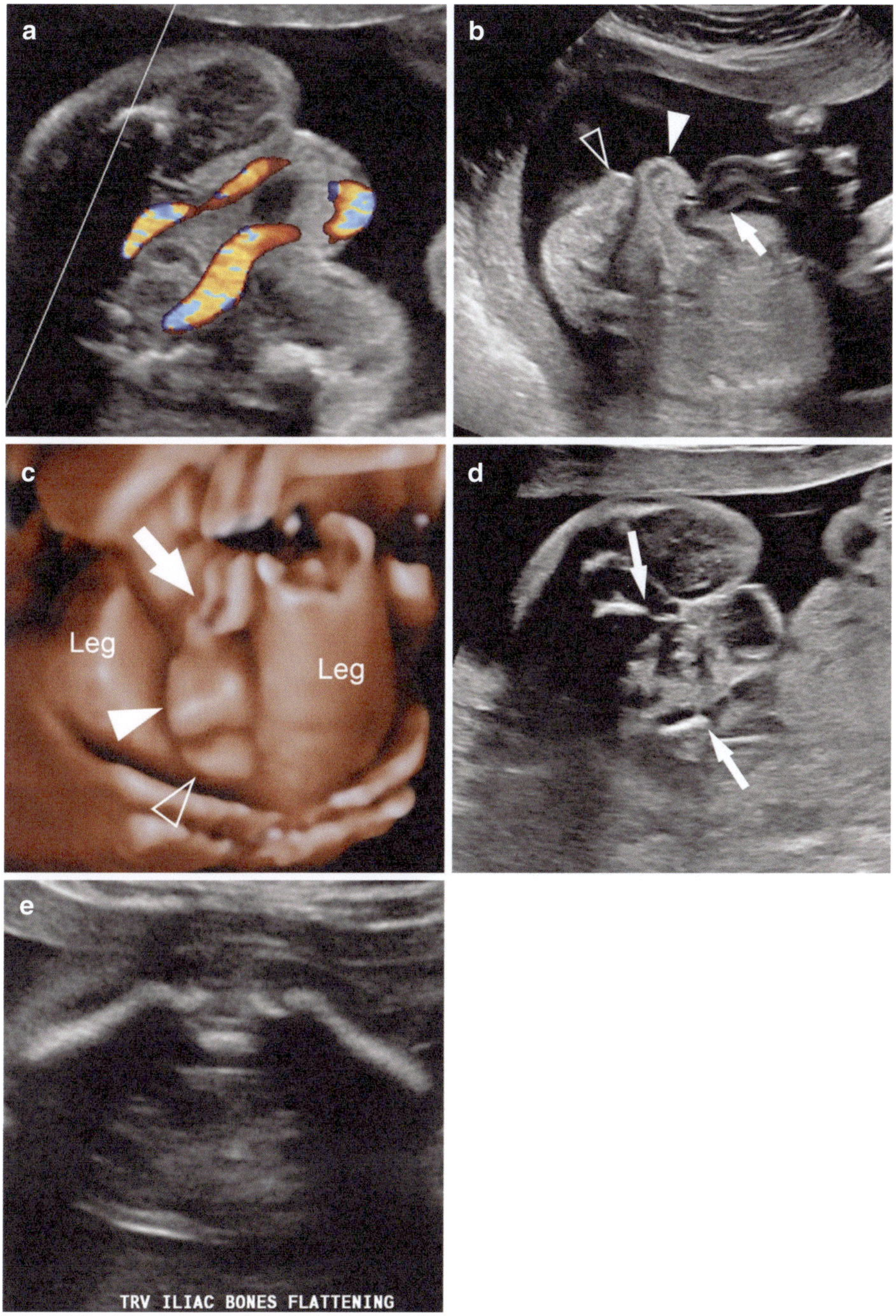
a
b
c
Leg
Leg
d
e
TRV ILIAC BONES FLATTENING

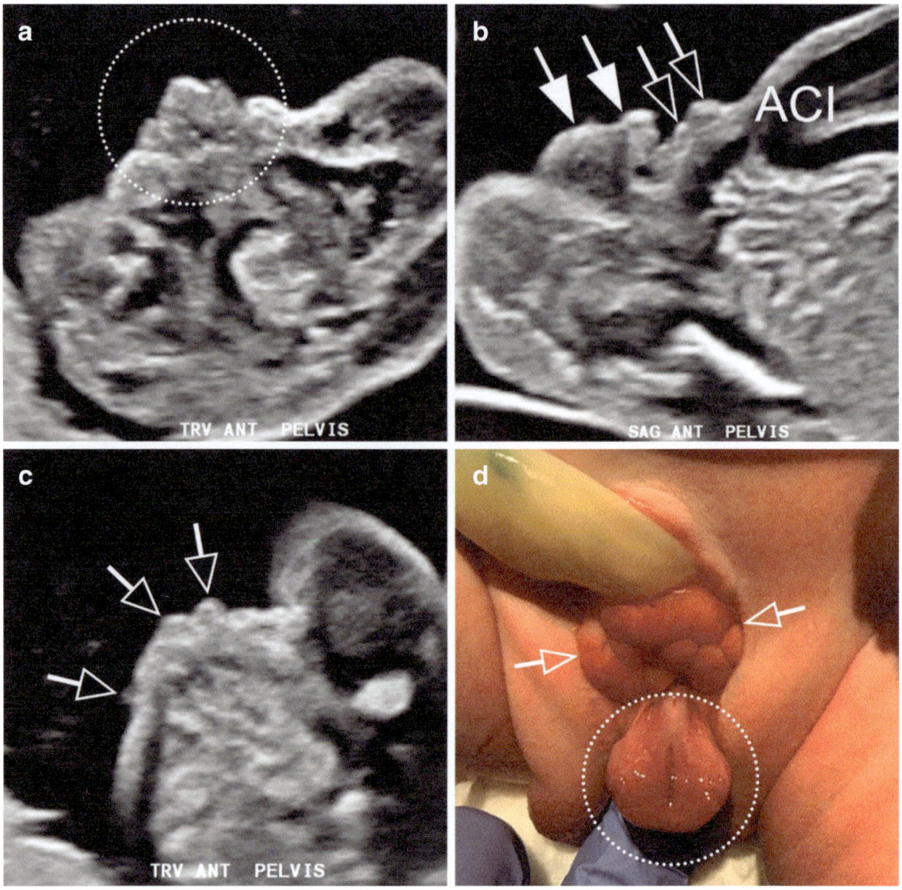

Fig. 4.4 US findings of the abnormal external genitalia and irregular bladder mucosa in classic bladder exstrophy at 19 weeks gestation. (**a**) Transverse grayscale image of the external genitalia reveals an abnormal ambiguous appearance of the genitalia (circle). (**b**) Sagittal grayscale image through the lower abdomen demonstrates a ventral wall defect between the abdominal cord insertion (ACI) and external genitalia (closed arrows). The defect has a lobulated and irregular surface (open arrows). (**c**) Transverse grayscale image of the infraumbilical defect further illustrates the irregular contour of the defect (open arrows), corresponding to the inflamed bladder mucosa. (**d**) Postnatal photograph reveals the lobulated exposed bladder mucosa (between open arrows) and abnormal male external genitalia with epispadias (circle)

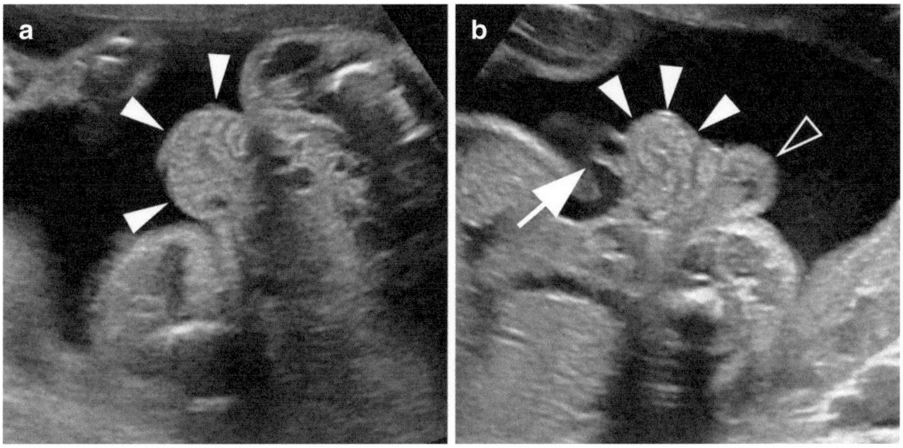

Fig. 4.5 Classic bladder exstrophy with ultrasound findings mimicking a bowel-containing omphalocele at 27 weeks gestation. (**a**) Transverse grayscale image of the abdomen demonstrates a protruding ventral wall defect containing non-dilated bowel (arrowheads). (**b**) Sagittal grayscale image reveals that the ventral wall defect (arrowheads) is infraumbilical and immediately below the ACI (arrow) and cephalad to the external genitalia (open arrowhead). The infraumbilical location and absence of a fluid-filled bladder on other images (not shown) are consistent with bladder exstrophy with a protruding bladder plate rather than an omphalocele

Cloacal Exstrophy

Cloacal exstrophy represents a more severe constellation of urogenital and gastrointestinal malformations and is considered by many to represent the most severe clinical entity on the bladder exstrophy-epispadias complex spectrum [11, 12]. In addition to bladder exstrophy, an omphalocele, imperforate anus, and spine abnormality are classically present, leading to the acronym by which this entity is also known—*o*mphalocele, bladder *e*xstrophy, *i*mperforate anus, and *s*pine anomalies (OEIS) complex. The acronym OEIS was originally coined as a mnemonic for the typical anomalies seen in cloacal exstrophy [13], and the terms "cloacal exstrophy" and "OEIS complex" should be considered synonymous [14]. It is also important to recognize that not all four components of classic cloacal exstrophy need to be present for its diagnosis [15]. Indeed, in one series of cloacal exstrophy, only 22.6% had all four components (OEIS), 32.8% had cloacal exstrophy without spine abnormalities (OIE), and 18% had cloacal exstrophy without omphalocele (EIS) [15]. Therefore, when making a prenatal diagnosis of cloacal exstrophy, it is likely best to specify which individual components are present (e.g., "Cloacal exstrophy, characterized by …"), as this will help optimize prenatal counseling, delivery planning, and neonatal management [16].

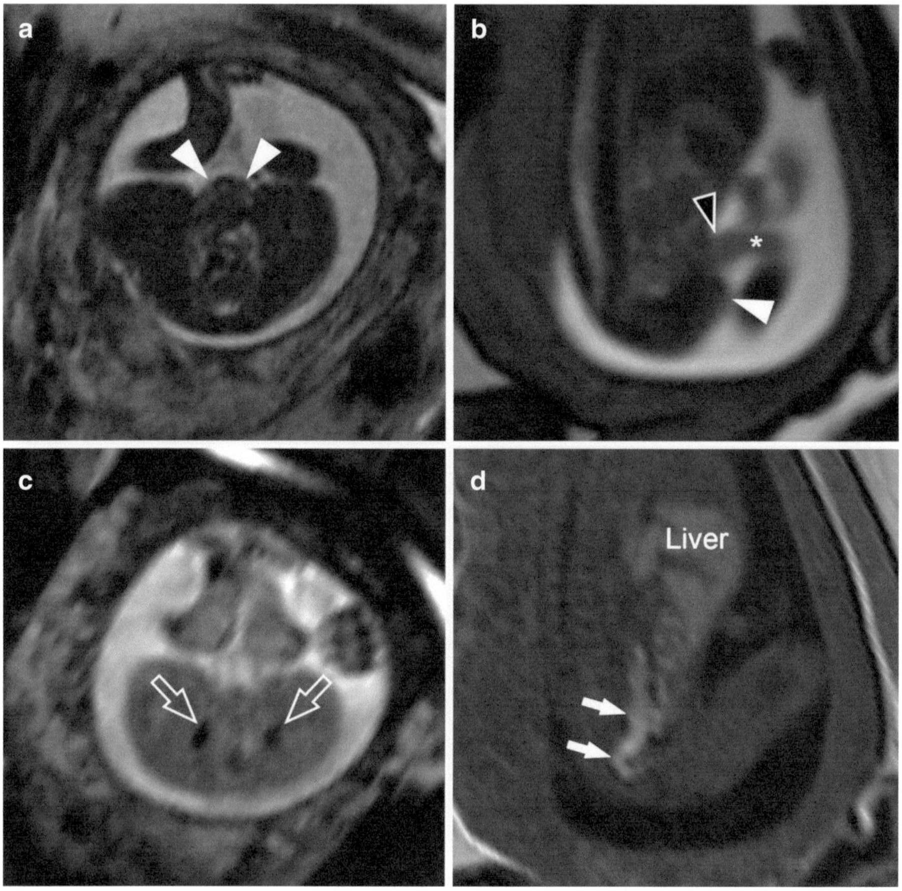

Fig. 4.6 MRI findings of classic bladder exstrophy at 22 weeks gestation. (**a**) Transverse FSE T2-weighted image (TR/TE ms, 1100/84) through the lower abdomen just below the level of the umbilical cord insertion demonstrates the absence of a fluid-filled bladder and a relatively small infraumbilical defect (arrowheads). (**b**) Sagittal SSFP image (TR/TE ms, 3.99/1.74) through the mid-abdomen demonstrates a ventral wall defect (arrowhead) located immediately below the level of a low ACI (black arrowhead) representing the exstrophied bladder. *, umbilical cord. (**c**) Transverse EPI image (TR/TE ms, 5841/50) through the lower bony pelvis demonstrates widening of the symphysis pubis (measured distance 1.2 cm). (**d**) Sagittal T1-weighted gradient echo image (TR/TE ms, 202/4.76) through the lower abdomen and pelvis demonstrates a normal course of the T1-hyperintense meconium (arrows) extending to the perineum, arguing against the presence of an imperforate anus/anorectal malformation. A fluid-filled bladder was not identified on any other sequences, and the constellation of findings is consistent with classic bladder exstrophy

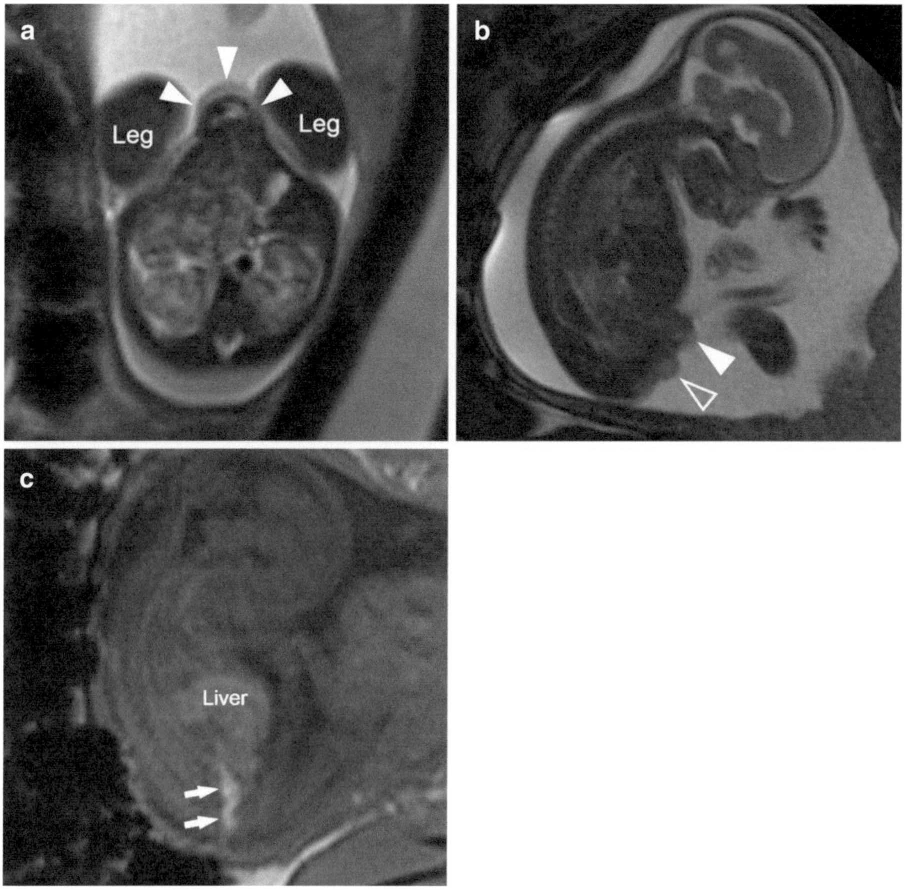

Fig. 4.7 MRI findings of classic bladder exstrophy at 21 weeks gestation (same case as Fig. 4.2). (**a**) Transverse FSE T2-weighted image (TR/TE ms, 1100/76) through the lower abdomen just below the level of the umbilical cord insertion demonstrates the absence of a fluid-filled bladder and a relatively small infraumbilical defect (arrowheads) protruding between the adducted legs. (**b**) Sagittal SSFP image (TR/TE ms, 4.18/1.92) through the mid-abdomen demonstrates a ventral wall defect (arrowhead) that was immediately below the level of the ACI (not shown) representing the exstrophied bladder and cephalad to the external genitalia (open arrowhead). (**c**) Sagittal T1-weighted gradient echo image (TR/TE ms, 209/4.76) through the lower abdomen and pelvis demonstrates a normal course of the T1-hyperintense meconium (arrows) extending to the perineum, which argues against imperforate anus/anorectal malformation. A fluid-filled bladder was not identified on any other sequences, and the findings are consistent with classic bladder exstrophy

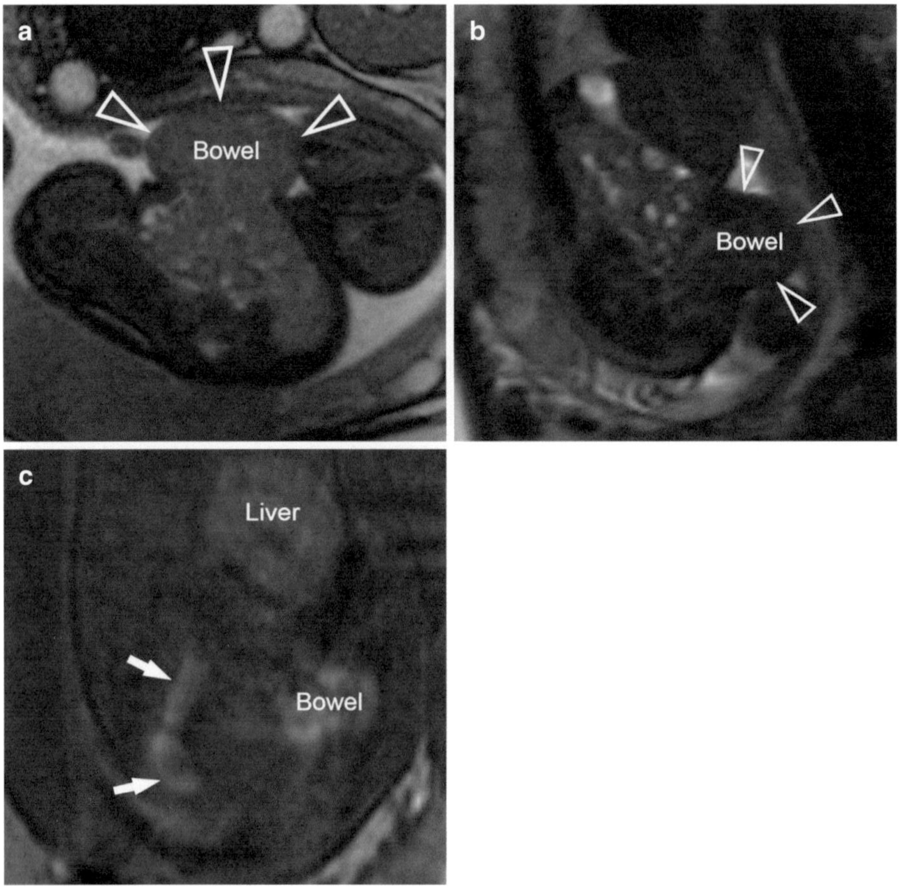

Fig. 4.8 MRI findings of classic bladder exstrophy at 21 weeks gestation with a large infraumbilical defect mimicking an omphalocele. (**a**) Transverse SSFP image (TR/TE ms, 4.05/1.65) through the lower abdomen just below the level of the umbilical cord insertion demonstrates the absence of a fluid-filled bladder and a large infraumbilical defect (arrowheads) containing bowel loops. (**b**) Sagittal FSE T2-weighted image (TR/TE ms, 1100/76) through the mid-abdomen demonstrates a large ventral wall defect (arrowheads) that was immediately below the level of the ACI (not shown) representing the exstrophied bladder with protruding bowel contained by the bladder plate. (**c**) Sagittal T1-weighted gradient echo image (TR/TE ms, 202/4.76) through the lower abdomen and pelvis demonstrates a normal course of the T1-hyperintense meconium (arrows) extending to the perineum, which argues against imperforate anus/anorectal malformation. Meconium-filled loops of the bowel are also noted within the large infraumbilical defect. No other findings on US or MRI were present to suggest cloacal exstrophy, and postnatal examination confirmed the presence of classic bladder exstrophy with a large infraumbilical defect mimicking an omphalocele

The characteristic prenatal imaging findings of cloacal exstrophy include those of bladder exstrophy, an omphalocele, an inability to identify a normal anal orifice, and a spinal abnormality (Fig. 4.9). In cloacal exstrophy, the primary prenatal ultrasound findings of bladder exstrophy are similar to isolated bladder exstrophy—an infraumbilical ventral wall defect, "absent" bladder, low abdominal cord insertion, and pelvic anomalies. However, it is important to recognize that the exstrophied bladder in cloacal exstrophy consists of two hemibladders that are separated by the cecal plate. Moreover, prolapsed ileum may extend from the cecal plate between the hemibladders and result in the characteristic "elephant trunk sign" (Fig. 4.10) [17]. Detection of an omphalocele can be challenging in the setting of the infraumbilical defect associated with bladder exstrophy, and especially if the omphalocele is small. Nevertheless, careful attention should be directed at the abdominal wall, and an omphalocele should be suspected if the ventral wall defect is observed to involve and/or extend above the level of the abdominal cord insertion (Fig. 4.9). An inability to document a normal anal dimple and/or the presence of a dilated rectum should raise strong suspicion for imperforate anus (Fig. 4.8) or anorectal malformation. Lastly, any spinal abnormality may be present. A closed spinal dysraphism (i.e., myelocystocele and lipomyelomeningocele) is considered a strict criterion for the classic diagnosis of cloacal exstrophy; however, the severity of spinal abnormalities may be mild and take the form of vertebral segmentation anomalies or a low conus medullaris (Figs. 4.10 and 4.11) [18].

Experienced sonologists are often capable of identifying the myriad abnormalities present in cloacal exstrophy; however, fetal MRI is a useful adjunct for clarifying or confirming the findings of cloacal exstrophy, especially in the setting of unfavorable fetal lie, anterior placenta, and/or maternal factors. Similar to ultrasound, a fluid-filled bladder will not be identified on T2-weighted MR images, and prolapse of the distal ileum between the exstrophied hemibladders may also be present. The ability of MRI to obtain a sagittal image of the abdominal wall regardless of fetal lie and maternal factors is helpful in assessing the relationship of the ventral wall defect to the abdominal cord insertion and whether a small omphalocele is present (Fig. 4.11). T1-weighted sequences nicely depict the course of meconium in the distal colon, and an inability to trace the meconium signal to the level of the perineum or an abnormal course of the meconium signal in the distal-most colon should raise concern for imperforate anus or other anorectal malformation (Figs. 4.11 and 4.12). Although major spine abnormalities associated with cloacal exstrophy, such as lipomyelomeningocele and myelocystocele, should be identifiable by ultrasound, MRI provides another opportunity to assess the fetal spine. T2-weighted sequences are especially helpful in identifying the cerebrospinal fluid-filled component of complex closed spinal dysraphisms (Figs. 4.11 and 4.12). Although the spatial resolution of MRI may not be optimal to identify subtle segmentation anomalies, MRI may help demonstrate the position of the conus medullaris, which will vary throughout gestation (Fig. 4.11) [19, 20].

Isolated Epispadias

Epispadias without bladder exstrophy represents a relatively minor malformation on the EEC spectrum. Prenatal diagnosis can be particularly challenging and may be overlooked, especially if the abnormality is mild or the external genitalia are not adequately assessed [7]. Ultrasound findings may include bifid penis/clitoris, absent genitalia, or simply an abnormal appearance of the external genitalia (Fig. 4.13) [7, 21]. MRI may not be able to further characterize the abnormality due to the small size of the involved anatomic structures and the modality's lower spatial resolution.

Exstrophy Variants

Variant presentations of the bladder exstrophy—epispadias complex are rare, occurring approximately ten-fold less frequently than the classic forms [22]. The clinical phenotypes of the exstrophy variants are wide-ranging, but a recent 40-year retrospective study from a high-volume center reported that the most common exstrophy variants (excluding cloacal exstrophy) were skin-covered bladder exstrophy (also termed "pseudoexstrophy") and epispadias with bladder prolapse; these atypical presentations accounted for 43% and 32% of the bladder exstrophy variants, respectively [23]. Variants of cloacal exstrophy also have been reported but are less common and reportedly accounted for 0.7% of cases in an older study from the same institution [24].

The prenatal imaging appearance of exstrophy variants can be confusing. Indeed, the identification of a fluid-filled bladder in skin-covered exstrophy variants may result in failure to consider exstrophy as a diagnostic possibility [25]. There is,

Fig. 4.9 24-week gestation fetus with cloacal exstrophy. (**a**) Transverse Color Doppler image of the pelvis at the expected level of the bladder demonstrates a single left umbilical artery, consistent with a two-vessel cord. No fluid-filled bladder is present, and none was identified throughout the course of the examination, consistent with bladder exstrophy. LT, left; RT right. (**b**) Sagittal grayscale image through the anterior abdomen demonstrates a large ventral wall defect with a covering membrane (arrows) containing most of the liver and multiple loops of bowel, consistent with a giant omphalocele. (**c**) A transverse grayscale image of the sacral spine reveals a fluid-filled, thick-walled, and skin-covered spinal dysraphism. A small focus of echogenic tissue representing macroscopic fat is also present, and the findings are consistent with a lipomyelomeningocele. (**d**) Sagittal grayscale image through the lumbosacral spine shows a low conus medullaris terminating at S2, consistent with a tethered cord. (**e**) Transverse grayscale image of the perineum demonstrates the absence of a normal anal "target" sign, consistent with imperforate anus (compare to Fig. 4.2e), consistent with anorectal malformation. (**f**) Sagittal grayscale images of the pelvis also confirm the absence of a normal rectosigmoid colon (compared to the Fig. 4.2f). The constellation of anomalies is consistent with cloacal exstrophy (aka OEIS syndrome)

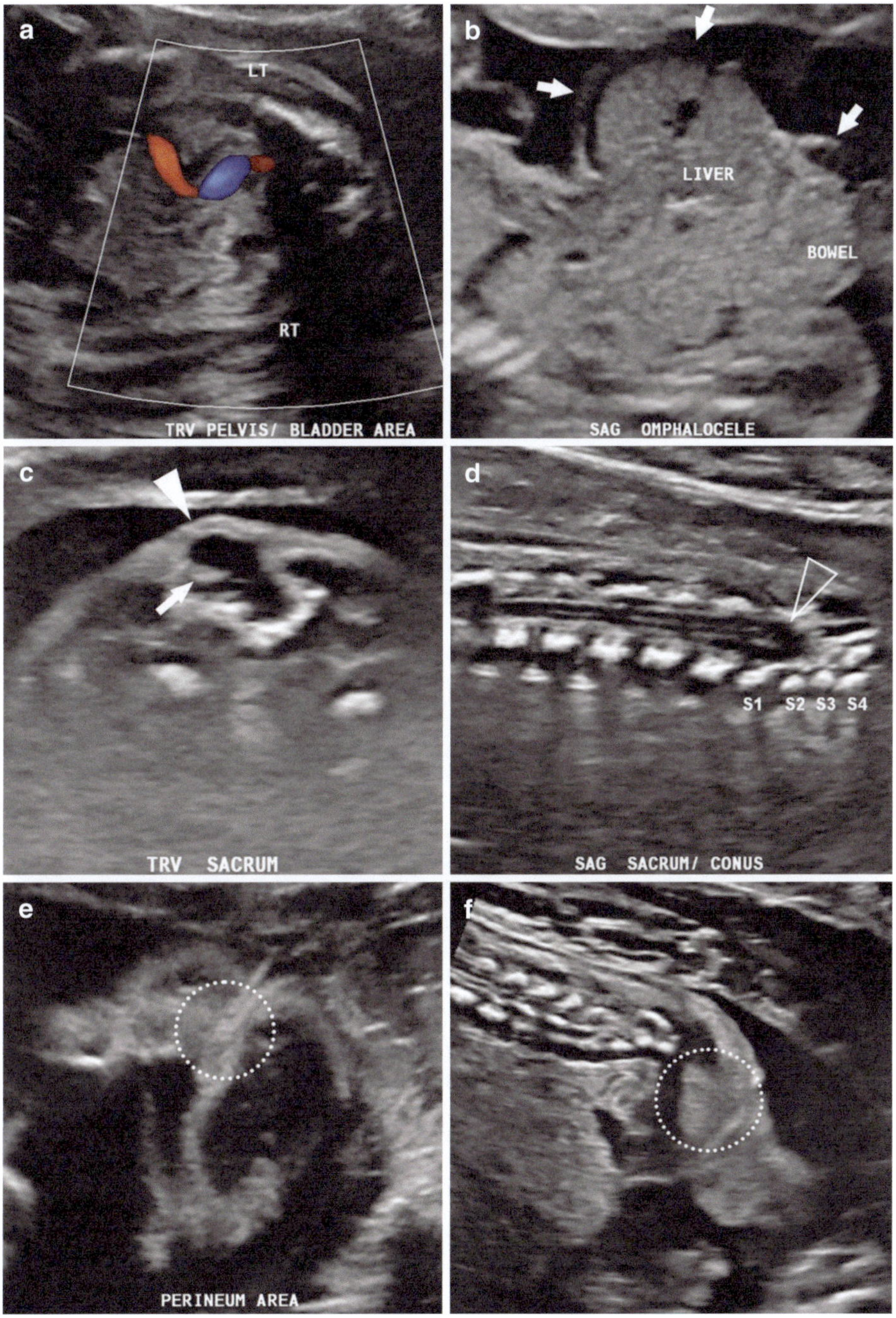
a
LT
RT
TRV PELVIS/ BLADDER AREA
b
LIVER
BOWEL
SAG OMPHALOCELE
c
TRV SACRUM
d
S1 S2 S3 S4
SAG SACRUM/ CONUS
e
PERINEUM AREA
f

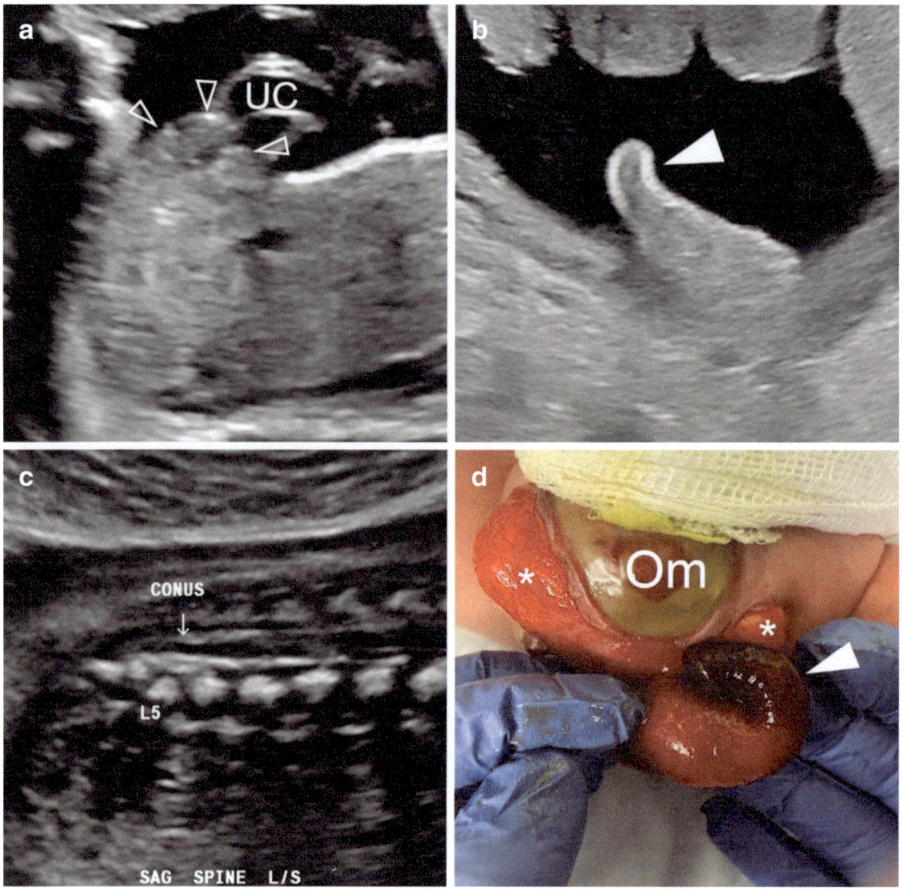

Fig. 4.10 KS. 30-week gestational age fetus with cloacal exstrophy. (**a**) Sagittal grayscale image through the lower abdomen demonstrates an infraumbilical ventral wall defect (open arrows). Although centered below the ACI, careful assessment reveals that the abdominal contents extend into the base of the umbilical cord (UC), consistent with a small omphalocele. (**b**) Transverse grayscale image through the ventral wall defect demonstrates a protruding tubular loop of bowel (arrowhead), consistent with prolapsed ileum ("elephant trunk" sign) that may be observed in cloacal exstrophy. (**c**) Sagittal grayscale image of the lumbosacral spine demonstrates a low conus medullaris terminating at L5. Segmentation anomalies of the lumbosacral spine were also present; however, no findings of a closed spinal dysraphism, such as lipomyelomeningocele or myelocystocele, were present. Spine anomalies associated with cloacal exstrophy may be mild or subtle as in this case. Additional prenatal findings consistent with cloacal exstrophy included non-visualized bladder and small bowel-containing omphalocele (not shown). (**d**) Postnatal photograph of the ventral wall defect demonstrates the prolapsed ileum (arrowhead) seen prenatally, which extends between the two hemibladders (*) and below the small omphalocele (Om)

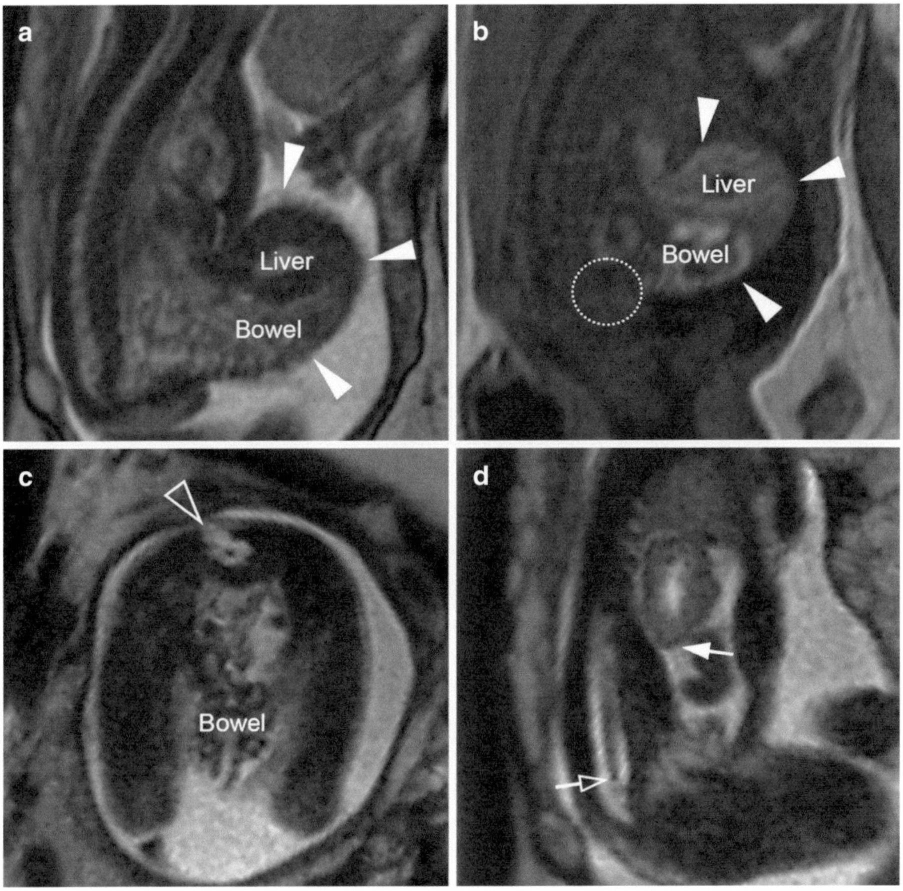

Fig. 4.11 24-week gestational age fetus with cloacal exstrophy (same case as Fig. 4.9). (**a**) Sagittal steady-state free precession image (TE/TR ms, 4.12/1.66) through the fetal body demonstrates a large membrane-covered ventral wall defect (arrowheads) containing most of the liver and multiple loops of bowel, consistent with giant omphalocele. (**b**) Sagittal T1-weighted image (TE/TR ms, 202/4.76) through the fetal body demonstrates the giant omphalocele containing the T1-hyperintense liver and meconium-filled bowel loops; however, no T1-hyperintense meconium is identified in the expected region of the rectum (circle), consistent with imperforate anus. (**c**) Transverse fast-spin echo T2-weighted image (TE/TR ms, 1100/78) through the pelvis reveals small skin-covered spinal dysraphism (open arrowhead), consistent with a lipomyelomeningocele. Bowel loops extending into the omphalocele are partially visualized. (**d**) Sagittal oblique fast-spin echo T2-weighted image (TE/TR ms, 1100/78) through the lower spine shows the conus medullaris (open arrow) terminating well below the inferior pole of the right kidney (arrow), in keeping with a low conus medullaris. Normally, the conus medullaris does not extend below the lower poles of the kidneys. A fluid-filled bladder was not identified on this MRI examination or on ultrasound, consistent with bladder exstrophy. The constellation of findings is consistent with cloacal exstrophy (OEIS syndrome)

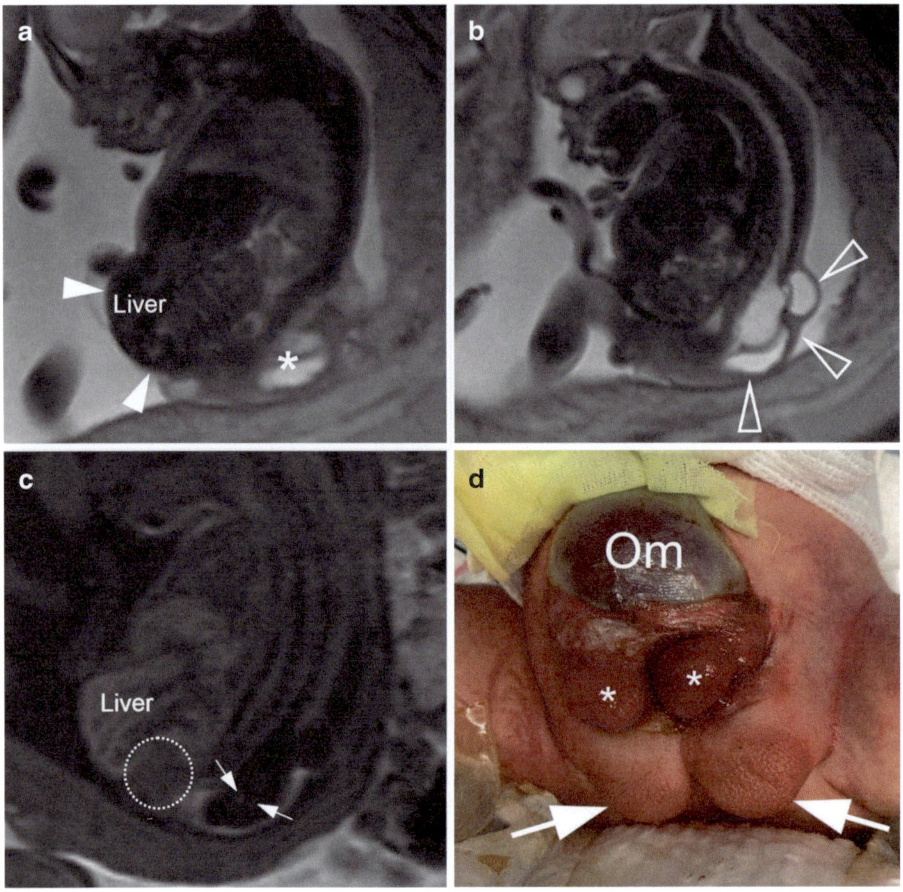

Fig. 4.12 28-week gestational age fetus with cloacal exstrophy. (**a**) Sagittal fast-spin echo T2-weighted image (TE/TR ms, 1100/76) through the fetal body demonstrates a moderately sized membrane-covered ventral wall defect (arrowheads) containing a portion of the liver, consistent with giant omphalocele. A complex spinal dysraphism is partially visualized (*). (**b**) Sagittal fast-spin echo T2-weighted image (TE/TR ms, 1100/76) through the spinal dysraphism depicts the large size and internal complexity of the defect. The combined MRI and ultrasound features were consistent with lipomyelomeningocele. (**c**) Sagittal T1-weighted image (TE/TR ms, 202/4.76) through the fetal body demonstrates the liver-containing omphalocele and the absence of T1 hyperintensity in the expected location of the rectum (circle), consistent with an imperforate anus. T1-hyperintense components (arrows) are also present within the spinal dysraphism sac, consistent with macroscopic fat and a lipomyelomeningocele. A fluid-filled bladder was not identified on this MRI examination or on ultrasound, consistent with bladder exstrophy. The constellation of findings is consistent with cloacal exstrophy (OEIS syndrome). (**d**) Postnatal photograph demonstrates two exstrophied hemibladders (*) between a bowel- and liver-containing omphalocele (Om) and bifid scrotum (arrows). A skin-covered spinal dysraphism and anal atresia were confirmed postnatally (not shown). A hindgut fistula was also present below the left hemibladder (not shown)

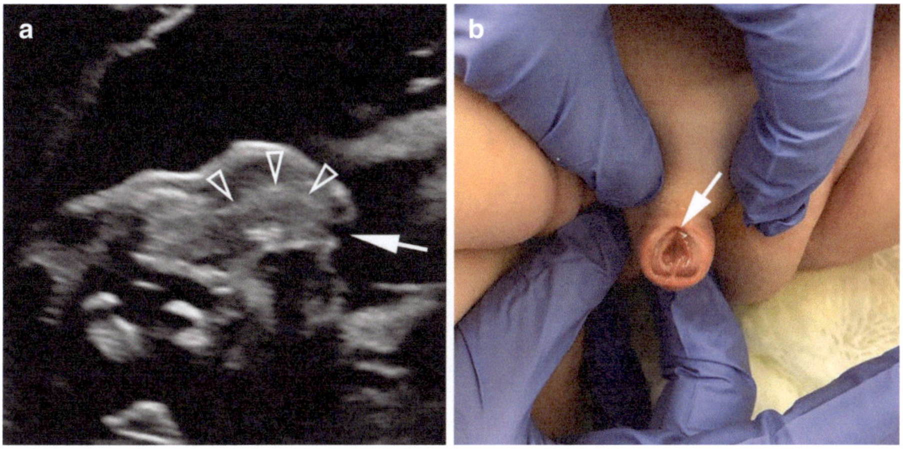

Fig. 4.13 Isolated epispadias. (**a**) Sagittal grayscale image of the external genitalia of a genetically proven male fetus at 25 weeks gestational age. There is a defect at the tip of the phallus (arrow), which is dorsal to the penile urethra (mildly hyperechoic line denoted by open arrowheads). The external genitalia was recognized as being abnormal, however, a diagnosis of epispadias was not made. (**b**) Clinical photograph of the external genitalia demonstrates a dorsal defect along the glans of the penis (arrow), consistent with epispadias and explaining the prenatal imaging findings

however, increasing recognition of the prenatal imaging findings in these variants, with multiple case reports now describing their imaging features [25–29]. Although a bladder may be present, the appearance of the urinary bladder in cases of skin-covered exstrophy variants is not normal. The bladder may extend into the base of the umbilical cord and mimic an allantoic cyst [25, 29], extend beyond the normal infraumbilical abdominal contour (Fig. 4.14) [26, 27], or communicate with the hindgut and contain echogenic debris [28]. Features common to almost all cases of exstrophy variants are low abdominal cord insertions and pubic diastasis [23, 30], and any abnormality of the bladder or other constellation of findings seen with the exstrophy spectrum should prompt assessment of the abdominal cord insertion, symphysis pubis, and bony pelvis (Fig. 4.14). The presence of a bladder anomaly should also prompt careful assessment for anomalies associated with cloacal exstrophy (e.g., omphalocele, anorectal malformation, spine anomaly) (Fig. 4.14) to ensure a more severe exstrophy variant is not overlooked.

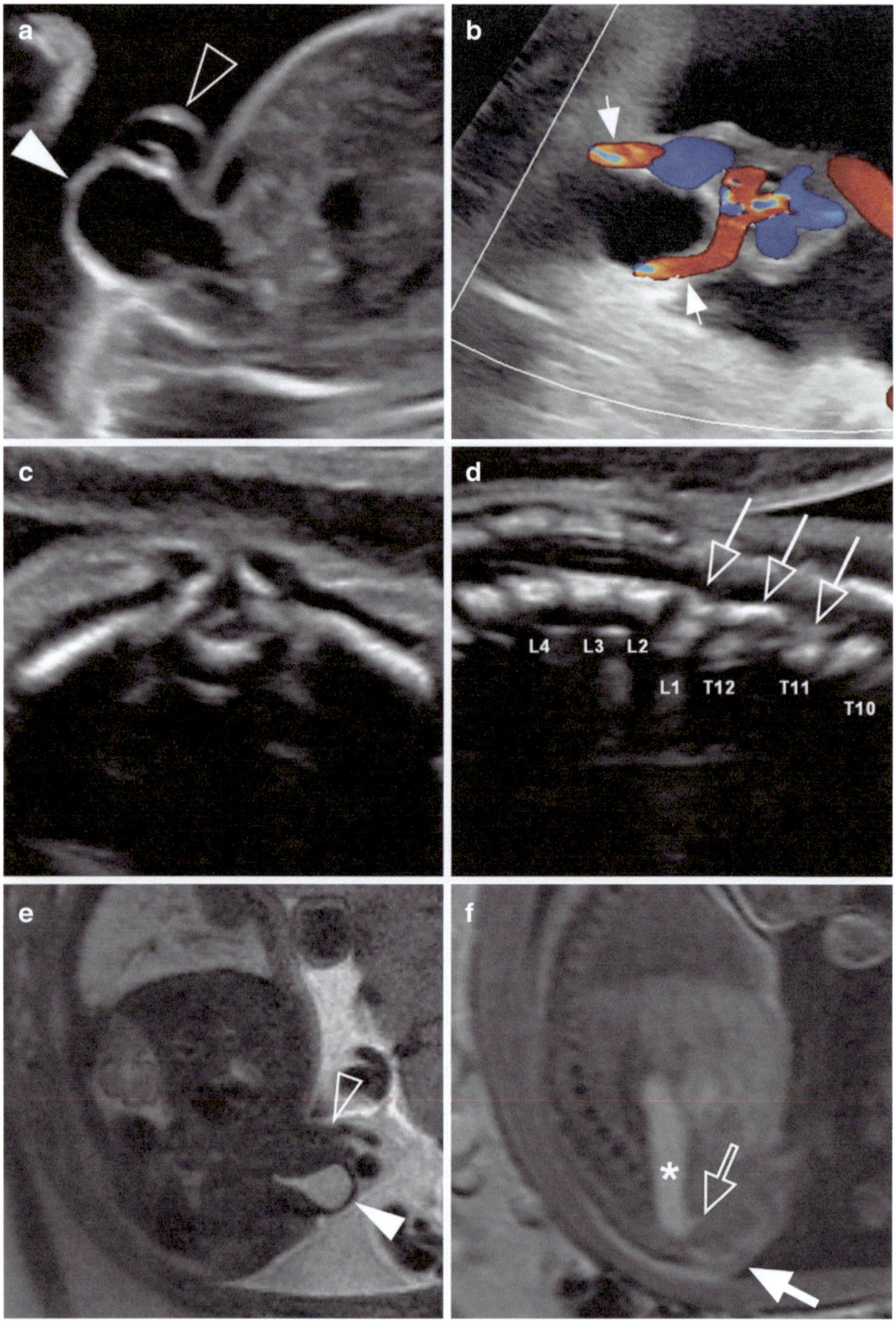
a
b
c
d
L4
L3
L2
L1
T12
T11
T10
e
f
*

Postnatal Imaging Findings

Postnatal imaging of a child with EEC is done to understand their anatomy prior to surgery and to assess postoperative changes and suspected complications. Radiography, fluoroscopy, renal scintigraphy, ultrasound (US), computed tomography (CT), and MRI each have a role in the care of these children. The type of imaging used depends on availability and the anatomic area of interest.

Urinary System

Although uncommon, congenital renal anomalies occur in a proportionally (1.6–9.1 times) higher number of patients with classic bladder exstrophy compared with the general population [31]. Among those with EEC, they are more commonly associated with cloacal exstrophy. In keeping with the goal of preserved renal function over the course of exstrophy repair, understanding the patient's urinary tract anatomy at birth and monitoring for changes during bladder reconstruction and ureteral reimplantation is of paramount importance. Renal size, location, and morphology can be assessed by US at baseline and after interventions (Fig. 4.15).

Complete primary repair of bladder exstrophy (CPRE) may expose the upper urinary tracts to higher pressure earlier in life, which may contribute to urinary tract dilation (UTD) and vesicoureteral reflux (VUR). Bladder pressure and compliance can be evaluated by video urodynamic studies, and UTD can be followed by renal US. Even after CPRE, high-grade UTD is uncommon [32] (Fig. 4.16). Similar to children without EEC, VUR can be evaluated either by voiding cystourethrography (VCUG) (Fig. 4.17) or, where available, contrast-enhanced voiding urosonography (ceVUS).

Fig. 4.14 30-week gestational age fetus with skin-covered cloacal exstrophy variant. (**a**) Sagittal grayscale image of the lower abdominal wall demonstrates a thick-walled fluid-filled defect (arrowhead) extending anteriorly from the abdomen just below the ACI (open arrowhead). (**b**) Transverse color Doppler image just below the level of the ACI reveals that the fluid-filled structure is midline and bordered by both umbilical arteries (short arrows), consistent with an abnormal bladder. (**c**) Transverse grayscale image of the iliac bones demonstrates flattening of the iliac bones, a finding typically observed in bladder exstrophy. (**d**) Sagittal grayscale image of the spine demonstrates disorganized vertebral bodies (arrows) at T11, T12, and L1. (**e**) Sagittal fast-spin echo T2-weighted image (TR/TE ms, 1100/78) demonstrates the fluid-filled bladder and ventral wall defect (arrowhead) inferior to the ACI (open arrowhead). (**f**) Sagittal T1-weighted gradient echo images (TR/TE ms, 204/4.76) demonstrate a meconium-filled rectum (*) that does not extend to the expected location of the perineum (arrow) but terminates abruptly with anterior angulation (open arrow). Although no omphalocele was observed on the ultrasound or MRI, the constellation of findings was interpreted as representing skin-covered bladder exstrophy on the spectrum of cloacal exstrophy (i.e., cloacal exstrophy variant). The diagnosis of a skin-covered cloacal exstrophy variant was confirmed postnatally

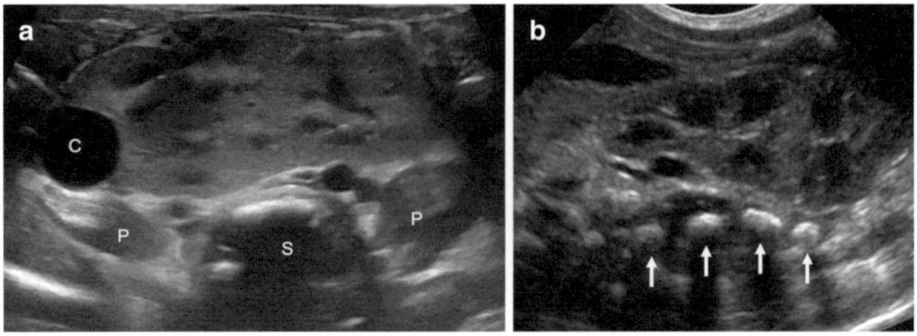

Fig. 4.15 Renal anomalies in the exstrophy-epispadias complex. (**a**) 2-day-old boy with covered exstrophy variant. Transverse midline grayscale image from a screening ultrasound (US) shows a midline pelvic, fused kidney with multiple cysts (C = largest cyst). S = spine; P = psoas muscle. (**b**) 3-day-old boy with cloacal exstrophy. Sagittal grayscale US image of the pelvis, to the right of the midline, shows the right kidney in an ectopic, pelvic position with normal morphology. Note the lower lumber spine and sacrum posterior to the kidney (arrows)

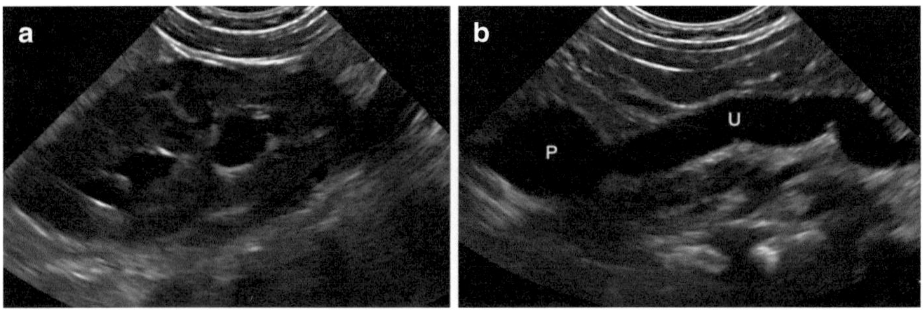

Fig. 4.16 UTD following bladder exstrophy repair. A 4-month-old boy with bladder exstrophy. 1 month after stage 1 repair, a sagittal grayscale ultrasound image of the left kidney (**a**) and left ureter (**b**) showed UTD including central calyceal dilation, renal pelvic (P) and ureteral (U) dilation developed. Initial renal bladder ultrasound was normal (not shown). The postoperative UTD ultimately resolved

In the setting of recurrent urinary tract infections, dimercaptosuccinic acid (DMSA) and mercapto-actyl-triglycine (MAG3) nuclear medicine exams can be valuable to assess renal parenchymal scarring and function. One series found that male patients were at greater risk for UTD, both presence and degree, as well as compromised renal function [32]. However, lower tract surgical and clinical status (e.g., ureteral reimplantation, continence, bladder pressure) and risk of high blood pressure were not associated with upper tract outcomes (e.g., dilation, function) [32, 33].

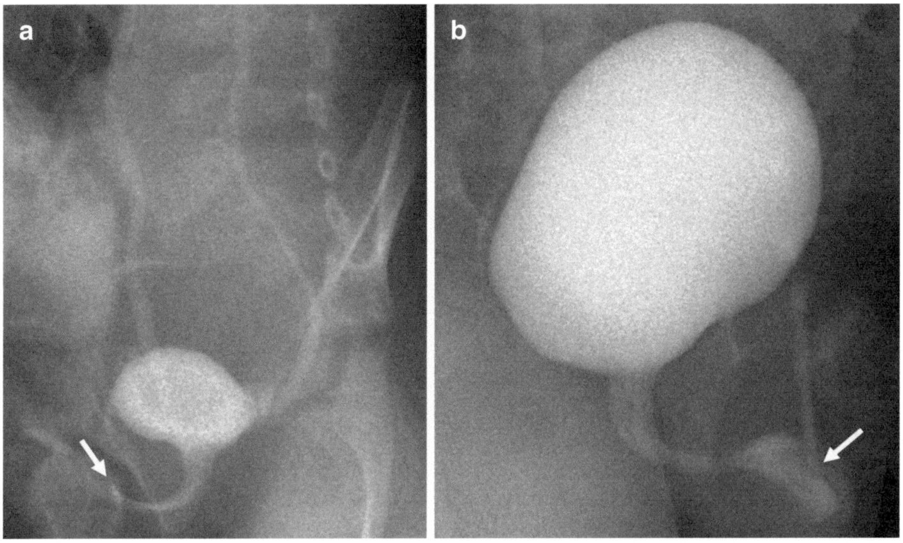

Fig. 4.17 Two boys with epispadias. (**a**) 2.5-year-old boy with epispadias. Right oblique fluoroscopic image from a voiding cystourethrogram (VCUG) shows bilateral vesicoureteral reflux (VUR), a smooth-walled bladder, and a shortened urethral length. The arrow indicates contrast at the distal end of the urethra. (**b**) Left oblique fluoroscopic image from a VCUG of a 7-month-old boy shows bilateral VUR, a smooth-walled bladder, and shortened urethral length. The arrow indicates the location of the meatus with contrast directed cephalad during the voiding phase

During closure of bladder exstrophy, ureteral stents and suprapubic cystostomy catheters are placed. Some centers perform "stentograms," where contrast is instilled through the ureteral stents by gravity into the upper tracts and ureteral drainage is assessed prior to removing the stents (Fig. 4.18). The contrast infusion is administered by gravity and is positioned at a height of 30 cm or less above the level of the kidneys so that it is administered at low pressure. A cystogram through the suprapubic catheter can demonstrate contrast extravasation, contour of the bladder, and bladder capacity (Fig. 4.19). Prior to reimplantation, the distal ureters have been described as having a "J-shape" [34]. The ureters are sometimes reimplanted at the time of primary closure and are more often reimplanted at the time of bladder neck reconstruction.

Fluoroscopic imaging can also be used to assess for complications, when suspected, including of the urethra, by retrograde urethrography or voiding cystogram. Following epispadias repair, the urethra may have an irregular appearance.

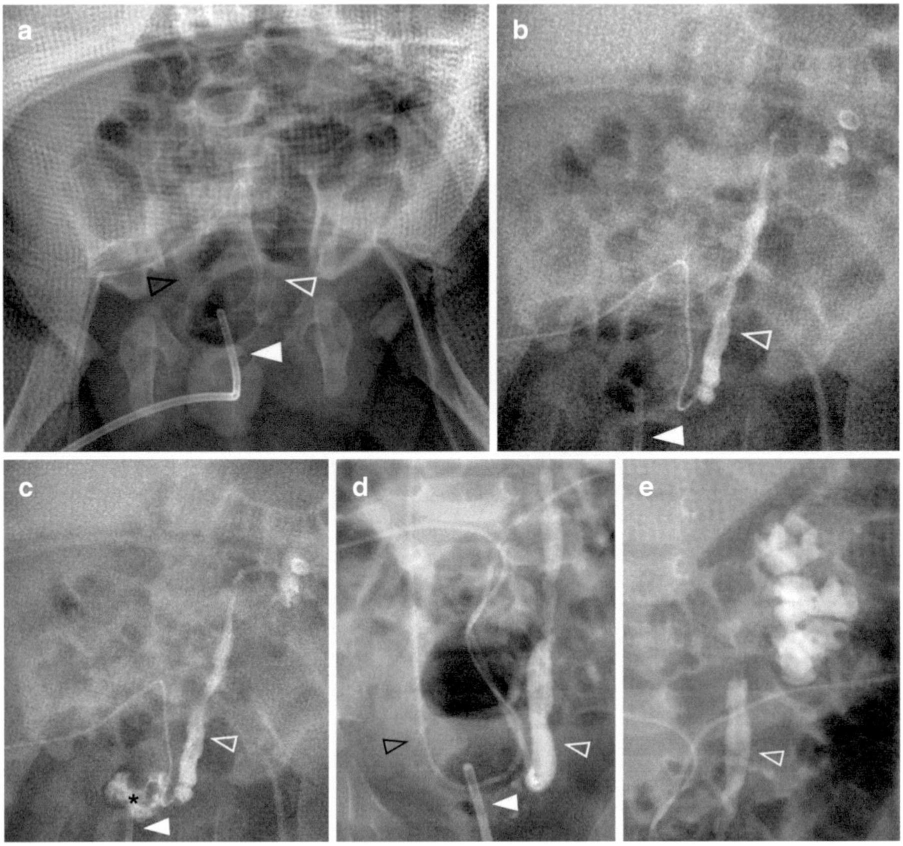

Fig. 4.18 Stentograms in two patients. (**a**) 4-month-old boy, 2 weeks after bladder exstrophy repair. Abdominal radiograph showing right ureteral stent (open black arrowhead), left ureteral stent (open white arrowhead), and transurethral bladder (solid white arrowhead) catheters are present. A cast is partially seen due to iliac osteotomies. (**b**) Fluoroscopic image from the left stentogram. Contrast is instilled into the left ureteral stent with filling of the left renal calyces and ureter (open white arrowhead). Transurethral bladder catheter (solid white arrowhead). (**c**) Moments later, the contrast is seen draining into the irregularly shaped bladder (asterisks). (**d**, **e**) 4-month-old girl, 2 weeks following bladder exstrophy closure with bilateral ureteral reimplantation. Right (open black arrowhead) and left (open white arrowhead) ureteral stents and a transurethral bladder catheter (solid white arrowhead) are present. Contrast was administered into the right stent with prompt contrast drainage into the bladder (not shown). Next, the contrast was administered to the left stent. There is left ureteral (open white arrowhead), renal pelvic, and calyceal dilation. No contrast drained into the bladder during the examination. A cast is seen over the upper abdomen

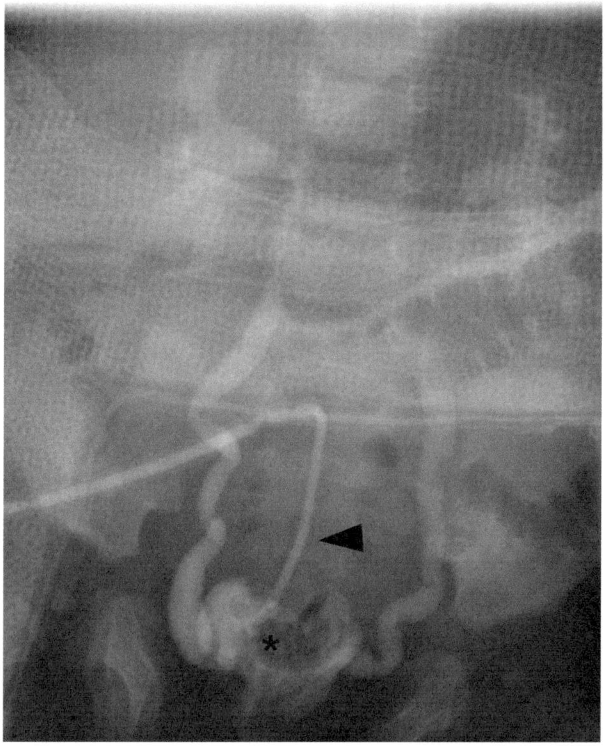

Fig. 4.19 Cystogram of a 3-month-old boy, 1 month following complete primary repair of exstrophy with bladder neck reconstruction. Contrast was instilled by gravity infusion into the suprapubic cystostomy catheter (black arrowhead). The irregularly shaped bladder (asterisks) fills with contrast. There is prompt right and left vesicoureteral reflux. A cast is present over the abdomen supporting iliac osteotomies

Musculoskeletal System

Radiography is an excellent tool to examine the skeletal system and is often the first radiologic imaging done on a child with EEC to assess pubic diastasis (Fig. 4.20). When cross-sectional imaging is indicated to evaluate the musculoskeletal anatomy, either MRI or CT can be used. Each modality has its advantages and disadvantages. While MRI is radiation-free, a young child usually requires sedation or anesthesia to remain still during image acquisition. However, MRI is preferred for soft tissue evaluation due to the high spatial resolution and better tissue contrast in those without external fixation hardware or MRI-incompatible implants. Even though CT exposes a child to radiation, current CT technology can obtain diagnostic images with low doses and can provide valuable information about the osseous pelvis. Three-dimensional (3D) reconstructions can be generated from either modality (Fig. 4.21). 3D-computerized and printed models can aid surgical planning, multidisciplinary care discussions, and patient and family education, especially in more complex or variant anatomy [35]. Some centers routinely perform dedicated imaging of the pelvis before and after surgical repair; however, there are no set guidelines [36].

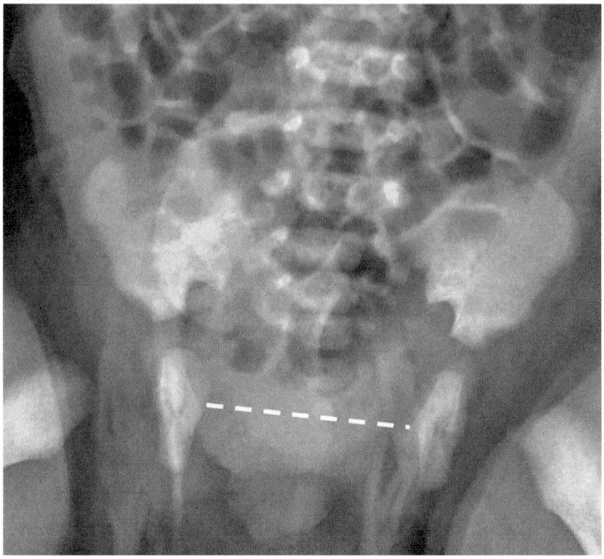

Fig. 4.20 Pubic diastasis assessment. Anterior posterior pelvic radiograph in a newborn boy with bladder exstrophy on day of life one. There is wide separation of the pubic symphysis (dashed line), consistent with pubic diastasis and a typical finding associated with bladder exstrophy

Imaging has afforded a better understanding of the pelvic musculoskeletal anatomy in children with EEC. Studies of CT and MRI of the pelvis prior to and following exstrophy repair have described the structure of the pelvis, including angular and linear distances between bones and pelvic floor muscles, as well as how the surgeries affect these anatomic relationships and the potential sequelae on pelvis shape, acetabular morphology, and continence [37, 38]. The focus of these studies is on classic bladder exstrophy (CBE), noting that within the EEC spectrum, the pelvic structure of children with epispadias is closer to normal, and those with cloacal exstrophy can have greater asymmetry between each side of the pelvis compared with CBE.

Children with CBE have shorter pubic bones, external rotation of the pelvis and retroversion of the acetabulae, as well as alteration in the muscles of the pelvic diaphragm, or levator ani muscle group [39–41]. The levator ani muscle group, including the iliococcygeus, pubococcygeus, and puborectalis sling muscles, is oriented in an anterior to posterior direction and attaches to the pubis and coccyx. The levator ani muscles are further supported through lateral attachments to the obturator internus muscles, which originate along the inferior aspect of the superior pubic ramus and insert on the greater trochanter of the femur. The muscular diaphragm supports the pelvic genitourinary anatomy and has sphincteric function. The levator ani in patients with CBE are wider and flatter than normal with increased dome-shaped contour, which is disproportionately pulled anteriorly. As a result, the puborectalis sling is not centered on the genitourinary structures and anus, which can affect continence [40, 41] (Fig. 4.22).

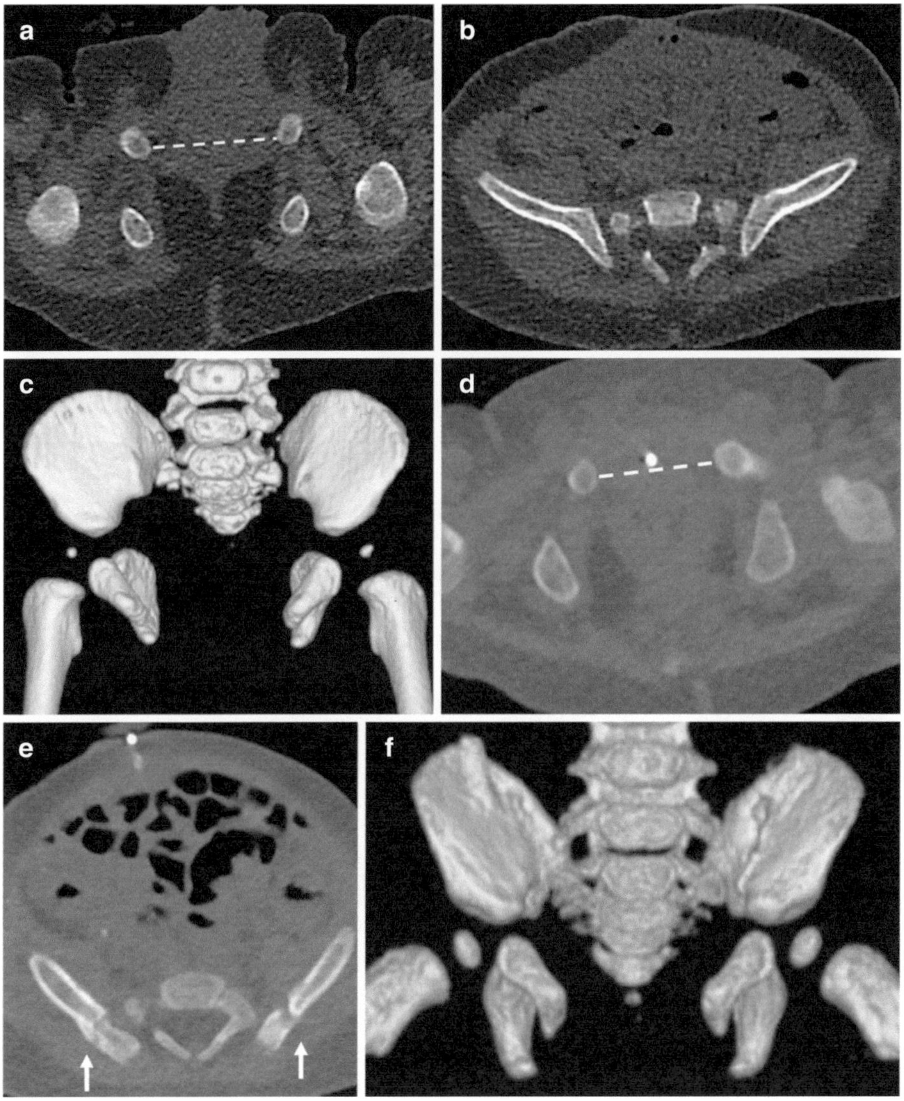

Fig. 4.21 CT of the pelvis of a boy with bladder exstrophy prior to and following stage 1 repair in bladder exstrophy. (**a**–**c**) Images from preoperative CT, at 3 months of age, with images at the level of the pubis (**a**) and S1 (**b**) showing the expected osseous configuration in a patient with bladder exstrophy. The pubic bones are shortened and pubic diastasis is present (dashed line). The pelvis is externally rotated with an "open-book" appearance. (**c**) 3D-reconstruction rendered from 2D-preoperative images. (**d**–**f**) One month following surgery, (**d**) the pubic bones are more approximated (dashed line), and (**e**) posterior iliac osteotomies have been done to help close the midline repair. Healing bone is present at the osteotomies (arrows). The cystostomy catheter is partially visualized in (**d**) and the cystostomy and right ureteral stent are partially visualized in (**d**) and (**e**). (**f**) 3D-reconstruction rendered from 2D-postoperative images

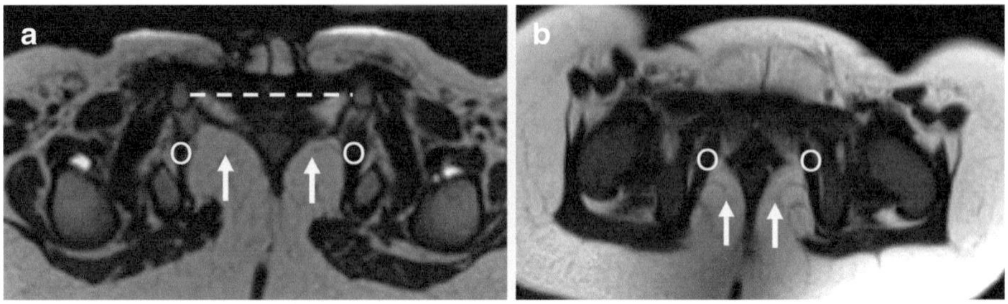

Fig. 4.22 Pelvic floor musculature in bladder exstrophy. Axial T2 SPACE MRI image of the pelvis (**a**) through the level of the pubic bones in an 11-month-old boy with skin-covered exstrophy variant compared to a normal infant (**b**). There is pubic diastasis (dashed line). The levator ani muscle group (arrows) is disproportionately positioned anteriorly. The rectum and urethra are relatively anterior. O = obturator internus muscles

Because of the origins and insertions of the pelvic floor musculature, it would follow that the skeletal differences in children with EEC would portend muscular differences. Analyzing musculoskeletal relationships along with the clinical outcomes may improve attainment of the surgical goals of abdominal wall closure and urinary continence while reducing morbidity [42]. However, understanding which musculoskeletal relationships correlate with continence has been challenging as children continue to grow and develop after surgery and normative relationships are not established. Those who have attained continence have been described as having a pelvic shape closer to that of age-matched unaffected children [43].

In order to reduce tension on the midline closure, the pubic bones are reapproximated. Depending on the age of the child at the time of surgery and the degree of diastasis, the pubis may be reapproximated with tension sutures alone in newborn infants or pelvic osteotomies in older infants and children. The consideration of which type of osteotomy is addressed in another chapter. Pubic diastasis is most commonly observed by radiographs in a newborn with classic bladder exstrophy or cloacal exstrophy. A transverse linear measurement between the midportion of the right and left pubic bones defines the distance of the diastasis. In skeletally immature children, only the ossified bone, and not the cartilage, is visible by radiograph. Diastasis can also be measured on CT and MRI. Following osteotomies, bone healing and hardware can be monitored by radiographs or CT.

Spine

Of children with EEC, those with cloacal exstrophy most commonly have spine anomalies associated with the OEIS complex, which may take the form of vertebral segmentation anomalies and/or closed (i.e., skin-covered) spinal dysraphisms. Radiography can depict vertebral anomalies, and spinal US is used as a first-line screening evaluation of the spinal cord (Figs. 4.23 and 4.24). Spine US in the neonate is a non-invasive, well-tolerated examination and readily detects anomalies of the spinal canal, which can be visualized commonly up to 6 months of age due to the timing of spine ossification [44]. It is ideally performed with the infant in the prone position. If additional imaging is warranted, a spine MRI can be obtained to further classify the anomaly, which can range from closed to open dysraphism (Fig. 4.24) [45].

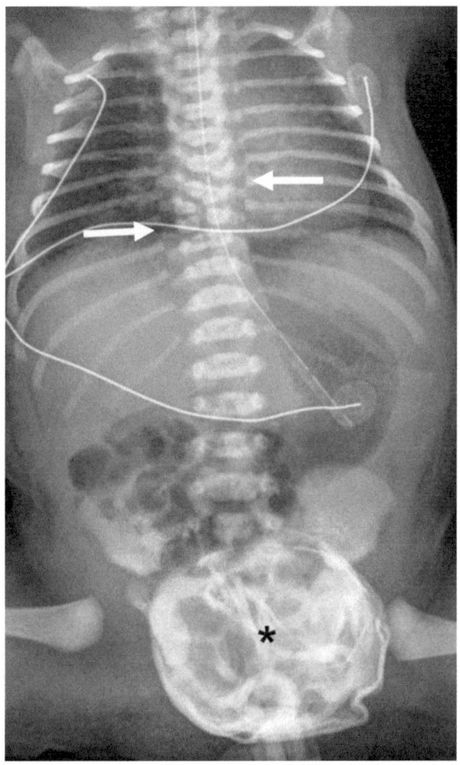

Fig. 4.23 Thoracoabdominal radiograph in a newborn girl with cloacal exstrophy shows mid-thoracic vertebral anomalies (arrows) and an omphalocele (asterisks) projecting over the pelvis

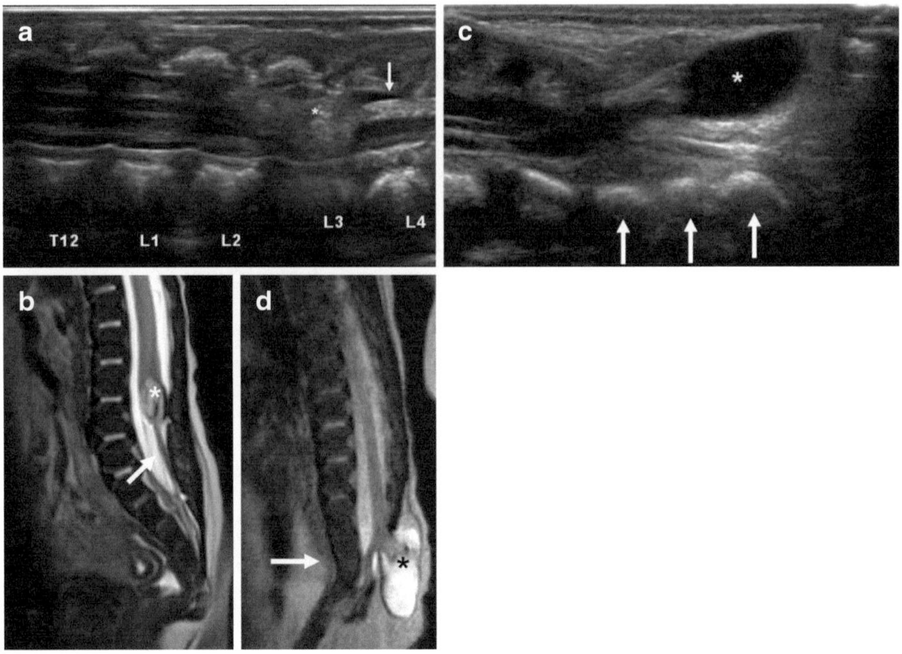

Fig. 4.24 Spine US and MRI in two patients with cloacal exstrophy. (**a**) Sagittal ultrasound (US) image of the spine with the infant in the prone position on the day of life 0. The vertebral levels are numbered. The low-lying conus is associated with a round, echogenic lesion (asterisk) suspicious for a lipoma. The filum terminale is thickened (arrow). These features are concerning for tethered cord. (**b**) Sagittal T2 TSE MRI images at 1 week of life, in the midline showing the same findings as seen in US. (**c**) Spine ultrasound of the second child on the day of life 3 with the conus and nerve roots communicating with a fluid-filled sac in the inferior soft tissues (asterisk) at the level of the hypoplastic sacrum (arrows). Skin overlies the fluid-filled sac. (**d**) Sagittal T2 TSE image of the spine just to the left of the midline at 1 month of age showing the abnormal configuration of the sacrum (arrow) and low-lying cord. On MRI tissue with fat signal characteristics was identified associated with the fluid-filled sac (asterisk), consistent with a lipomyelomeningocele

Conclusions

Prenatal and postnatal imaging are each important in the care of children with EEC but serve two distinct roles. Prenatal imaging primarily serves to make an accurate diagnosis in order to facilitate prenatal counseling and prepare for postnatal care. Postnatal imaging, however, helps to more completely define the child's anatomy and monitors for post-surgical complications. Understanding the prenatal imaging manifestations, pitfalls, associated anatomic anomalies, and potential complications of care strengthens the communication between the radiologist, urologist, and medical team.

References

1. American Institute of Ultrasound in Medicine. AIUM-ACR-ACOG-SMFM-SRU practice parameter for the performance of standard diagnostic obstetric ultrasound examinations. J Ultrasound Med. 2018;37(11):E13–24.
2. American Institute of Ultrasound in Medicine. AIUM practice parameter for the performance of detailed second- and third-trimester diagnostic obstetric ultrasound examinations. J Ultrasound Med. 2019;38(12):3093–100.
3. American Institute of Ultrasound in Medicine. AIUM practice parameter for the performance of detailed diagnostic obstetric ultrasound examinations between 12 weeks 0 days and 13 weeks 6 days. J Ultrasound Med. 2021;40(5):E1–16.
4. Gearhart JP, Ben-Chaim J, Jeffs RD, Sanders RC. Criteria for the prenatal diagnosis of classic bladder exstrophy. Obstet Gynecol. 1995;85(6):961–4.
5. Mirk P, Calisti A, Fileni A. Prenatal sonographic diagnosis of bladder extrophy. J Ultrasound Med. 1986;5(5):291–3.
6. Antomarchi J, Moeglin D, Laurichesse H, Combourieu D, Bigi N, Maisonneuve E, et al. The pubic diastasis measurement, a key element for the diagnosis, management, and prognosis of the bladder exstrophy. Fetal Diagn Ther. 2019;45(6):435–40.
7. Mallmann MR, Mack-Detlefsen B, Reutter H, Pohle R, Gottschalk I, Geipel A, et al. Isolated bladder exstrophy in prenatal diagnosis. Arch Gynecol Obstet. 2019;300(2):355–63.
8. Pakdaman R, Woodward PJ, Kennedy A. Complex abdominal wall defects: appearances at prenatal imaging. Radiographics. 2015;35(2):636–49.
9. Manganaro L, Antonelli A, Bernardo S, Capozza F, Petrillo R, Satta S, et al. Highlights on MRI of the fetal body. Radiol Med. 2018;123(4):271–85.
10. Marine MB, Forbes-Amrhein MM. Magnetic resonance imaging of the fetal gastrointestinal system. Pediatr Radiol. 2020;50(13):1895–906.
11. Weiss DA, Oliver ER, Borer JG, Kryger JV, Roth EB, Groth TW, et al. Key anatomic findings on fetal ultrasound and MRI in the prenatal diagnosis of bladder and cloacal exstrophy. J Pediatr Urol. 2020;16(5):665–71.
12. Dannull KA, Browne LP, Meyers MZ. The spectrum of cloacal malformations: how to differentiate each entity prenatally with fetal MRI. Pediatr Radiol. 2019;49(3):387–98.
13. Carey JC, Greenbaum B, Hall BD. The OEIS complex (omphalocele, exstrophy, imperforate anus, spinal defects). Birth Defects Orig Artic Ser. 1978;14(6B):253–63.
14. Carey JC. Exstrophy of the cloaca and the OEIS complex: one and the same. Am J Med Genet. 2001;99(4):270.
15. Feldkamp ML, Botto LD, Amar E, Bakker MK, Bermejo-Sánchez E, Bianca S, et al. Cloacal exstrophy: an epidemiologic study from the International Clearinghouse for Birth Defects Surveillance and Research. Am J Med Genet C Semin Med Genet. 2011;157C(4):333–43.
16. Coleman PW, Marine MB, Weida JN, Gray BW, Billmire DF, Brown BP. Fetal MRI in the identification of a fetal ventral wall defect spectrum. AJP Rep. 2018;8(4):e264–76.
17. Hamada H, Takano K, Shiina H, Sakai T, Sohda S, Kubo T. New ultrasonographic criterion for the prenatal diagnosis of cloacal exstrophy: elephant trunk-like image. J Urol. 1999;162(6):2123–4.
18. Goncalves LF, Hill H, Bailey S. Prenatal and postnatal imaging techniques in the evaluation of disorders of sex development. Semin Pediatr Surg. 2019;28(5):150839.
19. Coblentz AC, Teixeira SR, Mirsky DM, Johnson AM, Feygin T, Victoria T. How to read a fetal magnetic resonance image 101. Pediatr Radiol. 2020;50(13):1810–29.
20. Zalel Y, Lehavi O, Aizenstein O, Achiron R. Development of the fetal spinal cord: time of ascendance of the normal conus medullaris as detected by sonography. J Ultrasound Med. 2006;25(11):1397–401; quiz 1402.
21. Bronshtein M, Riechler A, Zimmer EZ. Prenatal sonographic signs of possible fetal genital anomalies. Prenat Diagn. 1995;15(3):215–9.
22. Valioulis I, Levard G, Lottmann H, Hameury F, Cendron J. A rare complex bladder exstrophy variant. BJU Int. 2000;86(3):398–400.

23. Maruf M, Benz K, Jayman J, Kasprenski M, Michaud J, Di Carlo HN, et al. Variant presentations of the exstrophy-epispadias complex: a 40-year experience. Urology. 2019;125:184–90.
24. Lowentritt BH, Van Zijl PS, Frimberger D, Baird A, Lakshmanan Y, Gearhart JP. Variants of the exstrophy complex: a single institution experience. J Urol. 2005;173(5):1732–7.
25. Overland MR, Oliver ER, Back SJ, Kolon TF, Shukla AR, Weiss DA. Prenatal presentation of a covered cloacal exstrophy variant; early diagnostic challenges within the broad spectrum of the exstrophy-epispadias complex. Urology. 2024;183:204–8.
26. Choi SM, Park T, Park JK, Shin JK, Choi WJ, Lee SA, et al. Pseudoexstrophy of the bladder diagnosed prenatally. Prenat Diagn. 2013;33(10):1002–3.
27. Rudzinska M, Bijok J, Tomaszewska K, Massalska D, Gastol P, Ostrowska J, et al. Skin-covered bladder exstrophy diagnosed antenatally. J Ultrasound Med. 2013;32(11):2043–5.
28. Ono K, Kikuchi A, Takagi K, Takahashi D, Yoshizawa K, Nishizawa S. Prenatal sonographic features of complete covered cloacal exstrophy. Ultrasound Obstet Gynecol. 2009;34(4):481–2.
29. Vinit N, Glénisson M, Chalouhi G, Salomon LJ, Millischer-Bellaiche AE, Beaudoin S, et al. Prenatal diagnosis of unusual variant of exstrophy-epispadias complex. Ultrasound Obstet Gynecol. 2023;62(1):155–6.
30. Sahoo SP, Gangopadhyay AN, Sinha CK, Gupta DK, Gopal SC. Covered exstrophy: a rare variant of classical bladder exstrophy. Scand J Urol Nephrol. 1997;31(1):103–6.
31. Stec AA, Baradaran N, Gearhart JP. Congenital renal anomalies in patients with classic bladder exstrophy. Urology. 2012;79(1):207–9.
32. Ellison JS, Ahn J, Shnorhavorian M, Grady R, Merguerian PA. Long-term fate of the upper tracts following complete primary repair of bladder exstrophy. J Pediatr Urol. 2017;13(4):394.e1–6.
33. Kanabolo D, Cain M, Brown M, Ahn J, Fernandez N, Halbach S, et al. Long term renal outcome and risk of elevated blood pressure in children undergoing complete primary repair of bladder exstrophy (CPRE). J Pediatr Urol. 2023;19(4):370.e1–7.
34. Pierre K, Borer J, Phelps A, Chow JS. Bladder exstrophy: current management and postoperative imaging. Pediatr Radiol. 2014;44(7):768–86; quiz 765.
35. Silvestro E, Kolon TF, Canning D, Serai SD, Carson R, Sze R, et al. Pediatric genitourinary 3D modeling and printing using multiphase postcontrast imaging segmentation. Urology. 2023;173:149–52.
36. Tekes A, Ertan G, Solaiyappan M, Stec AA, Sponseller PD, Huisman TA, et al. 2D and 3D MRI features of classic bladder exstrophy. Clin Radiol. 2014;69(5):e223–9.
37. Kenawey M, Wright JG, Hopyan S, Murnaghan ML, Howard A, Kelley SP. Can neonatal pelvic osteotomies permanently change pelvic shape in patients with exstrophy? Understanding late rediastasis. J Bone Joint Surg Am. 2014;96(16):e137.
38. Manyevitch R, Dunn E, Zaman MH, Maruf MN, Benz K, Clennon EK, et al. Volumetric and acetabular changes in the bony pelvis associated with primary closure of classic bladder exstrophy. J Pediatr Urol. 2020;16(6):832.e1–9.
39. Sponseller PD, Bisson LJ, Gearhart JP, Jeffs RD, Magid D, Fishman E. The anatomy of the pelvis in the exstrophy complex. J Bone Joint Surg Am. 1995;77(2):177–89.
40. Stec AA, Pannu HK, Tadros YE, Sponseller PD, Fishman EK, Gearhart JP. Pelvic floor anatomy in classic bladder exstrophy using 3-dimensional computerized tomography: initial insights. J Urol. 2001;166(4):1444–9.
41. Williams AM, Solaiyappan M, Pannu HK, Bluemke D, Shechter G, Gearhart JP. 3-Dimensional magnetic resonance imaging modeling of the pelvic floor musculature in classic bladder exstrophy before pelvic osteotomy. J Urol. 2004;172(4 Pt 2):1702–5.
42. Tourchi A, Inouye BM, Di Carlo HN, Young E, Ko J, Gearhart JP. New advances in the pathophysiologic and radiologic basis of the exstrophy spectrum. J Pediatr Urol. 2014;10(2):212–8.
43. Gargollo PC, Borer JG, Retik AB, Peters CA, Diamond DA, Atala A, et al. Magnetic resonance imaging of pelvic musculoskeletal and genitourinary anatomy in patients before and after complete primary repair of bladder exstrophy. J Urol. 2005;174(4 Pt 2):1559–66; discussion 1566.
44. Dick EA, de Bruyn R, Patel K, Owens CM. Spinal ultrasound in cloacal exstrophy. Clin Radiol. 2001;56(4):289–94.
45. Kumar N, Chatur C, Balani A, Bisharat M, Tahir Z, Johal N, et al. Patterns of spinal cord malformation in cloacal exstrophy. J Neurosurg Pediatr. 2021;28:1–8.

Surgical Considerations: Indications and Timing for Surgery (Defining Outcomes and Expectations of Exstrophy Repair)

5

Pramod P. Reddy

Introduction

The exstrophy-epispadias complex (EEC) is a spectrum of complex congenital anterior midline abdominal wall defects arising from mesodermal abnormality and can involve the genitourinary tract, the bony pelvis, pelvic floor musculature, and in cases of cloacal exstrophy, the gastrointestinal tract.

There are three main clinical phenotypes of EEC:

- Epispadias (penopubic, penile, and glandular). The incidence is 1:117,000 in males and 1:484,000 in females [19].
- Classic bladder exstrophy (BE). The incidence is 1 in 10,000–50,000 births, with a male-to-female ratio of 2.3:1 [27].
- Cloacal exstrophy. The incidence is 1 in 200,000–400,000 with higher rates in females [13].

This chapter will address the evolution of the timing of surgical intervention and also define the clinical outcomes impacted by the timing of surgery in cases of classic BE. The management of epispadias and cloacal exstrophy will be discussed in subsequent chapters.

The management of BE has undergone significant evolution and transition as we have gained a better understanding of the pathophysiology of the condition, surgical and anesthetic considerations in the care of newborn babies and infants, and critical review of clinical outcomes. The literature demonstrates that over the past 150 years, we have gone from managing children with BE in a nonsurgical manner to a

P. P. Reddy (✉)
Division of Pediatric Urology, Cincinnati Children's, Cincinnati, OH, USA
e-mail: pramod.reddy@cchmc.org

A. R. Shukla, R. S. Joshi (eds.), *Bladder Exstrophy and Epispadias*,
https://doi.org/10.1007/978-3-031-91238-2_5

condition managed with urinary diversion to the contemporary treatment that involves either a staged reconstruction or a single-stage repair [18].

H. H. Young reported the first successful repair of BE with primary bladder closure in 1942. His patient, a young girl, was able to achieve urinary continence; however, his results were not replicated by other surgeons of this era, and so surgical efforts were directed toward urinary diversion in children born with BE [52].

In 1977, Dr. Jeffs reported the outcomes of the modern staged repair of BE (MSRE), and for the next 20 years, this was adopted as the standard of care for BE [23].

In 1998, Dr. Mitchell reported the outcomes of his primary complete reconstruction of BE technique (CPRE), which had evolved from his primary penile disassembly technique for epispadias [18, 20, 35].

Until 2005, BE was considered a urological emergency and required repair within the first 72 h of life. The criteria for the emergent repair of BE included having a clinically stable newborn with an adequate bladder template and a pubic diastasis <4 cm. It was felt that in such cases, the repair could be performed successfully in a tension-free manner without the need for an osteotomy, thereby rendering the repair less complex.

The premise for this approach was that the hormone relaxin would permit tension-free approximation of the pubic diastasis without the need for osteotomies. The role of relaxin in neonates has since been refuted. Relaxin is a hormone that is not active or needed in neonates. Its functions are mainly related to facilitating physiological changes in the female body during pregnancy and labor.

The extent and severity of the BE phenotype that the child is born with will influence both the type of repair undertaken and also the timing of the repair. There has been a defined move away from emergency repair of BE to a more planned elective/delayed repair to allow for the patient to be optimized for this complex reconstructive procedure.

The concept of a planned elective/delayed repair was initially reserved for infants who were deemed to have unfavorable anatomy (i.e., a bladder plate that was too small) or if the surgeon experienced in surgical management of BE was not available [2, 3]. The observation that waiting to repair BE in infants was not associated with an increased incidence of polypoid formation or loss of bladder plate compliance, coupled with the benefits of improved infantile cardiopulmonary physiology and enhanced maternal-child bonding with earlier breastfeeding, has allowed the concept of the elective/delayed repair of BE to become the preferred management strategy for a number of surgeons [16, 29, 33]. The elective/delayed strategy for BE repair allows for better patient selection and safer management and does not negatively influence the final outcome of the management of BE [14].

The timing of the surgical repair is a complex decision, must be individualized for each patient, and take into account the patient's anatomy (i.e., size of the bladder plate) and medical comorbidities, parents' preference, and the availability of a surgical team with expertise in managing BE. The ultimate goal is to offer timely multidisciplinary care for the child with BE in order to provide the best possible long-term outcome.

Any discussion of the timing of elective surgical procedures for the repair of a congenital anomaly, such as BE, is inherently based on at least two assumptions with regard to the psychological impact of care on the child [45]:

1. The surgery has the potential to affect a significant change in the development of the patient, psychologically or physiologically. There is no question that surgical repair of a child born with BE directly impacts them both physiologically and psychologically—while it is mostly a positive impact, as the child grows, societal expectations of their reconstructed anatomy may cause adverse psychological impact.
2. The procedure has a differential impact on the patient at various stages of their life. The child with a closed BE has the chance for their bladder to cycle and grow, enabling them to achieve social continence later in their childhood and functional genitalia as adults.

In general, from the viewpoint of emotional development, the period from 6 weeks to approximately 15 months appears to be a relatively less difficult time for surgery on children [45].

The parents of a child born with BE may experience a significant psychological impact that can influence their relationship with the child with BE and their interpersonal relationships with their spouse and other children. McCollum has described that parents often experience fear, grief, anger, anxiety, bitterness, and aversion in varying degrees when faced with a child who is not "perfect" [32].

In the era before prenatal diagnosis was available, Fineman found that parents of children with BE first responded with horror, withdrawal, and guilt and then followed with attempts at coping, usually based on denial and displacement. They also expressed their feelings that the genital anomaly of the child was related to a weakness or deficiency in their own reproductive system [15].

When BE is diagnosed prenatally, it offers an opportunity to alleviate a lot of parental anxiety through education of the nature and etiology of the condition, preparing the parents for how their baby will appear and allowing them to discuss treatment options leading to shared decision-making with regard to the nature of the repair and timing of surgery.

There are currently three widely accepted surgical techniques deployed by surgeons worldwide to treat children born with BE [22]:

- Modern staged repair of BE (MSRE)
- Complete primary repair of BE (CPRE)
- Radical soft tissue mobilization (RSTM) also known as the Kelly procedure [6, 25]

The choice of surgical technique by the surgeon also factors into the timing of surgery. Generally, if performing either the CPRE or the RSTM (Kelly procedure), the surgeon may choose the elective/delayed repair rather than the early repair.

Regardless of the choice of procedure or the timing of the surgery, we do recommend the following steps to protect the exposed bladder from injury until the BE is closed:

- Replace the plastic clamp that is used to occlude the umbilical stump of the neonate with a silk ligature. This prevents the clamp from rubbing against the bladder mucosa and traumatizing the bladder plate.
- Cover the exposed bladder plate with a barrier; reports have described using Tegaderm or Saran wrap.
- Frequent irrigation of the exposed bladder plate, to keep the urothelium from drying out.

Early/Neonatal Repair (<28 Days)

Early repair typically involves surgical intervention in the neonatal period within the first few weeks of life (<28 days). This approach offers several advantages:

- Decreased risk of infection from the bladder plate being exposed.
- Protection of the exposed bladder mucosa with reduced polyp development and decreased inflammation.
- Early restoration of bladder storage function, cycling, and improved compliance of the bladder plate can result in better bladder dynamics and growth [20].
- In some cases, it might obviate the need for osteotomies that reduce the morbidity of the repair and also the length of stay in the hospital.
- Aesthetic and psychological benefits. Early repair of the BE results in a more normal-appearing abdominal wall and external genitalia of the affected infant, preventing psychological distress that the parents might experience when changing the diaper of a child with BE.

The disadvantages of early repair include:

- The inability of the mother to hold the infant and lack of skin-to-skin contact disrupts the normal bonding between the child and their mother. Data regarding emotional development indicate that the most important first step is adequate bonding to the mother [34]. The accessibility of the child to the mother especially during the first several weeks after birth is critical for normal bonding. When surgery is undertaken early/neonatal repair, it disrupts this process. Normal bonding has also been shown to be beneficial in the infantile pain response. Okonkwo et al. have shown higher levels of comfort and lower pain scores after delayed repair of BE in the infants who were breastfed early [17, 41, 46].
- Postop immobilization can disrupt the mother's ability to breastfeed the child. There is evidence that supports the benefits of early breastfeeding in decreasing respiratory and gastrointestinal infections; milk proteins have also been shown to be protective of the bladder urothelium by preventing the attachment, invasion,

and cytotoxicity of uropathogenic *E. coli* [16, 29]. The lack of breastfeeding could place the bladder at risk for increased infections.
- Neonates tend to be clinically malnourished, and this can impact their wound-healing ability, potentially resulting in a higher risk of wound complications, i.e., infections, fistulae, and dehiscence.
- These repairs are typically performed before the child has undergone the "Mini-puberty"; this places the genitalia at higher risk of injury due to the more delicate vascularity.
- The neonate's physiology is still adapting to its independence from placental circulation, the pulmonary and cardiac reflexes are still immature, and the impact of a prolonged general anesthetic on the central nervous system is still poorly understood [39]. Collectively these facts can negatively impact the peri-operative recovery of the infant [10, 36].
- Neonates that have undergone surgical procedures shortly after birth have been shown to react to later exposures to noxious stimuli with a heightened behavioral response, which can predispose them to behavioral issues later in life [49].
- The use of intravenous and oral opiates early in life has been associated with gastrointestinal motility issues later in life [41].

Elective/Delayed Repair (>28 Days)

The purposeful scheduling of the repair of BE as a scheduled case beyond the first month of life is considered an elective/delayed repair. The term elective is better used to describe this pathway rather than allow for the parental perception that the child's care is being delayed.

The benefits of elective/delayed repair (>28 days) include:

- Opportunity for the parents to be appropriately counseled and enable them to participate in shared decision-making. Permits an unbiased, informed consent process.
- Anesthesia and regional analgesia are safer in the older infant compared to the neonate. The largest number of peri-operative complications related to either respiratory or cardiac issues occur in the newborn [10, 36].
- Permits growth of the child—the bladder plate has been shown to grow as the child grows. Genital growth is important if considering a combined primary repair (CPRE) to reduce potential for harm to genital tissue.
- Improved nutrition. Newborns have a higher caloric requirement than healthy children (approx. 110–135 kcal/kg/day). This is due to increased energy consumption due to thermoregulation, work of feeding, digestion, etc. For preterm infants, the requirement is even higher. Subjecting a newborn child to a major reconstructive procedure without the ability to optimize their nutritional needs will potentially cause a more profound catabolic state in the postoperative period with a theoretically greater risk of wound complications.

- Improved physiology and development/maturation of vital organs that make the patient more tolerant of the stress of a major reconstructive procedure [22].
- Permits time for maternal-child bonding, which reduces parent anxiety and also may positively impact normal psychosocial development of the child [34, 45].
- Allows the child to go through mini-puberty, thereby allowing for hormone-mediated improved vascularity of the genitalia and also growth of the child, specifically the genitalia, potentially reducing the risk of injury during surgery.
- Potentially makes the bladder plate larger and more malleable because the bladder plate increases in size along with somatic growth and possibly because of constant stretching of the bladder plate by the positive intra-abdominal pressure [14, 28].
- Concomitant inguinal hernia repair may be a safer procedure in the older child with fewer recurrences and reduced injury to the blood supply of the testis [1, 22].
- Ossification of pelvic bones enables options for postoperative immobilization if needed after osteotomy (i.e., external fixator and spica cast). It is important to note that the elective repair does not commit the child to requiring osteotomies for a successful repair [22, 38].
- Alignment of familial schedules with surgical scheduling.
- Involvement of an appropriate and experienced multidisciplinary surgical team.

The disadvantages of elective/delayed repair (>28 days) include:

- Prolonged exposure of the bladder mucosa may increase the risk of polyp formation and also make the bladder plate less pliable. However, Roesch et al. have demonstrated that postponing the bladder closure is not associated with any histologically or immunohistochemically detectable premalignant changes. Rosch et al. characterized the histology of polyps and mucosal biopsies excised during early and elective/delayed closure and compared them. He showed that only active inflammation was different between the two groups. There was no difference in the presence of fibrosis or severe active inflammation between the two groups [42, 43].
- Development of squamous metaplasia of the bladder plate—however, it should be noted that on followup endoscopic assessment after bladder closure, most of the metaplasia is macroscopically resolved [14]. This has been our experience also when we have performed cystoscopic assessment of our patients with elective/delayed closure—most of the metaplastic changes documented at the time of initial closure have resolved as early as 1 year postop.
- Baradaran et al. hypothesized that the prolonged exposure of the bladder plate to the ex vivo environment might increase the risk of infections due to colonization of the urothelium with uropathogenic enteric bacteria [3]. However, there are numerous reports that with the appropriate use of peri-operative antibiotics, there is actually not an increased risk of infections in patients undergoing elective/delayed repair.

- Parental anxiety of caring for a child with unrepaired BE is prolonged. Some parents have reported anxiety with diaper changes and also the inability to allow other caregivers to participate in diaper changes or bathing their child due to the visual nature of the BE deformity.
- Delaying the child's time to surgery may be perceived by the parents as prolonging the child's defective state and may add to crystallizing of any disruption in family relationships that the child's condition may have produced [45]. It is imperative to ensure that the parents have access to psychological counseling and support during this difficult time.

Table 5.1 demonstrates the key differences between the pros and cons of early/neonatal repair versus elective/delayed repair of BE. These are important issues that need to be discussed with the parents at the time of surgical consultation to ensure

Table 5.1 Comparison of early/neonatal repair of BE versus elective/delayed repair of BE

Early/neonatal repair of BE	Elective/delayed repair of BE
Birth to 28 days of life	>28 days of life
May not need osteotomies	Can be performed without osteotomies
Bladder plate is usually healthier with fewer polyps	Bladder plate may grow but may also develop polyps, which make closure challenging at times
Reduced risk of infected/colonized bladder plate	Bladder plate is colonized by time of closure
Early restoration of bladder physiology, important to note that bladder cycling may not occur until bladder neck procedure performed	Bladder plate may become less pliable and result in smaller bladder capacity, unless performing CPRE as bladder neck procedure will allow early cycling
Genitalia more prone to injury	Mini-puberty improves vascularity and growth of the genitalia
Increased risk of anesthetic complications given immature cardiac and pulmonary reflexes	General and regional anesthesia is safer in the older infant
Neonatal malnourishment impairs wound healing	Permits time to optimize the child's nutritional status and wound healing
Reduced risk of peri-op blood transfusion	Most patients will require blood transfusion, especially if undergoing osteotomies
Pelvic bones are mostly cartilaginous, limiting options for postop immobilization	Pelvic bones are ossified, and this allows enhanced options for postop immobilization of the pelvic ring
Increased rate of wound complications, i.e., bladder prolapse and dehiscence	Reduced rates of bladder prolapse and wound dehiscence
Delayed time to maternal-child bonding can increase parental anxiety	Prolonged time with visible defect can cause parental anxiety
Delayed time to breastfeeding	Permits normal maternal-child bonding and breastfeeding to occur
Urgent nature of repair prevents shared decision-making	Allows parents to better understand nature of condition and permits shared decision-making
Parents may not be able to choose surgical team	Parents can choose surgical team and align schedules

that they have all of the relevant data to make shared decisions with the surgical team and to provide informed consent.

Complications of Early Versus Elective/Delayed Repair of BE

A major factor to consider when deciding on the timing and nature of surgical repair for a child born with BE is the safety of the procedure and clinical outcomes, and this will aid in counseling the parents on the optimal clinical pathway for their child.

Ferrara et al. have demonstrated that in their cohort of patients, the timing of primary closure did not influence the eventual bladder capacity [14]. In the absence of any proven improvement in eventual bladder capacity, understanding the complication rate of early versus elective/delayed repair will aid in determining the choice of timing of surgery.

When considering the safety of the procedures, the risk of anesthesia has to be discussed with the family, as it varies significantly between the neonate and the infant. Other complications to bear in mind include wound infections, wound dehiscence, prolapse of the bladder, and urethral outlet/bladder neck obstruction. Morrill et al. reviewed a cohort of patients at their institution that had either undergone neonatal/early repair or an elective/delayed repair of BE and compared the complication rates [37]. See Table 5.2 for a summary of their data.

The total complication rate was higher for the elective/delayed repairs (58%) compared to a rate of 48.2% for the early/neonatal repairs. The majority of the complications in both groups were Clavien I–II.

The most common complication was unplanned postoperative blood transfusion at a rate of 38% for the elective/delayed repair and 26.3% for the early/neonatal repairs, which is not unexpected, as there is a higher incidence of pelvic osteotomies and associated surgical blood loss in the elective/delayed repair group. If blood transfusions were excluded from the analysis, the overall complication rate for the elective/delayed group declined to 28% and 34.7% for the early/neonatal repairs.

There were five cases of wound dehiscence in the early/neonatal group, and three of these patients required reoperation, whereas there were none in the elective/delayed group.

These data are compelling for the safety and efficacy of the elective/delayed group given that one of the most common indications at the authors' institution for postponing the early/neonatal repair was an inadequate bladder plate (<3 cm in diameter).

There are numerous studies that have demonstrated the importance of a successful primary closure in optimizing the bladder capacity and subsequent urinary continence as well as protection of renal function [9, 42].

Table 5.2 Thirty-day postoperative complications: early/neonatal (95 Pts) vs. elective/delayed (50 Pts) repair of BE [37]

Variable, *n* (%)	Early (neonatal)	Elective (delayed)	*P*-value
Closure technique—MSRE	95 (100%)	38 (76%)	
Closure technique—CPRE		12 (24%)	
Any complication	46 (48.4%)	29 (58%)	0.298
Complication w/o transfusion	33 (34.7%)	13 (26%)	0.349
Clavien I–II complications	40 (42.1%)	27 (54%)	0.292
Wound dehiscence	2 (2.1%)		
Wound infection	1 (1%)	1 (2%)	
Febrile UTI	5 (5.3%)	1 (2%)	
Pyelonephritis	8 (8.4%)	1 (2%)	
Urinary fistula	1 (1%)	3 (6%)	
Non-GU infection	2 (2.1%)	3 (6%)	
Other	5 (5.3%)	2 (4%)	
Postoperative transfusion	25 (26.3%)	19 (38%)	0.34
Clavien III complications	7 (7.4%)	1 (2%)	0.263
Wound dehiscence	3 (3.2%)		
Bowel obstruction		1 (2%)	
Non-GU infection	1 (1%)		
Other	3 (3.2%)	1 (2%)	
Clavien IV complications	3 (3.2%)	1 (2%)	
Non-GU infection	1 (1%)	1 (2%)	
Other	2 (2%)		

While the main emphasis of this discussion regarding the timing of surgery is to point out the pros and cons of early/neonatal repair of BE versus elective/delayed repair, we do need to point out the harm that can occur if the repair of BE is postponed beyond infancy. It is not unusual for children in low-resource countries to present at much older ages. In some cases of very delayed presentation, the bladder plate may be irreversibly injured, and in such cases, the best primary surgical intervention might be to proceed with a cystectomy and urinary diversion. There is also the negative psychosocial impact of living with a malformation beyond the age of 3 years, when peer relationships have begun to become important, and also the child may be in settings where sexual comparisons may occur, i.e., washrooms. Delay of surgery beyond the age of 3 years also prolongs the period of actual as well as perceived abnormality by the child and causes a distortion of their body image, since their body image at this age is derived from the feedback of their primary caretakers—both of these can cause long-term psychological impact on the individual [45].

It is important to assess each case and personalize the care for the individual patient, and there is anecdotal evidence of children as old as 13 years undergoing a successful CPRE with minimal morbidity and excellent clinical outcomes including a 2-h dry interval.

Disadvantages of postponing surgery beyond a year of life:

- Psychological impact—emotionally most children can be expected to tolerate undergoing surgical procedures without massive disruption of normal psychological development until the age of approximately 8 months, or the emergence of "stranger anxiety."
- Irreversible changes to the bladder plate with inflammatory polyp development and loss of compliance. These bladder plates do not grow and can cause upper tract injury if closure is attempted.
- Higher probability that the child will end up with a urinary diversion rather than reconstruction of the BE.

Parental Expectations After Repair of BE

The expectations of the parents can be divided into short-term and long-term outcomes.

In the short term, the parents expect that their child's surgery will be successful with minimal complications, i.e., wound infections, failure of the repair, and dehiscence or fistula, and provide a normal cosmetic appearance of their child's abdomen and genitalia.

Long-term expectations are more functional and include that their child will be able to achieve urinary continence, void per urethra, have minimal UTIs, and have no kidney injury. Later in life, parents expect their child will have typical sexual function and fertility. Most parents are also focused on the psychosocial impact of being born with BE on their child's body image, as shown in Fig. 5.1.

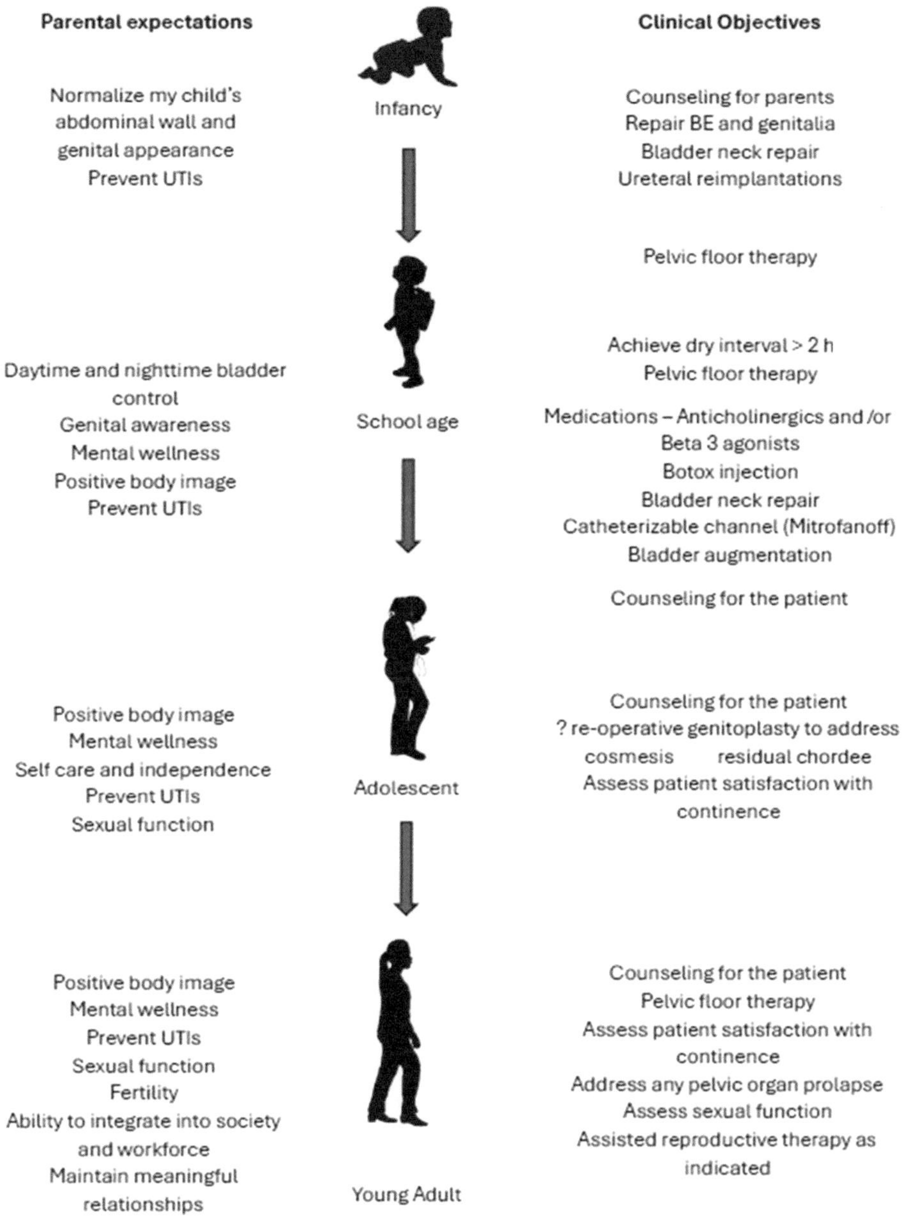

Fig. 5.1 Parental expectations by age of patient with BE and clinical objectives

Clinical Outcomes After Repair of BE

There is a significant worldwide lack of uniform clinical outcomes for this patient cohort, partly due to the dearth of multicenter studies with an adequate number of patient to achieve statistical significance and precisely defined patient-reported outcomes using validated instruments [42].

Defining clinical outcomes of surgery for children born with BE is critically important, as it is only when we have universally accepted definitions guided by the inputs from patients (patient-reported outcomes) with BE that we will truly be able to track how well our management strategies are working. It is also imperative that these outcomes be tracked at multiple intervals throughout the patient's lifetime, as change is the only constant that we can expect when monitoring a chronic health condition, such as BE, where there are age-dependent clinical outcomes.

The pediatric and adult outcomes of patients with BE are of critical importance when counseling an expectant couple with a prenatal diagnosis, as these data may impact the family's decision whether or not to proceed with the pregnancy.

In the following section, a few of the currently identified and tracked clinical outcomes that might be impacted by the timing of surgery will be presented. In the future standardization of healthcare practices, the proactive collection and analysis of data obtained from quality-of-life reports and screening questionnaires related to mental health, urinary continence, sexual function, and fertility should be included. This will enable us to significantly enhance the overall quality of care while reducing the cost and burden of care provided to individuals with BE.

Successful Initial Repair of BE

This is an important outcome and can be defined as the absence of wound dehiscence, bladder prolapse, or urinary fistula following the surgical procedure to close the defect. Successful repair has better long-term bladder, kidney, and continence outcomes; a positive impact on the psychological well-being of the patient and their parents; and has been documented to be less of a financial burden.

Morrill et al. have demonstrated a higher incidence in the rate of dehiscence of the initial repair of BE in those patients who underwent early/neonatal repair compared to the elective/delayed cohort [37].

The impact of a failed initial repair is significant. Gearhart et al. have demonstrated that the mean age at reoperation of children who had failed their initial closure was 1.14 years; this is the additional time that the parents have to manage their child's abnormal anatomy, and this has been shown to add to the stress of the parents [21].

Numerous studies have demonstrated that patients that require reoperative repair of BE have smaller bladder capacities, significantly lower rates of urethral continence, and a higher rate of requiring bladder augmentation or urinary diversion [40]. Joshi et al. have demonstrated in their cohort that patients who required reoperative repair had a higher incidence of CKD and kidney injury, and while this did not reach statistical significance, it points to the importance of a successful initial repair [24].

The hospital charges related to the reoperative care have to be factored into the impact of the failed initial repair, and this can be substantial and add to the burden of care that the parents have to face [21].

Psychological Impact on the Patient with BE

The correction of genital abnormalities before the age of 3 years in both genders has been shown to have a positive impact on the child's psychological development and body image, as the repair is completed before peer relationships and sexual comparisons have not yet evolved [45]. There is a higher rate of successful bladder and abdominal wall closure in the elective/delayed repair cohort, and this will positively impact the child.

Psychological Impact on the Parents of a Child with BE

In the neonatal period, parents who were not expecting a child with this diagnosis might require crisis intervention. All parents of a baby born with BE deserve to be provided with psychological support to work through their emotions, as this will facilitate attachment to the child and prevent later serious psychiatric problems [47].

The correction of genital abnormalities before the age of 3 years in both genders has been shown to be beneficial for the parents, in which it limits the period of time during which they have a child who appears "abnormal." Although the surgery may not eliminate all of their concerns, it affirms the conditions correctability and provides them with hope for their child's future [11, 45].

Bladder Growth

It is believed that early bladder closure results in better bladder cycling and improved bladder growth. Baradaran et al. have studied the impact of the timing of repair of BE on eventual bladder growth [3]. In their cohort, the indications for the elective/delayed repair were either a small-bladder template or delayed referral to a center of excellence for BE repair. They demonstrated that patients undergoing elective/delayed repair due to a small-bladder plate had an overall smaller bladder capacity, 36 mL smaller than their cohort of neonatal repair. However, they also demonstrated that the rate of annual bladder growth was not statistically different between the two groups. It is important to note here that regardless of the timing of the initial repair of BE, it is the timing of the bladder neck repair that ultimately influences the bladder's ability to cycle and grow. Most surgeons that have adopted the elective/delayed repair usually perform the CPRE technique, which permits the cycling of the bladder much sooner than those patients undergoing either the MSRE or the RSTM techniques.

Urinary Continence

Urinary continence does not appear to be directly impacted by the timing of surgery in current clinical series. The impact of the continence status is related to the outcome of the initial repair, with children that require reoperation demonstrating lower rates of urinary continence with their native urinary tract and a higher incidence of bladder augmentation or urinary diversion in this group.

Urinary continence is the most common adult concern of patients who had undergone childhood repair of BE; in one series, it affected 39% of the study cohort [4]. Urinary continence has been defined as voluntary control of the bladder with the ability to safely store urine (without harm to the upper tracts) and empty the bladder when needed. Dr. Dana Weiss will discuss in a later chapter the more appropriate outcome for patients with BE, which might be the length of the dry interval, i.e., duration of urinary storage in the bladder without leakage at rest or with activity.

Urinary continence is significantly influenced by cultural norms, which dictate the acceptable age at which it should be acquired and the duration of the dry interval. In most communities, social continence is defined as being able to hold urine and stay dry for up to 3 h during the daytime and up to 8 h overnight.

Patients with BE often require multiple extensive surgical procedures to achieve continence. The challenge with fully understanding the data about this clinical outcome lies in the variation in the definition of continence (i.e., duration of dry interval, voiding via urethra, or does it also include patients on CIC who have an acceptable dry interval?) and the duration of the study period [30]. Unarguably, the most important aspect of continence is the patient's satisfaction with their continence, and its impact on their QoL is the most important metric.

Up to 70% of patients with BE have been shown to require either bladder augmentation or urinary diversion [48]. The ability to void spontaneously via the urethra has only been reported in 14–25% of adults with BE and a continent reconstruction, with the remainder of patients having to rely on catheterization to empty their bladder [4, 8, 31]. Continence status has been shown to be comparable in adults with BE [12].

It is also important to note that urinary continence is not a static outcome and is dynamically influenced by age, body habitus, and general health of the individual. Short-term continence has rates of success as high as 80–90%, but as the patients age and are followed beyond childhood, the long-term continence rates decrease significantly. The ongoing anatomical and physiological changes associated with aging have been shown to impact the achievement of dry intervals in patients with BE. In the children, there does appear to be a positive impact, with patients who have been followed into their early adolescence demonstrating bladder growth and urinary storage function that permits dry intervals. Woodhouse et al. have demonstrated the opposite influence of aging beyond childhood into adulthood; in their series, they demonstrated that of the 23% of their pediatric patients who were voiding normally, only 5% of them continued to be able to do so beyond adolescence [51].

Patient-reported outcomes have shown that only 40% of adults with BE have sustained perineal dryness [51]. There was no difference between continent and incontinent adults with regard to social or sexual parameters, stone formation, incidence of UTIs, or kidney injury [12].

Modifications to existing surgical techniques, a better understanding of bladder cycling during childhood after repair of BE, and improved understanding of pelvic floor dysfunction in this patient cohort may positively impact continence rates in the future. There are already patients benefiting from early referral for pelvic floor physiotherapy/urotherapy. Up to 37% of study patients have been reported to achieve urinary continence, and 61% show improvement of incontinence after completion of pelvic floor rehabilitation programs [50].

Preservation of Kidney Function and Prevention of UTIs

Unlike patients with cloacal exstrophy, where congenital renal anomalies are common, most children with BE are born with two healthy kidneys. Given the abnormal intramural ureteral anatomy, there is a high incidence of vesicoureteral reflux (VUR). Patients who are continent tend to have clinically significant VUR, with a higher incidence of pyelonephritis and kidney scarring noted in this cohort [7]. There is no direct impact of the timing of surgery on the child's kidney health; rather, this is a function of the health of the lower urinary tract that has been shown to be improved in series of children who have undergone elective/delayed repair of their BE.

Ben-Chaim et al. reported that up to 50% of their adult cohort of patients with BE had experienced pyelonephritis and 18% had been diagnosed with epididymitis [5]. This is similar to the data presented by de Jesus et al., which was a questionnaire-based study of 50 adults with BE. Recurrent UTIs were reported by 64% of their patients, and 40% of them developed kidney scars and progressed to chronic kidney disease [12]. Joshi et al. in a more contemporary series with 72 patients with a median followup of 4 years after repair of BE have demonstrated a 5% incidence of CKD stage 2 or higher based on eGFR and a 30.4% incidence of kidney scarring by DMSA. There was a higher incidence of CKD in those patients who had undergone a reoperative repair of BE [24]. Roth et al. have recently published on a series of 197 patients with BE that underwent primary bladder repair, and they reported a 1.5% incidence of end-stage kidney disease (ESKD), compared to a rate of 0.003% in the general population at comparable ages. In their cohort, there was a 2% incidence of CKD 3 or higher in the pediatric age group, and this increased to 8% in the adult patients [44].

In adult women with BE who were able to achieve pregnancy, none of them had any deterioration of the kidney function as a result of the pregnancy [26].

In summary, once the bladder has been closed in patients with BE, there is an ongoing risk to the upper tracts irrespective of the nature or timing of the repair that these patients have undergone. Anecdotal observations have suggested that those children who have undergone elective/delayed repair with CPRE have better kidney health outcomes, as they have usually undergone ureteral reimplantations at the initial repair.

It is recommended that kidney function and upper tract monitoring be performed at regular intervals for all patients who have undergone repair of BE; furthermore, since some of the impact of CKD may not be manifest until they are adults, a proper transition of their care to adult providers is mandatory for their safety.

Conclusions

The management of BE continues to evolve as we gain better understanding of the impact of the nature of the repair and timing of the repair. Historical teaching in the management of BE has favored the early/neonatal repair of BE; however, more contemporary management is increasingly trending toward the elective/delayed repair of BE. The use of elective/delayed repair is associated with a higher incidence of osteotomies and blood transfusions. The majority of complications associated with the elective/delayed closure are of low Clavien-Dindo grade. Families should be counseled about the differences between early/neonatal versus elective/delayed repairs and that there is an increased possibility of minor, conservatively managed complications and the likelihood of a blood transfusion with osteotomy [37]. Given the dynamic impact of aging on clinical outcomes, such as continence, sexual function, fertility, and mental wellness, it is imperative that all patients with BE should be appropriately transitioned as adults to specialists with expertise in managing these conditions. This will ensure not only their safety but also permit ongoing monitoring of their clinical outcomes. Future studies that include quality-of-life metrics and patient-reported outcomes are needed to investigate the long-term complications, rate of kidney injury, continence, and sexual outcomes for patients who have undergone elective/delayed repair of BE.

References

1. Ahn JJ, Shnorhavorian M, Katz C, Goldin AB, Merguerian PA. Early versus delayed closure of bladder exstrophy: a National Surgical Quality Improvement Program Pediatric analysis. J Pediatr Urol. 2018;14(1):27.e21–5.
2. Baradaran N, Cervellione RM, Stec AA, Gearhart JP. Delayed primary repair of bladder exstrophy: ultimate effect on growth. J Urol. 2012a;188(6):2336–41.
3. Baradaran N, Stec AA, Schaeffer AJ, Gearhart JP, Mathews RI. Delayed primary closure of bladder exstrophy: immediate postoperative management leading to successful outcomes. Urology. 2012b;79(2):415–9.
4. Bazinet A, Filfilan A, Mokhtari N, Lenfant L, Elghoneimi A, Chartier-Kastler E. Adult patients treated for bladder exstrophy at a young age: what are their current demands? Can Urol Assoc J. 2024;18:E187–93.
5. Ben-Chaim J, Jeffs RD, Reiner WG, Gearhart JP. The outcome of patients with classic bladder exstrophy in adult life. J Urol. 1996;155(4):1251–2.
6. Ben-Chaim J, Hidas G, Wikenheiser J, Landau EH, Wehbi E, Kelly MS, McLorie GA, Khoury AE. Kelly procedure for exstrophy or epispadias patients: anatomical description of the pudendal neurovasculature. J Pediatr Urol. 2016;12(3):173.e171–6.
7. Braga LH, Lorenzo AJ, Jrearz R, Bagli DJ, Salle JL. Bilateral ureteral reimplantation at primary bladder exstrophy closure. J Urol. 2010;183(6):2337–41.

8. Capolicchio G, McLorie GA, Farhat W, Merguerian PA, Bagli DJ, Khoury AE. A population based analysis of continence outcomes and bladder exstrophy. J Urol. 2001;165(6 Pt 2):2418–21.
9. Chan DY, Jeffs RD, Gearhart JP. Determinants of continence in the bladder exstrophy population: predictors of success? Urology. 2001;57(4):774–7.
10. Cohen MM, Cameron CB, Duncan PG. Pediatric anesthesia morbidity and mortality in the perioperative period. Anesth Analg. 1990;70(2):160–7.
11. Ellens REH, Bakula DM, Mullins AJ, Scott Reyes KJ, Austin P, Baskin L, Bernabe K, Cheng EY, Fried A, Frimberger D, Galan D, Gonzalez L, Greenfield S, Kolon T, Kropp B, Lakshmanan Y, Meyer S, Meyer T, Mullins LL, Nokoff NJ, Palmer B, Poppas D, Paradis A, Yerkes E, Wisniewski AB, Wolfe-Christensen C. Psychological adjustment of parents of children born with atypical genitalia 1 year after genitoplasty. J Urol. 2017;198(4):914–20.
12. Eyer de Jesus L, Dekermacher S, Pippi-Salle JL. Bladder exstrophy: we need to improve. A lot. J Pediatr Urol. 2022;18(1):38.e1–38.e11.
13. Feldkamp ML, Botto LD, Amar E, Bakker MK, Bermejo-Sanchez E, Bianca S, Canfield MA, Castilla EE, Clementi M, Csaky-Szunyogh M, Leoncini E, Li Z, Lowry RB, Mastroiacovo P, Merlob P, Morgan M, Mutchinick OM, Rissmann A, Ritvanen A, Siffel C, Carey JC. Cloacal exstrophy: an epidemiologic study from the International Clearinghouse for Birth Defects Surveillance and Research. Am J Med Genet C Semin Med Genet. 2011;157C(4):333–43.
14. Ferrara F, Dickson AP, Fishwick J, Vashisht R, Khan T, Cervellione RM. Delayed exstrophy repair (DER) does not compromise initial bladder development. J Pediatr Urol. 2014;10(3):506–10.
15. Fineman AD. Preliminary observations on ego development in children with congenital defects of the genitourinary system. Am J Orthopsychiatry. 1959;29(1):110–8; discussion 118–120.
16. Frank NM, Lynch KF, Uusitalo U, Yang J, Lonnrot M, Virtanen SM, Hyoty H, Norris JM, TEDDY Study Group. The relationship between breastfeeding and reported respiratory and gastrointestinal infection rates in young children. BMC Pediatr. 2019;19(1):339.
17. Friedrichsdorf SJ, Goubert L. Pediatric pain treatment and prevention for hospitalized children. Schmerz. 2021;35(3):195–210.
18. Grady RW, Mitchell ME. Newborn exstrophy closure and epispadias repair. World J Urol. 1998;16(3):200–4.
19. Grady RW, Mitchell ME. Management of epispadias. Urol Clin North Am. 2002;29(2):349–60, vi.
20. Grady RW, Carr MC, Mitchell ME. Complete primary closure of bladder exstrophy. Epispadias and bladder exstrophy repair. Urol Clin North Am. 1999;26(1):95–109, viii.
21. Hesh CA, Young E, Intihar P, Gearhart JP. The cost of failure: the economic impact of failed primary closure in classic bladder exstrophy. J Pediatr Surg. 2016;51(8):1312–6.
22. Hofmann A, Haider M, Promm M, Neissner C, Badelt G, Rosch WH. Delayed primary closure of bladder exstrophy without osteotomy: 12 year experience in a safe and gentle alternative to neonatal surgery. J Pediatr Surg. 2022;57(10):303–8.
23. Jeffs RD. Functional closure of bladder exstrophy. Birth Defects Orig Artic Ser. 1977;13(5):171–3.
24. Joshi RS, Eftekharzadeh S, Shukla AR, Ramji J, Hingorani SR, Canning DA, Pippi-Salle JL, Merguerian P, DeFoor WR Jr, Frazier JR, Weiss DA, Reddy PP. Kidney function outcomes in patients after complete primary repair of bladder exstrophy and penopubic epispadias: results from the international bladder exstrophy consortium. J Pediatr Urol. 2023;19(1):34.e31–9.
25. Kelly JH, Taghavi K, Mushtaq I. Justin H. Kelly and his procedure for bladder exstrophy and epispadias. J Pediatr Surg. 2022;57(2):314–21.
26. Krisiloff M, Puchner PJ, Tretter W, Macfarlane MT, Lattimer JK. Pregnancy in women with bladder exstrophy. J Urol. 1978;119(4):478–9.
27. Lattimer JK, Smith MJ. Exstrophy closure: a followup on 70 cases. J Urol. 1966;95(3):356–9.
28. Lee SL, Beyer TD, Kim SS, Waldhausen JH, Healey PJ, Sawin RS, Ledbetter DJ. Initial nonoperative management and delayed closure for treatment of giant omphaloceles. J Pediatr Surg. 2006;41(11):1846–9.

29. Lin AE, Autran CA, Espanola SD, Bode L, Nizet V. Human milk oligosaccharides protect bladder epithelial cells against uropathogenic Escherichia coli invasion and cytotoxicity. J Infect Dis. 2014;209(3):389–98.
30. Lloyd JC, Spano SM, Ross SS, Wiener JS, Routh JC. How dry is dry? A review of definitions of continence in the contemporary exstrophy/epispadias literature. J Urol. 2012;188(5):1900–4.
31. Maruf M, Manyevitch R, Michaud J, Jayman J, Kasprenski M, Zaman MH, Benz K, Eldridge M, Trock B, Harris KT, Wu WJ, Di Carlo HN, Gearhart JP. Urinary continence outcomes in classic bladder exstrophy: a long-term perspective. J Urol. 2020;203(1):200–5.
32. McCollum A. Coping with prolonged health impairment in your child. New York: Little Brown and Co, Inc; 1975.
33. Michelet D, Brasher C, Kaddour HB, Diallo T, Abdat R, Malbezin S, Bonnard A, Dahmani S. Postoperative complications following neonatal and infant surgery: common events and predictive factors. Anaesth Crit Care Pain Med. 2017;36(3):163–9.
34. Minde KK, Marton P, Manning D, Hines B. Some determinants of mother-infant interaction in the premature nursery. J Am Acad Child Psychiatry. 1980;19(1):1–21.
35. Mitchell ME, Bagli DJ. Complete penile disassembly for epispadias repair: the Mitchell technique. J Urol. 1996;155(1):300–4.
36. Morray JP, Geiduschek JM, Ramamoorthy C, Haberkern CM, Hackel A, Caplan RA, Domino KB, Posner K, Cheney FW. Anesthesia-related cardiac arrest in children: initial findings of the Pediatric Perioperative Cardiac Arrest (POCA) Registry. Anesthesiology. 2000;93(1):6–14.
37. Morrill CC, Manyevitch R, Haffar A, Wu WJ, Harris KT, Maruf M, Crigger C, Di Carlo HN, Gearhart JP. Complications of delayed and newborn primary closures of classic bladder exstrophy: is there a difference? J Pediatr Urol. 2023;19(3):249.e241–8.
38. Mushtaq I, Garriboli M, Smeulders N, Cherian A, Desai D, Eaton S, Duffy P, Cuckow P. Primary bladder exstrophy closure in neonates: challenging the traditions. J Urol. 2014;191(1):193–7.
39. Nasr VG, Davis JM. Anesthetic use in newborn infants: the urgent need for rigorous evaluation. Pediatr Res. 2015;78(1):2–6.
40. Novak TE, Costello JP, Orosco R, Sponseller PD, Mack E, Gearhart JP. Failed exstrophy closure: management and outcome. J Pediatr Urol. 2010;6(4):381–4.
41. Okonkwo I, Bendon AA, Cervellione RM, Vashisht R. Continuous caudal epidural analgesia and early feeding in delayed bladder exstrophy repair: a nine-year experience. J Pediatr Urol. 2019;15(1):76.e71–8.
42. Promm M, Roesch WH. Recent trends in the management of bladder exstrophy: the Gordian knot has not yet been cut. Front Pediatr. 2019;7:110.
43. Roesch W, Bertz S, Ebert AK, Hofstaedter F. Mucosal changes in the exstrophic bladder: is delayed timing of reconstruction associated with premalignant changes? ESPU annual meeting. Antalya, Turkey. 2010.
44. Roth J. End-stage and chronic kidney disease in classic bladder exstrophy. A. P. Pediatric Urology Midwest; 2024.
45. Schultz JR, Klykylo WM, Wacksman J. Timing of elective hypospadias repair in children. Pediatrics. 1983;71(3):342–51.
46. Shah PS, Herbozo C, Aliwalas LL, Shah VS. Breastfeeding or breast milk for procedural pain in neonates. Cochrane Database Syst Rev. 2012;12(12):CD004950.
47. Stjernqvist K, Kockum CC. Bladder exstrophy: psychological impact during childhood. J Urol. 1999;162(6):2125–9.
48. Szymanski KM, Fuchs M, McLeod D, Rosoklija I, Strine AC, VanderBrink B, Whittam B, Yerkes E, Gargollo PC, Pediatric Urology Midwest Alliance. Probability of bladder augmentation, diversion and clean intermittent catheterization in classic bladder exstrophy: a 36-year, multi-institutional, retrospective cohort study. J Urol. 2019;202(6):1256–62.

49. Taddio A, Katz J. The effects of early pain experience in neonates on pain responses in infancy and childhood. Paediatr Drugs. 2005;7(4):245–57.
50. van Geen FJ, Nieuwhof-Leppink AJ, Wortel RC, de Kort LMO. Bladder exstrophy-epispadias complex: the effect of urotherapy on incontinence. J Pediatr Urol. 2024;20:645.e1–5.
51. Woodhouse CR, North AC, Gearhart JP. Standing the test of time: long-term outcome of reconstruction of the exstrophy bladder. World J Urol. 2006;24(3):244–9.
52. Young HH. Exstrophy of the bladder: the first case in which a normal bladder and urinary control have been obtained by plastic operations. Surg Gynecol Obstet. 1942;74:729–37.

Complete Primary Repair of Bladder Exstrophy and Epispadias

6

Karl F. Godlewski, Michael E. Mitchell, Dana A. Weiss, and Aseem R. Shukla

The challenge of surgically reconstructing bladder exstrophy patients such that they are volitionally void, are continent and have cosmetically normal-appearing genitalia has perplexed pediatric urologists for decades. The sheer rarity of the condition, 1 in 10,000 to 50,000 live births, and severity of the phenotypic changes to normal anatomy in the pelvis make this reconstruction a significant undertaking. The bladder exstrophy and epispadias complex represents a spectrum of disease. The degree of anatomic and physiological derangement is thought to be directly correlated with the timing of the embryological insult; specifically, the earlier the embryological insult, the more severe the anomaly. Although many theories exist regarding the true embryological cause of this disease process, premature loss of the infra-umbilical membrane is a commonly accepted hypothesis [1]. The anomaly may be considered as part of a continuum ranging from mild forms of balanitic or distal epispadias to penopubic epispadias to classic bladder exstrophy, and, finally, cloacal exstrophy. Although each patient has a unique phenotype, there are common and reproducible features among all patients within this spectrum that support this theory. As surgeons, we aim to anatomically reconstruct "normal" anatomy with the hopes of

Supplementary Information The online version contains supplementary material available at https://doi.org/10.1007/978-3-031-91238-2_6.

K. F. Godlewski · D. A. Weiss · A. R. Shukla
Children's Hospital of Philadelphia, Philadelphia, PA, USA
e-mail: godlewskk1@chop.edu; WeissD1@chop.edu; ShuklaA@chop.edu

M. E. Mitchell (✉)
Children's Hospital of Philadelphia, Philadelphia, PA, USA

Children's Hospital of Wisconsin, Medical College of Wisconsin, Milwaukee, WI, USA

A. R. Shukla, R. S. Joshi (eds.), *Bladder Exstrophy and Epispadias*,
https://doi.org/10.1007/978-3-031-91238-2_6

establishing "normal" physiology; however, the more severely distorted the anatomy (earlier the embryologic insult), the more difficult it is to achieve this result.

Generations of surgeons have conjectured about the optimal surgical technique for treatment of bladder exstrophy, which has led to the development of various approaches, many of which are discussed in other chapters. Until the 1950s, cystectomy and ureterosigmoidostomy were the commonly accepted methods for managing these patients. In 1966, Lattimer as well as Tsakagiannes and Williams published their results with complete repair of bladder exstrophy [2–4]. Though initial results were promising, upper tract deterioration and recurrent urinary tract infection pushed many to continue performing ureterosigmoidostomy or adopting a staged approach to closure.

A more modern complete primary repair of bladder exstrophy (CPRE) was initially described by Grady and Mitchell in 1999 [5]. This alternative to the popular staged approach was predicated on the belief that early introduction of bladder outlet resistance facilitates "bladder cycling" and creates an environment where bladder growth and development can occur more reliably. Despite exstrophic bladders being abnormal both histologically and physiologically at birth, Mitchell felt that with the appropriate early physical stimulus (cycling), even exstrophic bladders could be rehabilitated and function normally. Differing from the planned staged approach, which may or may not achieve bladder cycling initially, the CPRE offers an opportunity to achieve bladder growth and successful outcomes regardless of bladder plate size, potentially with a single surgery.

The surgery, performed during infancy (6–12 weeks) and in conjunction with pelvic osteotomies to reduce the abdominal wall tension during closure, includes bladder closure, anatomic bladder neck tailoring with or without ureteral reimplantation, penile disassembly, epispadias repair and umbilicoplasty. It is critical to fashion an appropriate level of resistance at the bladder neck to allow for bladder cycling and growth at safe storage pressures that do not put the upper tracts at risk of deterioration. Striking such a delicate balance in a single surgery can seem daunting or unachievable; however, adhering to the core principles of the CPRE reconstruction can facilitate success in this repair.

Although many bladder exstrophy patients are now referred to tertiary, high-volume exstrophy centers with expert surgeons, this chapter will detail each critical step of the CPRE and provide a roadmap for surgeons to follow in practice.

Male Bladder Exstrophy and Epispadias Repair

Assessment of Anatomy and Preparation

There is considerable variation in size and degree of epithelialization/metaplasia of the bladder plate as well as volume of bladder polyps among bladder exstrophy patients. These variables rarely if ever prevent a CPRE in primary cases. After general anesthesia is administered, an epidural is typically placed for postoperative pain control. The surgeon then performs a full body preparation with betadine and

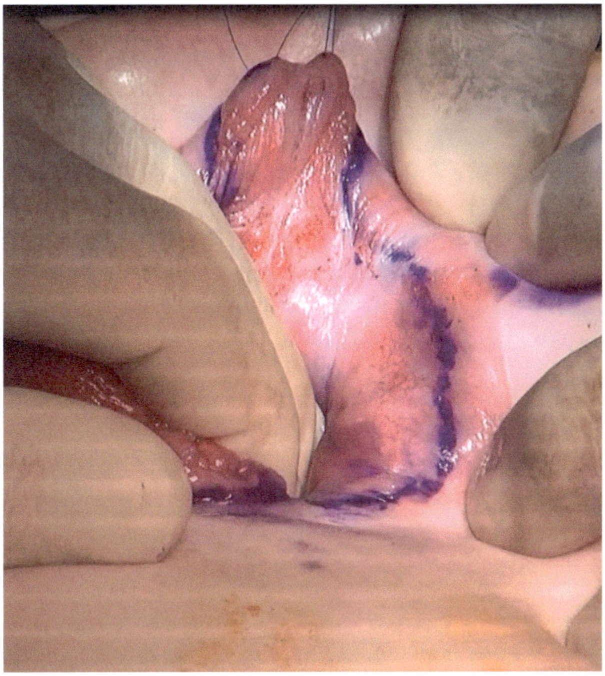

Fig. 6.1 Circumferential marking around bladder and urethral plate leaving paraexstrophy skin to use in skin closure if necessary. Medial aspects of pubic bones have also been marked

identifies important landmarks. A stay suture is placed transversely through each hemiglans of the penis to facilitate exposure. The ureteral orifices are identified and catheterized with 4 French (Fr) feeding tubes; these tubes are secured with an absorbable suture (5–0 chromic). Marks are made along the medial aspects of each pubic symphysis, and the bladder neck region (longitudinal fibers midway between the ureteral orifices and the verumontanum) is identified. A neoumbilicus site is marked in the midline 1-finger breadth above the ASIS. Any large bladder polyps are excised and closed with a running absorbable suture (5–0 Monocryl). Marks are made around the perimeter of the bladder, bladder neck and urethral plate leaving some paraexstrophy skin on the abdominal wall, which can be excised at the end of the procedure if necessary, to avoid excessive tension on the skin closure (Fig. 6.1). The triangular fascial defect cephalad to the bladder plate at the site of the former umbilical stump is marked with an inverted V to be used as handle during the initial dissection.

Incision and Initial Dissection

Incisions begin at the most cephalad extent above the triangular fascial defect (inverted V marking line) and are carried around the marked borders of bladder and urethral plate with either a knife or pinpoint electrocautery. At the level of the triangular fascial defect, the incisions are deepened and the obliterated umbilical vessels are identified and ligated. A stay suture is placed through the umbilical stump, and with traction, the peritoneum is identified and carefully swept off the bladder dome, and lateral aspects of the bladder plate. As the incisions are deepened circumferentially, the rectus fascia is identified laterally first utilizing the abdominal wall fat as a marker for the appropriate level of dissection. Alternatively, the dissection can begin at the level of the pubic symphysis where a similar fat layer exists and progressed in a cephalad direction. Regardless of approach, once the rectus fascia is identified, it is critical to precisely identify where the medial edge of fascia and abdominal rectus muscle meet the detrusor muscle to avoid inappropriately thinning the detrusor or excising rectus muscle with the bladder during the dissection. Insertion of a finger inside the bladder to invert it, during this dissection, can improve visualization of the plane between the detrusor, fascia and rectus muscle. Identification of a second "fat" plane, when the perivesical fat is noted, establishes that a correct plane between the detrusor muscle and rectus fascia has been identified and dissection will next encounter the intersymphyseal bands.

Dissection of Intersymphyseal Bands and Urethral Plate

Once the bladder is released from its attachments to the lateral fascia and rectus muscle cranially, at the level of the pubic symphysis, intersymphyseal bands will be encountered. With upward traction on the bladder, a plane lateral to the bladder neck and poster-medial to the pubic symphysis is developed bluntly. Release of these intersymphyseal bands is one of the most critical aspects of the dissection, as it will allow for a tension-free bladder neck and posterior urethral closure and enable placement of the bladder neck and posterior urethra in a more orthotopic location deep in the pelvis. This dissection is typically safest to perform after the corpora, and its neurovascular bundles have been identified following the ventral penile dissection and partial penile disassembly.

Dissection of Corpora Cavernosa and Spongiosum

An incision is carried out with a fresh scalpel blade or fine-tip cautery on the dorsal surface of the epispadias penis parallel to the exposed urethral plate beginning at the presumed bladder neck location. This incision is carried ventrally onto the ventral skin, transversely, parallel to the corona. The penis is degloved noting that in bladder exstrophy, the neurovascular bundles are placed laterally on the corpora and can be adherent to the thin shaft skin proximally. With adequate exposure of the corpora, a plane is developed between the corpora cavernosa and the urethral plate's underlying spongiosum, by beginning dissection ventrally using sharp dissection and bipolar electrocautery as needed. Gentle rolling and lifting of the corpora laterally can facilitate exposure of the correct plane—just along Buck's fascia over the

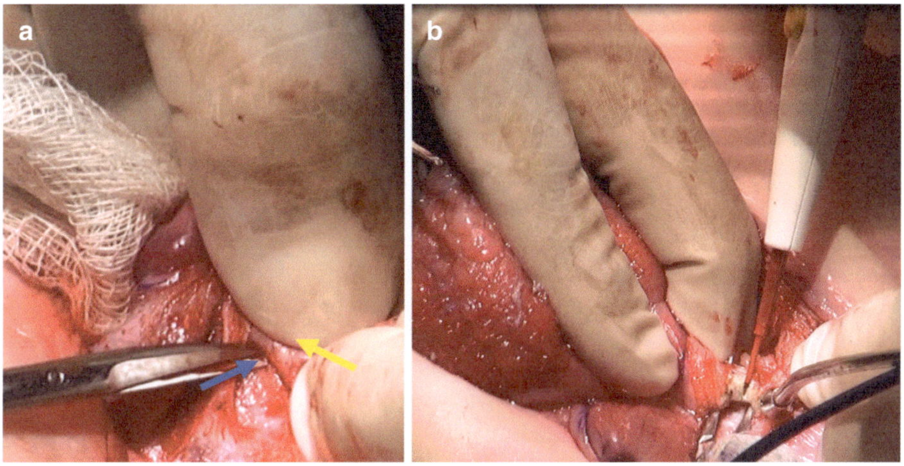

Fig. 6.2 (**a**) Penile disassembly (spongiosum—blue arrow; corporal body—yellow arrow). (**b**) Dissection of intersymphyseal bands that tether the bladder neck anteriorly

corpora cavernosa—to release the spongiosum off the corpora without injury to the urethral or corporal blood supply (Fig. 6.2a). The dissection is systematically carried proximally to where the corpora split and along the curvilinear corporal body toward the incised urethral plate dorsally. Much of the dissection can be carried out ventrally; however, a dorsal approach is useful to complete the circumferential dissection again utilizing mostly sharp dissection and bipolar electrocautery as needed. The dorsal dissection must be medial and parallel to the neurovascular bundle to prevent injury. Ultimately, once the corpora are free of spongiosum in one area, a vessel loop is passed around the corporal body and another around the urethral plate for improved retraction and the dissection is carried proximally toward the prostate and distally toward the glans. Presently, we do not routinely disassociate the urethral plate from the glans unless there is a significant dorsal chordee from a short urethral plate tethering the penis as we have found that once the corpora are rotated and approximated, the chordee typically resolves. If the urethral plate is disassociated from the underlying corpora, then the right and left hemiglans are left in continuity to minimize the risk of postoperative glans ischemia. The dissection progresses until the urethral plate and underlying spongiosum are dissociated from the corpora on either side from the glans distally to the prostate proximally. With traction on the hemiglans holding stitch, the ipsilateral intersymphyseal bands, corporal body and neurovascular bundle can be easily identified and the intersymphyseal bands incised safely (Fig. 6.2b). The use of a Pena muscle stimulator can be helpful to differentiate fibrous intersymphyseal bands, which need to be released, from pelvic floor musculature, which should be left intact.

Bladder Neck Reconstruction, Bladder/Urethral Closure

The aforementioned initial dissection that has now fully mobilized the bladder from its intersymphyseal attachments and separated the corpora cavernosa from the urethral plate maintains the natural width of the urethral plate along with the exposed bladder neck. Approximation of the bladder neck and urethra in continuity may commence at this point. However, to create appropriate outlet resistance to facilitate bladder growth, we recommend tailoring the bladder neck. First, the bladder neck is identified between the verumontanum and ureteral orifices by its characteristic longitudinal ridges or striations. The width of the bladder neck as measured at the point of the striations is typically 25 mm to 30 mm. We tailor the bladder neck at this point to 2–3 mm wider than the urethral plate (to around 18 mm) and then flare the incision laterally and distally into the bladder. The excess mucosa at the edge of the bladder neck tailoring is de-epithelialized preserving the underlying detrusor muscle (Fig. 6.3). The bladder neck is then closed in an interrupted fashion using imbricating 4–0 polydioxanone suture (PDS), which is not tied initially to provide exact visualization of the mucosal edge. Each suture incorporates a substantial amount of serosa and detrusor with minimal mucosa to decrease the risk of fistula by rolling the mucosa inward. Once the bladder neck region is approximated, the feeding tubes are individually externalized through the bladder, fascia and skin lateral to the incision and secured at the skin with a 3–0 nylon suture. An 8.5 French (Fr) Dawson-Mueller suprapubic tube is also placed through a lateral skin incision into the dome of the bladder to provide maximal decompression. When necessary, purse-string sutures are placed on the external surface of the bladder around the tubes to prevent urinary leakage postoperatively. Lastly, a 7 Fr round Jackson-Pratt (JP) drain is

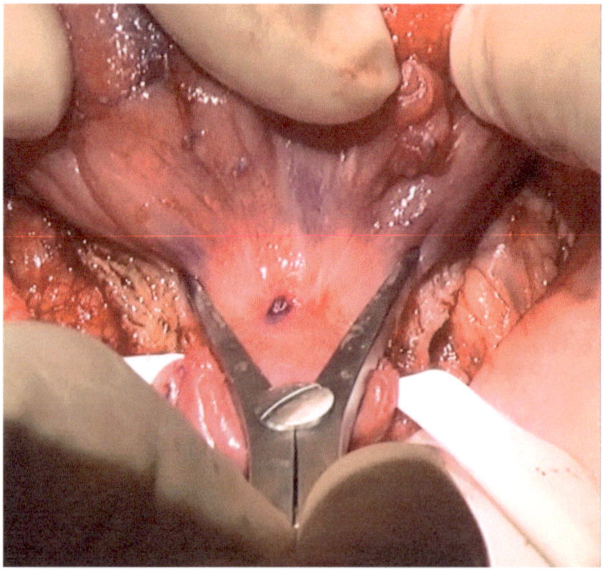

Fig. 6.3 Tailored bladder neck to 18 mm with excess mucosa excised leaving behind detrusor muscle. Verumontanum is marked in the midline

placed in the urethra and sutured to the back wall of the bladder mucosa with a 5–0 chromic suture to prevent dislodgement. The umbilical stump can be excised at this time and the remainder of the bladder closed in an interrupted imbricating fashion incorporating minimal mucosa using 3–0 PDS. The urethra is tubularized over the 7 Fr round JP using 5–0 PDS proximally and 6–0 PDS distally in an interrupted fashion. A small piece of Alloderm is then sutured atop the bladder neck (interrupted 5–0 Vicryl) and posterior urethral closure, putatively to reduce the risk of fistula formation at the most vulnerable location of the urethral and bladder neck repair, prior to pubic bone approximation (Fig. 6.4).

Pubic Bone Closure

Adequate exposure of the pubic bones is essential for accurate suture placement during pubic bone approximation. The anterior subcutaneous tissues should be elevated such that the superior and medial edges of the bone can be easily identified. A horizontal mattress #1 or 0 PDS suture is placed through the bone to allow for the knot and portions of the suture that cross midline to be anterior and away from the bladder neck and posterior urethral closure. A small segment of lateral glanular epithelium on each respective hemiglans is denuded/excised to aid in monitoring glans ischemia during closure. Closure of the pubic bones is performed after pelvic osteotomies have been completed utilizing manual reduction of the pubic diastasis to facilitate good approximation. If blood flow to the glans is compromised (no bleeding from the cut edges of glans), the pubic stitch is removed and replaced with slightly less tension. Throughout the remainder of the procedure, the glans should

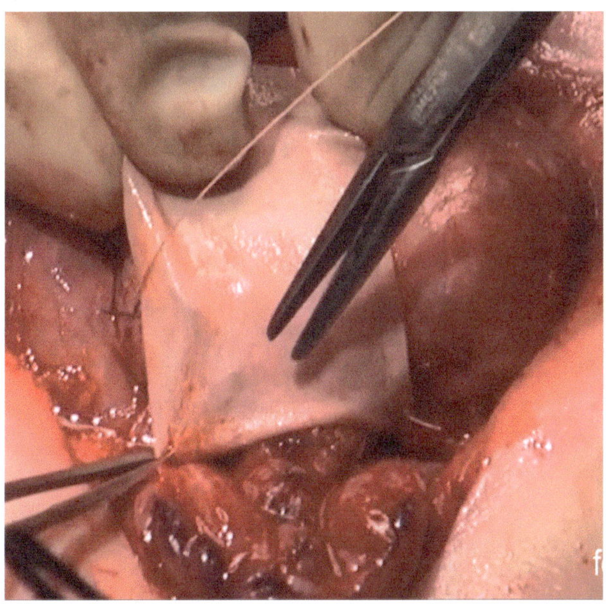

Fig. 6.4 Acellular dermal matrix being placed the over bladder neck, proximal urethra and bladder suture line

be inspected to ensure it remains well perfused. Alternatively, others have utilized intraoperative laser angiography for monitoring glans perfusion intraoperatively [6]. Indocyanine green (ICG) is administered intravenously at a dose of 1 mg per 10 kg body weight and binds tightly to plasma proteins and remains confined within vasculature with a half-life of approximately 2–3 min. Relative perfusion is assessed using the SPY Elite system (Stryker, Kalamazoo, MI) comparing glans perfusion to a control (thigh skin). No threshold currently exists for acceptable or inadequate glans perfusion after penile disassembly and closure, although future studies may elucidate a cutoff for relative glans perfusion that prevents penile injury.

Glansplasty and Corporal Cavernosa Approximation

Once adequate perfusion to the glans has been confirmed after pubic bone approximation, the remainder of the closure can be completed. The corpora cavernosa are approximated dorsally using interrupted 4–0 PDS sutures to gently externally rotate (proximally and along midshaft) to correct chordee and slightly internally rotate (distally) to facilitate glans closure. The lateral edges of the glanular epithelium are trimmed as needed to avoid a dorsal cleft in the glans after closure, and the glans is closed with an interrupted subcuticular 6–0 PDS suture avoiding excessive closure and tension distally to prevent meatal stenosis of the neourethra.

Abdominal Wall Closure and Penile Shaft Skin Coverage

Rectus fascia is closed with the interrupted figure-of-eight 2–0 PDS sutures. The subcutaneous tissue is then approximated using 4–0 Vicryl ensuring symmetric alignment of the skin edges. Skin is closed using interrupted subcuticular 5–0 Monocryl sutures. Excess paraexstrophy skin can be excised at this point if there is no tension on the closure. Penile shaft skin coverage can be difficult, and various methods have been described including reverse Byars skin flaps, buttonhole and ventral rotational flap. The reverse Byars flaps and buttonhole techniques both often lead to a cosmetically imperfect appearance due to dorsal suture line scarring after a Byars flap, and excess lateral shaft skin with the buttonhole. PippiSalle described the ventral rotational skin flap which rotates the ventral shaft skin 90° on a dartos pedicle moving the shaft skin suture line to a more lateral position [7]. Regardless of the technique for shaft skin coverage, anchoring sutures along the proximal penile shaft should be placed to prevent shaft skin from intussuscepting over the glans and burying the penis.

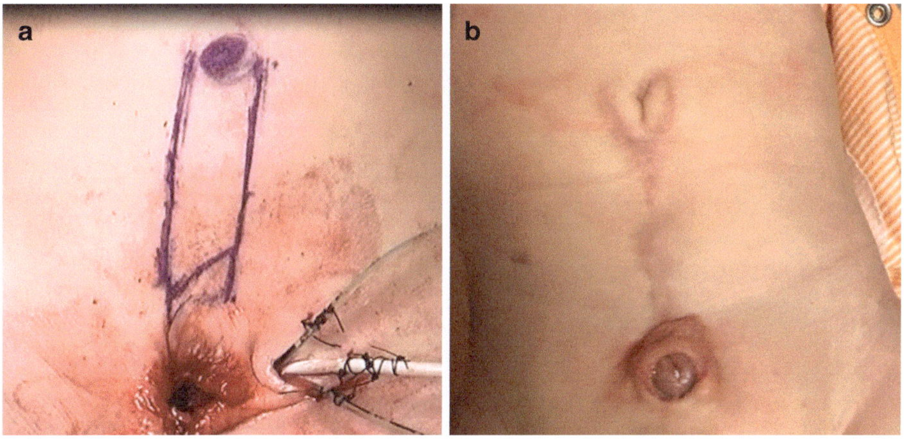

Fig. 6.5 (**a**) Marking for rhomboid rotational flap umbilicoplasty. (**b**) 6 months postoperatively

Umbilicoplasty

Similar to penile shaft skin coverage, many methods exist for creating a neoumbilicus. We have found that cosmetically we achieve the most pleasing and reproducible results utilizing a rotational rhomboid skin flap (Fig. 6.5). The center of the desired neoumbilicus is marked, and a rhomboid strip of skin and subcutaneous tissue approximately 1.5 cm wide is raised off the fascia and curved around itself in a counterclockwise direction. The medial edge is sutured to the fascia transforming the width of the flap into the depth of the umbilicus. A small fascial defect is typically left in the center of the umbilicus. Alternatively, others have described full-thickness skin grafting and Z-shaped or trapezoidal flaps to create a deep-seated neoumbilicus.

Immobilization

Postoperative immobilization optimizes pelvic stabilization and healing. Inadequate immobilization can lead to failure of the bladder closure, bladder prolapse and fistula formation. Multiple techniques for postoperative immobilization exist including mummy wraps, spica casts, internal fixation and external fixation with or without Buck's traction. The age of the child and comfort of the orthopedic surgeon should be weighed when selecting an appropriate immobilization technique. As external fixation or internal pinning can be difficult given the limited bone integrity in children less than 1 year of age, we use bivalved spica casts, or, more recently, molded adjustable braces for postoperative immobilization. In the first 5 days postoperatively, movement is limited to once-daily skin checks to minimize any disruption in bone healing. The cast or brace is typically kept in place for a minimum of 6 weeks when X-rays are obtained to assess bone union.

Female Bladder Exstrophy and Epispadias Repair

Incision and Initial Dissection

In a similar fashion to males, the ureteral orifices are intubated with feeding tubes and secured with absorbable suture and larger polyps on the bladder plate are excised and oversewn. Incision lines are then marked along the perimeter of the bladder, umbilical stump scar, bladder neck and urethral plate. The neoumbilicus is marked in the midline one-finger breadth above the superior aspect of the anterior superior iliac spine. Incisions are then made using cutting current electrocautery circumferentially, and caudally, these incisions are just lateral to the urethral plate and medial to clitoral tissue. Care should be taken to maximize the width of the urethral plate as the urethral plate distal to the bladder neck can contract if the incision is carried too medially. Wide incision lines will also facilitate an eventual more normal urethral meatus caliber without injuring erectile tissue. These incisions are then deepened, and dissection was carried in a cephalad-to-caudad direction identifying and separating detrusor muscle and fascia in the aforementioned fashion. Once the bladder is released from the fascia, the intersymphyseal bands can be identified caudally at the level of the pubic symphysis.

Dissection of Intersymphyseal Bands and Urethral Plate

As described in males, intersymphyseal bands are encountered caudally and must be released fully as they tether the bladder neck and urethral plate anteriorly and prevent adequate closure and placement of the bladder into an orthotopic location deep in the pelvis. With careful blunt dissection along the lateral bladder wall, perivesical fat guides the plane of dissection posterior to the intersymphyseal bands at the pubis. The intersymphyseal bands are then carefully incised and released using the medial aspect of the pubic tubercle and a sound in the vagina as anatomic markers. Dissection is typically performed along the medial border of the pubis to avoid injury to the vagina and clitoral body. A Pena muscle stimulator is helpful to differentiate fibrous bands from pelvic floor musculature in order to incise all tethering fibrous bands without harming the pelvic floor musculature. With all bands released, the bladder neck should approximate with no tension. The posterior aspect of the urethral plate is fused to the anterior vaginal wall and this connection should be maintained.

Urethral Plate Dissection

Incisions along the lateral borders of the urethral plate should maximize the width of the distal and proximal urethral plate to avoid any tension during closure. The lateral edges should be carefully dissected as both the clitoral body and vagina are in close proximity (lateral and posterior, respectively).

Y-V Vaginoplasty and Labiaplasty

In female exstrophy patients, the vagina is anteriorly displaced and should be repositioned into a more orthotopic location via vaginoplasty. The lateral urethral plate incisions are continued in a caudal direction, down and around the vaginal introitus and then inferiorly along the midline of the perineum for approximately 5–10 mm. The distance the vagina is able to be advanced posteriorly depends, in part, on the location of the anus. The incision around the vaginal introitus is deepened through dermis, but a partial or total vaginal or urogenital mobilization is not necessary as the degree to which the vagina is being advanced inferiorly is minor. The posterior vaginal lip is then advanced inferiorly into the perineum to the vertex of the caudal incision with a series of interrupted 4–0 PDS sutures. The labia majora are also more anteriorly positioned and should be mobilized along their lateral border and advanced posteriorly alongside the vagina, effectively elongating them and locating the labia in approximation of the vaginal introitus. The labia can be secured again with either 5–0 or 4–0 PDS sutures to the lateral perineal skin and medial vaginal introitus. These maneuvers elongate the vaginal introitus and reposition it posteriorly to provide a more appropriate cosmetic introital appearance (Fig. 6.6).

Bladder Neck Reconstruction, Bladder Closure, and Urethroplasty

The bladder neck region is identified via longitudinal striations and is measured. In infants, the bladder neck is tapered to 18 mm by de-epithelializing the bladder mucosa laterally and salvaging the underlying detrusor muscle. The proximal urethral plate is not narrowed during tapering, and the incisions at the bladder neck are gently flared out into the bladder to provide additional resistance in an effort to promote continence. The bladder neck is closed with robust interrupted subcuticular sutures of 4–0 PDS inverting the mucosa into the lumen. The urethroplasty is performed in a similar fashion using interrupted subcuticular 5–0 PDS suture proximally and 6–0 PDS or Maxon distally. The bladder closure is completed with interrupted 3–0 PDS suture. Prior to bladder closure, a suprapubic catheter is placed and externalized through the skin laterally along with the ureteral stents. Sutures to mature the urethral meatus to the clitoris and labia are then preplaced with 5–0 PDS and tagged as visualization will be difficult after pubic bone approximation. Alloderm is again used as a secondary coverage layer over the bladder neck and urethra and is secured atop the closure using interrupted 5–0 Vicryl sutures.

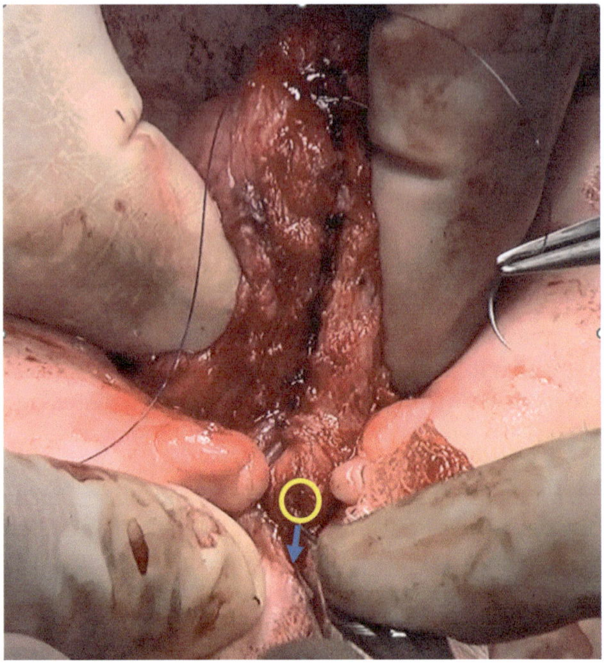

Fig. 6.6 Y-V vaginoplasty where the vagina is partially mobilized and advanced inferiorly to a more orthotopic position. The yellow circle indicates vaginal introitus. The blue arrow indicates the distance it was advanced inferiorly

Pubic Bone Approximation and Fascial Closure

A small area of the medial clitoral epithelium is denuded sharply until bleeding is observed in preparation for the pubic bone closure—the bleeding from the denuded tissue will serve as a sentinel of clitoral vascularity during pubic reapproximation. The pubis is then manually rotated inward and medially to bring the pubic bones together, and a #1 or 0 PDS suture is used in a horizontal mattress fashion to approximate the bones in a similar fashion as in boys. During this process, the denuded clitoris is examined to ensure there is good perfusion and bleeding after approximation. If there is concern or a lack of good perfusion to the clitoral bodies, then the suture is removed and the closure is repeated with slightly less correction of the diastasis. The preplaced sutures that mature the urethral meatus to the medial aspect of each hemiclitoris are then tied. The fascial closure is then completed in an interrupted fashion using 2–0 PDS in a figure-of-eight fashion.

"Grady Monsplasty"

Given the aberrant anatomy, in order to provide a more normal introital appearance to females with bladder exstrophy, a monsplasty is critical. Without an appropriate dorsal clitoral hood, the clitoral bodies can appear more prominent and can often be seen diverging from the midline. The Grady monsplasty is performed by first marking two symmetrical incisions superior to the clitoral bodies in an oblique fashion extending at a 45° angle in downward direction. These incisions are made with Bovie electrocautery and through the dermis until fat is visible. Next, the medial or inner edges of the incised skin are closed using simple interrupted 5–0 Monocryl sutures. Once the medial cut edges are approximated (creating the underside of the clitoral hood), the more lateral skin edges are approximated using simple interrupted subcuticular 5–0 Monocryl completing the outer or more superior aspect of the clitoral hood. Of note, during this process the clitoral bodies are not sutured to one another in the midline to avoid injury via either devascularization or nerve entrapment.

Abdominal Wall Closure and Umbilicoplasty

The umbilicus is created in a similar fashion to males using a rotational rhomboid flap. Once this is completed, the subcutaneous tissues of the skin are approximated using interrupted 4–0 Vicryl and the skin is closed in an interrupted fashion using 5–0 Monocryl. Vaseline gauze is applied over the wound.

Complications

Success with the initial repair is paramount as a failed initial closure often portends worse outcomes in terms of bladder growth and continence [9–11]. Balancing the risks of upper tract deterioration with outlet resistance, bladder cycling and growth as well as the creation of a cosmetically pleasing genital appearance can obviously be difficult. Complications after bladder exstrophy repair vary including bladder dehiscence, bladder prolapse, outlet obstruction, urethral stricture, genital soft tissue loss, UTIs, upper tract deterioration, vesicocutaneous or urethrocutaneous fistula.

In 2005, Borer et al. reported on a cohort of 23 patients (16 males and 7 females) who underwent primary CPRE from 1996 to 2004 [8]. They noted 6 of 23 (26%) had a total of 8 complications. Vesicocutaneous fistula was noted in 2 males, and urethrocutaneous fistula was noted in 6 patients (5 males and 1 female). Many of these fistulae closed spontaneously with bladder decompression, and only one vesicocutaneous fistula and one urethrocutaneous fistula required formal repair. The Multi-Institutional Bladder Exstrophy Consortium (MIBEC) published their short-term outcomes in 2017 on 22 classic bladder exstrophy patients. Of 10 females and 12 males, 6 of 10 females experienced a complication—5 pyelonephritis and 4 urinary retention (bladder outlet obstruction), 2 temporary CIC, 1 vesicostomy and 1 bladder rupture, while 3 of 12 males had a complication—1 pyelonephritis and 2 urethrocutaneous fistulae. Notably in this series, no patients developed bladder dehiscence after closure which was favorable compared to the past publications [8, 12–16]. Pelvic osteotomies and aggressive dissection of the intersymphyseal bands help to create a tension-free bladder closure and pubic bone approximation allowing the bladder and urethra to be placed deep into the pelvis likely decreasing the risk of dehiscence. However, the rate of bladder outlet obstruction in females after CPRE was increased compared to prior publications. Hypotheses as to the potential causes included direct denervation or surgical injury to the vasculature of the bladder neck or urethra, too much tapering of the bladder neck relative to the urethral width and bladder size, or compartment syndrome from excessive pubic bone approximation and acute tapering of the bladder neck during reconstruction. As a result of these observations, we propose that excessive tightening of the pubic diastasis—creating "kissing" pubic bones—should be avoided and erectile body (glans/clitoris) perfusion used as an indicator for how tightly to approximate the bones. Furthermore, the proximal urethra should never be narrowed or tapered and creating a gentle transition from the bladder neck to bladder will avoid acute changes in luminal caliber that could lead to obstruction.

Recurrent febrile urinary tract infections and pyelonephritis are common among bladder exstrophy patients postoperatively (22–50%), as many of these patients, not surprisingly, have vesicoureteral reflux (VUR) after closure [17–20]. The small capacity, often high pressure, bladder and abnormal ureteral insertions (entering more inferior and lateral) with minimal submucosal tunnels lead to the high rate of VUR in these patients.

One option to mitigate the risk is concurrent ureteral reimplantation at the time of the CPRE. Whether or not reimplantation is performed at the time of exstrophy closure is often dictated by the size and quality of the bladder plate, and is typically performed in a cephalotrigonal manner [21]. When the bladder plate is small or has excessive polyps, ureteral reimplantation may not be feasible. Jarosz et al. published the MIBEC experience with bilateral cephalotrigonal reimplantation at the time of CPRE in 15 patients and found that there was a significant decrease in rates of postoperative VUR, number of refluxing renal units and subsequent ureteral surgery in the treatment group versus those that underwent CPRE alone. There was also a reduction in the incidence of recurrent pyelonephritis and dilating reflux in these patients, but it did not reach clinical significance. A larger cohort of bladder exstrophy patients from an international collaboration in Ahmedabad, India, were analyzed comparing outcomes in CPRE with and without ureteral reimplantation. Ramji et al. found similar results noting a significantly decreased rate of VUR postoperatively (45% vs 82%; $p = 0.007$) with persistent VUR after reimplantation being more often unilateral and lower in grade. This group also reported a significantly larger bladder capacity in the reimplanted cohort; however, this could be attributed to a larger bladder plate size at the time of initial closure which allowed for ureteral reimplantation [22]. Dickson published the Manchester UK experience with reimplantation and reported similar results with bilateral ureteral reimplantation, albeit at the first stage of MSRE [23]. Although ureteral reimplantation may not be possible in all children with bladder exstrophy, it can significantly reduce the grade of reflux postoperatively and need for future ureteral surgery and should be considered in those patients at highest risk of pyelonephritis, namely, females with a suitable bladder plate.

Partial or complete penile skin, glanular or corporal tissue, loss is a rare, yet devastating, potential complication after penile reconstruction in male exstrophy patients and is likely a result of direct or indirect maneuvers that cause ischemia or poor venous outflow. Reconstruction after such an event is problematic and exponentially more difficult requiring neophallus creation in severe cases. Husmann et al. reported on 9 male patients evaluated for penile injuries following CPRE at two institutions over a 7-year time period. All of these patients underwent complete penile disassembly during their exstrophy repair. Each of these patients suffered loss of at least 1 hemiglans with or without corresponding corporal or penile skin loss [24]. Cervellione et al. reported on 28 exstrophy cases with penile tissue loss, 23 of which occurred after CPRE. In this cohort, 19 of 23 did not undergo pelvic osteotomy at the time of closure [25]. Similarly, Kasprenski et al. reviewed institutional experience with 1337 bladder exstrophy patients, identifying 26 with penile loss. The majority of these patients were closed in the neonatal period, and only 54% had osteotomy at the time of initial closure [26].

As most bladder exstrophy closures now occur in a delayed fashion outside the initial newborn period, osteotomies confer the ability to perform an adequate pubic bone approximation without creating a pelvic compartment syndrome which could jeopardize perfusion of the penile tissues. In addition to osteotomy, it is crucial to be cognizant of the location of the pudendal vasculature during dissection and assess, and reassess, glans perfusion before, during and after pubic bone approximation to prevent penile soft tissue injury. Doing so in a diligent manner will prevent many, if not all, penile soft tissue complications after male exstrophy repair. Lastly, complete penile disassembly is not necessary in all boys with bladder exstrophy and should only be considered in those where the urethral plate significantly tethers the penis dorsally. In these cases, attempting to preserve the bridging tissue between each hemiglans can potentially decrease the risk of ischemia. Failure to recognize or act on poor glans perfusion intraoperatively can lead to irreversible devastating consequences during recovery [23]. By incorporating the rigorous observation of glanular perfusion, osteotomies and willingness to leave pubic bones slightly separated at the time of exstrophy closure, we have not experienced loss of hemiglans nor corporal injury in our series of consecutive classical bladder exstrophy repairs through the MIBEC endeavor.

Children with bladder exstrophy typically possess normal renal function and upper tracts. However, bladder closure and outlet reconstruction can potentially expose the upper tracts to elevated pressures transmitted from the bladder which, in addition to the known high incidence of VUR after closure, puts the upper tracts at risk of damage. The US-India Multi-institutional Bladder Exstrophy Collaboration retrospectively looked at renal outcomes in 104 patients who underwent CPRE. They found 19% had eGFR <90, and 30% had scarring on DMSA; however, on neither scarring, VUR status nor continence status predicted the presence of eGFR <90 [28]. In a single institution retrospective review, Ellison et al. described long-term upper tract outcomes and risk of renal deterioration after CPRE. They evaluated 30 patients with a minimum of 5 years of follow-up and found that, overall, hydronephrosis was common (53%) after closure; however, the incidence of high-grade hydronephrosis was low. Notably, significantly more males had hydronephrosis compared to females; 14 vs 2 ($p < 0.001$), respectively. Furthermore, no significant differences were noted in creatinine or eGFR between patients that were continent and incontinent or those with and without reimplantation [29]. Shnorhavorian et al. also found similar results, albeit with shorter term follow-up [13]. As with any type of exstrophy repair, upper tract deterioration is more likely if the bladder outlet is too restrictive for urinary flow, if the bladder itself is hypotonic or atonic leaving large residuals or if continence is achieved but the child does not focus on intentional timed voiding. But overall, surgeons may be reassured that despite the reported high incidence of hydronephrosis in exstrophy patients after closure, single-stage CPRE does not predispose patients to undo risk of upper tract deterioration compared to other surgical techniques for bladder exstrophy closure.

Volitional voiding and continence may be the holy grail of bladder exstrophy reconstruction; however, it remains an elusive outcome to achieve reliably for any surgeon, regardless of approach. An important consideration in the journey to, and quest for, continence is the virtue of patience. After initial closure, we recommend a more observational approach to continence as we have seen many children improve over time. Although some children will need additional surgeries to achieve dryness with patience and appropriate conservative interventions, many can also improve greatly without major reconstruction.

Conclusion

The contemporary complete repair of bladder exstrophy, as described above, is a reproducible technique to successfully reconstruct a bladder exstrophy defect while reconstructing the bladder neck and complete urethra in situ, while conveying a low risk of dehiscence and while offering the possibility that one major surgical intervention may anatomically begin the child's journey toward volitional voiding and continence. Despite this stated goal of complete repair, a substantial subset of patients still require additional procedures after CPRE to achieve continence and address complications—for which risk factors for additional surgeries and poor outcomes are currently being investigated. We have adopted a conservative approach in monitoring children with bladder exstrophy for an extended period of time—possibly up to puberty—prior to performing irreversible procedures such as bladder neck closure and bladder augmentation to achieve "dryness." Our "patience" is predicated on the observation that in some patients, maturation of the pelvic floor augmented with physical therapy can help achieve volitional voiding per the native urethra in a significant number of patients. Furthermore, adhering to the core surgical principles discussed in this chapter—performing osteotomies at the time of closure, aggressive release of intersymphyseal bands and monitoring erectile body perfusion during pubic bone approximation—will hopefully allow future surgeons to replicate results seen in our modern cohorts and limit previously characterized complications associated with CPRE and all exstrophy repairs writ large.

References

1. Ambrose SS, O'Brien DP 3rd. Surgical embryology of the exstrophy-epispadias complex. Surg Clin North Am. 1974;54(6):1379–90.
2. Lattimer JK, Smith MJ. Exstrophy closure: a follow-up on 70 cases. J Urol. 1966;95:356–9.
3. Tsajaguabbes E. Total exstrophy of the urinary bladder: complete anatomical and functional restoration. Hell Cheirourgike. 1964;11:300–6.
4. Williams DI, Savage J. Reconstruction of the exstrophied bladder. Br J Surg. 1966;53:168–73.
5. Grady RW, Mitchell ME. Complete primary repair of exstrophy. J Urol. 1999;162(4):1415–20.
6. Kaefer M, Saad K, Gargollo P, Whittam B, Rink R, Fuchs M, Bowen D, Reddy P, Cheng E, Jayanthi R, Pediatric Urology Midwest Alliance (PUMA). Intraoperative laser angiography in bladder exstrophy closure: a simple technique to monitor penile perfusion. J Pediatr Urol. 2022;18(6):746.e1–7.
7. Pippi Salle JL, Jednak R, Capolicchio JP, França IM, Labbie A, Gosalbez R. A ventral rotational skin flap to improve cosmesis and avoid chordee recurrence in epispadias repair. BJU Int. 2002;90(9):918–23.
8. Borer JB, Gargollo PC, Hendren HW, Diamond DA, Peters CA, Atala A, Grant R, Retik AB. Early outcome following complete primary repair of bladder exstrophy in the newborn. J Urol. 2005;174:1674–9.
9. Meldrum KK, Mathews RI, Nelson CP, Gearhart JP. Subspecialty training and surgical outcomes in children with failed bladder exstrophy closure. J Pediatr Urol. 2005;1(2):95–9.
10. Gearhart JP, Ben-Chaim J, Sciortino C, Sponseller PD, Jeffs RD. The multiple reoperative bladder exstrophy closure: what affects the potential of the bladder? Urology. 1996;47(2):240–3.
11. Novak TE, Costello JP, Orosco R, Sponseller PD, Mack E, Gearhart JP. Failed exstrophy closure: management and outcome. J Pediatr Urol. 2010;6(4):381–4.
12. Gargollo PC, Borer JG, Diamond DA, Hendren WH, Rosoklija I, Grant R, et al. Prospective follow-up in patients after complete repair of bladder exstrophy. J Urol. 2008;180:1655–70.
13. Shnorhavorian M, Grady RW, Andersen A, Joyner BD, Mitchell ME. Long-term follow-up of complete primary repair of exstrophy: the Seattle experience. J Urol. 2008;180:1615–20.
14. Baradaran N, Stec AA, Schaeffer AJ, Gearhard JP, Mathews RI. Delayed primary closure of bladder exstrophy: immediate postoperative management leading to successful outcomes. Urology. 2012;79(2):415–9.
15. Ellison JS, Shnorhavorian N, Willihnganz-Lawon K, Grady R, Merguerian PA. A critical appraisal of continence in bladder exstrophy: long-term outcomes of the complete primary repair. J Pediatr Urol. 2016;12(4):205.
16. Inouye BM, Lue K, Adelwahab M, DiCarlo HN, Young EE, Tourchi A, et al. Newborn exstrophy closure without osteotomy: is there a role? J Pediatr Urol. 2016;12(1):51.e1–4. https://doi.org/10.1016/j.jpurol.2015.07.010. [Epub 2015 Sep 5].
17. Mathews R, Hubbard JS, Gearhart JP. Ureteral reimplantation before bladder neck plasty in the reconstruction of bladder exstrophy: indications and outcomes. Urology. 2003;61(4):820–4.
18. Garat JM, de la Peña E, Caffaratti J, Villavicencio H. Prevention of vesicoureteral reflux at the time of complete primary repair of the exstrophy-epispadias complex. Int Urol Nephrol. 2004;36(2):211–2.
19. Tourchi A, Di Carlo HN, Inouye BM, Young E, Gupta A, Abdelwahab M, Gearhart JP. Ureteral reimplantation before bladder neck reconstruction in modern staged repair of exstrophy patients: indications and outcomes. Urology. 2015;85(4):905–8.
20. Braga LH, Lorenzo AJ, Jrearz R, Bagli DJ, Salle JL. Bilateral ureteral reimplantation at primary bladder exstrophy closure. J Urol. 2010;183(6):2337–41. https://doi.org/10.1016/j.juro.2010.02.032. Epub 2010 Apr 18.
21. Canning DA, Gearhart JP, Peppas DS, Jeffs RD. The cephalotrigonal reimplant in bladder neck reconstruction for patients with exstrophy or epispadias. J Urol. 1993;150(1):156–8.

22. Ramji J, Weiss DA, Romao RLP, Eftekharzadeh S, Shah J, Frazier JR, Reddy PP, Merguerian PA, Pippi Salle JL, Canning DA, Joshi RS, Shukla AR. Impact of bilateral ureteral reimplantation at the time of complete primary repair of bladder exstrophy on reflux rates, renogram abnormalities and bladder capacity. J Pediatr Urol. 2021;17(3):393.e1–7.
23. Dickson AP. The management of bladder exstrophy: the Manchester experience. J Pediatr Surg. 2014;49(2):244–50. https://doi.org/10.1016/j.jpedsurg.2013.11.031. Epub 2013 Nov 16.
24. Husmann DA, Gearhart JP. Loss of the penile glans and/or corpora following primary repair of bladder exstrophy using the complete penile disassembly technique. J Urol. 2004;172(4 Pt 2):1696–700. discussion 1700–1.
25. Cervellione RM, Husmann DA, Bivalacqua TJ, Sponseller PD, Gearhart JP. Penile ischemic injury in the exstrophy/epispadias spectrum: new insights and possible mechanisms. J Pediatr Urol. 2010;6(5):450–6.
26. Kasprenski M, Maruf M, Davis R, Jayman J, Benz K, Michaud J, Di Carlo H, Dunn EA, Gearhart JP. Penile disassembly in complete primary repair of bladder exstrophy: time for re-evaluation? Urology. 2020;137:146–51.
27. Lazarus J. Penile loss following complete primary repair of bladder exstrophy. J Pediatr Urol. 2009;5(6):519–20. https://doi.org/10.1016/j.jpurol.2009.03.021. Epub 2009 May 8.
28. Joshi RS, Eftekharzadeh S, Shukla AR, Ramji J, Hingorani SR, Canning DA, Pippi-Salle JL, Merguerian P, DeFoor WR Jr, Frazier JR, Weiss DA, Reddy PP. Kidney function outcomes in patients after complete primary repair of bladder exstrophy and penopubic epispadias: results from the international bladder exstrophy consortium. J Pediatr Urol. 2023;19(1):34.e1–9.
29. Ellison JS, Ahn J, Shnorhavorian M, Grady R, Merguerian PA. Long-term fate of the upper tracts following complete primary repair of bladder exstrophy. J Pediatr Urol. 2017;13(4):394.e1–6.

7 The Modern Staged Repair of Classic Bladder Exstrophy

Chad B. Crigger and John P. Gearhart

Introduction

The exstrophy-epispadias complex (EEC) represents a spectrum of congenital anomalies ranging from epispadias to classic bladder exstrophy (CBE) and, most severely, cloacal exstrophy (CE). This spectrum of complex congenital defects is among the most challenging conditions practicing pediatric urologists and surgeons may encounter. Several techniques exist, including the complete primary repair of exstrophy (CPRE) and Kelly Repair, among others; however, this chapter will focus on the modern staged repair of exstrophy (MSRE).

The staged technique, championed by Robert Jeffs of the Johns Hopkins Hospital (Baltimore, MD) and Jean Cendron (Paris, France), has been refined through the years and has yielded outcomes that withstand the test of time and against which all modern outcomes are compared. Broadly, the stages refer to the surgical sequence for CBE, where the first stage involves closure of the bladder and repositioning the posterior urethrovesical unit deep within the pelvis while also reducing the pubic diastasis, with or without pelvic osteotomy. Additionally, the urethra is closed as distally as the penile skin allows in males. The second stage is to close the urethra and completely repair the epispadias defect. Once repaired, all patients are placed in a program that allows close follow-up to assess bladder growth coupled with gauging emotional readiness. Once patient maturation is appropriate, patients undergo the final stage, continence surgery, typically paired with ureteral reimplantation.

What follows is the contemporary implementation of this technique, along with pertinent tips and tricks, where applicable, to ensure success in exstrophy closure.

C. B. Crigger · J. P. Gearhart (✉)
Jeffs Division of Pediatric Urology, The Brady Urological Institute, Johns Hopkins Hospital, Baltimore, MD, USA
e-mail: jgearha2@jhmi.edu

A. R. Shukla, R. S. Joshi (eds.), *Bladder Exstrophy and Epispadias*, https://doi.org/10.1007/978-3-031-91238-2_7

Additionally, future directions in this technique and the latest research gains will be added to the text at times to enhance understanding.

Prenatal Diagnosis

Despite rapid advances in fetal ultrasonography (fUS) and other imaging modalities, only 47% of patients are diagnosed prenatally [1, 2]. Though the first prenatal diagnosis of CE occurred in 1985, the first screening criteria for prenatal diagnosis of CBE would come a decade later when major and minor criteria were proposed [3, 4]. For CBE, five imaging findings were identified: (1) failure to visualize the bladder on fUS, (2) a lower abdominal bulge representing the exstrophied bladder, (3) a demure penis with anteriorly displaced scrotum, (4) low umbilical insertion, and (5) increased pubic diastasis or widening of the iliac crests [4].

The challenge is even greater for fUS diagnosis of CE, which classically relies on three key findings: (1) A sizeable midline infraumbilical abdominal defect, (2) lumbosacral myelomeningocele, and (3) inability to visualize the urinary bladder [5]. This list was further refined by delineating diagnostic criteria as either major or minor findings [3]. Seen in >50% of cases, it constituted a major criterion and included non-visualization of the bladder (91%), a large midline infraumbilical anterior wall defect or cystic anterior wall structure (82%), omphalocele (77%), and myelomeningocele (68%). Minor criteria were those seen in <50% of cases and included lower extremity defects (23%), renal anomalies (23%), ascites (41%), widened pubic arches (18%), narrow thorax (9%), hydrocephalus (9%), and a single umbilical artery (9%). Even with these diagnostic criteria, only an estimated 15% of patients have been diagnosed prenatally on fUS alone, as findings may be incompletely identified as isolated omphalocele, CBE, or other midline defects.

The recent introduction of fetal magnetic resonance imaging (fMRI) in prenatal diagnosis has added a valuable adjunct in evaluating EEC. Compared to fUS, fMRI provides superior anatomical detail when a bladder is not identified and may also aid in assessing the presence or absence of an omphalocele, associated spinal defects, and gender when not readily identified with fUS.

Recently, Weiss et al., in a multi-institutional study, identified key anatomic findings on fUS and fMRI to assess their respective validity in prenatally diagnosing CBE and CE [1]. Between 2001 and 2018, they identified 21 patients who had prenatal imaging. CBE was the postnatal diagnosis in 14 and CE in the remainder. Fifteen of twenty-one patients had both fUS and fMRI available for review, and the median gestational age for evaluation by prenatal imaging was 25 weeks. Of the 16 fUS with initial interpretations available, the original prenatal diagnosis was correct in 12 cases, yielding a 69% sensitivity of fUS. All 4 cases of incorrect prenatal diagnoses of CE were later determined to be CBE. Of the 18 fMRIs included in the analysis, 16 of 18 diagnoses aligned (83% sensitivity), and the two incorrect prenatal CE diagnoses were reclassified as CBE. These misdiagnoses were attributed to a large protruding bladder plate with bowel loops posteriorly imitating an omphalocele containing bowel. They concluded that identification of the point of umbilical cord insertion on both fUS and fMRI was prudent to differentiate between CBE and CE given the abdominal wall defects.

The importance of a correct and early prenatal diagnosis cannot be overstated. In the largest single institution series on prenatal diagnosis of CE to date assessing fUS trends, Morrill and colleagues found a 78.6% rate of prenatal diagnosis ($n = 44$), while 21.4% ($n = 12$) were diagnosed postnatally [6]. Importantly, patients diagnosed prenatally were more likely to undergo closure at exstrophy centers of excellence (72.1% vs. 33.3%, $p = 0.020$), and primary closures that occurred at these specialized centers were significantly more likely to be successful compared to outside hospitals without the designation (90.9% vs. 50.0%, $p = 0.002$). Similar findings parallel this data in unpublished but presented data for CBE as well [2].

Anatomic Anomalies

Bony Pelvis and Pelvic Floor Considerations

Anomalies of the bony pelvis and the requisite pubic diastasis are the hallmark of EEC. Utilizing three-dimensional (3D) computed tomography (CT) of the bony pelvis in exstrophy patients and elucidating abnormalities, Sponseller et al. modernized our understanding of the characteristic widening of the pubic symphysis. Most notably, two broad categories of abnormalities were identified—rotational and dimensional anomalies (Table 7.1) [7]. Compared to age-matched controls, in CBE, the posterior pelvis is externally rotated an average of 12 degrees on each side, while the anterior pelvis is externally rotated an average of 18 degrees. Added to this rotational difference, the pubic rami are 30% shorter, which, combined with a retroverted acetabulum, leads to an average diastasis of 4.8 centimeters (cm) in CBE. These defects are even more exaggerated in CE patients, with an overall 43% decrease in bony length in the entire pelvis, with an average pubic diastasis greater than 6 cm and an increased likelihood of asymmetry between the right and left sides of the pelvis [7]. For clarity, mild diastasis is less than 4 cm, moderate diastasis is between 4 and 6 cm, and extreme diastasis is anything >6 cm.

Table 7.1 Anomalies of the exstrophy pelvis

Rotational	Dimensional
External rotation of the posterior pelvis/iliac wings	Increased pubic diastasis
External rotation of the anterior pelvic segment	Shortened anterior pubic segment (30%)
Coronal rotation of the sacroiliac joint	Increased intertriradiate cartilage distance
Acetabular retroversion	
Convergence of iliac wings	
Femoral retroversion	

The rotational and dimensional anomalies of the aforementioned bony pelvis directly impact the maldevelopment of the pelvic floor. Pelvic floor 3D-CT imaging of children with exstrophy revealed that the levator ani muscles are positioned more posteriorly (68% posteriorly/32% anteriorly) compared to age-matched controls (52% posteriorly/48% anteriorly) [8]. In addition to being more posteriorly oriented, the levator ani is also less concave. Another consequence of the bony pelvis deformities manifested in the pelvic floor is the more flattened puborectalis compared to its usual conical shape. The paucity of anterior pelvic floor musculature and the lack of a conical shape drive the surgical technique in reconstructing the bony pelvis and pelvic floor, which positions the posterior urethrovesical unit deep within the pelvis. This technique is discussed separately below.

It is critical to have a clear understanding of all anatomic anomalies prior to closure, particularly with CE, given the multitude of major multisystem defects. Specific commentary on each system impacted is beyond the scope of this chapter; however, all pressing gastrointestinal, neurological, and genitourinary concerns should be addressed prior to definitive surgical intervention.

Initial Evaluation and Management

Typically, the pediatric urology team is at least aware of the child's arrival, particularly if a prenatal diagnosis was made. However, the diagnosis of EEC alone does not necessarily require delivery at an exstrophy center of excellence. *In the delivery room, the umbilical cord should be tied with 2–0 silk as close to the abdominal wall as possible rather than occluding it using the usual umbilical stump clamps.* It is important to remember that the exposed bladder mucosa is usually pink and smooth but friable. Minimizing trauma—using silk suture to occlude the umbilical stump, for instance—will help protect the delicate mucosa from undue trauma or excoriations and the development of bladder polyps. Keeping the bladder moist with sterile saline irrigation and covering the bladder mucosa using non-adhesive film such as Saran Wrap can prevent abrasions from the diaper and the mucosa from drying out. Such care can be performed at each diaper change.

Determining Suitability for Immediate Closure

Successful closure relies on careful assessment of the size and potential functional capacity of the detrusor muscle. Often, examination under anesthesia allows full assessment of the bladder template, free of Valsalva manipulation from the newborn crying or moving. If the child is robust, without any more pressing medical concerns (rarely the case for CE), then immediate closure within 72 h may be considered in CBE. An ideal bladder template is one that is at least 3 × 3 cm and free of polyps [9]. Additionally, some conditions may force closure in a delayed manner, including penoscrotal duplication, ectopic bowel, and significant bilateral hydronephrosis.

Regarding pelvic osteotomy—typically, the greater the bladder template, the wider the resultant diastasis, and the greater the need for osteotomy. Generally, if closure is attempted within 72 h of birth, osteotomy is not required unless diastasis is over 4 cm or the pelvis demonstrates poor malleability [10]. Anatomically, the inherent laxity of the sacroiliac ligaments in the first 72 h of life allows closure of the defect without undue tension. If conditions are not perfect or resources cannot be mobilized quickly enough, then closure should be delayed several weeks to months to allow optimization of bladder mucosa and surgical teams.

Immediate vs Delayed Closure

Historically, CBE closure occurred as soon as it was safe for the child to undergo anesthesia, as success rates were deemed better, and due to concerns for poor eventual bladder growth in delayed closure. Recent publications challenge this notion and reflect a greater shift in closure practices.

Baranadan et al. were among the first to assess the impact of delayed primary repair of CBE on bladder capacities. The authors evaluated 33 patients who underwent delayed exstrophy closure due to small bladder templates (n = 18) or due to late referral (n = 15) and compared outcomes to 82 patients who underwent closure at a median of 2 days of life. The authors found that delayed closures did have smaller bladder capacities (36 cc smaller in the poor template group and 29 cc smaller in the late referral group), but the rate of bladder growth did not differ [11]. In short, children with smaller templates will have smaller capacities, but the rate of growth in capacity is not affected. Additionally, children with smaller templates are less likely to undergo bladder neck reconstruction (BNR) and more likely to need bladder neck transection (BNT).

With the safety of delaying primary closure to allow a demure bladder template to grow, without jeopardizing the growth rate, Wu and colleagues sought to determine if a threshold exists beyond which it is too late to delay. The authors assessed bladder capacities in successful neonatal (e.g., ≤28 days old) or delayed (e.g., >28 days old) closures. Additionally, time points for closure and bladder capacity measurements were stratified by quartiles, with the second and fourth quartiles representing 4–6 months and beyond 9 months, respectively [12]. Based on this, the authors found that the appropriate time to close an exstrophy patient is as early as possible (first quartile) or delayed between 6 and 9 months (third quartile), but that the most significant declines in capacity occurred at 4–6 months and beyond 9 months [12].

Though primary closure can safely be delayed, within reason, the decision to do so should be approached delicately. With recent trends in exstrophy closure shifting to a more delayed approach with success, associated complication rates remained unanswered. Ahn et al. (2018) assessed 62 patients who underwent primary exstrophy closure, of which 44 (71%) were delayed. Mean anesthesia and operative times were greater in the delayed closure group (4–120 days of life), which also had more concurrent procedures (e.g., inguinal hernia repair, osteotomies) compared to early closure (defined as surgery at 0–3 days of life). When comparing 30-day complications, the delayed closure group had a higher 30-day complication rate, mostly due to a greater need for blood transfusion (57% vs. 11%); however, wound dehiscence also occurred more in the delayed group as well (6/44, 14% vs. 0/18, 0%). A review of the national data available during the study period ranging from 1999 to 2010 confirmed a rapid trend toward delayed closure in this cohort (71% vs. 27%) [13].

Surgical Reconstruction

Soft Tissue Closure: Bladder, Posterior Urethra, and Abdominal Wall

Soft tissue reconstruction begins with careful consideration of the bladder and urethral template coupled with the perceived laxity of the abdominal wall. Of note, preoperative testosterone supplementation is utilized as an adjunct for males to enhance penile and urethral closure.

Beginning at the level of the anterior superior iliac spine in the midline at the level of the expected umbilicus, a "V"-shaped incision is made with a midline extension caudally to the cephalad aspect of the bladder template. The incision is then carried circumferentially, paralleling the border of the bladder mucosa, taking great care to not violate or harm delicate mucosa. This is extended caudally along the inferior aspect of the bladder template until a strip of mucosa 2 cm wide is created at the extent of the distal trigone. This strip is continued distally below the verumontanum to the midshaft of the penis in males, depending on available skin, or to the level of the vaginal orifice in females. In males, the urethral groove and posterior urethral length may be inadequate, necessitating elevation of paraexstrophy skin flaps and transection of the urethral plate for urethral lengthening according to the manner described by Duckett [14–16].

With the template outlined and sharply dissected, a plane is established between the rectus fascia and the bladder. Gentle blunt dissection, often with a moistened Kittner, peels the peritoneum off the bladder. This, along with doubly ligating and dividing the umbilical vessels, allows the bladder to be placed deep within the pelvis without any undue tethering. The created plane is continued caudally, *following the rectus fascia as a guide*, until the urogenital diaphragm fibers and pubis are encountered bilaterally. One trick the authors employ is to utilize a double-pronged wide skin hook and insert it into the bone to apply lateral traction. Doing so accentuates the urogenital diaphragm fibers. *These fibers must be radically dissected, typically with electrocautery, down to the levator hiatus in the pelvic floor in their entirety*. Failure to fully dissect these fibers may result in: (1) a posterior vesicourethral unit that is brought anteriorly into an unsatisfactory position for later Cantwell-Ransley epispadias repair and (2) an increased likelihood of failed primary closure [14].

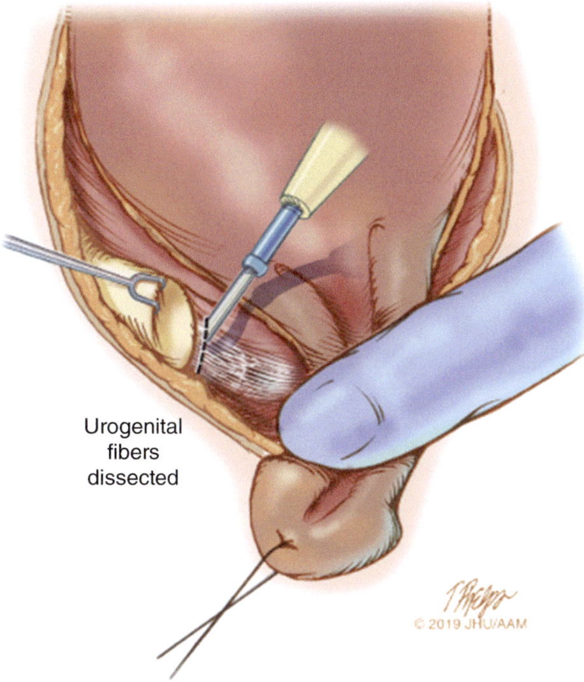

Fig. 7.1 Radical dissection of urogenital diaphragm fibers. Complete release of these pelvic floor fibers is necessary to appropriately place the posterior urethrovesical unit and bladder deep within the pelvis. Failure to dissect these fibers completely was shown to increase the failed closure rate [17]

The importance of radical dissection of all urogenital diaphragm fibers was eloquently demonstrated by Davis et al. in identifying 93 failed primary CBE closures referred to the authors' institution (Fig. 7.1) [17]. In review of operative notes of the primary closure, compared to intraoperative findings during re-closure, urogenital fibers were completely intact bilaterally at the time of repeat closure in 74 patients (79.6%). Interestingly, no patients had urogenital diaphragm fibers intact unilaterally. Similarly, others have utilized the advantages of 3D-MRI imaging preoperatively to assess pelvic floor anatomy, overlayed intraoperatively with BrainLab (Munich, Germany) to guide intraoperative dissection and ensure complete dissection of urogenital diaphragm fibers (Fig. 7.2) [18, 19].

With the bladder template dissected freely from all possible tethering tissues, the mucosa and muscle of the bladder, bladder neck, and urethra are closed, and the entire unit is easily placed deep within the pelvis. Prior to closure of the bladder, each ureteral orifice is cannulated with a 5 Fr feeding tube that is externalized via a small window in the dome of the bladder through which the feeding tubes (acting as urethral stents) and a nonlatex suprapubic Malecot catheter are brought. These tubes will allow the bladder to heal while continuously draining the bladder of urine. These various tubes will remain in place until ultrasonography coupled with clamping trials of the suprapubic Malecot demonstrate that they may be safely removed. This is discussed under postoperative management.

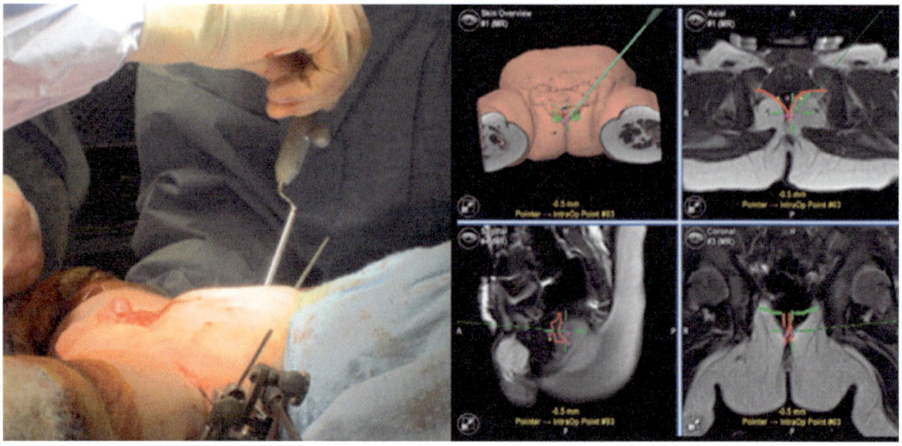

Fig. 7.2 MRI-guided anatomic dissection utilizing BrainLab. MRI reconstruction of the pelvic floor anatomy has shown great promise in guiding anatomic dissection and aiding in successful closure

Pressure is then applied to the greater trochanters bilaterally, bringing the pubic bones into midline apposition. A horizontal mattress suture, typically a No. 2 nylon, is placed at the junction where the rectus fascia inserts onto the dorsal pubic bone, securing the pubic closure into position (Fig. 7.3). The fascia is then closed, and skin flaps are elevated to aid in cosmesis. At the cephalad aspect of the midline incision, prior to closing the fascia entirely, all drainage tubes are brought to the skin surface. Utilizing the "V"-shaped flap created at the initial midline incision beginning the case, this flap is fixed to the abdominal fascia, and formal umbilicoplasty is performed in the manner described by Hanna [20]. The key steps of soft tissue closure are detailed in Fig. 7.4a–h [14].

Soft tissue reconstruction of CE parallels that of CBE. Approximation of the hemibladders posteriorly converts the defect from CE to CBE. This is achieved by dissection of the lateral aspects of the bladder halves from the abdominal wall and closure in the midline [21]. Orthotopic reconstruction via placement of the bladder and posterior urethra deep into the pelvis remains a crucial factor in successful surgical reconstruction. Approximation of the widened pelvis aids in this goal, permitting abdominal wall and urinary tract reconstruction; however, this usually requires pelvic osteotomies and fixation in a staged fashion, as will be described later in this chapter.

Unlike in CBE, the large abdominal wall defect found in CE presents a significant challenge in tension-free abdominal wall reconstruction. Failure to consider tension at the time of closure may impact rates of successful closure and fistula formation. Bioprosthetic materials such as Alloderm (Allergan, Branchburg, NJ) have shown great promise in bridging the gap in lack of abdominal wall tissue while providing a tension-free closure [22]. Additionally, Alloderm has been used as an

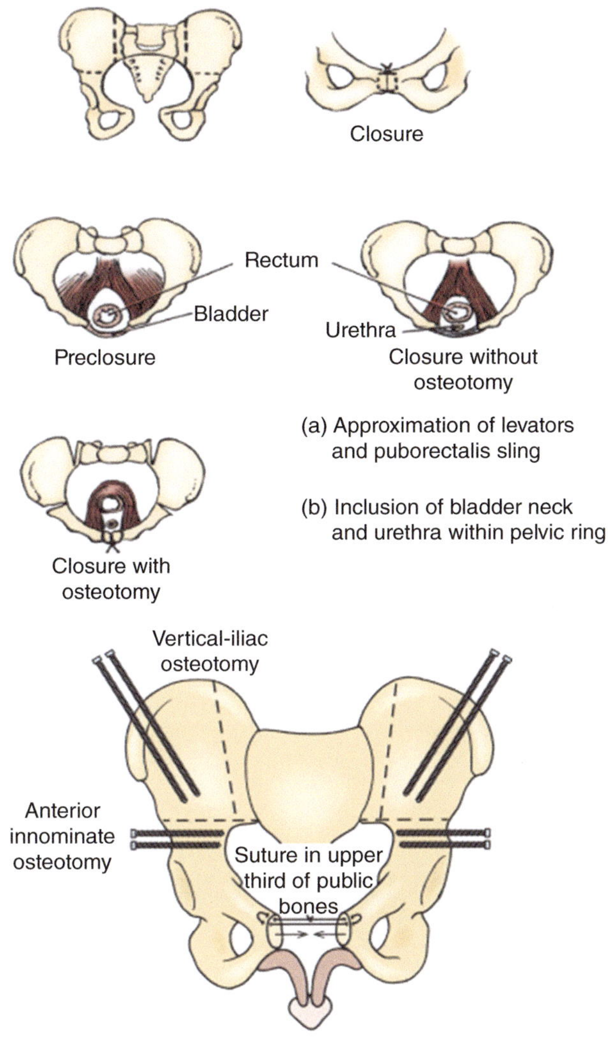

Fig. 7.3 Pelvic reconstruction. The combined posterior vertical iliac osteotomy and anterior innominate osteotomy reconfigure the pelvis and aid in soft tissue closure. At the authors' institution, it is seen as a critical adjunct in successful closures when utilized

adjunct to decrease penopubic fistulization through coverage of the interpubic stitch at the time of urinary tract reconstruction [23].

The Role of Osteotomy

As aforementioned, the open pelvic ring is a hallmark of the EEC, and as such, osteotomy has emerged as a critical factor in successful closure in most children with CBE and is indicated in all children with CE at the time of bladder closure [14, 24]. Osteotomy corrects the wide pubic diastasis and allows for orthotopic positioning of the bladder and posterior urethra as deep as possible within the pelvis while

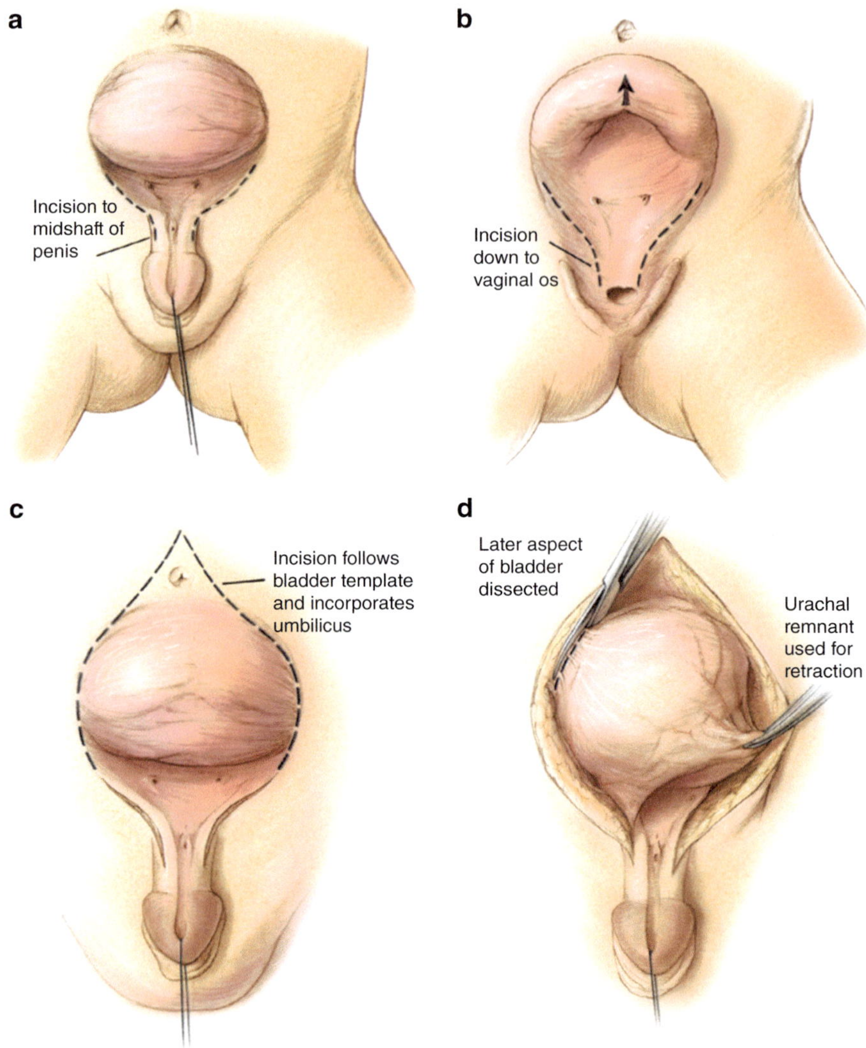

Fig. 7.4 (**a**–**h**) Soft tissue reconstruction in MSRE. Complete mobilization of the bladder so that the bladder may be closed without undue tension

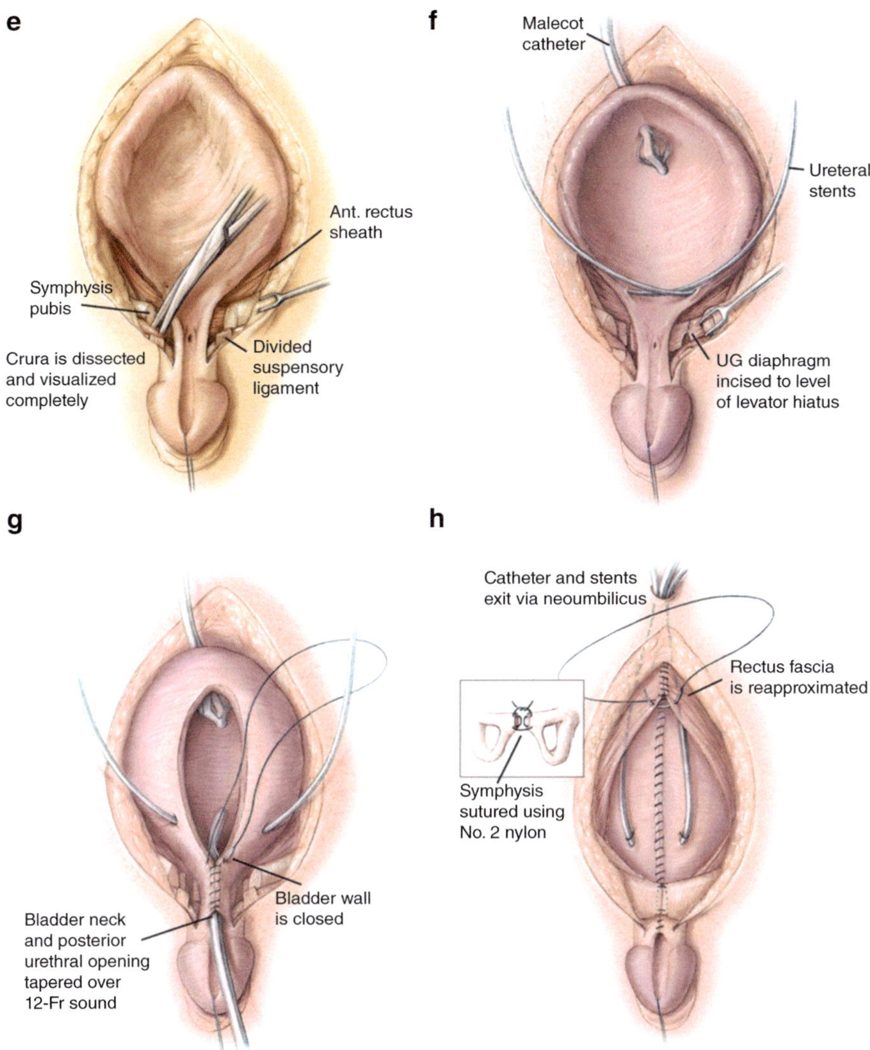

Fig. 7.4 (continued)

also facilitating bladder and abdominal wall reconstruction with minimal tension. Reducing undue tension correlates with improved outcomes, mainly decreased rates of dehiscence and postoperative ventral hernias. Additionally, osteotomy in the CE patient has been found to reduce the likelihood of significant complications from 89% in patients closed without osteotomy to 17% in children closed with osteotomy [25]. This was confirmed in a large series of 80 CE patients that reported 91% successful exstrophy repairs with osteotomy performed at the time of closure [26]. Finally, osteotomy allows repositioning of the pelvic floor musculature more anteriorly to support the bladder neck and potentially aid in eventual urinary control in epispadias and CBE patients.

The timing of osteotomy is critical. *In CBE patients younger than 72 h old, if examination under anesthesia demonstrates malleable pubic bones that are* ***easily*** *brought to the midline, the patient may undergo closure without osteotomy, but with appropriate postoperative immobilization.* Beyond this age, combined osteotomies (as described below) are recommended. Osteotomies are also recommended for pubic diastasis greater than 4 cm, even if closure is planned before 72 h of life, and should be mandated in all CE closures [14].

Though several types of pelvic osteotomies exist, the combined bilateral anterior innominate and posterior vertical iliac osteotomies are the preferred method at the authors' institution and are coordinated with bladder closure at the time of CBE closure, or in an approach coined the Dual-Staged Pathway (DSP) for CE [27, 28]. A benefit of the combined osteotomy in the supine position is the added benefit of not needing to reposition the patient prior to bladder and abdominal wall closure. Avoiding a posterior approach reduces the risk of damaging any spinal or neurovascular structures. Additionally, in CE, pelvic osteotomies allow gradual pelvic reduction with external fixation 2–3 weeks prior to bladder and abdominal wall closure (DSP). This is often utilized in instances of extremely wide pubic diastasis (>10 cm) and was even successfully used in one patient with a pubic diastasis of 16 cm [27]. At the authors' institution, external fixation and modified Buck's traction are maintained for 4 weeks in CBE closures and 6 weeks in CE closures to ensure adequate healing. In our experience, this immobilization technique provides exceptional results with a 3.8% failure rate in primary closures, compared to 65.7% for immobilization with a spica cast [29].

Trends in osteotomy use for CE closures have drastically changed in the post-1990, or "modern," era of exstrophy. Haney et al. found that the combined osteotomy approach has increased in prevalence over time, with the posterior approach significantly decreasing [30]. Additionally, lower limb immobilization has increased overall, with Buck's traction becoming the most common. Finally, multi-staged procedures have increased over time while single-staged approaches have significantly decreased (Table 7.2).

Table 7.2 Comparisons of closure outcome success rates by management of CE during primary closure

	All			AH		OH	
	Success	Univariate *p*-value	Multivariate *p*-value	Success	Univariate *p*-value	Success	Univariate *p*-value
Osteotomy		0.007	0.473		0.343		0.023
None	15 (41.7%)			2 (66.7%)		13 (39.4%)	
Any	66 (77.6%)			39 (88.6%)		27 (65.9%)	
Osteotomy type		<0.001	0.272		0.230		0.043
Combined	36 (90.0%)			33 (89.2%)		3 (100%)	
Posterior	16 (76.2%)			4 (100%)		12 (70.6%)	
Anterior	14 (60.9%)			2 (66.7%)		12 (60%)	
Immobilization		<0.001	<0.001		0.085		0.007
Bryant's	17 (81%)			8 (88.9%)		9 (75.0%)	
Buck's	35 (92.1%)			29 (93.5%)		6 (85.7%)	
Spica	16 (36.4%)			1 (50.0%)		15 (35.7%)	
Fixation		<0.001	0.977		0.614		0.064
None	39 (54.2%)			9 (81.2%)		30 (49.2%)	
External fixation	43 (86.0%)			32 (88.9%)		11 (78.6%)	
Staged		0.001	0.145		0.343		0.136
Single	16 (45.7%)			2 (66.7%)		14 (43.8%)	
Multi	65 (77.4%)			39 (88.6%)		26 (65%)	

From Haney et al. with permission [30]

Immobilization Techniques

Osteotomies are vital to pelvic and bladder reconstruction; however, immobilization of the healing pelvis and lower extremities significantly aids in each closure's success. It is important to realize, though, that not all immobilization techniques are equally effective.

Zaman et al. demonstrated the impact of pelvic immobilization techniques on the outcomes in primary and secondary CBE closures in a large cohort of CBE patients [31]. Review of these patients revealed that 343/476 (72.1%) patients with primary closures and 92/101 (91.1%) patients who underwent secondary closures achieved success. Primary closures were categorized by technique and included the MSRE, CPRE, or others (e.g., Kelly repair, Erlangen repair), with a multitude of immobilization techniques ranging from Buck's traction with external fixation and Bryant's traction to spica casting or Velcro pelvic binder, among others. Specifically, the authors found that in primary closures, Buck's and Bryant's traction achieved the highest success (95.0% and 79.3%, respectively), whereas spica casts had the lowest success rate (49.6%) (Table 7.3). These findings supported the existing literature demonstrating superior Buck's traction, followed by Bryant's traction, with little support for less stringent immobilization methods such as mummy wraps or spica casts [32].

Haffar et al. recently demonstrated how the combination of pelvic and lower extremity immobilization may be protective against bladder closure failure. A total of 747 closure events were reviewed—597 primary closures (79.9%) and 150 reclosures (20.1)—revealing limb immobilization was used in 627 (83.9%) of closure events [33]. Successful closures were associated generally with osteotomy use ($p < 0.0001$) and limb immobilization ($p < 0.0001$). When comparing the impact of various osteotomy and immobilization types on primary closures, the authors found that the combined osteotomy offered 7.22 greater odds of success compared to posterior osteotomy alone, and Buck's traction had 4.91 greater odds of success compared to spica casting and 11.05 greater odds of success compared to mummy wrapping. Similar significant trends were found among secondary closures. Interestingly, patients who received only external fixation without any limb immobilization were successful in 66.7% of cases, while patients who received any form of dual (defined as pelvic and limb) immobilization had successful closures in 92.9% of cases. Finally, among patients with lower limb immobilization without traction (e.g., spica, mummy wrapping, or knee immobilization), pelvic immobilization through external fixation was associated with increased success (Table 7.3a, b).

Despite the evidence supporting osteotomy and immobilization, some patients still are closed without osteotomy, immobilization, or both. Immobilization has been utilized in every closure at the authors' institution, so this study population represented an entirely referred population. In total, 56 closure events representing 47 unique patients were identified, with 13 closure events being secondary closures. Overall, the primary closure failure rate was 83.7% (36/43), and the secondary closure failure rate was 9/13, or 69.2%, underscoring the importance of pelvic osteotomy and lower limb immobilization [34]. Admittedly, pelvic osteotomy with postoperative immobilization does imply an extended hospital stay; however, the drastic reduction in failure rates is worthwhile for patients, families, and overall future success.

Table 7.3 (**a**, **b**) Comparison of outcomes of various pelvic and lower extremity immobilization techniques

(**a**)

Immobilization technique	Primary closure			Repeat closure		
	Total (%)	Authors' institution	Referring institution	Total (%)	Authors' institution	Referring institution
Bryant's	134 (79.3)	92 (95.8)	42 (57.5)	12 (75)	11 (91.7)	1 (25)
Buck's traction + EF	95 (95.0)	71 (96.1)	22 (91.7)	73 (97.3)	68 (97.1)	1 (100)
Spica cast	69 (49.6)	–	69 (49.6)	6 (66.7)	–	6 (66.7)
Mummy wrap	23 (57.5)	–	23 (57.5)	1 (100)	–	1 (100)
Other[a]	22 (78.6)	9 (1)	13 (68.4)	–	–	–
p-value		0.925	0.007		0.587	0.456

(**b**)

Method of immobilization	Total closures			Closures with osteotomy			Closures without osteotomy		
	Total no. ($n = 597$)	No. failed	% Failed	Total no. ($n = 411$)	No. failed	% Failed	Total no. ($n = 186$)	No. failed	% Failed
External fixation with no lower limb immobilization	33	11	33.3	31	10	32.3	2	1	50
External fixation with any form of lower limb immobilization	184	13	7.1	174	11	6.3	10	2	20
External fixation with spica casting/ mummy wrapping	42	14	33.3	39	12	30.8	3	2	67
Spica casting with no external fixation	148	81	54.7	74	30	40.5	74	51	68.9
No form of immobilization	87	60	69.0	20	10	50	67	50	74.6

[a]lesser known or used methods of immobilization

Complications of Osteotomy and Immobilization

Though osteotomy is a tool heavily relied upon for successful closure, it and immobilization techniques are not without risks. Generally, osteotomies are associated with a greater requirement for blood transfusions, as well as longer anesthetic and operative times. Reported complications of osteotomy and immobilization include surgical pin site infections, transient femoral nerve palsies, traction or compression injuries including injury to the lateral femoral cutaneous nerve, osteomyelitis, or erosion of orthopedic hardware [35–37].

Khandge et al. recently sought to characterize and evaluate orthopedic complications in newborn (<28 days of life) vs. delayed (>28 days of life) closures [38]. 186 patients underwent newborn closure, while 100 patients underwent delayed closure. Although relatively common, the rate of blood transfusions did not differ (37.7% newborn cohort vs. 42.6% in delayed cohort, $p = 0.68$) between groups. Overall, orthopedic complications were uncommon in this cohort, impacting 1.7% (5/286), with 3 (2.4%) complications in the newborn group and 2 (2.3%) in the delayed group. The authors concluded that pelvic osteotomy may safely be performed even in newborn patients.

Until recently, no direct comparison in the rate of orthopedic complications between CBE and CE closures existed. Sholklapper et al. assessed a total of 146 patients, 109 of whom were CBE and 37 CE. As expected, there were significant differences in patient characteristics, including median age at primary closure (68 days vs. 597 days), diastasis width (4 cm vs. 6.1 cm), and osteotomy at the time of closure (99.1% vs. 75.7%) [39]. There were no significant differences by gender, osteotomy technique, or hip immobilization technique. Success was achieved in 104/109 (95.4%) of CBE closures and 36/37 (97.3%) of CE closures. Any complication was experienced in 38.5% and 56.8% of CBE and CE patients, respectively, though this did include the need for blood transfusion. There was a significant difference in orthopedic complications, with 4.6% and 16.2% for CBE compared to CE, though there was no significant difference in severe grade III or higher complications between cohorts based on the Clavien-Dindo classification system. The most common complications cited were pin site infections requiring debridement. Overall, the complications were likely to be less severe, grade I or II. Thus, while complications were more likely in this cohort than previously reported, the overwhelming majority were minor in nature and easily treated.

Epispadias Repair

Though a successful primary closure is at the forefront of exstrophy care, considerable attention is given to the cosmesis of the external genitalia. Recall that at the time of primary closure, the urethral plate is closed distally as far as available skin will allow. Typically, this is to the level of the midshaft of the penis. In delayed primary closures, testosterone enanthate is used as an adjunct 5 weeks and 2 weeks prior to closure to facilitate penile skin coverage. Epispadias repair typically occurs 6–12 months after a successful bladder closure, and in males with either isolated epispadias or those presenting for the second stage of repair in MSRE, the modified Cantwell-Ransley repair has been utilized at the authors' institution since 1988 [40]. The details of this technique are well documented in the literature [14].

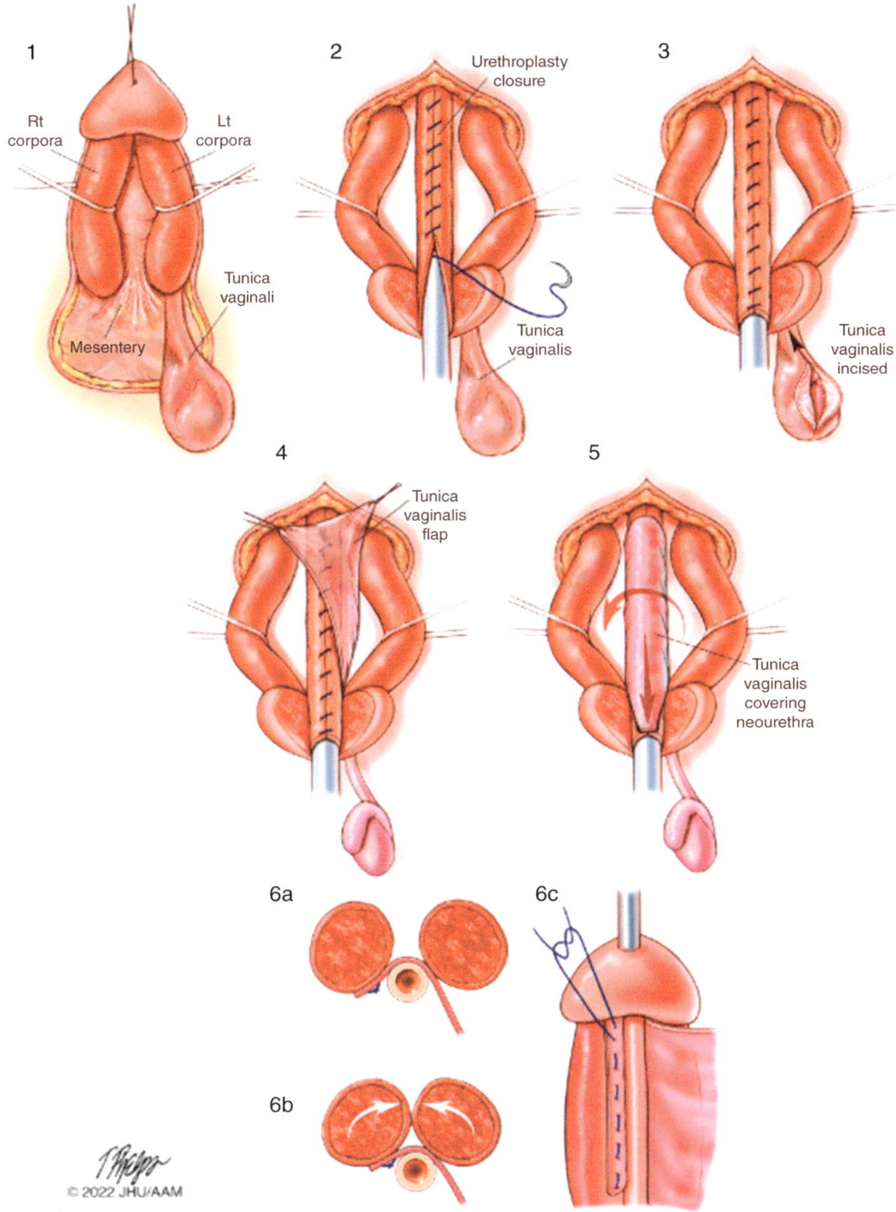

Fig. 7.5 (1–6b) Tunica vaginalis flap for additional coverage in epispadias repair. (From Campbell-Walsh-Wein, with permission [41])

Aiming to create a neourethral channel that is easily catheterizable and acceptable in cosmetic appearance and a penis that is ultimately functional with a glandular or near-glandular urethra combine to make epispadias repair a nuanced reconstructive task. A modern iteration of the previously published modified Cantwell-Ransley repair involves the application of a tunica vaginalis flap for epispadias repair (Fig. 7.5, 1–6b) [41]. By providing a healthy, vascularized tissue flap as an adjunct, the authors demonstrated durable protection against fistula development in EEC patients who failed prior epispadias repair and in primary repair of patients with isolated complete male epispadias.

Outcomes and Complications

Incremental improvements, continuously updated through the years, have resulted in a dramatic improvement in the success of urinary reconstruction. Restoring functional anatomy with the goal of achieving eventual urinary continence remains the focus of the reconstructive team. To this effect, the two most reliable predictors of future urinary continence are the size of the bladder template at birth and a successful primary closure, regardless of the technique used.

In their large series, Surer et al. reinforced the importance of a successful primary closure. Sixty-eight patients, 57 male and 11 female, underwent a modified Young-Dees-Leadbetter BNR, of which 57 (83%) were continent per urethra, 9 (13%) required clean intermittent catheterization, and 2 developed a severe posterior urethral stricture requiring revision [42]. Urinary retention was the most encountered complication, but cases were successfully managed via a combination of catheter dilation and prolonged suprapubic tube drainage.

If the posterior urethral obstruction persists and jeopardizes renal function, surgical correction is warranted. One technique employed by the authors includes the modified Tanagho flap, in which an anterior detrusor flap is rotated to cover the incised portion of the posterior urethral stricture [43]. In the small reported series, with an even split being closed via MSRE and CPRE, all patients with CBE who underwent proximal urethral reconstruction in this fashion remained stricture-free at the cost of postoperative urinary incontinence. At a mean follow-up of 9.9 years, half subsequently underwent elective BNT to achieve continence.

The existing literature regarding successful primary closures demonstrates that the rate of continence is higher, and the onset earlier, compared to those patients who require re-closure [44, 45]. In assessing the long-term impact of failed closures, Novak et al. reported on CBE patients who underwent more than one attempt at closure. Specifically, the authors found that the likelihood of having a sufficient bladder capacity for BNR fell to 60%, and the overall chance of voided continence was a meager 17% [46]. Interestingly, sub-analysis of this group revealed that, at the time of primary attempted closure, 80% of patients did not have an osteotomy, perhaps demonstrating the importance of securing soft tissue reconstruction through appropriate reconstruction of the bony pelvis.

Regardless of the surgical approach utilized, successful primary bladder closure is the primary goal. A failed primary closure is devastating for the patient and family, and the implications are significant. Patients who experience a failed primary closure are subject to more operations and general anesthetic exposure. Though a failed bladder closure negatively impacts ultimate urinary continence in CBE, the impact on continence specifically is less pronounced in patients with CE, as most of these patients require additional continence procedures regardless of the primary outcome [47, 48]. The ramifications extend beyond the additional operations to include financial morbidity.

In analyzing the cost of failure, Hesh et al. reviewed 162 CBE patients and found that simply having a failed primary closure increased total charges by $19,677 [49]. Similarly, Goldstein et al. assessed the cost of primary vs. failed CE closure in terms of continence and found that a successful primary repair of CE costs approximately $196,000 to reach continence, while the cost to achieve continence rises to $407,000 after a failed primary closure [48].

Failed urinary reconstruction in children with exstrophy is significant as it may lead to blunted bladder growth and loss of the bladder template, which may make it increasingly difficult, if not impossible, to achieve continence. This, along with the financial impact, should motivate reconstructive surgeons to use every tool at their disposal—from osteotomy to radical tissue dissection of the urogenital fibers and methods of immobilization—to achieve a successful closure the first time.

Achieving Urinary Continence

The third and final surgery in the MSRE pathway is the continence procedure paired with the urinary antireflux procedure. Despite successful closures conferring dry intervals alone in a limited number of patients, the overwhelming majority of patients will require some sort of outlet procedure to achieve continence. It is the practice at the authors' institution that children undergo yearly ultrasonography to assess for any upper tract deterioration and yearly (or at least every other year) cystoscopy and cystogram so that growth in bladder capacity can be meticulously tracked. Additionally, all patients treated at the authors' institution are started on antibiotic prophylaxis for likely de novo vesicoureteral reflux (VUR).

The target capacity prior to BNR is 100 mL, as sub-analysis in patients who underwent successful primary closure for CBE, followed by epispadias repair and BNR, had a greater likelihood of being dry if the last measured capacity was at least 100 mL [50, 51]. However, prior to any surgical intervention, children and families undergo intense pre-surgical counseling, including assessment by a child psychologist with a background in pediatric urology, along with pelvic floor physiotherapy to assess emotional and maturational readiness to participate in a postoperative voiding (or catheterization) program. "Graduation" from such a program prior to surgery entails 6 months of intensive and regular exposure with the voiding improvement program (VIP) team.

Ureteral reimplantation is performed utilizing either a Cohen transtrigonal technique or cephalotrigonal reimplantation if the ureter must be moved above the trigone [52]. The modified Young-Dees-Leadbetter is employed for the BNR and involves marking an approximately 1.5 cm-wide and 3 cm-long strip of mucosa posteriorly running proximally from the posterior urethra. Bladder mucosa lateral to this is denuded, leaving only detrusor remaining. These laterally created detrusor muscle triangles are then tightly wrapped and sewn around a small catheter, typically 8-Fr [42].

A review of 95 patients who underwent all stages of MSRE by a senior surgeon at the authors' institution demonstrated that of the 67 patients with BNR and a minimum of 5-year follow-up available, 47 (70%) are continent and voiding per urethra without the need for augmentation or intermittent catheterization, and another seven patients (10%) were at least socially continent (daytime dryness of at least 3 h), while the remaining 13 (19%) were wet [53].

A much larger series including 432 patients treated between 1975 and 2017 provides an update to the existing literature. All 432 patients underwent successful bladder closure (71.5% primary, 28.5% repeat) and a urinary continence procedure [54]. At last follow-up, 162 (37%) underwent BNR, 76 (18%) underwent BNR with augmentation cystoplasty (AC) or continent catheterizable stoma (CCS), and bladder neck transection (BNT) with CCS was performed in 173 (40%) patients, and 18 underwent other procedures. Continence was assessed after a median follow-up of 7.2 years from the first continence procedure and found that after isolated BNR, 91 of 142 patients (64%) were continent, and 124 of 133 patients (93%) who underwent BNT with CCS were continent. These findings showed that most patients with CBE require reconstructive procedures to achieve continence.

Typically, continence procedures are performed in CBE patients around age 7, while CE patients are continent at a median of 11 years of age [55]. Due to the greater degree of complexity involved in CE, as it is more of a multisystem defect, additional procedures are often required, and CE patients require a median of 2 (range 1–4) urinary continence procedures to achieve a dry interval greater than 3 h [55].

Adjuncts to continence, AC and CCS, present unique complications, including mucus overproduction from various incorporated bowel segments, bladder calculi, chronic bacterial colonization, and epithelial polyps. Other long-term issues arise from AC, including chronic metabolic acidosis and, less likely, carcinoma [56, 57]. With time, the stoma created for CUD may stenose, prolapse, necrose, or leak, requiring revision [57]. Methods and techniques for managing these complications are the topic of current research, with exciting results to share soon.

Proposed Follow-Up

Patients along the EEC spectrum, their families, and the treating medical and surgical teams develop a special bond that is unique in medicine. After urinary tract and abdominal wall reconstruction and possible subsequent epispadias repair, the focus in management shifts to protecting the upper urinary tracts at all costs. Typically, at the author's institution, any evidence of reflux is assessed with yearly cystograms and cystoscopy while tracking bladder growth. Bladder capacity, urodynamics, and

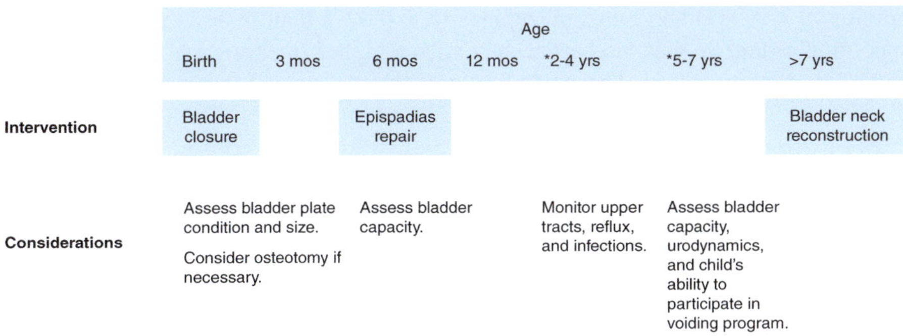

Fig. 7.6 Proposed timeline from birth to continence for the patient with CBE. (From Campbell-Walsh-Wein, with permission [14])

the child's ability to participate in their own care are assessed in school-aged children (at least 5–7 years old) (Fig. 7.6). Additionally, the child's readiness to participate in their own care, through the evaluation of dexterity and maturity, is a prerequisite to BNR [14]. This timeline is shifted later in CE patients, and usually the reconstructive discussion centers on BNT with CCS.

Future Directions

For decades, research in the care of patients across the spectrum of the EEC focused on improvements in surgical techniques to drive better outcomes. Initially, the challenge was restoring form and function while ensuring survival, particularly in CE, while contemporary research focuses on improving quality of life across the lifespan of the exstrophy-epispadias patient. Thanks to advances in research and resulting successes, these children are active and productive adults, with many now entering middle-aged or later adulthood. The field of congenital transitional urology, though practiced for years without an official designation, now attracts such a number of patients that it demands closer attention, moving from a niche patient population to an established discipline.

Exemplifying this, consideration of the whole patient as they age is important, even when considering how interventions during infancy may impact adulthood. Haney et al. assessed the prevalence of opioid and benzodiazepine use in 2627 adult patients with the EEC (337 with CE, 1854 with CBE, and 436 with epispadias [E]) [58]. Overall, EEC patients had a significantly higher opioid prescription rate compared to non-EEC controls: 55.5% of CE, 56.4% of CBE, and 41.1% of E vs. 0.3% of non-EEC ($p < 0.0001$). The prevalence of these medications increased accordingly across the spectrum with E patients having the lowest likelihood and CBE patients the greatest. In CBE specifically, females were more likely to be prescribed opioids ($p = 0.039$) and benzodiazepines ($p = 0.027$) than males. Across the EEC spectrum, older age was also associated with a higher likelihood of opioid or benzodiazepine prescription. These two findings, female sex and increasing age, mirror the US population, as both female sex and increasing age are associated with higher rates of prescriptions, chronic diagnoses, and surgical procedures. Understanding the potential increased risk for substance abuse or the likelihood for more procedures in the EEC population throughout the lifespan can help clinicians best treat these patients from infancy well into adulthood.

Building on the body of knowledge, nomograms are being developed to serve as tools in predicting outcomes, providing a tailored, personalized approach to EEC care. The recently developed mucosal violation index (MVI) has provided a framework for predicting outcomes and complications—specifically fistula rate—in patients who undergo BNT [59]. The authors found that in 192 CBE patients, 23 developed a fistula and that predictors of failed BNT included a wider pubic diastasis at the time of primary exstrophy closure, a failed exstrophy closure, or having undergone three or more bladder surgeries (defined as mucosal violations [MVs]) prior to BNT. In fact, on multivariate logistic regression, the impact of MVs conferred a per-violation odds ratio of 5.1 ($p < 0.0001$) of failure (reference). The effect of MVs was even more pronounced in 35 CE patients, where 11 (31.4%) failed. In this CE cohort, patients with 2 or more MVs prior to BNT experienced a 47.4% fistula rate ($p = 0.0252$), underscoring the increased magnitude of this anomaly [59, 60]. Taken together, these results reiterated the importance of a successful initial primary closure and of minimizing surgeries and trauma to the bladder to achieve the best outcomes.

Finally, sexual health outcomes and improvements in techniques to increase sexual satisfaction are the subject of intense and growing research. In males, the penis is 50% shorter and 30% wider, and while they may interact well socially, 71% express concerns about the appearance of their genitalia and feel it negatively impacts romantic relationships [61]. Harris et al. evaluated 28 EEC males with a median age of 18.3 years who underwent penile lengthening and cosmetic reconstruction using either tissue expansion (TE), skin grafting (SG), or neophalloplasty (NP). The authors found that the overall penile perception score (PPS) increased significantly from 4.5 to 7.5 ($p = 0.0034$), indicating favorable improved views, with NP reconstructed patients reporting the greatest improvement in self-perception, as would be expected [62]. Prior to any intervention, only 9 patients engaged in sexual intercourse, which increased to 17 patients after reconstruction. Finally, 23 patients were dissatisfied or very dissatisfied with penile length, with 18 reporting improvement in length post-intervention ($p = 0.0002$) [62]. This cohort demonstrated how the focus of EEC care is shifting to improve quality of life across the age spectrum.

As the vagina is anteriorly displaced and shorter, EEC females also require careful consideration regarding their sexual health outcomes. While 75–90% of females with exstrophy engage in sexual activity, only 67% report sexual satisfaction, indicating a large percentage of women who face sexual dysfunction. Typically, the introitus and vagina must be reconstructed to allow placement of feminine products, including tampons, or even to adequately allow for penetrative intercourse [63]. Utilizing the Female Sexual Function Index, or FSFI, Canalichio et al. found that women with exstrophy scored lower across all domains in the FSFI, including desire, arousal, and lubrication [64]. Though EEC affects males at a rate of 3-to-1, research and improvements in the quality of life for women along the EEC spectrum deserve just as much focus and attention.

Conclusion

The EEC remains one of the most challenging diagnoses for reconstructive surgeons, owing to its inherent rarity. Add to this the infrequency with which it is seen and operated on, and the complex can easily overwhelm. However, several surgical techniques now exist to allow these children to not only survive infancy but also lead long and productive lives. The MSRE, championed at the authors' institution, remains the most commonly used method for closure and the technique against which others are compared. It is our hope that, regardless of the technique utilized, careful consideration of the bony pelvis, with a low threshold to perform pelvic osteotomies followed by lower limb immobilization, along with aggressive soft tissue mobilization, remains at the forefront of the reconstructive surgeon's mind and arsenal.

Dedication This chapter is dedicated to the extraordinary talent and humility of Douglas A. Canning, MD, a leader in exstrophy care who completed his pediatric urology training at Johns Hopkins in Baltimore, MD, before ultimately becoming Professor and Chief of Pediatric Urology at Children's Hospital of Pennsylvania in Philadelphia, PA. His legacy lives on in the trainees lucky enough to learn from him, in colleagues he helped mentor, and in the countless lives he touched caring for patients and their families. His calm, thoughtful, and kind nature is sorely missed.

References

1. Weiss D, Oliver E, Borer J, Kryger JV, Roth E, Groth T, et al. Key anatomic findings on fetal ultrasound and MRI in the prenatal diagnosis of bladder and cloacal exstrophy. J Pediatr Urol. 2020;6(5):665–71. https://doi.org/10.1016/j.jpurol.2020.07.024.
2. Prenatal diagnosis of classic and cloacal exstrophy: room for improvement. Presented by Dr. Alex Hirsch at 81st Mid-Atlantic section, American Urological Association, October 20th, 2023.
3. Austin PF, Homsy YL, Gearhart JP, Porter K, Guidi C, Madsen K, Maizels M. The prenatal diagnosis of cloacal exstrophy. J Urol. 1998;160(3.2):1179–81. https://doi.org/10.1097/00005392-199809020-00061.

4. Gearhart JP, Ben-Chaim J, Jeffs RD, et al. Criteria for the prenatal diagnosis of classic bladder exstrophy. Obstet Gynecol. 1995;85:961.
5. Meizner I, Bar-Ziv J. In utero prenatal ultrasonic diagnosis of a rare case of cloacal exstrophy. J Clin Ultrasound. 1985;13(7):500–2. https://doi.org/10.1002/jcu.1870130714.
6. Morrill C, Haffar A, Crigger C, Black M, Jelin A, et al. A single-institutional experience with prenatal diagnosis of cloacal exstrophy: room for improvement. J Pediatr Surg. 2023;58(10):1949–53.
7. Sponseller PD, Bisson LJ, Gearhart JP, Jeffs JD, Magid D, Fishman E. The anatomy of the pelvis in the exstrophy complex. J Bone Joint Surg Am. 1995;77(2):177–89. https://doi.org/10.2106/00004623-199502000-00003.
8. Stec A, Pannu HK, Tadros YE, Sponseller PD, Fishman EK, Gearhart JP. Pelvic floor anatomy in classic bladder exstrophy using 3-dimensional computerized tomography: initial insights. J Urol. 2001;166(4):1444–9. PMID: 11547108.
9. Gearhart JP, Jeffs RD. The bladder exstrophy-epispadias complex. In: Walsh PC, et al., editors. Campbell's urology. 3rd ed. Philadelphia: WB Saunders; 1998. p. 1939.
10. Inouye BM, Tourchi A, Di Carlo HN, Young EE, Gearhart JP. Modern management of the exstrophy-epispadias complex. Surg Res Pract. 2014;2014:587064. https://doi.org/10.1155/2014/587064.
11. Baradaran N, Cervellione RM, Stec AA, et al. Delayed primary repair of bladder exstrophy: ultimate effect on growth. J Urol. 2012;188(6):2336–41.
12. Wu W, Maruf M, Manyevitch R, Davis R, Harris KT, et al. Delaying primary closure of classic bladder exstrophy: when is it too late? J Pediatr Urol. 2020;16(834):e1–834.e7.
13. Ahn J, Shnorhavorian M, Katz C, Goldin AB, Merguerian PA. Early versus delayed closure of bladder exstrophy: a national surgical quality improvement program pediatric analysis. J Pediatr Urol. 2018;14(1):27.e1–5.
14. Gearhart JP, Di Carlo HN. Exstrophy-epispadias complex. In: Partin AW, Dmochowski R, Kavoussi L, Peters CA, Wein AJ, editors. Campbell-Walsh-Wein urology. 12th ed. Philadelphia: Elsevier; 2020. p. 528–80.
15. Purves JT, Gearhart JP. Complications of radical soft-tissue mobilization procedure as a primary closure of exstrophy. J Pediatr Urol. 2008;4:65–9.
16. Duckett JW. Use of paraexstrophy skin pedicle grafts for correction of exstrophy and epispadias repair. Birth Defects Orig Artic Ser. 1977;13:171.
17. Davis R, Maruf M, Dunn E, Di Carlo HN, Gearhart. The role of anatomic pelvic dissection in the successful closure of bladder exstrophy: an aid to success. J Pediatr Urol. 2019;15(5):559.e1–7.
18. Dunn EA, Kasprenski M, Facciola J, Benz K, Maruf M, et al. Anatomy of classic bladder exstrophy: MRI findings and surgical correlation. Curr Urol Rep. 2019;20(9):48.
19. Di Carlo H, Tekes A, Gearhart JP. V7-01 intraoperative MRI-guided navigation of the pelvic floor during exstrophy closure. J Urol. 2017;197(4):e823.
20. Hanna MN. Reconstruction of the umbilicus during functional closure of bladder exstrophy. Urology. 1986;27:340.
21. Gearhart JP, Jeffs RD. Techniques to create urinary continence in the cloacal exstrophy patient. J Urol. 1991;146(2.2):616–8.
22. Davis R, Stewart D, Maruf M, Lau H, Gearhart JP. Complex abdominal wall reconstruction combined with bladder closure in OEIS complex. J Pediatr Surg. 2019;54(11):2408–12. https://doi.org/10.1016/j.jpedsurg.2019.03.022.
23. Henderson GC, North AC, Gearhart JP. The use of alloderm as an adjunct in the closure of the bladder-cloacal exstrophy complex. J Pediatr Urol. 2011;7(1):44–7. https://doi.org/10.1016/j.jpurol.2010.02.209.
24. Mathews R, Jeffs RD, Reiner WG, Docimo S, Gearhart JP. Cloacal exstrophy improving the quality of life: the Johns Hopkins experience. J Urol. 1998;6(2):2452–6.
25. Ben-Chaim J, Peppas DS, Sponseller PD, Jeffs RD, Gearhart JP. Applications of osteotomy in the cloacal exstrophy patient. J Urol. 1995;154(2.2):865–7. https://doi.org/10.1097/00005392-199508000-00146.

26. Phillips TM, Salmasi AH, Stec A, Novak T, Gearhart JP, Mathew J. Urological outcomes in the omphalocele exstrophy imperforate anus spinal defects (OEIS) complex: experience with 80 patients. J Pediatr Urol. 2013;9(3):353–8. https://doi.org/10.1016/j.jpurol.2012.04.017.
27. Mathews R, Gearhart JP, Bhatnagar R, Sponseller P. Staged pelvic closure of extreme diastasis in the exstrophy-epispadias complex. J Urol. 2006;176(5):2196–8. https://doi.org/10.1016/j.juro.2006.07.058.
28. Jayman J, Michaud J, Maruf M, Trock B, Kaspresnski M, et al. The dual-staged pathway for closure in cloacal exstrophy: successful evolution in collaborative surgical practice. J Pediatr Surg. 2019;54(9):1761–5.
29. Benz KS, Jayman J, Maruf M, Baumgartner T, Kasprenski M, Friedlander DA, et al. Pelvic and lower extremity immobilization for cloacal exstrophy bladder and abdominal closure in neonates and older children. J Pediatr Surg. 2018;53(11):2160–3.
30. Haney NM, Crigger C, Sholklapper T, Mudalegundi S, Griggs-Demmin A, et al. Pelvic osteotomy in cloacal exstrophy: a changing perspective. J Pediatr Surg. 2022;11(19):1–6.
31. Zaman M, Kasprenski M, Maruf M, Benz K, Jayman J, et al. Impact of pelvic immobilization techniques on the outcomes of primary and secondary closures of classic bladder exstrophy. J Pediatr Urol. 2019;15(4):382.e1–8.
32. Meldrum KK, Baird AD, Gearhart JP. Methods of pelvic and extremity immobilization following bladder exstrophy closure: associated complications and impact on surgical success. Urology. 2003;62:1109.
33. Haffar A, Morrill C, Crigger C, Sponseller PD, Gearhart JP. Fixation with lower limb immobilization in primary and secondary exstrophy closure: a saving grace. J Pediatr Urol. 2023;19(2):179.e1–7.
34. Haffar A, Hirsch A, Morrill C, Crigger C, Sponseller PD, Gearhart JP. Classic bladder exstrophy closure without osteotomy or immobilization: an exercise in futility? Urology. 2023;181:128. Online ahead of publication: https://linkinghub.elsevier.com/retrieve/pii/S0090429523007823.
35. Kelly D. Campbell's operative orthopaedics. 14th rev ed. Philadelphia: Elsevier; 2021. p. 1186e230.
36. Zaman MH, Davis R, Maruf M, DiCarlo H, Gearhart JP. Exploration of practice patterns in exstrophy closures: a comparison between surgical specialties using a national and institutional database. Urology. 2019;131:211e6.
37. Maruf M, Jayman J, Kasprenski M, Benz K, Feng Z, Friedlander D, et al. Predictors and outcomes of perioperative blood transfusions in classic bladder exstrophy repair: a single institution study. J Pediatr Urol. 2018;14(5):430.e1e6.
38. Khandge P, Wu W, Hall S, Manyevitch R, Sullivan B, et al. Osteotomy in the newborn classic bladder exstrophy patient: a comparative study. J Pediatr Urol. 2021;17(4):482.e1–6.
39. Sholklapper T, Crigger C, Haney N, Khandge P, Wu W, Sponseller PD, Gearhart JP. Orthopedic complications after osteotomy in patients with classic bladder exstrophy and cloacal exstrophy: a comparative study. J Pediatr Urol. 2022;18(5):586.e1–8.
40. Surer I, Baker LA, Jeffs RD, et al. The modified Cantwell-Ransley repair in exstrophy and epispadias: 10-year experience. J Urol. 2000;164:1040.
41. Sholklapper T, Crigger C, Haney NM, Harris TGW, Gearhart JP. Application of tunica vaginalis flap for epispadias repair in the epispadias-exstrophy complex. Urology. 2023;171:190–5.
42. Surer I, Baker LA, Jeffs RD, et al. Modified Young-Dees-Leadbetter bladder neck reconstruction in patients with successful primary bladder closure elsewhere: a single institution experience. J Urol. 2001;165:2438.
43. Guan H, Sholklapper T, Crigger C, Haney NM, Harris TGW, Gearhart JP. Modified Tanagho flap in bladder exstrophy: novel application of a tested technique. J Pediatr Urol. 2023;19(1):37.1–7.
44. Oesterling JE, Jeffs RD. The importance of a successful initial bladder closure in the surgical management of classical bladder exstrophy: analysis of 144 patients treated at the Johns Hopkins Hospital between 1975 and 1985. J Urol. 1987;137:258.

45. Husmann DA, McLorie GA, Churchill BM. Closure of the exstrophic bladder: an evaluation of the factors leading to its success and its importance on urinary continence. J Urol. 1998;142:522.
46. Novak TE, Costello JP, Orosco R, et al. Failed exstrophy closure: management and outcome. J Pediatr Urol. 2010;6:381.
47. Davis R, Sood A, Maruf M, Singh P, Kasprenski M, Di Carlo HN, Gearhart JP. The failed bladder closure in cloacal exstrophy: management and outcomes. J Pediatr Surg. 2019;54(11):2416–20.
48. Goldstein SD, Inyoue BM, Reddy S, Lue K, Young EE, Abdelwahab M, et al. Continence in the cloacal exstrophy patient: what does it cost? J Pediatr Surg. 2016;51(4):622–5.
49. Hesh CA, Young E, Intihar P, et al. The cost of failure: the economic impact of failed primary closure in classic bladder exstrophy. J Pediatr Surg. 2016;51(8):1312–6.
50. Gearhart JP, Jeffs RD. State of the art reconstructive surgery for bladder exstrophy at the Johns Hopkins Hospital. Am J Dis Child. 1989;143:1475.
51. Chan DY, Jeffs RD, Gearhart JP. Determinates of continence in the bladder exstrophy population after bladder neck reconstruction. Urology. 2001;165:1656.
52. Canning DA, Gearhart JP, Peppas DS, et al. The cephalotrigonal reimplant in bladder neck reconstruction for patients with exstrophy or epispadias. J Urol. 1992;150:156.
53. Baird AD, Nelson CP, Gearhart JP. Modern staged repair of bladder exstrophy: a contemporary series. J Pediatr Urol. 2007;3(4):311–5.
54. Maruf M, Manyevtich R, Michaud J, Jayman J, Kasprenski M, et al. Urinary continence outcomes in classic bladder exstrophy: a long-term perspective. J Urol. 2020;203:200–5.
55. Maruf M, Kasprenski M, Jayman J, Goldstein S, Benz K, Baumgartner T. Achieving urinary continence in cloacal exstrophy: the surgical cost. J Pediatr Surg. 2018;53(1):1937–41.
56. Surer I, Ferrer F, Baker L, Gearhart JP. Continent urinary diversion and the exstrophy-epispadias complex. J Urol. 2003;169(3):1102–5.
57. Woodhouse CR, North AC, Gearhart JP. Standing the test of time: long-term outcome of reconstruction of the exstrophy bladder. World J Urol. 2006;24(3):244–9.
58. Haney NM, Li O, Agrawal P, Kohn TP, Sholklapper T, Crigger C, DiCarlo HN, Gearhart JP. Prevalence of opiod and benzodiazepine use in adult patients with the exstrophy-epispadias complex. J Pediatr Urol. 2023;19(562):e1–562.e8.
59. Harris TGW, Crigger C, Sholklapper T, Khandge P, Yang R, Redett R, Gearhart JP. The impact of repeated bladder surgeries on successful bladder neck closure in classic bladder exstrophy: the role of mucosal violations. J Pediatr Urol. 2023;19(4):372.e1–6.
60. Crigger C, Harris TGW, Sholklapper T, Haffar A, Morrill C, Nasr I, Yang R, Redett R, Gearhart JP. Mucosal violations and their effect on successful bladder neck closure in cloacal exstrophy. J Pediatr Surg. 2023;58:2313.
61. Harris KT, Namdarian B, Gearhart JP, Wood D. Long term outcomes in classic bladder exstrophy – the adult picture. J Pediatr Urol. 2023;20:157.
62. Harris TGW, Khandge P, Wu W, Leto Barone AA, Manyevitch R, et al. Sexual health outcomes after penile reconstruction in the exstrophy-epispadias complex. J Pediatr Urol. 2022;18(6):747–55.
63. Sinatti C, Waterschoot M, Roth J, Van Laecke E, Hoebeke P, Spinoit AF. Long-term sexual outcomes in patients with exstrophy-epispadias complex. Int J Impot Res. 2021;33:164–9.
64. Canalichio KL, Ahn J, Artigas P, Oelschlager AM, Rowe C, Merguerian P, et al. Patient-reported outcomes in adult females with bladder exstrophy: a study of long-term sexual, reproductive and urinary outcomes using social media. J Pediatr Urol. 2020;16(5):567.e1–7.

The Kelly Procedure

8

Navroop S. Johal, Mehak Sehgal, and Imran Mushtaq

Introduction

Bladder exstrophy (BEX) represents a significant reconstructive challenge for the paediatric surgeon and urologist. The incidence of BEX is 1 in 46,000 live births and is twice as common in males compared with females [1]. In the past, children born with this condition were condemned to poor outcomes and, for many, an unfortunate quality of life, with little prospects for education, employment and relationships. Even today in some countries these outcomes remain the reality for patients with bladder exstrophy. Nevertheless, early diagnosis, prompt initial management and novel surgical reconstructive techniques have resulted in reduced morbidity and significant improvements in the long-term quality of life.

There are several factors involved in the success of managing a patient with bladder exstrophy, and it is not solely based upon a successful operative closure in the neonatal period, even though we know that children requiring a redo closure fare less well in terms of urinary continence [2]. It is paramount that treatment is undertaken by a bladder exstrophy specialist who has an understanding of the altered anatomy and appreciates the evolution of bladder development, increase in capacity and function throughout childhood and into adulthood. The bladder exstrophy specialist should be part of a bladder exstrophy multi-disciplinary team comprising one

Supplementary Information The online version contains supplementary material available at [https://doi.org/10.1007/978-3-031-91238-2_8].

N. S. Johal · M. Sehgal · I. Mushtaq (✉)
Department of Paediatric Urology, Great Ormond Street Hospital for Children NHS Foundation Trust, London, UK

A. R. Shukla, R. S. Joshi (eds.), *Bladder Exstrophy and Epispadias*,
https://doi.org/10.1007/978-3-031-91238-2_8

or more urology nurse specialists, psychologist, gynaecologist and orthopaedic specialist. In the United Kingdom, bladder exstrophy care has been centralised to two centres for the last 20 years, with the main objective having been to improve outcomes. It is also essential that there exists a pathway for children with bladder exstrophy to transition to an adult or adolescent urologist, and for that individual to possess the same appreciation for the condition and most importantly to have a thorough understanding of the previous surgeries that would have been undertaken.

It is without doubt that Justin Kelly made one of the most noteworthy contributions to the management of children with BEX when he first described in 1971 'a procedure for lengthening the phallus in boys with exstrophy of the bladder', which we now understand universally as the 'Kelly procedure' [3]. It is somewhat ironic that a small spelling mistake in his surname on that publication has kept this paper concealed from those seeking a better understanding of his operation, which still remains somewhat of an enigma if it has not been witnessed it in person. Justin Kelly first encountered patients with BEX during his fellowship training in Boston where he worked with Robert Gross in the late 1960s [4]. He encountered many patients with disappointing clinical outcomes whom at the time were undergoing a cystectomy and ureterosigmoidostomy. Although they were continent of urine, it was evident that the older male patients with BEX were psychologically scarred by the short penile length and reportedly some males were committing suicide [4]. Justin Kelly undertook a detailed anatomical dissection of the male genitalia in the autopsy room and conceptualised a new technique that would enhance and 'normalise' the anatomy. He initially proposed the procedure to lengthen the penis in male patients with bladder exstrophy [3]. He described the identification and mobilisation of the neurovascular pedicle within Alcock's canal that supplied each of the corporal bodies and a method for detaching the corporal bodies from their attachment to the ischiopubic ramus (Fig. 8.1). This manoeuvre would allow the corporal bodies to come into approximation and move out of the pelvis, thereby enhancing the visibility of the penis. Over time Justin Kelly modified and further refined the technique, both when he returned to Melbourne, Australia, and subsequently at Great Ormond Street Hospital for Children, London. By the time he was working in London, the Kelly procedure had already matured from a penile lengthening to a continence procedure, by virtue of the fact that the exposure achieved by the radical dissection allowed an orthotopic reconstruction of the bladder neck and an external urethral sphincter mechanism.

At our institution for the past 20 years, the surgical pathway for bladder exstrophy, for both males and females, has comprised a neonatal bladder closure without osteotomy followed by a Kelly procedure at 12–18 months of age. The bladder neck is constructed in a more gentle manner and provides a fixed outlet resistance for a gradual increase in bladder capacity over the ensuing years. This is supplemented with a more dynamic outlet resistance achieved through the implementation of nurse-led biofeedback therapy once the child is 6–8 years of age. Patients are monitored with ultrasound imaging of the urinary tract, non-invasive and invasive urodynamic evaluation into late adolescence before transitioning to the adult urology services.

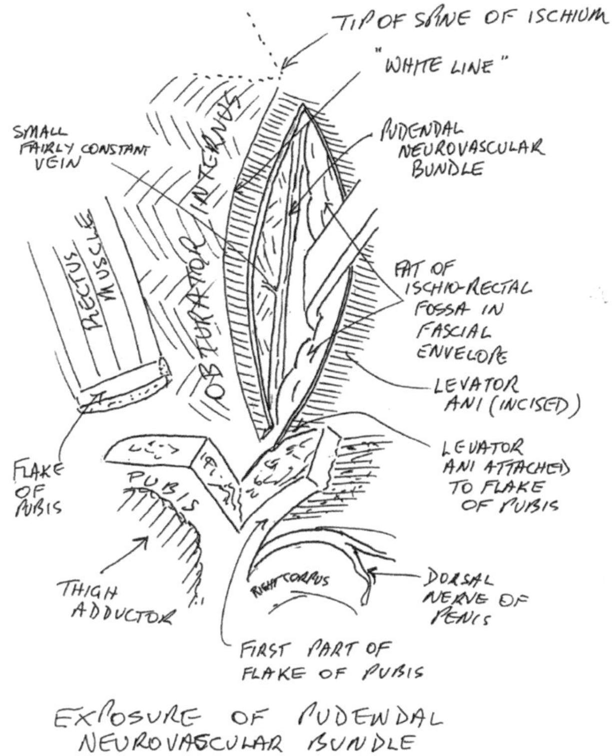

Fig. 8.1 Original hand drawing by Justin Kelly of the identification and exposure of the pudendal neurovascular bundle

Operative Steps of the Kelly Procedure in Males (Video 1)

As mentioned above, all our BEX patients undergo bladder closure in the early neonatal period, with high successful closure rates without the need to perform pelvic osteotomy [5]. To achieve a tension free bladder closure, it is essential to release the bladder detrusor from the rectus muscles laterally, extending down distally to just above and lateral to the verumontanum in boys and the vaginal opening in girls. At this level, posteriorly will be encountered the 'tight' interpubic bands, also known as intersymphyseal bands, which need to be fully divided on each side in order for the construction of the bladder neo-meatus, which should be close fitting on a 8 Fr urethral stent. Despite this somewhat radical dissection at the time of initial bladder closure, we do not encounter difficulty with further dissection in this region at the time of the Kelly procedure.

In his original publications of this operation, Justin Kelly described it as a 'radical soft tissue mobilisation', but those who have adopted this technique prefer to address it as a Kelly procedure. Just as the name has altered a little, the key components have done so also. For example, ureteric reimplantation and creation of a hypospadiac urethral meatus are no longer considered by many as mandatory for success in terms of continence and cosmesis. In our opinion, a Kelly procedure should, however, comprise the following key steps:

- Radical mobilisation of the pelvic musculature and corpora
- Identification and preservation of the pudendal neurovascular bundles
- Construction of an orthotopic bladder neck

Deconstruction: Opening Midline Wound and Degloving of Penis

A 4/0 Prolene suture is placed through the glans to aid retraction. The skin incision marked along the previous incision, encircling the urethral neo-meatus and then extending to either side of the urethral plate and meeting ventrally in region of the frenulum of the penis. The previous lower midline wound is opened and deepened to the level of the rectus muscle. The skin and subcutaneous tissues are raised extensively to achieve a full exposure of the rectus muscle and pubic tubercles. The rectus is incised in the midline taking care to avoid, if possible, a breach in the peritoneum. It is also desirable to not breach the bladder, which is often adherent to the under surface of the rectus muscle. The incision continues around the penile shaft skin leaving a mucosal cuff below the glans. The penis is fully degloved to expose lateral and ventral surfaces of the corporal bodies. This dissection should continue proximally along the corporal bodies to expose their attachment to the ischiopubic ramus. In this region, a triangular area of bulbospongiosum and overlying muscle will come into view. The bulbospongiosus muscle runs horizontally between the ischiopubic rami, over the surface of each corporal body and meeting in the midline. The preservation of this muscle is vital as it will be used to create an external urethral sphincter.

The bladder should be separated from the rectus muscle, taking care not to damage the detrusor muscle. The dissection should continue inferiorly towards the trigone and area of the verumontanum, until the point is reached where the attachment of the corpora to the ischiopubic ramus is visualised. It is essential to preserve an adequate amount of detrusor muscle in the region of, and proximal to, the verumontanum, as this will be utilised for the placement of the sutures in the construction of the bladder neck.

Identification of Pudendal Neurovascular Bundle

Before the corpora is detached from the ischiopubic ramus, the pudendal neurovascular bundle (artery, veins and nerve) to each corpora should be localised. The first step is to expose the pelvic muscular floor (levator ani) by retracting the bladder

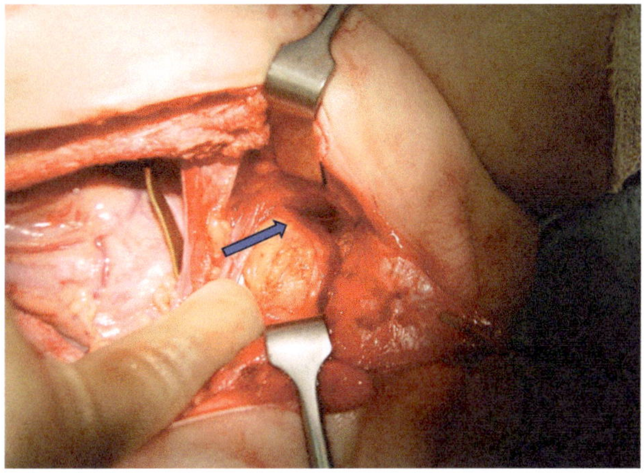

Fig. 8.2 Operative image demonstrating location of pudendal neurovascular bundle

medially, going deep into the pelvis until the ischial spine can be localised by palpation. The neurovascular bundle runs within Alcock's canal, which lies beneath the pelvic floor musculature. The pelvic floor is opened with bipolar cautery along an imaginary line that extends from the first point of union between the corpora and the ischiopubic ramus anteriorly to the ischial spine posteriorly. Once incised, the underlying ischiorectal fat is retracted inferiorly until the neurovascular bundle can be seen through the fascia of Alcock's canal. The pudendal vein usually receives a tributary from the obturator internus through a small perforation in the fascia of Alcock's canal. This 'constant' vein is a helpful landmark for the localisation of Alcock's canal and the pudendal neurovascular bundle within. The overlying fascia is incised along its length exposing the neurovascular bundle (Fig. 8.2). Once identified, attention then moves to detachment of the corporal bodies.

Detachment of Corpora and Release of the Penis

The corpora need to be fully released medially from the ischiopubic rami. Monopolar cautery is used to make an incision approximately 5 mm above and lateral to the attachment of the corpora to the pubic bone, extending through the periosteum/perichondrium to the surface of the bone. Using a periosteal elevator and/or an artery forceps, the corpora is peeled off the pubic bone in an inferior direction with a flake of ischium and pubis, exposing the underlying white-coloured perichondrium. Care must be taken to always keep the neurovascular bundle in sight, and as the separation advances the neurovascular bundle will be seen to enter the tail of the corpora. Moving posteriorly from this point, dissection and division of fibrous attachments of the corpora lateral to the neurovascular bundle will release the corpora entirely (Figs. 8.3 and 8.4).

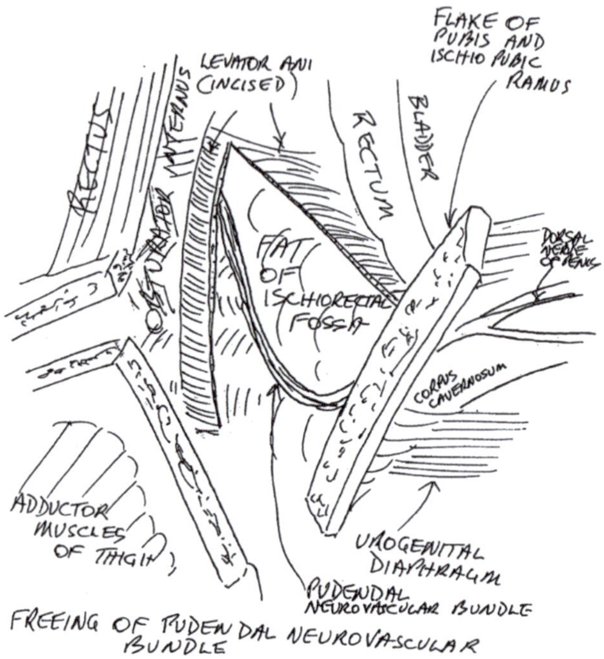

Fig. 8.3 Original hand drawing by Justin Kelly showing the fully detached corporal body and released pudendal neurovascular bundle

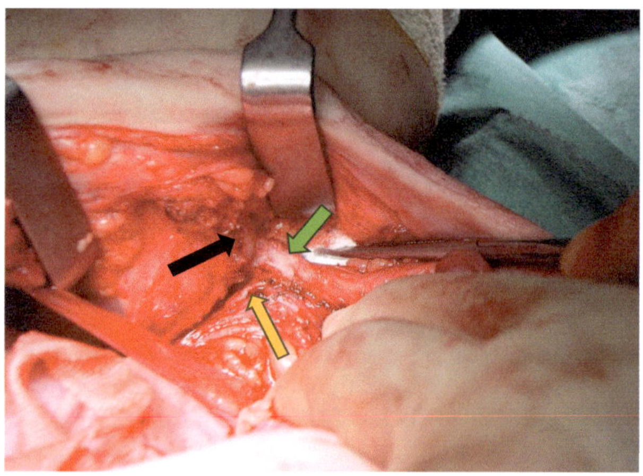

Fig. 8.4 Operative image demonstrating detachment of corpora from ischiopubic ramus (black arrow), flake of pubis (green arrow) and pudendal nerve (yellow arrow)

Disassembly of Corpora and Urethral Plate

Using either sharp dissection or monopolar needle cautery (set at level 8 or 10), the 2 corpora are separated from the dorsally placed urethral plate. The corpora are not detached from the glans distally. The separation of the corpora from the urethral plate is often a bloodless dissection and extends proximally only as far as the region of the prostate gland. This landmark is often heralded by the onset of brisk bleeding from the venous plexuses at the base of the prostate, which is easily controlled with bipolar cautery.

Tension-Free Bladder Neck Construction

The bladder is opened in the midline proximally from the urethral neo-meatus. The ureteric orifices are cannulated with a 4 or 6 Fr feeding tubes, and if required a Cohen type ureteric reimplantation is performed. The location for the construction of the bladder neck is just proximal to the verumontanum, an area that exhibits characteristic longitudinal linear folds (Fig. 8.5). Triangles of bladder mucosa are marked and removed, and a 1- or 2-layer tension-free orthotopic bladder neck reconstruction is performed over an 8 Fr silicone stent with interrupted 4/0 Monocryl sutures. We do not use a measure of the width of the remaining urethral plate, nor do we measure the final circumference of the reconstructed bladder neck. Instead, we use our judgement and experience to aim that first layer of sutures captures an adequate amount of detrusor muscle to ensure that the urethral stent can be moved with a degree of resistance. The proximal end of the catheter is secured within the bladder with a 6/0 Monocryl suture. A 10 or 12 Fr suprapubic catheter is inserted into the bladder for postoperative drainage. The bladder is closed with a single layer with interrupted 4/0 Monocryl sutures. Ureteric stents, when used, can be brought out through the midline closure or laterally through separate puncture sites.

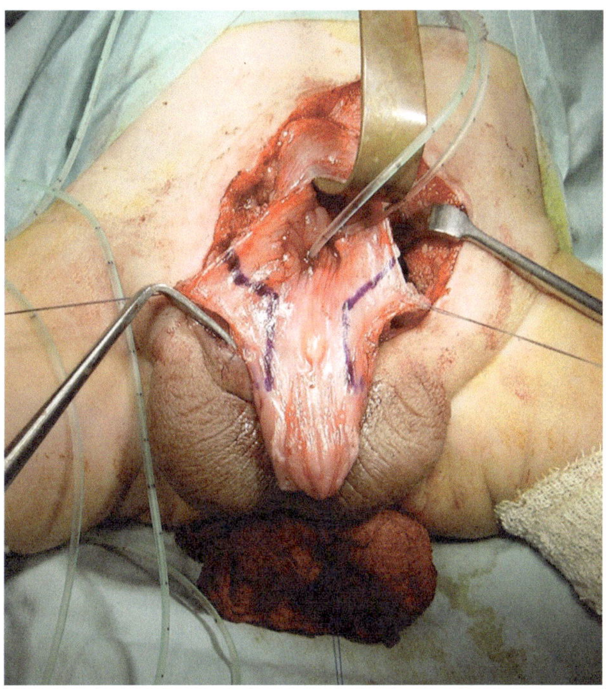

Fig. 8.5 Operative image showing orthotopic location of bladder neck construction, with marked mucosal triangles for excision

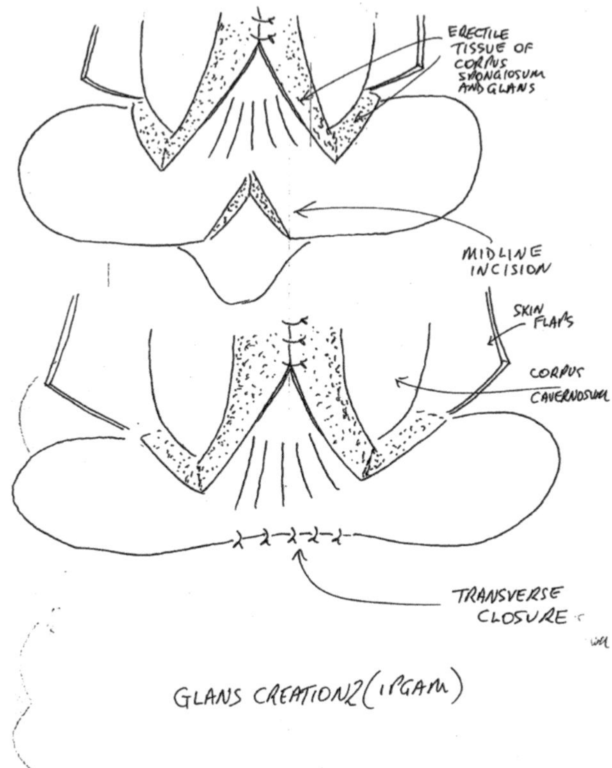

Fig. 8.6 Original hand drawing by Justin Kelly showing the IPGAM procedure

Urethral Reconstruction and Glans Closure

The urethral plate is tubularised with interrupted 5/0 or 6/0 PDS sutures on the existing 8Fr silicone urethral stent. An IPGAM procedure is performed distally to form a more ventrally placed urethral meatus (Fig. 8.6). Triangles of mucosa are excised from the dorsal aspect of the glans, lateral to the central urethral plate. The glans is reconstructed over the urethra with 1 or 2 layers of interrupted 6/0 PDS sutures. The urethra is retracted ventrally, and the corporal bodies are approximated in the midline with 1 or 2 layers of interrupted 5/0 PDS sutures, either with or without a rotation of the corpora to correct the dorsal chordee.

Wound Closure and Penile Skin Reconstruction

The rectus muscle closed in layers commencing with interrupted 2/0 Vicryl for the rectus muscle and 0 or 1 Vicryl for symphyseal region. The skin is closed in 2 layers, with Vicryl for the subcutaneous fat and Monocryl for skin. An umbilicoplasty can be performed at the skin closure stage if requested by the family. Skin coverage of the penis is always a challenge, and excision of the dartos tissue from the penile skin can facilitate this step. Anchoring sutures between the dartos tissue and the base of the corpora can enhance the visible penile length. The urethral stent is secured to the glans penis with 4/0 Prolene. A compression dressing is placed around the reconstructed penis.

Kelly Procedure in Females (Video 2)

The basic tenets of the procedure are the same as in the male patient. The incision continues inferiorly to expose both the clitoral corporal bodies leaving intact the labia minora skin flaps. This enables subsequent clitoral hood skin reconstruction following the bladder neck and urethral reconstruction. As in the male, the pelvic muscular floor is exposed in the extraperitoneal plane to access the neurovascular bundle, the obturator internus muscle and the superior aspect of the levator ani below and lateral to the vagina. Each clitoral body is separated from the surrounding fat of the labium majus. As in the male, the clitoral bodies can be detached from the ischiopubic ramus with identification and mobilisation of the pudendal neurovascular bundles. However, this step is not always necessary and is determined by the degree of pubic diastasis, which if significant can hinder a tension free bladder neck construction and approximation of the clitoral bodies. After the bladder neck is reconstructed, the muscle of the urogenital diaphragm below and lateral to the vagina can be used as a wrap over the bladder neck and urethral repair. The abdomen is closed as in the male. The mons pubis is constructed by approximation of the subcutaneous fat from either side to achieve a good cosmetic appearance.

Postoperative Management

Postoperatively the patient can return to the in-patient ward and can commence feeds almost immediately. Postoperative analgesia is delivered via an indwelling epidural catheter for the initial 4–5 days, which we have previously shown results in a reduced hospitalisation following primary closure [5]. Broad spectrum intravenous antibiotics such as co-amoxicav are continued for 48 h and then converted to an oral dose for a total of 7 days after which prophylactic dose antibiotics are administered. If the patient has undergone ureteric reimplantation, the ureteric catheters are removed after 7 days. The penile compression dressing is removed on day 7, the urethral stent on day 14 and the suprapubic catheter after day 21 once effective urethral voiding is established.

Complications and Outcomes

In our experience, major complications following a Kelly procedure are rare. Glans ischaemia and atrophy are widely muted as a potential complication, supposedly related to the mobilisation of the pudendal neurovascular bundle. Over the past

20 years, the exstrophy team has performed in excess of 400 Kelly procedures and has witnessed hemi-glans atrophy in 2 patients. Less serious and more common complications would include urethrocutaneous fistula formation, penile skin dehiscence, infrapubic incisional hernia and urethral meatal stenosis. Factors responsible for good outcomes are a high volume of cases (related to centralisation of BEX surgery to 2 centres in United Kingdom), collaborative working arrangements, specialist anaesthesia and postoperative analgesia, and highly experienced specialist urology nursing care.

Our institution made a conscious decision 25 years ago to seek an alternative surgical strategy for children with BEX, having concluded that the staged approach of neonatal bladder closure, Cantwell-Ransley epispadias repair and Young-Dees bladder neck reconstruction was not conferring good outcomes. The Kelly procedure was introduced and became the operation of choice for all BEX cases within a few years and has remained so to this day. We are highly satisfied with the improved penile cosmetic outcomes, reduced bladder augmentation rates and a significant increase in the number of patients who can achieve spontaneous urethral voiding without the need for continence pads or underwear. We are required to submit annual outcome data to the national funding organisation for highly specialised services, such as BEX care, and the number of children who are dry by day and voiding per urethra at 5 years of age is 50–60%. We know that this figure increases with age and specifically with biofeedback therapy, which commences at around 8 years of age. We remain confident that the decision we made to adopt the Kelly procedure for our BEX patients was correct and that it has provided our cohort of patients with improved outcomes.

It is wrong in our view to simplify urinary continence in terms of dryness by day and night, because in BEX patients it is a much more complex issue, that should take into account voiding intervals and fluid intake. There is a wide diversity of phenotypes in BEX, and outcomes are unpredictable and at times unexpected. To compare the outcomes of BEX surgeries and institutions by means of urinary continence is divisive and overlooks many other health outcome measures, which are equally and, in some cases, more important.

The Kelly procedure is not complex, but does require a high surgical skillset, courage and a large cohort of patients to become proficient. We are confident that the centralisation of BEX care that we have witnessed in the United Kingdom and that is now underway with the establishment of consortia in the United States will continue to enhance our understanding of what are the right goals and aspirations in the management of BEX.

References

1. Siffel C, Correa A, Amar E, Bakker MK, Bermejo-Sanchez E, Bianca S, Castilla EE, Clementi M, Cocchi G, Csaky-Szunyogh M. Bladder exstrophy: an epidemiologic study from the international clearinghouse for birth defects surveillance and research, and an overview of the literature. Am J Med Genet. 2011;157:321–32.
2. Burki T, Hamid R, Duffy P, Ransley P, Wilcox D, Mushtaq I. Long-term followup of patients after redo bladder neck reconstruction for bladder exstrophy complex. J Urol. 2006;176(3):1138–41. discussion 1141–2
3. Kelley JH, Eraklis AJ. A procedure for lengthening the phallus in boys with exstrophy of the bladder. J Pediatr Surg. 1971;6(5):645–9.
4. Kelly JH, Taghavi K, Mushtaq I, Justin H. Kelly and his procedure for bladder exstrophy and epispadias. J Pediatr Surg. 2022;57(2):314–21.
5. Mushtaq I, Garriboli M, Smeulders N, Cherian A, Desai D, Eaton S, Duffy P, Cuckow P. Primary bladder exstrophy closure in neonates: challenging the traditions. J Urol. 2014;191(1):193–7.

Scrotoperineal Approach to Bladder Exstrophy Repair

9

S. N. Kureel, Archika Gupta, and Kanoujia Sunil

Introduction

Bladder exstrophy is one of the most serious urological birth defects involving the lower abdominal wall, bladder, urethra, and penis with certain associated anomalies and mostly normal upper tracts. The classic description of this birth defect was given by O'Neill as "if one blade of a pair of scissors were passed through the urethra of a normal person; the other blade was used to cut through the skin, abdominal wall, anterior wall of the bladder and urethra, and the symphysis pubis; and the cut edges were then folded laterally as if the pages of a book were being opened" [1] (Fig. 9.1). Trendelenburg in 1906 described that despite the severity of the defect, all neurophysiological components necessary for continence are present in exstrophy [2]. Therefore, any strategy/approach for reconstruction must aim to create a low-pressure reservoir of adequate capacity, create an outlet, reconstruct the bladder neck with internal sphincter, and reconstruct the striated muscle of the external sphincter with preserved innervation. While aiming for satisfactory continence, it is of paramount importance that upper tracts do not suffer any damage from high pressure or the inevitable vesicoureteric reflux. Reconstruction of the outlet must be aimed at creating dynamic resistance with capacity to relax on command of the pontine micturition center and remain contracted in the filling phase to avert leakage of urine (Fig. 9.2). Therefore, outlet reconstruction should be accomplished such that innervation

Supplementary Information The online version contains supplementary material available at https://doi.org/10.1007/978-3-031-91238-2_9.

S. N. Kureel (✉) · A. Gupta
Department of Pediatric Surgery, King Geroge's Medical University, Lucknow, India

K. Sunil
Chandan Institute of Pediatric and Neonatology, Lucknow, India

A. R. Shukla, R. S. Joshi (eds.), *Bladder Exstrophy and Epispadias*, https://doi.org/10.1007/978-3-031-91238-2_9

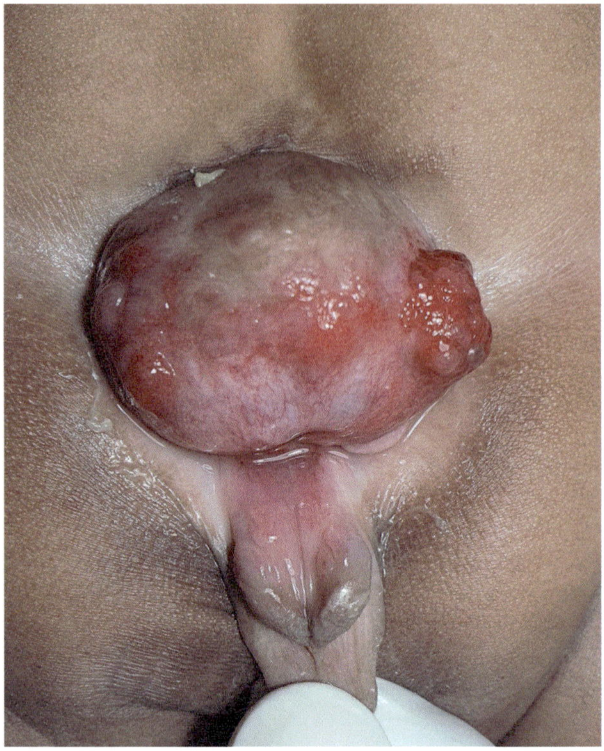

Fig. 9.1 Classic exstrophy bladder (male) showing open bladder plate with epispadias with preputial hood on ventral aspect of glans penis

remains preserved. Other desirable goals are preservation of the cavernosal nerve and an adequately sized phallus (Fig. 9.3). The technique of radical corporal detachment for penile lengthening must ensure absolute preservation of the neurovascular bundle of corpora and vessels supplying the glans.

The task of bridging the abdominal wall defect is achieved by bringing the recti toward the midline after doing the osteotomy [3–5]. The aesthetic appearance is further enhanced with umbilicoplasty, abdominoplasty, and penile skin coverage (Fig. 9.3).

The ***midline scrotoperineal approach of bladder exstrophy reconstruction with innervation-preserving sphincteroplasty and radical corporal detachment*** realizes all the aforementioned goals [6–8].

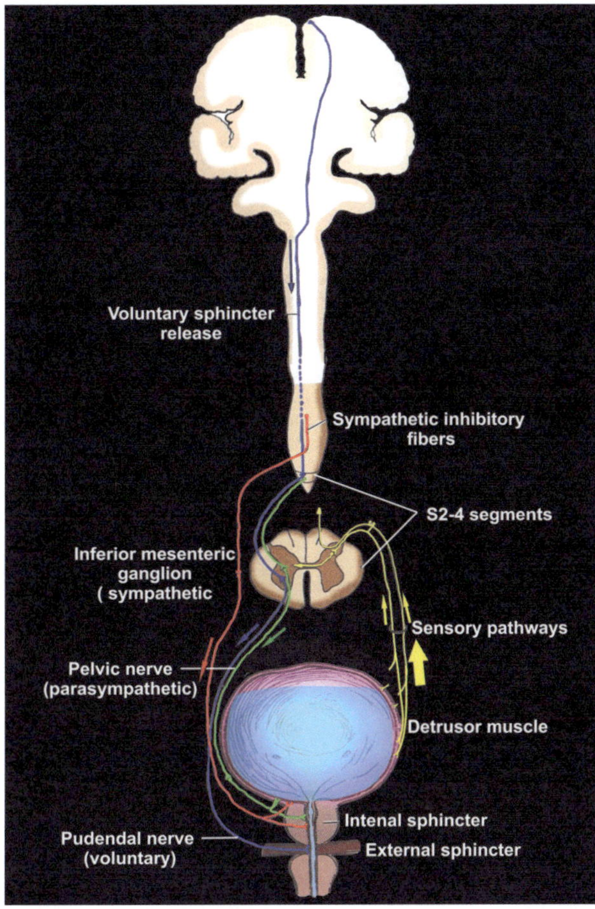

Fig. 9.2 Schematic diagram to show salient points of normal micturition. The filling phase under control of sympathetic (red) and emptying under control of parasympathetic (green). It is controlled by paracentral lobule of cerebral cortex through sacral micturition center (S2, 3, 4)

A brief review of the relevance of surgical anatomy, especially in the context of bladder exstrophy here, would be useful in understanding the technical nuances of the procedure. This would include:

1. Anatomy of the bony pelvis
2. Anatomy of the urogenital diaphragm in exstrophy
3. Anatomy of fascial planes and vessels in the epispadiac penis
4. Relevant anatomical details of open bladder-plate

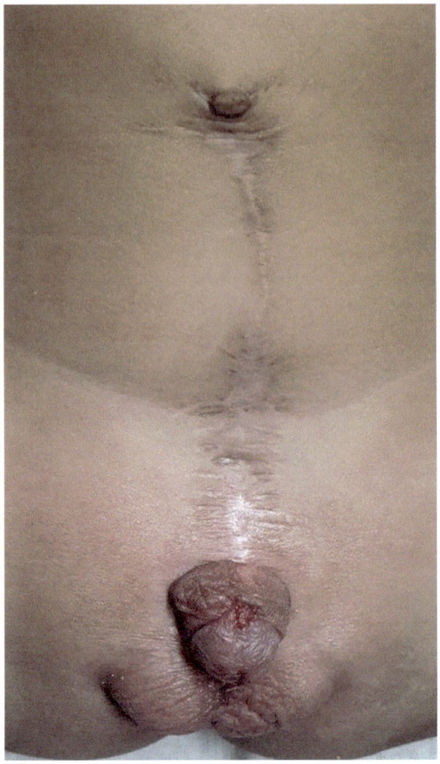

Fig. 9.3 Appearance after reconstruction of bladder exstrophy showing adequate-sized phallus, umbilicus, and well-aligned lower abdominal skin crease

Anatomy of Bony Pelvis

The bony configuration of the pelvis in bladder exstrophy has been described by Sponseller and associates using computerized tomography (CT) pelvis and three-dimensional reconstruction [9]. In a cross-sectional view of the bony pelvis at the level of acetabulum and triradiate cartilage, the intertriradiate distance is the length of an intertriradiate line joining the triradiate cartilage of the right and left sides across the pelvic cavity. This line also divides the pelvis into anterior and posterior segments (Fig. 9.4). There has been shown to be a mean external rotation of 12 degrees in the posterior pelvis on each side, retroversion of the acetabulum, a 31% increase in intertriradiate distance, a mean 18° external rotation of the anterior pelvis, and a 30% shortening of superior pubic rami compared to the control population. This shortening of superior pubic rami along with external rotation of the pelvis contributes to a varying degree of diastasis of the pubic symphysis. Our study on diastasis of the pubic bone in patients with bladder exstrophy has demonstrated that the shape of the gap between the ischiopubic rami, where the urogenital diaphragm is located, varies from rectangular to trapezoid [10] (Fig. 9.5a, b). Stec et al. have described that the sacrum in exstrophy patients has a 42.6% larger volume and 23% more surface area compared to the control population [11].

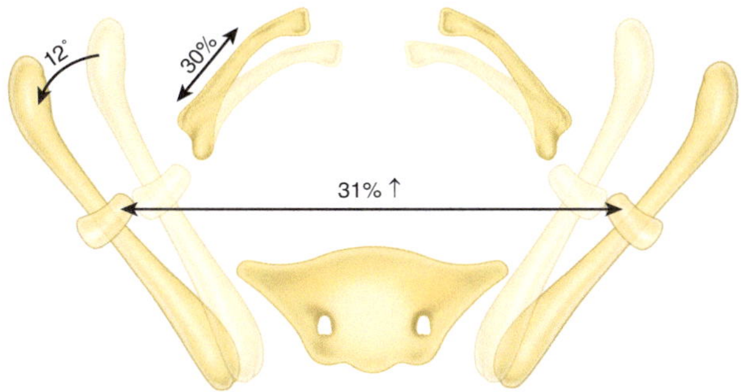

Fig. 9.4 Shows the magnitude of external rotation of pelvis, retroversion of acetabulum, increased intertriradiate distance, and external rotation of anterior pelvis with shortened superior pubic rami. Abnormal anatomy (*yellow*) is superimposed with normal anatomy of cross-section of pelvis (*ochre yellow*)

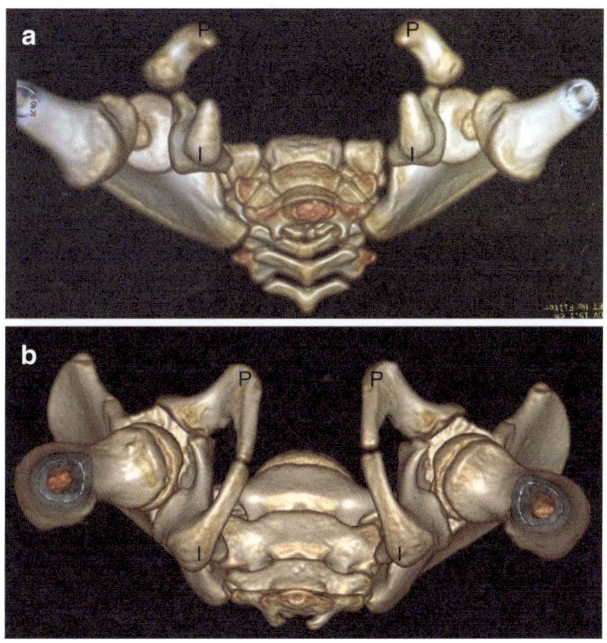

Fig. 9.5 (**a**) Three-dimensional image of CT pelvis perineal view showing rectangular shape of space between ischiopubic rami. I—medial and lowermost point of ischial tuberosity; P—Superior and medialmost point of pubic bone. (The cartilaginous segment of ischiopubic ramus is not ossified.). (**b**) Three-dimensional image of CT pelvis perineal view showing trapezoid shape of space between ischiopubic rami. I—Medial and lowermost point of ischial tuberosity; P—Superior and medialmost point of pubic bone

Anatomy of Urogenital Diaphragm in Bladder Exstrophy

It has been conclusively demonstrated that all the normal muscles of the urogenital diaphragm are present in patients with bladder exstrophy [12]. Normally, the urogenital diaphragm between bilateral ischiopubic rami and the base of the urogenital triangle is triangular. However, in bladder exstrophy, the urogenital diaphragm may be trapezoid or rectangular depending upon the degree of pubic diastasis [10]. The

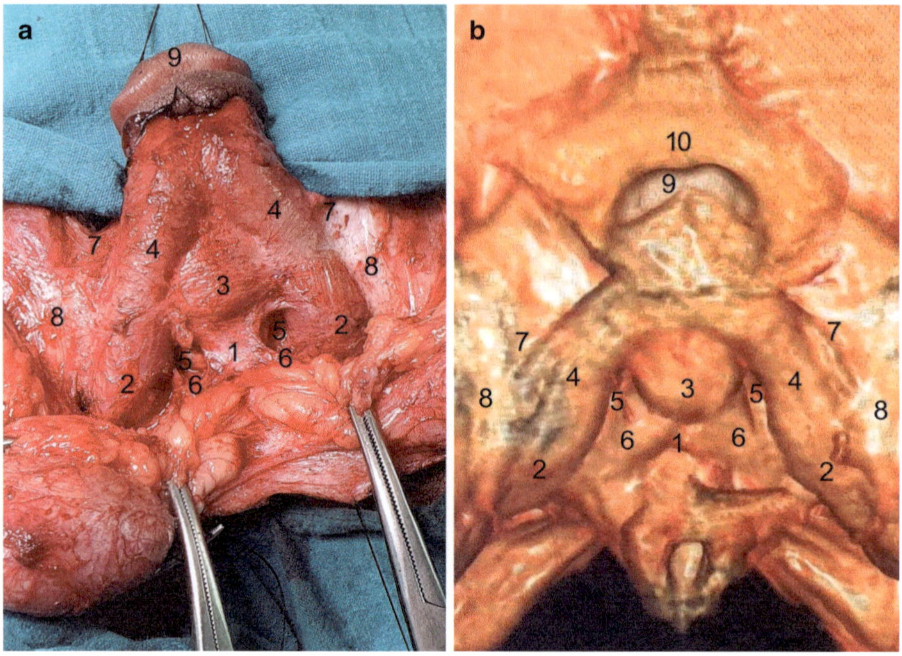

Fig. 9.6 (**a**) Muscle of urogenital diaphragm in bladder exstrophy as seen during exposure via scrotoperineal approach: (1) perineal body, (2) ischiocavernosus muscle, (3) bulbospongiosus muscle, (4) corpora cavernosa, (5) triangular space containing sphincteric branch of perineal nerve, (6) superficial transverse perinei muscle, (7) intersymphyseal band, (8) ischiopubic ramus, and (9) glans. (**b**) Muscle of urogenital diaphragm in bladder exstrophy as seen in volume-rendered CT imaging: (1) perineal body, (2) ischiocavernosus muscle, (3) bulbospongiosus muscle, (4) corpora cavernosa, (5) triangular space containing sphincteric branch of perineal nerve, (6) superficial transverse perinei muscle, (7) intersymphyseal band, (8) ischiopubic ramus, (9) glans, and (10) bladder plate

perineal body is present in the center of the base of the urogenital diaphragm. The corpora cavernosa are attached to ischiopubic rami, and the root of the corporal body is covered with ischiocavernosus muscle on both sides. Between the corpora cavernosa, the corpus spongiosum in the midline supports the dorsal urethral plate. Distally the corpus spongiosum is attached to the glans, while the proximal part is expanded as a bulb. The proximal-most part of corpus spongiosum is covered with bulbospongiosus muscle, which is attached to the perineal body (Fig. 9.6a, b). The bulbospongiosus muscle is continuous with the striated urethral sphincter fibers, which lay open on the cranial aspect of the bulbospongiosus muscle, flanking the urethral plate at the verumontanum. Superficial transverse perinei muscles at the base of the urogenital diaphragm are attached to the perineal body in the midline and laterally to the ischiopubic ramus near the ischial tuberosity (Fig. 9.6b). The potential triangular space between the medial surface of the ischiocavernosus muscle, the lateral aspect of the bulbospongiosus muscle, and the superior border of the transverse perinei muscle is somewhat accentuated in bladder exstrophy (Fig. 9.6a,

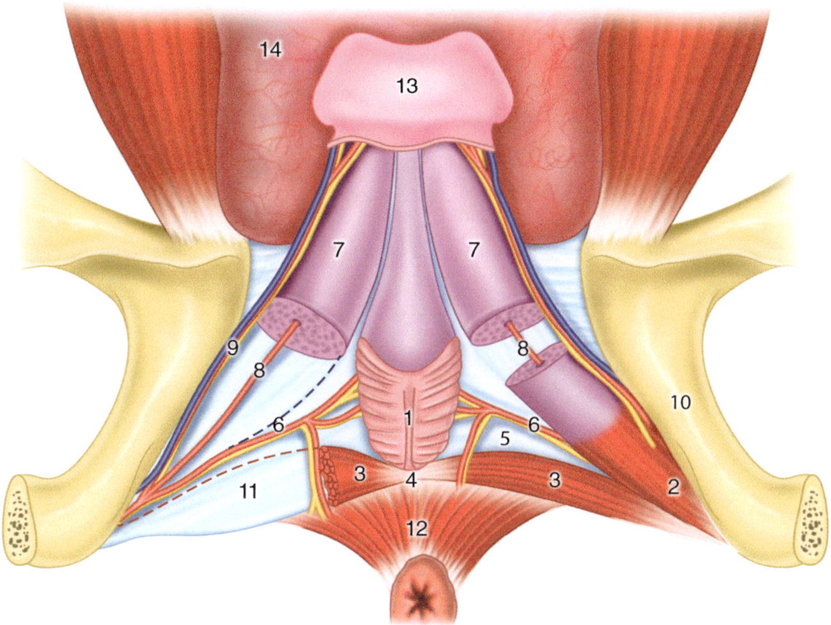

Fig. 9.7 Schematic diagram of panoramic view of undersurface of urogenital diaphragm in classic male exstrophy bladder showing muscles of urogenital diaphragm: (1) bulbospongiosus muscles, (2) ischiocavernosus muscles, and (3) superficial transverse perinei muscle, all attached to (4) the central perineal body. (5) Triangular space between (1) bulbospongiosus, (2) ischiocavernosus, and (3) superficial transverse perineal muscle containing (6) branches of perineal artery and nerves, including sphincteric branches. On the right side, proximal (7) corpora cavernosa, (2) ischiocavernosus muscle, and most of (3) superficial transverse perinei muscle, and on the left side middle part of (7) corpora cavernosa are shown as removed to show (8) deep artery of penis and course of (9) dorsal penile artery and nerves along the lateral aspect of (7) corpora after leaving the inner edge of (10) ischiopubic ramus. Deep to the perineal membrane shadow of (11) deep transverse perinei. (12) External anal sphincter, (13) glans, and (14) bladder plate

b). It is in this space that the sphincteric branches of the perineal nerve and artery course toward the bulbospongiosus muscle and the external urethral sphincter. The course of this nerve and vessel is parallel to the medial aspect of the ischiocavernosus muscle (Fig. 9.7). Therefore, by maintaining the plane of dissection close to the medial surface of the ischiocavernosus muscle, injury to this nerve and vessel can be avoided. This is the "safe plane of dissection" for corporal-urethral separation in this region. Another important anatomical detail to remember is that the pudendal vessels and nerve branch out as dorsal penile vessels and nerve after exiting Alcock's canal. They form the neurovascular bundle on the dorsolateral aspect of the distal part of the corpora cavernosa. Proximally, the neurovascular bundle runs along the *inner* edge of the ischiopubic ramus and then courses into Alcock's canal (Fig. 9.7). The surgical significance of this detail is that by entering the subperiosteal plane along the *outer* edge of the ischiopubic ramus for radical corporal detachment and

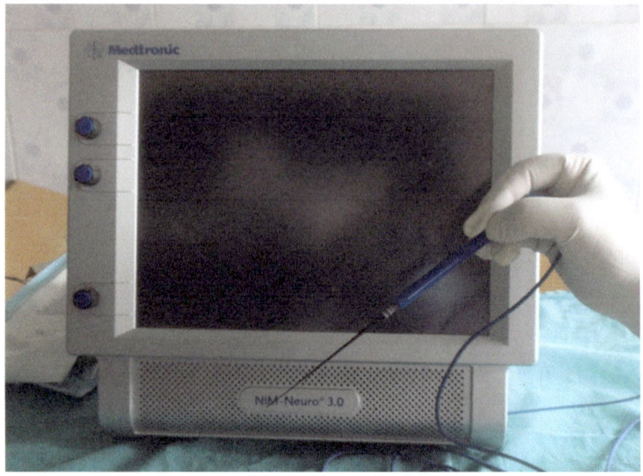

Fig. 9.8 The nerve locator probe is used to locate the sphincteric branch of the perineal nerve and other nerves

maintaining this subperiosteal plane onto the medial aspect of ischiopubic ramus, the preservation of neurovascular bundle is almost guaranteed despite radical corporal detachment down and even beyond its root. Additionally, the cavernous nerve is also preserved. All nerves can be identified using a nerve locator (Fig. 9.8).

Anatomy of Fascial Planes and Vessels in Epispadiac Penis

The anatomy of fascial planes and vessels and their surgical significance in epispadias have been published earlier by us [13]. The anatomy of fascial planes and vessels is shown in the schematic diagram (Fig. 9.9). The urethral plate lies on the dorsal side and continues to the tip between both the hemi glans. On the ventral side, the penile skin on either side of the median raphe runs up to the scrotal rugosities proximally and to the outer preputial skin distally. From the preputial edge, the inner preputial skin continues to the subcoronal sulcus, with a midline frenulum (Fig. 9.10). Penile skin and dartos are supplied by a pair of axial vessels from external pudendal vessels on both sides. The inner preputial skin has a double blood supply from preputial dartos vessels and from ultrafine branches of dorsal penile vessels, which branch out just before it enters the substance of the glans (Figs. 9.9, 9.11, and 9.12). A layer of loose areolar tissue lies between the penile dartos and the Buck's fascia over the corpora. The corpora cavernosa are encased in a double-layered tunica albuginea, whose fibers are oriented longitudinally in the outer layer and circularly in the inner layer. The outer longitudinal layer of the tunica albuginea of the corpora cavernosa is somewhat deficient medially onto the surface facing and flanking the wedge of corpus spongiosum. The neurovascular bundle runs parallel and lateral to the urethral plate on the dorsolateral aspect of the tunica albuginea and enters the glans substance distally. The corpus spongiosum is encased in a single ultrathin layer of tunica albuginea. The Buck's fascia encasing the corpora cavernosa splits to envelop the neurovascular bundle dorsolaterally and fuses again into one layer medial to the neurovascular

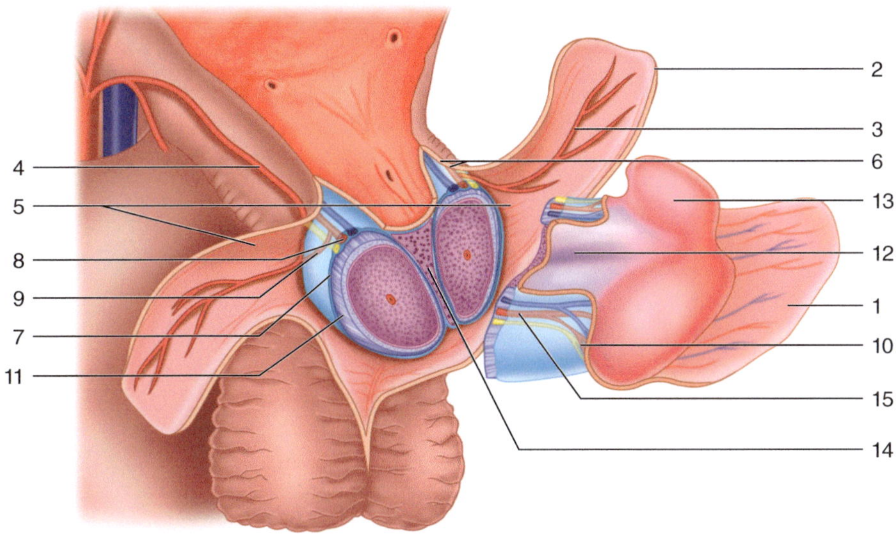

Fig. 9.9 Schematic diagram showing arrangement of fascial planes and course of blood vessels and collateral branches in epispadiac penis. (1) Inner preputial skin split off the (2) outer preputial skin-dartos along with ventral penile skin-dartos, degloved, and bifurcated as two lateral flaps. (3) Axial vessels from (4) external pudendal vessels seen running in (5) dartos fascia of both halves of ventral preputial skin. The middle segment of the shaft of the epispadiac penis is shown as removed to show details of the anatomic arrangement of the fascial plane. (6) Skin and dartos at proximal shaft penis, (7) Buck's fascia surrounding corpora, blending with ultrathin tunica albuginea of corpus spongiosum and splitting to envelop (8) dorsal penile vessels and nerves, (9) branches from dorsal penile vessels perforating into dartos and communicating with branches of axial vessels, (10) at coronal sulcus, terminal branches of dorsal penile artery entering glans give branch to prepuce and communicate with terminal branches of axial vessels of dartos, (11) tunica albuginea—double layer on the lateral side and single layer on the medial side, (12) dorsal open urethral plate (middle of urethral plate schematically removed to show anatomic layers), (13) glans, (14) wedge-shaped corpus spongiosum, and (15) terminal branches of dorsal penile vessels lateral to urethral plate deep to Buck's fascia

bundle. Medially it fuses with the ultrathin tunica albuginea of the corpus spongiosum to form one layer (Fig. 9.9). On the dorsal side, there is a layer of lamina propria underneath the urethral plate. This lamina propria and urethral plate receive their blood supply through the wedge of corpus spongiosum (Fig. 9.9).

The relevant points of surgical significance are that:

(i) since inner preputial skin has a dual blood supply, it remains viable even when split off the outer preputial skin-dartos and is useful in the skin cover [7].
(ii) The axial blood supply of the penile skin-dartos complex ensures the viability of both halves when it is bifurcated in the midline to be used for penile skin cover [7] (Fig. 9.11).
(iii) Buck's fascia can be disrupted in the margin between the neurovascular bundle and the urethral plate. Working in a subfascial plane on the tunica albuginea, corporal-urethral separation can be performed without compromising the vascularity of the corpus spongiosum [13].

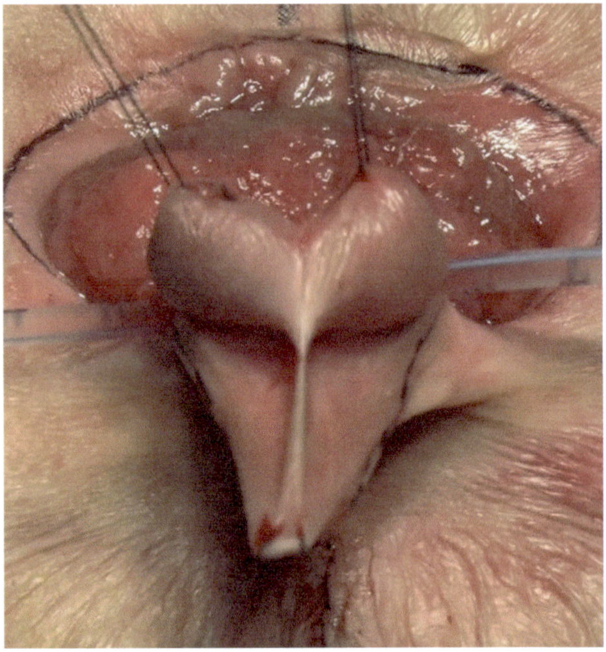

Fig. 9.10 Frenulum between the ventral midpoint of the corona and inner preputial mucosa

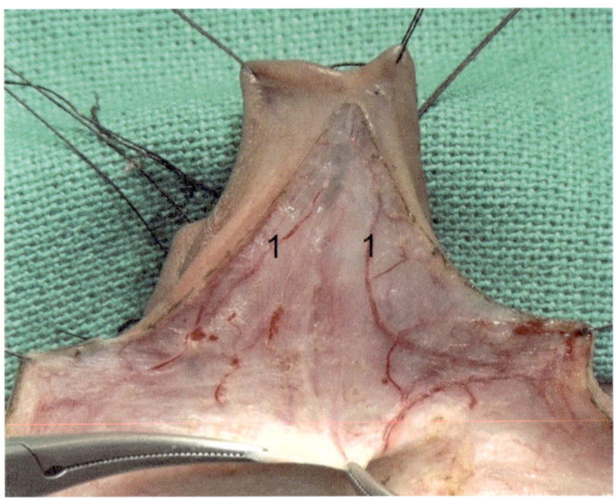

Fig. 9.11 Axial vessels (1) seen in the penile skin dartos complex on each side of the midline

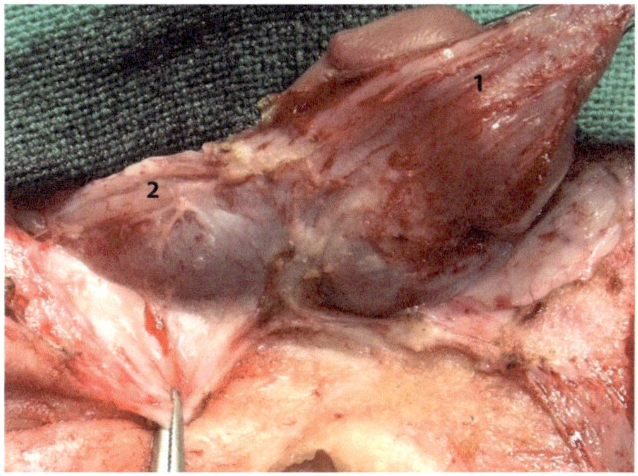

Fig. 9.12 Ultrafine straight vessels (1) supplying the inner preputial mucosa skin coming from (2) dorsal penile vessels

Relevant Anatomical Details of Open Bladder Plate

Since lower abdominal mesenchymal structures are lateralized in bladder exstrophy, pubic bone diastasis is present with variable interpubic distance. Seeking attachment to pubic crest, rectus abdominis muscles diverge, leaving a midline gap of variable size. The wide and stretched linea alba bifurcates to follow the medial edge of rectus abdominis down to the pubic tubercle and merges with the anterior rectus sheath laterally (Fig. 9.13). The posterior rectus sheath is present only up to the arcuate line. Beyond this level, the extraperitoneal space behind the posterior bladder wall contains loose areolar tissue, fat, and sometimes aberrant branches of the inferior epigastric vessels (Fig. 9.14). The edge of the bladder plate mucosa is attached to the skin of the abdominal wall, while the detrusor underneath the mucosa is attached to the bifurcated linea alba at the medial edge of the rectus muscle. Intersymphyseal bands are present on either side between the open bladder neck and the pubic bone laterally. Caudally, the intersymphyseal band extends up to the anterior edge of the levator muscle and lies in intimate contact with the root of the corpora cavernosa and its neurovascular bundle (Fig. 9.13). The autonomic perivesical plexus and perivesical fascia lie on the posterior aspect of the bladder plate. The obliterated umbilical arteries course on the posterior aspect of the bladder plate toward the midline (Fig. 9.15). Sometimes, the superior vesical artery may arise from the root of the obliterated umbilical artery. The blood supply to the detrusor comes from the inferior vesical artery, a branch of the anterior/posterior division of the internal iliac artery (Fig. 9.16).

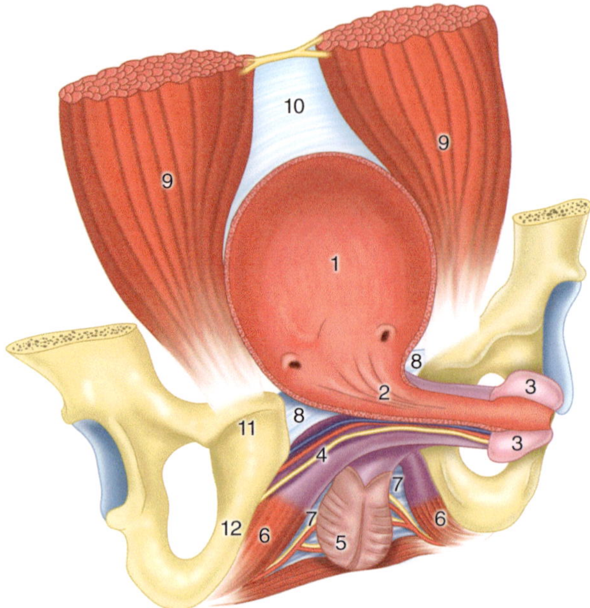

Fig. 9.13 Schematic diagram showing anatomical facts of open bladder neck (1) open bladder plate, (2) verumontanum, (3) open glans, (4) neurovascular bundle on corpora cavernosa, (5) bulbospongiosus muscle of urogenital diaphragm, (6) ischiocavernosus muscle, (7) sphincteric branch of perineal nerve, (8) intersymphyseal band, (9) rectus muscle, (10) stretched linea alba, (11) pubic bone, and (12) ischiopubic ramus

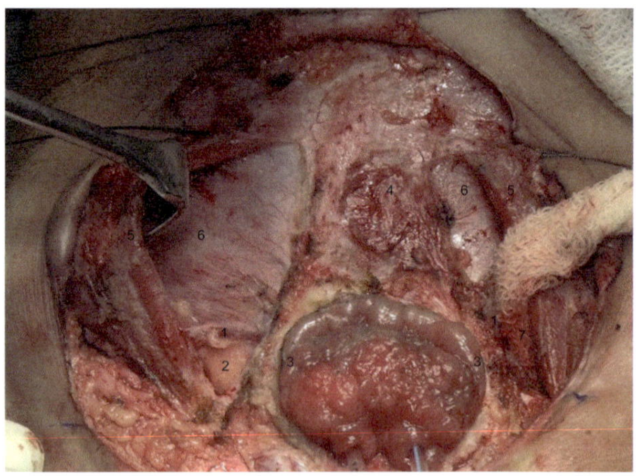

Fig. 9.14 Operative picture showing (1) arcuate line, (2) extraperitoneal fat below, (3) bladder plate margin, (4) stretched linea alba, (5) rectus muscle, (6) posterior rectus sheath, and (7) roller gauze placed in extraperitoneal space

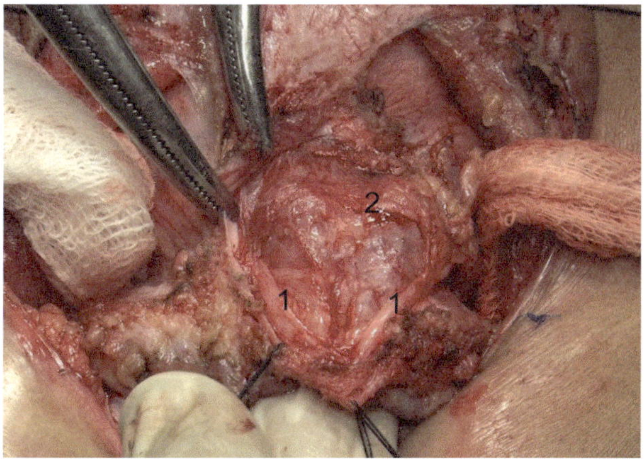

Fig. 9.15 Mobilized bladder plate showing (1) obliterated umbilical artery on the posterior aspect of corpora and (2) fold of peritoneum

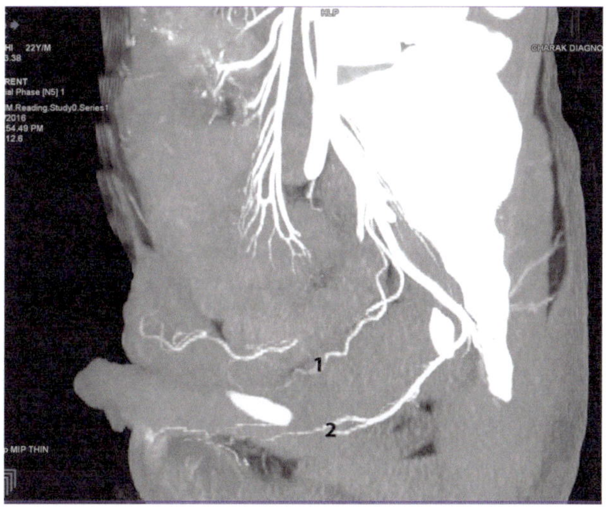

Fig. 9.16 CT angiogram MIP image showing (1) inferior vesical artery and (2) pudendal artery

Technical Details of Bladder Exstrophy Reconstruction Using Midline Scrotoperineal Approach

Preoperative Evaluation and Preparation

A baseline renal nuclear scan to record preoperative renal anomalies, renal function, and absence of renal scarring is done for comparison on follow-up after surgery (Fig. 9.17).

A plain CT of the pelvis with a volume-rendered three-dimensional image of the CT pelvis is obtained to evaluate the pelvic configuration in anterior, superior, perineal, and oblique views (Fig. 9.18a–d). This helps in planning the osteotomy.

At our center, surgical repair is undertaken at 10–12 weeks of age after a reliable evaluation of the upper tract by nuclear study is obtained after 6 weeks of age.

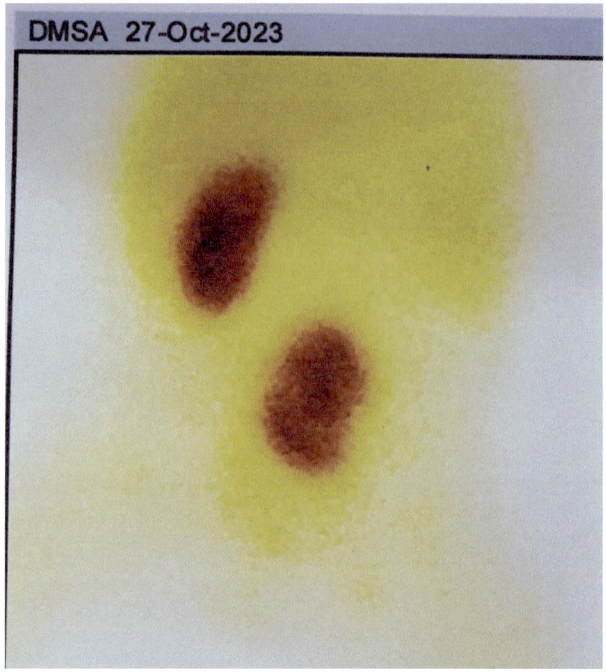

Fig. 9.17 Preoperative radionuclear scan for the upper tract showing ectopic location of the left kidney

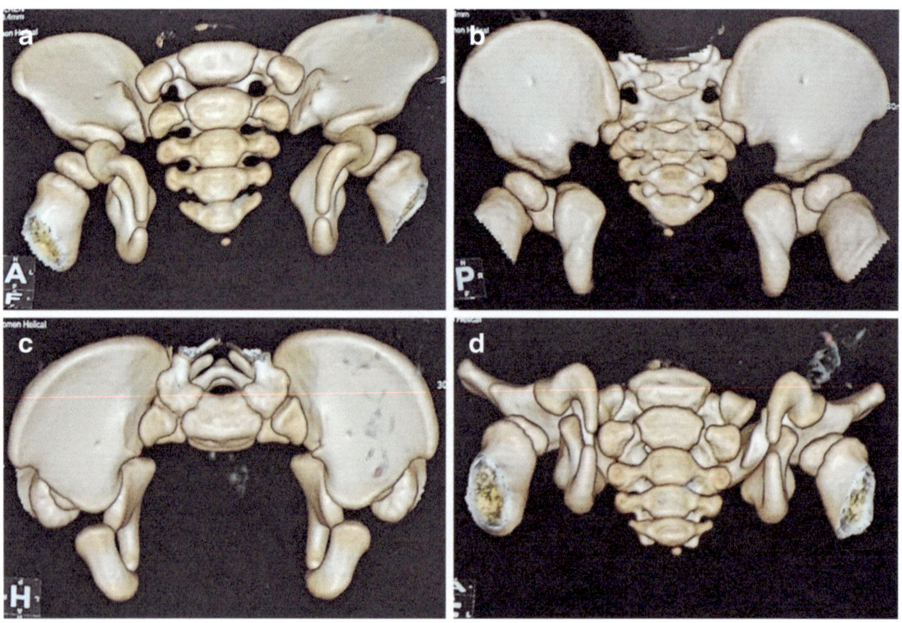

Fig. 9.18 Preoperative CT pelvis volume rendered image. (**a**) Anterior view, (**b**) posterior view, (**c**) superior view, and (**d**) perineal view showing complete perineal configuration

A mild laxative 12 hours prior to surgery and a digital rectal examination before shifting the patient into the operating room ensure an empty rectum at the time of surgery.

Anesthesia

General anesthesia with relaxant is administered with lines for measurement of blood pressure, central venous pressure, probes for temperature maintenance with $ETCO_2$ monitoring with continuous ECG monitoring. An epidural catheter is placed for postoperative analgesia.

Patient Positioning and Draping

The patient is placed in a supine position. The thighs up to the knee joints are draped in sterile leggings, and the rectum is packed with sterile roller gauze. The sterile drapes are anchored in the midline to the base of the urogenital triangle.

Incision

At the level of the transtubercular line, a midline trapezoid flap is marked for umbilicoplasty [8] (Fig. 9.19a). Incision lines are drawn along the ventral midline from the tip of the trapezoid flap to the bladder plate and from here along the margin of the bladder plate up to the bladder neck (Fig. 9.19a, b). From the bladder neck, incision lines are drawn along the margin of the urethral plate up to the tip of the glans on both sides (Fig. 9.19b).

Stay sutures are placed lateral to the margin of the urethral plate at the tip of the glans. Feeding tubes are placed in ureteric orifices and connected to a reservoir for urine output measurement.

The edge of the prepuce is marked and held with stay sutures (Fig. 9.19c). The median raphe of scrotum from the base of the urogenital triangle and the median raphe of penile skin up to the edge of the prepuce are also marked (Fig. 9.19d).

Bladder Plate Mobilization

Using fine needle-tip cautery, the umbilicoplasty flap is raised. A plane is developed in the subcutaneous plane superficial to the anterior rectus sheath by passing long artery forceps down to the pubic bone on both sides (Fig. 9.20a, b). Vesicocutaneous continuity is disrupted with the help of fine needle-tip cautery up to the bladder neck and root of the penis (Fig. 9.20c).

Near the root of the penis, the penile dartos is carefully dissected off to expose the root of the corpora (Fig. 9.20d).

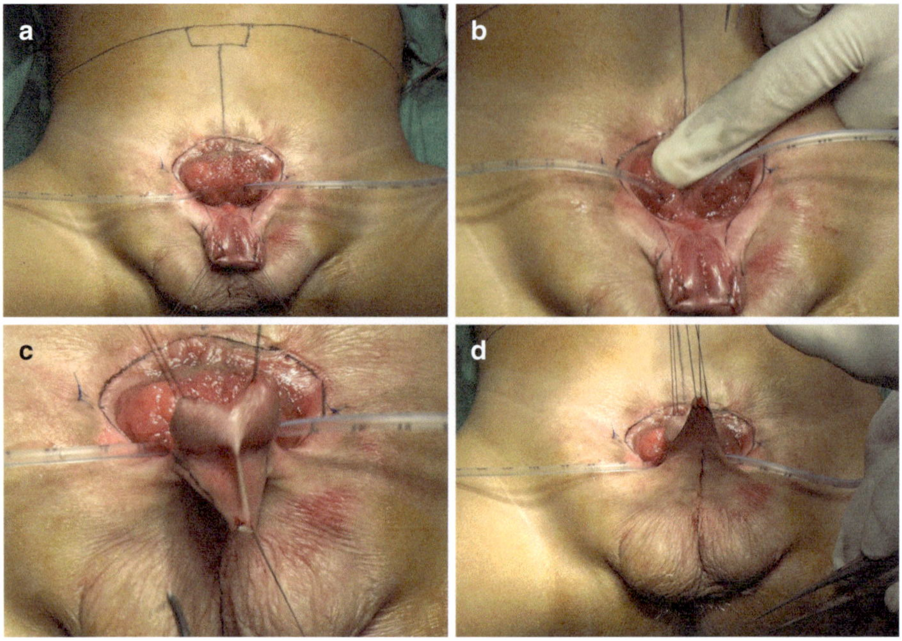

Fig. 9.19 (**a**) Incision plan including incision for trapezoid umbilicoplasty flap at the level of transtubercular line, incision along the bladder plate, and incision along the urethral plate; (**b**) Close-up view of incision line at proximal urethra and the glans. (**c**) Incision line along the preputial edge. (**d**) Scrotoperineal view showing the incision line along the median raphe

Along the medial edge of the rectus abdominis muscle, the continuity of anterior rectus sheath to linea alba is disrupted down to the pubic tubercle to expose the posterior rectus sheath on both sides (Fig. 9.21a).

Below the arcuate line, where extraperitoneal fat and loose areolar tissue are present, an extraperitoneal plane is easily created with the help of a roller gauze (Fig. 9.21b).

This plane is maintained, keeping the obliterated umbilical artery toward the bladder plate to mobilize the bladder plate (Fig. 9.21c).

The peritoneum is swept off till the ureterovesical junction without disturbing the autonomic neural plexus along the periureteric sheath. At this point, the vas deferens can also be seen (Fig. 9.21d).

While the area of the bladder dome can be mobilized in this extraperitoneal plane, complete mobilization of the plate needs division of intersymphyseal bands, which is to be done after exposure of the urogenital diaphragm.

Exposure of Urogenital Diaphragm

Four pairs of stay sutures are placed on both sides of the median raphe at the penoscrotal junction, anterior surface of the scrotum, posterior surface of the scrotum, and one in between. Exerting traction and countertraction across the stay sutures,

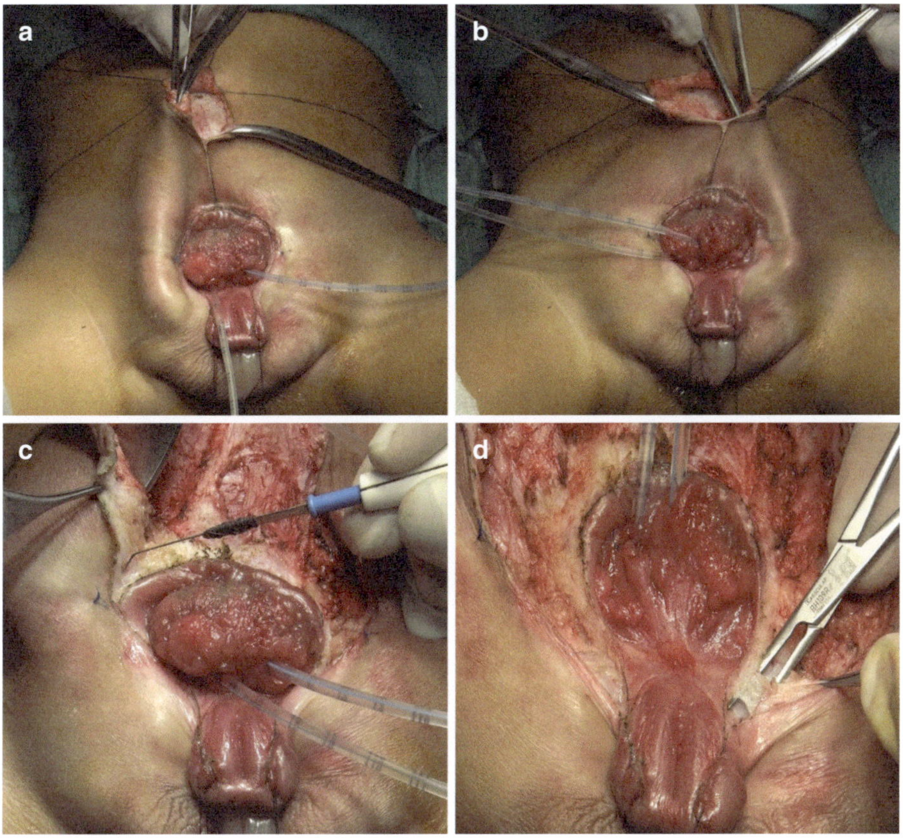

Fig. 9.20 (**a**, **b**) through the window of the umbilicoplasty flap in the subcutaneous plane; the prefascial plane is developed down to the pubic bone on both sides of the bladder plate; (**c**) vesicocutaneous continuity is disrupted with needle tip cautery; (**d**) near the root of the penis, subcutaneous tissue (penile dartos) is carefully dissected and divided, sparing the underlying root of corpora with neurovascular bundle

the scrotal septum is bisected precisely in the midline with needle tip cautery (Fig. 9.22a). Here, an avascular plane is visible as a 0.5 mm wide white line (Fig. 9.22b). The scrotal septal vessels lateral to the midline plane are seen and preserved to maintain clear visibility of the urogenital diaphragm.

The dissection along the white line is continued over the median raphe of penile skin and prepuce. The penile dartos is bisected precisely in the midline over the loose areolar tissue covering Buck's fascia. The axial vessels of penile skin dartos strips can be seen here on both sides of the midline (Fig. 9.22c).

Near the root of the penis on both sides of the midline, an avascular subdartos plane is created (Fig. 9.22d).

The dissection along the edge of the prepuce is started, separating the inner preputial skin from the outer skin, keeping the preputial dartos toward the outer preputial and penile skin. This separation is continued to the subcoronal sulcus on the

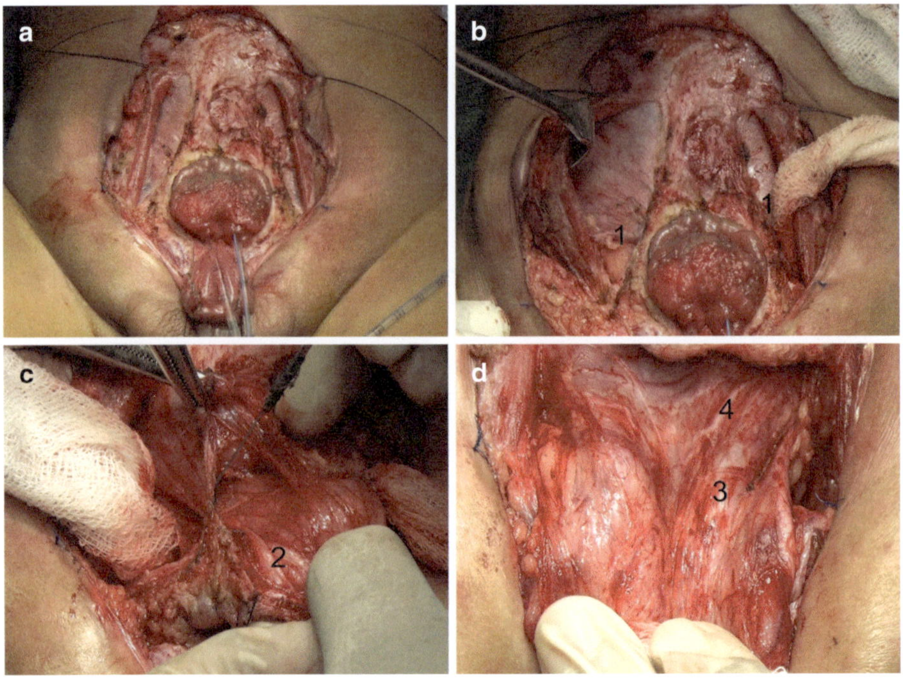

Fig. 9.21 (**a**) Along the medial edge of rectus, continuity of anterior rectus sheath to linea alba is disrupted down to the pubic tubercle; (**b**) below the (1) arcuate lines, the extraperitoneal plane is created by roller gauze packing; (**c**) the bladder plate is mobilized in extraperitoneal plane, keeping (2) umbilical artery toward bladder plate. (**d**) Complete sweeping of peritoneum up to (3) uretero-vesical junction and (4) vas with spared autonomic neural plexus

ventral side and to the urethral plate margins dorsolaterally on both sides (Fig. 9.23a, b). Ventral penile skin dartos are bifurcated in the midline to create strips of penile skin dartos complex (Fig. 9.23c).

Proximally in the middle of the corpora, disruption of vascular connectivity between the neurovascular bundle and axial vessels of the penile skin-dartos complex is needed for complete lateral reflection of the penile skin-dartos complex (Fig. 9.23d).

The dissection in the avascular subdartos plane on the ventral aspect of the corpora is continued proximally, taking care to avoid invading the bulb of the urethra in the midline and the tunica albuginea of the corpora bilaterally (Fig. 9.24a). Dissection with fine needle tip cautery in the same avascular plane will expose the bulbospongiosus muscle in the midline and ischiocavernosus muscle at the root of corpora (Fig. 9.24b). On the medial aspect of the ischiocavernosus muscle, the safe innervation-preserving plane is identified as shown in Fig. 9.24c, d. The posterior scrotal vessels are identified and preserved while exiting the safe plane.

For better delineation of the anterior edge of the ischiopubic ramus, the fascia on the muscles of the adductor compartment adjacent to the ischiopubic ramus is reflected (Fig. 9.25a, b).

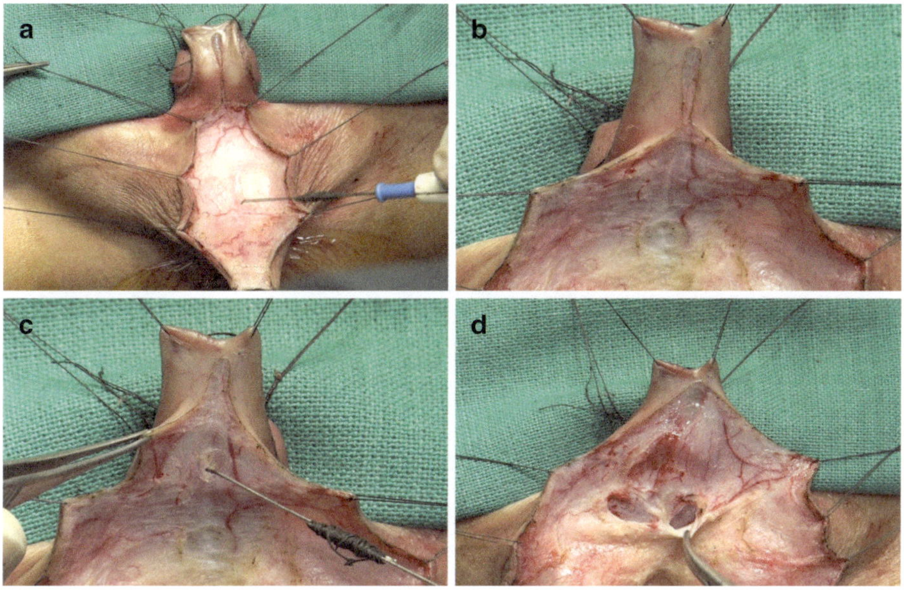

Fig. 9.22 (**a**) The scrotal septum is being bisected in midline avascular plane, (**b**) which is visible as a white line in midline, (**c**) axial vessels of penile skin dartos are seen on both sides of the midline, and (**d**) near the root of the penis, an avascular subdartos plane is created on both sides of the midline

The course of the neurovascular bundle can now be visualized on the dorsolateral aspect of the corpora all the way proximally to the edge of the pubic ramus. The intersymphyseal band is identified between the bladder plate margin and pubic bone, above and adjacent to the corpora and neurovascular bundle. The band is lifted over an artery forceps and released on both sides till the anterior edge of the levator ani muscle is visible (Fig. 9.26a, b). This completes the bladder mobilization.

Radical Corporal Detachment

With fine needle tip cautery, the periosteum along the anterior edge of the ischiopubic ramus is incised, taking care not to invade the adjacent corpora. On the medial border of the pubic bone, a U-shaped incision is made over the periosteum of the anterior and posterior aspects of the pubic bones (Fig. 9.27a). A controlled, forceful downward push with a mounted swab will separate the corporal body off the ischiopubic ramus in the subperiosteal plane without any insult to the neurovascular bundle (Fig. 9.27b–d).

Complete radical detachment of corpora cavernosa will also expose the anterior edge of the levator ani muscle, obturator surface of obturator internus muscle, and medial aspect of ischial tuberosity, as shown in Fig. 9.27d. At this stage, the osteotomy is planned.

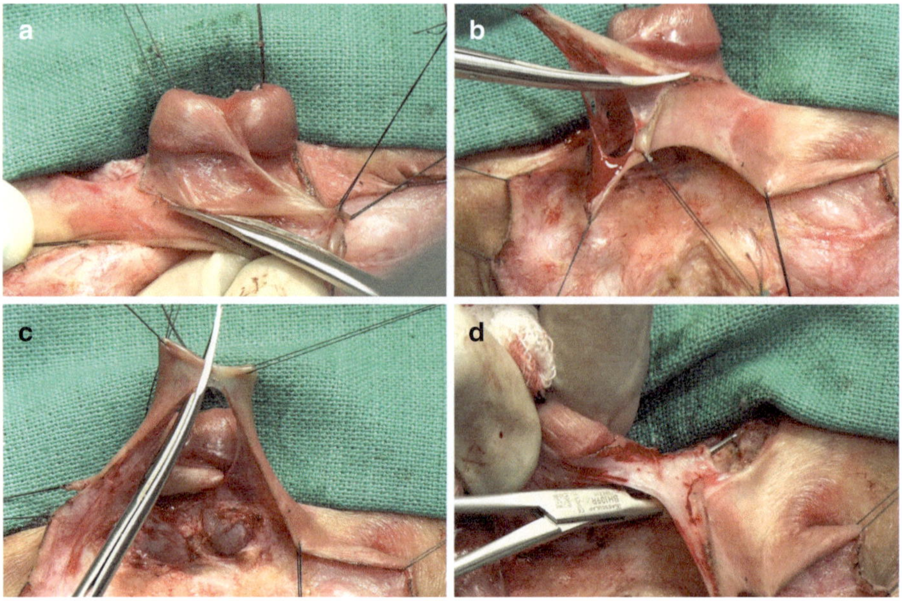

Fig. 9.23 (**a**, **b**) Inner preputial skin is split off outer preputial skin dartos up to subcoronal sulcus; (**c**, **d**) ventral penile skin-dartos complex is bifurcated in the midline and reflected laterally after disconnecting tiny bridging vessels from the neurovascular bundle

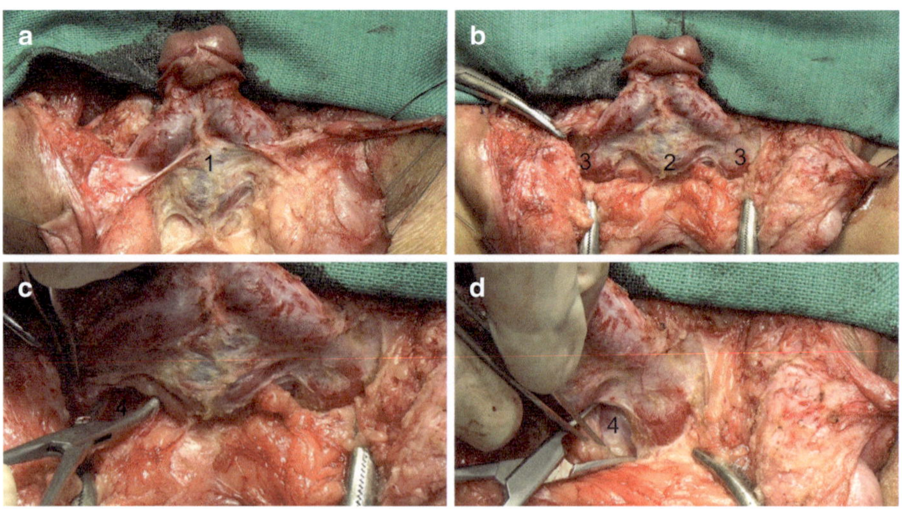

Fig. 9.24 (**a**) Staying in the subdartos plane, continued dissection exposes the (1) bulb of the penis and tunica albuginea of corpora; (**b**) Further dissection exposes (2) bulbospongiosus muscle and (3) ischiocavernosus muscle; (**c**, **d**) close views showing the (4) safe plane

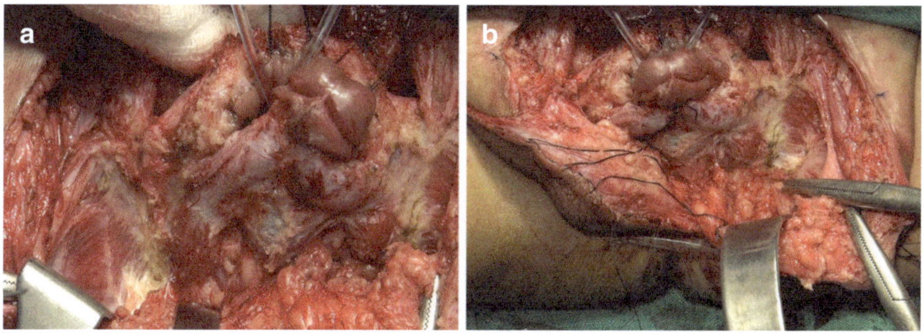

Fig. 9.25 (**a**, **b**) Fascia on the muscle of the adductor compartment adjacent to the ischiopubic ramus is reflected for precise delineation of the anterior edge of the ischiopubic ramus

Fig. 9.26 (**a**, **b**) The intersymphyseal band is lifted on artery forceps and released up to the anterior edge of the levator ani muscle

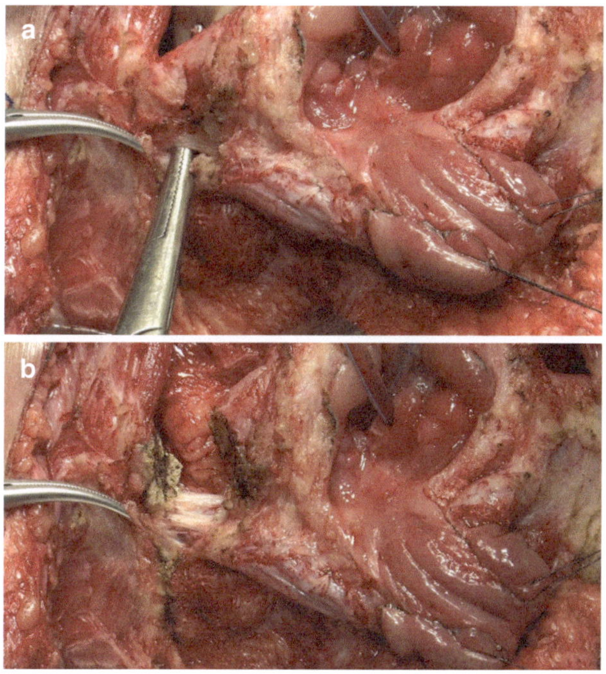

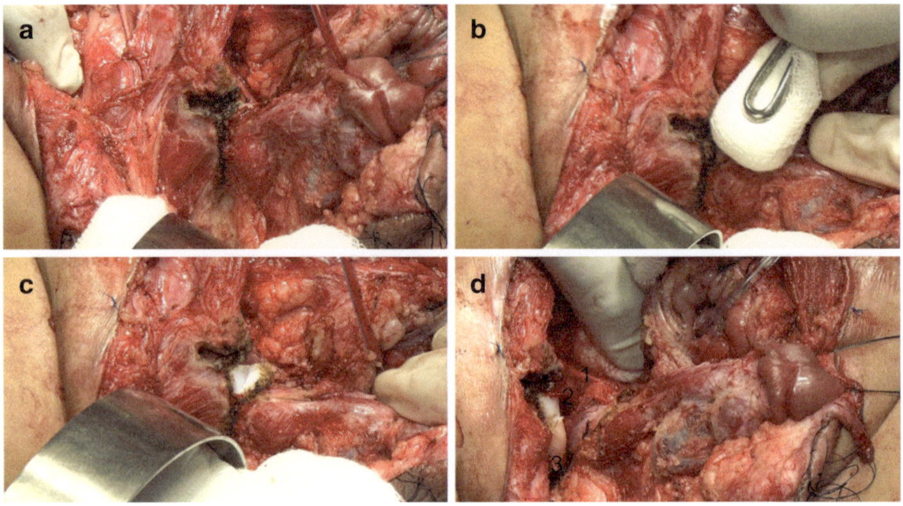

Fig. 9.27 (**a**) Periosteum along the anterior edge of the ischiopubic ramus and medial border of pubic bone is incised, (**b**) a forceful downward push with a mounted swab, (**c**) the subperiosteal plane of radical corporal detachment is created, and (**d**) radical corporal detachment is completed, exposing (1) levator muscle, (2) obturator internus muscle, and (3) medial aspect of ischial tuberosity

Osteotomy

At our center, osteotomy is an essential step of exstrophy repair to bring pubic bones toward the midline and facilitate midline closure of the linea alba and rectus muscle over the reconstructed bladder. The choice of osteotomy can be either ischiopubic osteotomy or transverse innominate osteotomy, depending on the extent of the gap between the pubic bones and the shape of the urogenital diaphragm.

Ischiopubic Osteotomy

Ischiopubic osteotomy is selected in those cases where the urogenital diaphragm is trapezoid or square and the interpubic distance is not very wide. Sites of ischiopubic osteotomy on the superior pubic ramus and ischial tuberosity are shown in Fig. 9.28a. A notch is made on the exposed medial aspect of the ischial tuberosity using a bone drill (Fig. 9.28b). Superior and inferior flaps of periosteum are reflected on the pelvic surface of the superior pubic ramus, above the obturator canal. The superior pubic ramus is cut transversely through and through with a bone drill (Fig. 9.28c). The pubic bones can now be approximated toward the midline using a bone approximator (Fig. 9.28d). Partial tenotomy of adductor longus muscle attachment toward the pubis on both sides further facilitates midline approximation of pubic bones and helps prevent recurrent pubic bone diastasis.

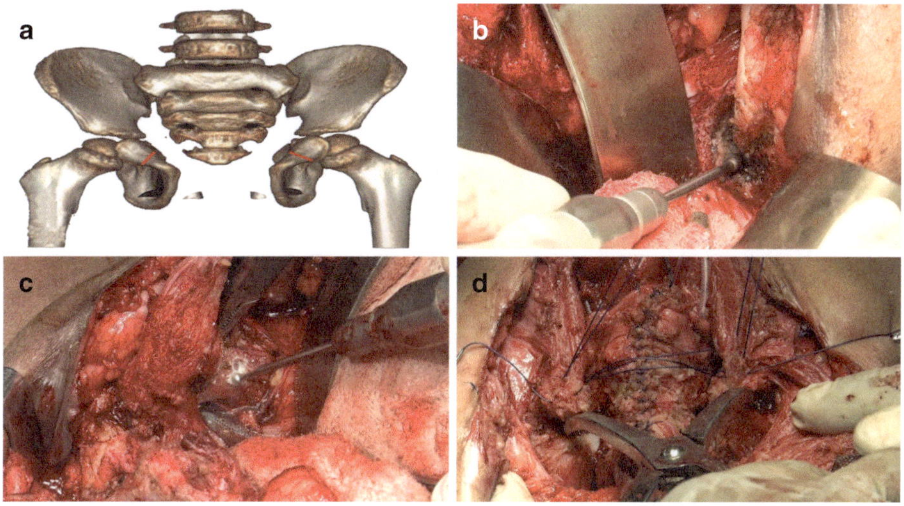

Fig. 9.28 (**a**) Three-dimensional CT image of bony pelvis showing the site of bone cut on superior pubic ramus; a wedge of bone removed from the medial aspect of ischial tuberosity is shown. (**b**) Operative picture showing creation of a notch on medial aspect of ischial tuberosity (left side) with the help of a bone drill. (**c**) Operative picture showing the cutting of superior pubic ramus (right side) with the help of a bone drill above the obturator canal. (**d**) Bone-holding forceps are used to bring pubic bones toward midline. Sutures (1/0 polygalactin) are preplaced

Transverse Innominate Osteotomy

In cases with a rectangular-shaped urogenital diaphragm and a very wide gap between pubic bones, a transverse innominate osteotomy is preferred without any additional skin incision. The line of osteotomy extends from the greater sciatic notch to the anterior inferior iliac spine (Fig. 9.29a, b). A roller gauze packing medial to the greater sciatic notch before cutting the bone displaces the sciatic nerve medially and provides a cushion between the greater sciatic notch and the sciatic nerve. This maneuver prevents the possibility of osteotome-induced injury to the sciatic nerve. Pubic bone approximation is done with two or three sutures of 1-0 or number 1 polygalactin. The radical corporal detachment done earlier prevents the inevitable retraction of the penis when the pubic bones are approximated.

With either osteotomy, there is no need for external fixators, limb immobilization, or plaster casts.

Corporal-Urethral Separation

Safe corpora-urethral separation with preservation of the neurovascular bundle and sphincteric branch of the perineal nerve, bulb of the urethra, periprostatic plexus, cavernous nerve, vascularity of corpus spongiosum and urethral plate, and

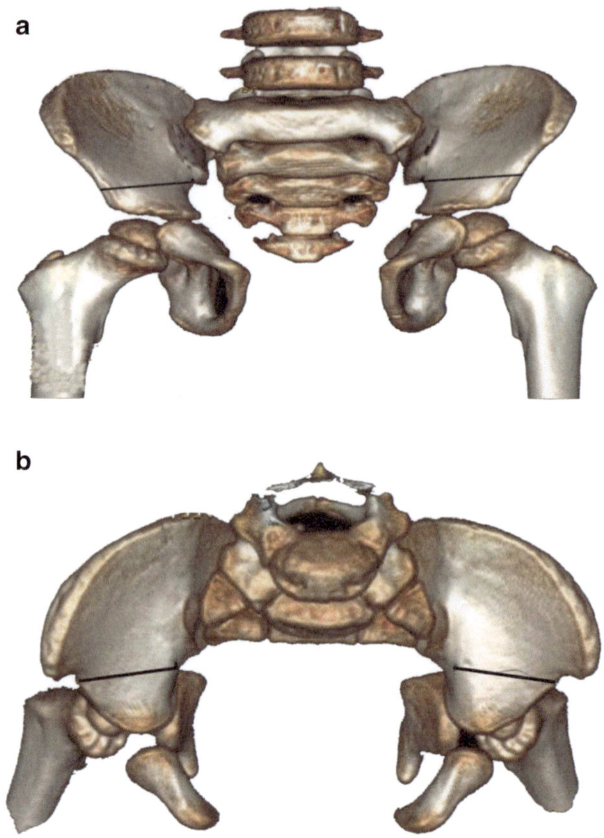

Fig. 9.29 (**a**, **b**) Three-dimensional CT image of bony pelvis showing the line of osteotomy from greater sciatic notch to anterior inferior iliac spine

vascularity of the corpus cavernosa and glans is the key to further reconstruction for continence.

Staying in the subfascial plane of Buck's fascia medial to the neurovascular bundle and lateral to the margin of the urethral plate, corpora are separated off the central wedge of corpus spongiosum and urethral plate (Fig. 9.30a, b).

Proximally, the dissection continues in the safe plane, preserving the innervation of the rhabdosphincter, and the corpora are separated off the external urethral sphincter, bulb, posterior urethra, bladder neck, and periprostatic plexus (Fig. 9.30c, d).

Reconstruction

An area vertically between the ureteric orifice and verumontanum with width equal to the width of the proximal urethral plate at verumontanum is marked for the bladder neck. Lateral triangular mucosal patches from the margin of the bladder neck are excised on both sides as shown in Fig. 9.31a.

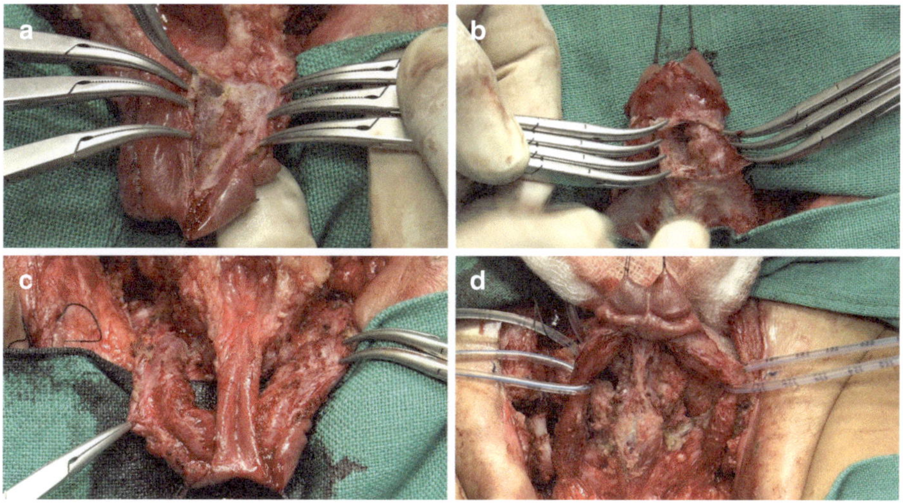

Fig. 9.30 (**a**) The subfascial plane entered medial to neurovascular bundle and lateral to urethral plate margin; a wedge of corpus spongiosum is separated off the medial aspect of corpora cavernosa. (**b**) Working in the subfascial plane from the ventral side, dissection continues to enter the plane created from the dorsal side. (**c**) Working in the subfascial plane on corpora toward bladder neck; posterior urethra, bulb, and bladder neck are separated off the corpora, preserving the vessels and periprostatic plexus. (**d**) On the ventral side, working in the safe plane, both limbs of the bulbospongiosus and adjacent external urethral sphincter are separated off the corpora with preserved innervation

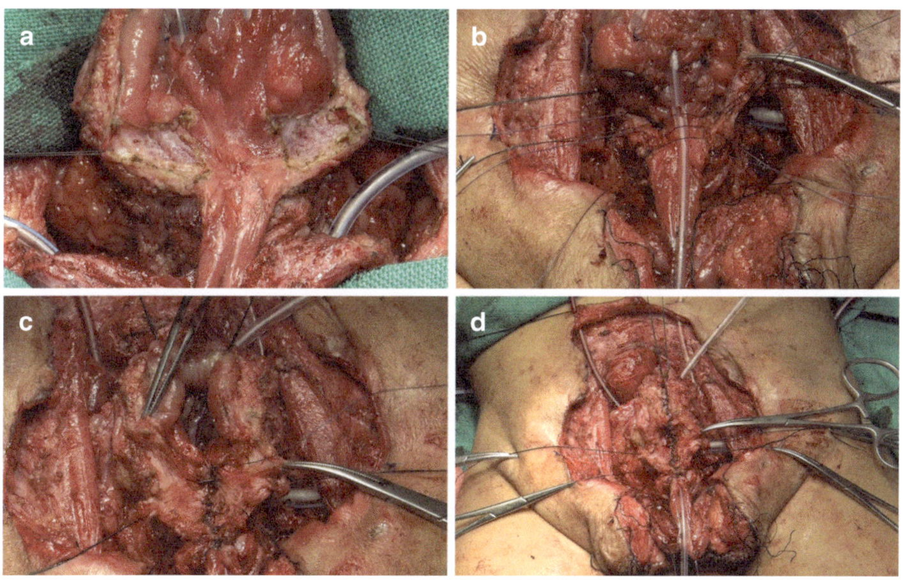

Fig. 9.31 (**a**) A triangular mucosal patch from the bladder plate margin is excised, keeping area of width equal to posterior urethra length between ureteric orifices and verumontanum, (**b**, **c**) 4/0 polygalactin sutures are placed across the bladder over the feeding tube and tied off for anatomical bladder neck reconstruction, and (**d**) the bladder is closed with ureteric stent, vesical stent, and urethral stent in place

If bladder capacity permits, ureters are mobilized and reimplanted either in a submucosal or extramucosal fashion [14, 15].

In preparation for anatomical bladder neck reconstruction without double breasting, three or four 4-0 polygalactin sutures are placed across the urethral plate over an 8 or 10 French feeding tube, incorporating the denuded detrusor at the bladder neck and tying it off (Fig. 9.31b, c) [16]. The bladder is closed with tubes for urethral drainage, bladder drainage, and bilateral ureteral drainage (Fig. 9.31d). Glansplasty is done by maintaining coronal alignment and fashioning a slit-like meatus after urethral tubularization (Fig. 9.32a).

The open limbs of the rhabdosphincter on both sides are anchored to the tubularized urethra, and the corpora are approximated in the midline dorsally (Fig. 9.32b, c).

Three sutures of polygalactin number 1-0 or number 1 are now placed across the cartilage of the pubic bone (Fig. 9.32d). A retropubic drain is placed, and the pubic bones and recti are approximated in the midline (Fig. 9.33a). The umbilicoplasty flap is tubularized, and the lowermost abdominal crease is approximated (Fig. 9.33b). The skin cover is completed by dorsal midline approximation of the bifurcated penile skin dartos and distal suturing to the dorsal subcoronal collar (Fig. 9.34a). A penoscrotal angle is created (Fig. 9.34b). Reverse advancement of the inner preputial skin provides cover to the ventral surface as shown in Fig. 9.34c. Lateral edges of inner preputial flaps and outer preputial skin strips are sutured (Fig. 9.34d). The scrotal median raphe is re-approximated (Fig. 9.35).

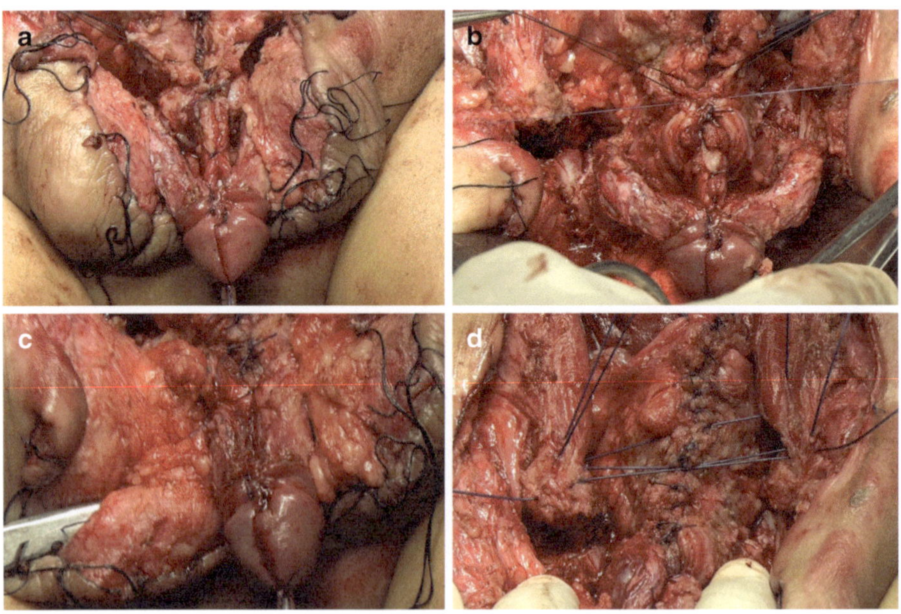

Fig. 9.32 (**a**) Glansplasty maintaining corporal alignment. (**b**) Open limbs of rhabdosphincter on both sides anchored to tubularized urethra. (**c**) Corpora approximated dorsal to tubularized urethra. (**d**) Polygalactin sutures preplaced across pubic bones

Fig. 9.33 (**a**) Pubic bones and recti approximated in the midline, (**b**) Umbilicoplasty flap tubularized and lower abdominal skin crease is aligned

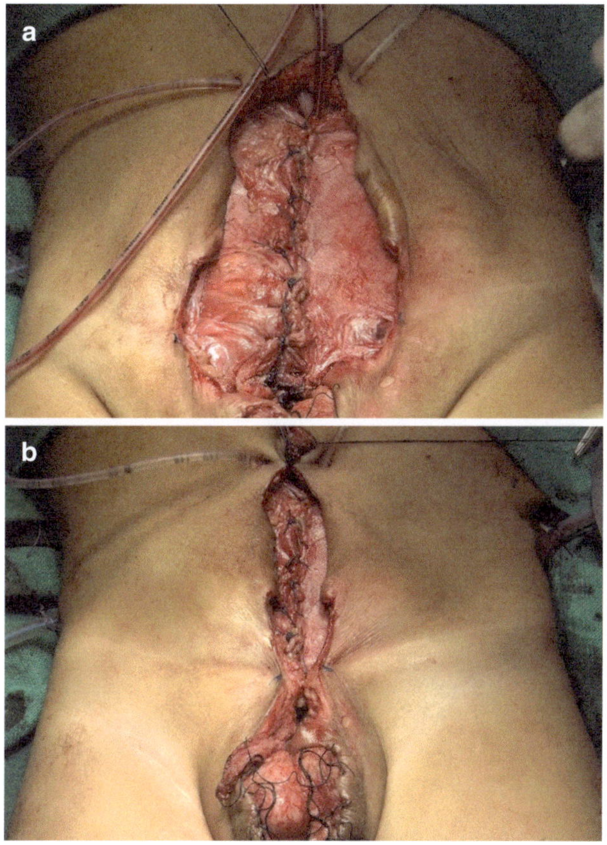

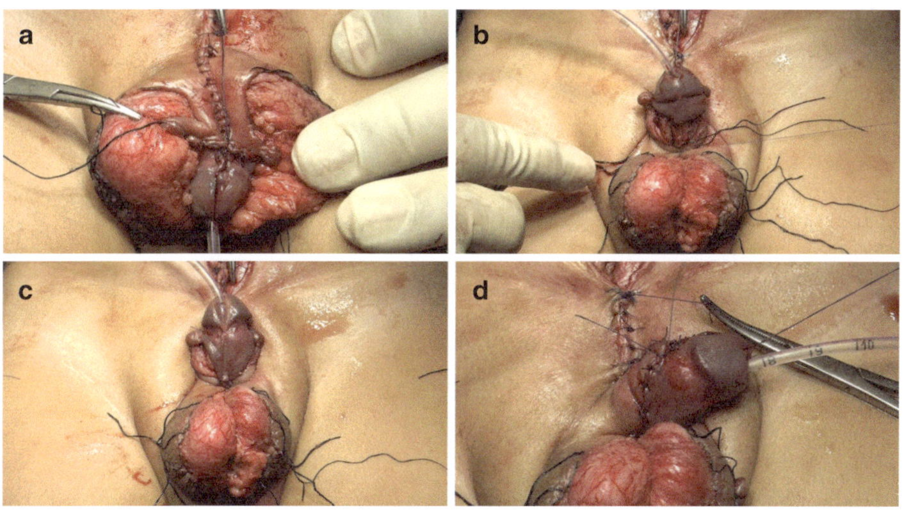

Fig. 9.34 (**a**) Bifurcated penile skin-dartos flaps approximated in dorsal midline providing dorsal cover to penile shaft, (**b**) Penoscrotal angle is created on ventral side, (**c**) Reverse advancement of inner preputial skin to provide ventral skin cover, (**d**) Joining the edges of dorsal and ventral flaps completes the penile skin cover

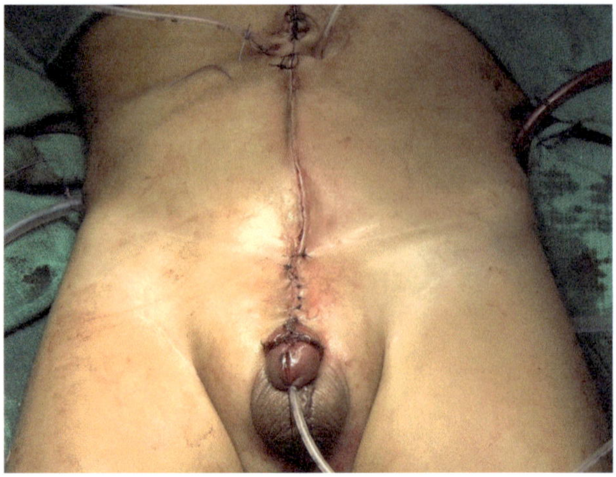

Fig. 9.35 Abdominal skin and scrotal skin reapproximated in midline

Postoperative Management

Postoperative analgesia is maintained by bupivacaine via epidural catheter as and when needed.

Ureteric catheters are removed by 12–14 days; suprapubic catheter is removed by day 18–19; and 48 hours after that, the urethral catheter is removed. Broad-spectrum injectable antibiotics are used for 10 days. After removal of the urethral catheter, spontaneous voiding occurs. In rare cases, the patient may need a sitz bath for 1–2 days.

Postoperative penopubic fistula occurs in about 50% of cases but usually heals spontaneously except for 1–2% who need repair after 6 months.

Follow-Up

Follow-up evaluation at 3 months, 6 months, and then yearly includes ultrasound for upper tract dilatation or thickening of the bladder and post-void residual urine volume. Yearly evaluation of serum creatinine and GFR is done and compared with preoperative baseline values. Continent patients who present with increased frequency are evaluated for urinary tract infection (UTI) with urine microscopy and culture and treated accordingly. An urodynamic study is done for the evaluation of bladder pressure. Based on the clinical status and urodynamic findings, oxybutynin and imipramine may be used to improve continence and preserve the upper tract by relaxing the bladder. Chemoprophylaxis is prescribed for those in whom antireflux surgery could not be done due to bladder plate condition.

Results

From 2004 to 2024, 241 cases of exstrophy-epispadias complex, ranging in age from 6 weeks to 24 years, were operated on. These included 173 male and 68 female patients. Out of these, 123 male patients with classical exstrophy and a good bladder plate underwent single-stage total reconstruction using a midline scrotoperineal approach with radical corporal detachment, innervation-preserving sphinctero-plasty, and bladder neck repair. Ureteric reimplantation was done whenever the supratrigonal area was not studded with multiple polyps. Forty cases of incontinent epispadias with good bladder capacity on cystogram (>60 ml) were also managed with the same protocol.

Ninety patients with a trapezoid-shaped urogenital diaphragm on 3-D CT pelvis received ischiopubic osteotomy, while 33 patients in whom the urogenital diaphragm was rectangular or square with a very wide gap between the pubic bones received transverse innominate osteotomy.

The outcome parameters assessed were:

1. Intraoperative complications
2. Immediate postoperative complications
3. Late complications
4. Urinary continence at 5-year follow-up
5. Upper tract status
6. Cosmetic outcome

1. *Intraoperative Complications*

   The transverse perinei muscle was found to be absent in seven patients. In one of these patients, minor invasion of the anterior wall of the rectum occurred, which was identified and repaired without subsequent complications.

   After approximation of pubic bone, compression of the corpora cavernosa was noted in three patients, which was identified intraoperatively, and the lowermost approximation suture of pubic bone was released to relieve the compression.

   After corporal-urethral separation, the urethral plate was usually adequate to take the meatus to the tip; however, in four patients, an unstretchable urethral plate mandated its division and the creation of a hypospadiac meatus.
2. *Immediate Postoperative Complications*

   In two patients, reexploration for intestinal obstruction was done around the 7th postoperative day. Postoperative ileoileal intussusception was the culprit, which was reduced, and the further course was uneventful.

   Two patients developed epididymo-orchitis, seven had superficial wound dehiscence, and penopubic fistula developed in 35 patients. All cases healed with conservative management, without the need for intervention.

   Three patients developed a ventral hernia secondary to the disruption of the midline-approximated linea alba; a secondary suturing without using a mesh was undertaken after 6 months. The subsequent appearance of the abdominal wall was normal with no recurrence.
3. *Late Complications*

   Recurrent UTI was noted in 40 patients in whom ureteric reimplantation was not done. After eradication of infection, a micturating cystourethrogram (MCU) revealed bilateral grade 2–3 reflux in all 40 patients. In one of these patients, left renal function as assessed on nuclear scan was reduced, necessitating ureteric reimplantation.

Mild hydroureteronephrosis was noted in 30 patients on follow-up ultrasound. But it was stable, and renal function did not deteriorate. These patients were started on oxybutynin.

There was no case of glans loss or penile loss.

4. *Urinary Continence*

   In 130 patients who have completed at least 5 years of follow-up after the repair, continence was evaluated with a voiding diary, dry interval at nighttime, dry interval at daytime, frequency of voiding, capacity to hold midstream micturition, uroflow, and video recordings of micturition captured on mobile by parents or patients themselves. Out of 130 patients operated on for bladder exstrophy and incontinent epispadias, 96 are continent with a dry interval of more than 2 hours in the daytime and 5 hours at night. Midstream holding and reinitiation of micturition could be demonstrated in 70 patients. Stress incontinence was seen in 60 patients and managed with medication.

5. *Bladder Capacity*

   Bladder capacity as assessed on ultrasound ranged from 80 to 110 ml in patients with dry intervals of more than 2 hours. Bladder capacity measured on MCU (done after eradication of infection in those patients who had recurrent UTI) ranged from 60 to 70 ml.

6. *Upper Tracts*

   Upper tracts were evaluated with follow-up ultrasound for hydronephrosis, bladder capacity, bladder wall thickness, and post-void residual urine volume at 3 months, 6 months, and yearly. A radionuclear scan was obtained yearly and compared with the preoperative baseline. Out of 163, unilateral deterioration of the upper tract was noted in one patient due to vesicoureteric reflux. There was no deterioration in GFR in the other 162 patients. The appearance of new cortical scarring was noted in six of the patients having vesicoureteric reflux, and modification of chemoprophylaxis was needed.

7. *Cosmetic Outcome*

   The aesthetic score was determined on a scale of 0–10, where a normal appearance of the lower abdominal wall and genitalia was scored 10 and boys with unoperated classic bladder exstrophy scored zero. Aesthetic scores ranged from 7 to 8 in 145 patients, while the parents of 18 patients were unsatisfied with the small size of the phallus.

Conclusion

Using the scrotoperineal approach, bladder exstrophy reconstruction can be done in a manner that preserves all the vascularity and innervation, with the creation of a dynamic outlet resistance and low-pressure bladder reservoir. Satisfying aesthetic and functional outcomes can be seen in more than two-thirds of patients.

References

1. Brock J III, O'Neill J Jr. Bladder exstrophy. In: O'Neill J, editor. Pediatric surgery. Philadelphia: WB Saunders; 1998. p. 1709–32.
2. Trendelenberg F. The treatment of ectopia vesicae. Ann Surg. 1906;44:981–9.
3. Gearhart JP, Forschner DC, Jeffs RD, et al. A combined vertical and horizontal pelvic osteotomy approach for primary and secondary repair of bladder exstrophy. J Urol. 1996;155:689–93.
4. Tomaszewski R, Pethe K, Koszutski T. Salter pelvic osteotomy in operative treatment in patients with bladder extrophy. Chir Narzadow Ruchu Ortop Pol. 2010;75:126–8.
5. Sunil K, Kureel SN, Gupta A, et al. IschioPubic osteotomy, a simple and effective technique for pelvic ring closure in repair of classic exstrophy bladder. J Indian Assoc Pediatr Surg. 2018;23(1):27–31.
6. Kureel SN, Gupta A, Kumar S, et al. A novel midline scroto-perineal approach facilitating innervation preserving sphincteroplasty and radical corporal detachment for reconstruction of exstrophy-epispadias. Urology. 2011;78(3):668–74.
7. Kureel SN, Gupta A, Singh CS, et al. A novel skin management scheme in surgery of epispadias undergoing Cantwell-Ransley repair: a technique to improve the aesthetics and minimize complications. Urology. 2013;82(6):1400–4.
8. Kureel SN, Rashid KA, Rawat J. Tubularized trapezoid flap neoumbilicoplasty—simple technique for umbilical reconstruction in bladder exstrophy. Urology. 2009;73(1):70–3.
9. Sponseller PD, Bisson LJ, Gearhart JP, et al. The anatomy of the pelvis in the exstrophy complex. J Bone Joint Surg Am. 1995;77:177.
10. Kanoujia Sunil, et al. Study of variations in configuration of bony pelvis and magnitude of pubic diastasis in exstrophy-epispadias in relation to type of anomaly in spectrum of exstrophy-epispadias complex- a prospective study – thesis submitted and accepted in 2017 for MCh Pediatric Surgery, King George's Medical University, Lucknow.
11. Stec AA, Pannu HK, Tadros YE, et al. Evaluation of the bony pelvis in classic bladder exstrophy using 3 D CT—further insights. Urology. 2001;58:1030.
12. Kureel SN, Gupta A, Gupta RK. Surgical anatomy of urogenital diaphragm and course of its vessels in exstrophy-epispadias. Urology. 2011;78(1):159–63.
13. Kureel SN, Gupta A, Singh CS, et al. Surgical anatomy of penis in exstrophy-epispadias: a study of arrangement of fascial planes and superficial vessels of surgical significance. Urology. 2013;82(4):910–6.
14. Gupta A, Kureel SN, Wakhlu A, et al. Bladder exstrophy: comparison of anatomical bladder neck repair with innervation preserving sphincteroplasty versus Young-Dees-Leadbetter bladder neck reconstruction. J Indian Assoc Pediatr Surg. 2013;18(2):69–73.
15. Gupta A, Kureel SN. Creation of effective antireflux mechanism without creation of submucosal tunnel in surgical correction of vesicoureteric reflux: myth or reality?-an experimental study. J Indian Assoc Pediatr Surg. 2014;19(1):17–21.
16. Sunil K, Gupta A, Chaubey D, et al. Technique of antireflux procedure without creating submucosal tunnel for surgical correction of vesicoureteric reflux during bladder closure in exstrophy. J Indian Assoc Pediatr Surg. 2018;23(2):70–3.

10 Surgical Management of Male Classic Bladder Exstrophy: The Toronto Approach

Joao Luiz Pippi Salle, Rodrigo L. P. Romao, and Michael Chua

Introduction

Bladder exstrophy represents one of the most challenging congenital anomalies within pediatric urology, often requiring multiple, meticulous surgical interventions and experience in order to achieve favorable long-term outcomes. Over the decades, the technique for the initial surgical closure of the exstrophy bladder has evolved, and modifications have been introduced, leading to significant improvements in the management and long-term prognosis of this complex condition.

The Toronto approach emerges as the accumulation of many advancements, aiming to address some of the shortcomings of previous surgical techniques and enhance the quality of life for affected individuals.

Supplementary Information The online version contains supplementary material available at https://doi.org/10.1007/978-3-031-91238-2_10.

J. L. P. Salle
Division of Urology, SickKids Hospital and Co-Director of the Center for Pelvic Reconstruction, Toronto, Canada
e-mail: pippi.salle@sickkids.ca

R. L. P. Romao (✉)
Division of Pediatric Urology, Division of Pediatric General and Thoracic Surgery, Hospital for Sick Children, University of Toronto, Toronto, ON, Canada
e-mail: rodrigo.romao@sickkids.ca

M. Chua
Division of Pediatric Urology, Hospital for Sick Children, University of Toronto, Toronto, ON, Canada
e-mail: michael.chua@sickkids.ca

A. R. Shukla, R. S. Joshi (eds.), *Bladder Exstrophy and Epispadias*, https://doi.org/10.1007/978-3-031-91238-2_10

Historical Context and Early Attempts at Primary Closure

The journey toward the development of effective surgical management for bladder exstrophy began with early attempts at primary closure. These initial endeavors often resulted in poor outcomes, predominantly due to the high incidence of postoperative infections [24]. The complexity of the condition, coupled with limited surgical expertise and technology at the time, contributed to the challenging nature of these early interventions.

Staged Repair and the Jeffs Proposal

Recognizing the limitations of primary closure, Dr. Robert D. Jeffs and Dr. J Cendron proposed a staged repair technique. At the initial primary closure, the approach was characterized by a deliberate decision not to attempt to create urethral resistance, opting instead for an open bladder neck to avoid the potential deterioration of the upper urinary tract [8, 17].

Following this protocol, males underwent epispadias repair around the age of one, followed by continence procedures as they reached school age, usually around 5 years. The treatment of epispadias involved internal rotation to correct dorsal penile curvature and the application of Byars' flaps for skin closure, laying the groundwork for subsequent interventions [25]. The patients remained incontinent until school age, when bladder neck reconstruction, following principles described by Young-Dees-Leadbetter, was performed [4]. They recognized early the importance of developing adequate bladder capacity after the initial primary closure and epispadias repair in order to achieve success [2, 15, 35].

The Mitchell and Grady Proposal: CPRE

Advances in neonatal medical and surgical care stimulated Michael E. Mitchell and Richard W. Grady to propose a simultaneous primary bladder closure and epispadias repair early in life, a procedure they called Complete Primary Repair of Exstrophy (CPRE) [13]. Despite its name, CPRE is almost never "complete," as it often results in hypospadias, which requires at least two additional surgical steps for the urethroplasty [24, 27, 33]. Initially, only minimal attempts to repair the bladder neck were made, a step later modified by the introduction of bladder outlet tailoring in order to increase urethral resistance and enhance bladder capacity [3, 14, 34].

This approach did, however, mirror the staged repair in terms of epispadias treatment and addressing incontinence, if present. A significant concern with CPRE is the risk of penile ischemia due to compartment syndrome; although rare, this is a catastrophic complication [9, 10, 21, 31]. Additionally, some patients experienced upper tract deterioration, particularly those with some degree of urethral resistance and improved bladder capacity. This deterioration can be accompanied by severe vesicoureteral reflux (VUR), hydronephrosis, and symptomatic UTIs [12].

The Toronto Approach: A Staged, Comprehensive Strategy Aiming for Improved Outcomes

The Toronto approach was developed as a modification of the staged repair and in response to some of the issues observed with CPRE.

Bilateral ureteral reimplantation (BUR) is performed at the time of exstrophy closure in a cephalad direction as previously described [7]. Tailoring/funneling of the bladder neck, aimed at generating some degree of early outlet resistance without significant obstruction as observed in patients with the Young-Dees-Leadbetter procedure and increasing the chances of continence in the future, is also undertaken. BUR significantly eliminates or at least downgrades reflux [30], reducing the chances of severe febrile UTIs and protecting the upper urinary tract [16]. Epispadias repair is carried out in a delayed fashion.

This approach prevents complications like penile ischemia seen with CPRE, protects the upper urinary tract, and potentially enhances bladder capacity [10]. Testosterone stimulation is administered before epispadias repair, which is performed later, around 9 months to 1 year of age. Epispadias repair is aimed at correcting the dorsal curvature with external corporal rotation, performing the urethroplasty and penile skin closure using a rotational penile skin flap rather than Byars' flaps, thereby avoiding midline dorsal scars, which can increase chances of recurrent dorsal curvature [26].

Rationale and Strategic Pillars

This approach is predicated on the understanding that bladder exstrophy is not a singular anomaly but a spectrum of disorders affecting the lower urinary tract, anterior abdominal wall, and pelvic bones. Reconstruction has a substantial impact on both lower and upper urinary tract function. The Toronto approach is designed to improve functional and cosmetic outcomes, offering a roadmap for reconstructing the bladder and external genitalia while preserving renal function and achieving urinary continence.

The rationale for early BUR is to provide room for gentle tailoring/funneling of the bladder neck to generate some degree of outflow resistance, following the natural striations observed in this area. Additionally, avoiding VUR reduces the risk of significant febrile UTIs [6, 16, 21]. Furthermore, urine stays in the bladder longer rather than refluxing freely into the upper urinary tract [18]. This coupled with increased outlet resistance potentially improves bladder capacity and continence in the long run [19, 30].

Technical Details and Innovations

Preoperative Assessment and Planning

Preoperative assessment includes baseline imaging studies, such as ultrasound, X-ray, and DMSA scans, to evaluate kidney, bladder, and pelvic bone anatomy. The orthopedic surgery team reviews pelvic X-rays in preparation for pelvic osteotomies.

While the Toronto approach was initially described in the neonatal period, it is currently performed electively, usually around 3–4 months of life. Although there are controversies about prolonged exposure of the bladder plate [1, 20, 22, 28, 36], many centers have switched to an elective surgical approach in recent years based on the following factors: exstrophy closure is not an emergency; the importance of bonding between family and baby allows breastfeeding to be established; take advantage of the early testosterone boost; time to assemble an experienced, consistent multidisciplinary team for surgical management; and increased risk of surgical and anesthetic complications in the neonatal period [29, 32].

Neonates with classic bladder exstrophy are admitted initially, and the bladder plate is covered with a plastic film (Saran Wrap). Prophylactic antibiotics are not given. The baby is allowed to feed early and can usually be discharged after a period of short observation and after the parents have been counseled about the care of the bladder plate and understand the future plans.

Surgical Procedures

First Stage: Bladder Closure, Ureteral Reimplantation, Bladder Neck Repair, Pelvic Osteotomy, Bilateral Inguinal Hernia Repair and Umbilicoplasty

Surgical Intervention, Lateral Dissection, and Approach to the Pubovesical Bands

Initially, the bladder plate characteristics are measured, including the area and depth of the defect, as well as the position of the ureteral orifices and the length of the urethral plate. The presence of polyps and bladder elasticity is documented. Large polyps should be removed.

After carefully incising the mucocutaneous junction, dissection is carried down laterally until the pre-vesical fat is identified on both sides. The dome is then dissected off the peritoneum using sharp and blunt dissection. The ligaments/bands between the urethro-vesical complex and the pubic bones are divided on both sides; this is preceded by proactive identification of the proximal aspect of the neurovascular bundle on either side to avoid its injury (Video 10.1). The future incisions for bladder neck tailoring are outlined with cautery (does not fade away with the manipulation) before proceeding with the ureteral reimplantation (Fig. 10.1).

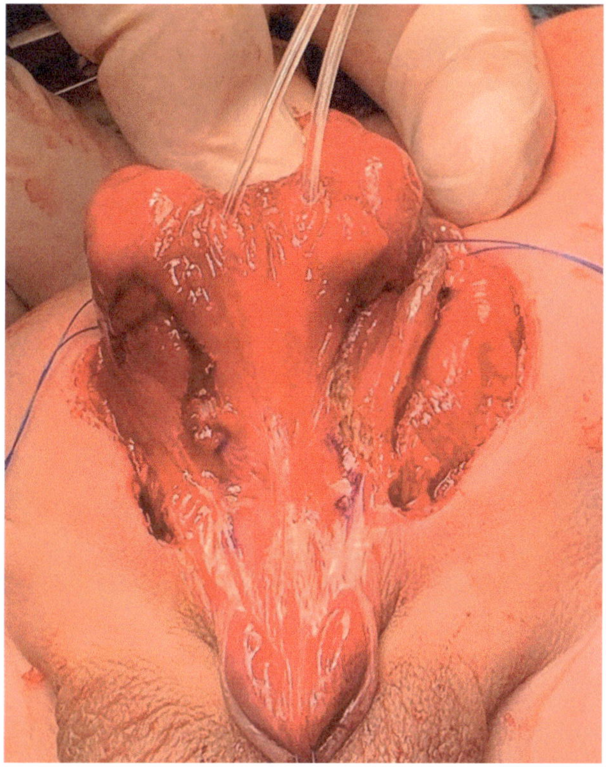

Fig. 10.1 The markings for future bladder neck tailoring

Bilateral Ureteral Advancement Reimplantation

Bilateral ureteral reimplantation is then performed to correct vesicoureteral reflux, a common issue in bladder exstrophy patients. The ureters are dissected circumferentially, and a submucosal tunnel is created in a cephalad direction, as previously described [7]. The anastomosis is performed with a fine, absorbable suture; one of the stitches is anchored to the detrusor for support (Fig. 10.2).

One must ensure that a feeding tube (3.5 or 5fr.) advances easily into the ureter after the reimplantation is completed. In some infants, the stent does not advance to the pelvis due to the presence of ureteral folds, which kink it and cause obstruction. It is essential to have good drainage; therefore, we obtain a retrograde pyelogram to ensure adequate stent position in the renal pelvis. The detrusor and mucosa are reapproximated at the original orifice site. Ureteral stents are inserted and externalized through the lateral bladder wall. They are usually secured in place with a purse-string suture to the bladder wall.

Bladder Neck Tailoring and Repair and Bladder Closure

Following BUR, attention is turned to the bladder neck. The goal is to create a funneled continence mechanism that effectively empties urine, aiming to increase resistance without obstruction. By doing so, there will be an increase in intra-vesical

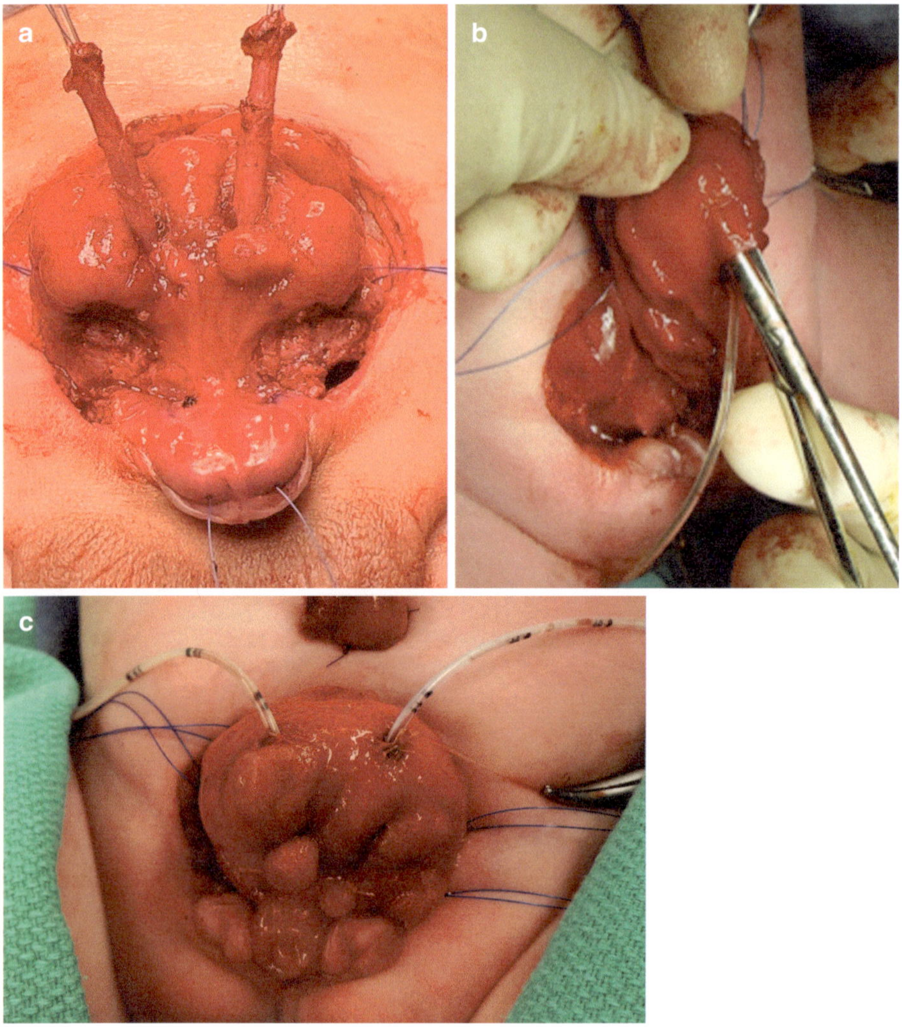

Fig. 10.2 Bilateral ureteral reimplantation at the time of primary exstrophy closure. (**a**) Ureters mobilized for reimplantation. (**b**) Submucosal tunnel developed in a cephalad orientation. (**c**) Reimplanted ureters improving exposure for tailoring and closing the bladder neck

pressure that stimulates bladder growth. This effect is achieved through meticulous reconstruction of the bladder neck, tailoring it following the striations often seen at the future outlet (Figs. 10.3 and 10.4).

The bladder neck is approximated using a long-standing absorbable suture with interrupted sutures over an 8fr urethral catheter. The sutures are laid in without tying to allow good visualization (Fig. 10.5). Each stitch is placed to carefully include a good muscle bite with a small amount of mucosa for apposition. The detrusor overlying lateral areas denuded of the mucosa is released from its attachments and used

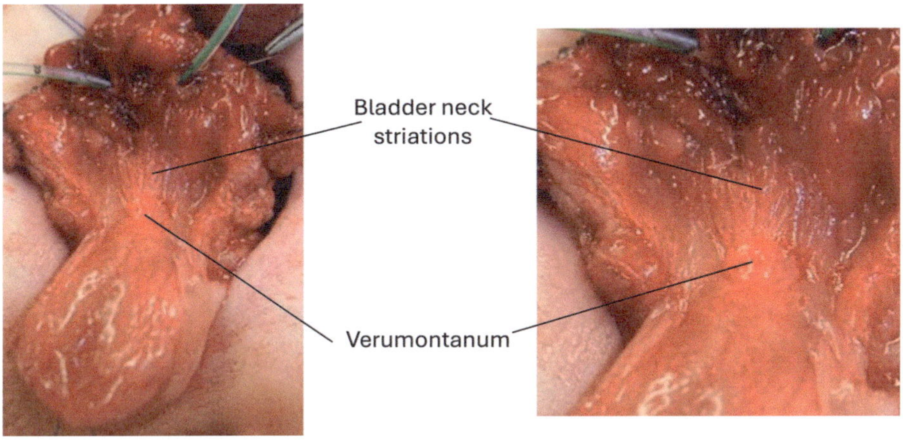

Fig. 10.3 Panoramic and zoomed-in view of the bladder neck striations and verumontanum prior to bladder neck tailoring

Fig. 10.4 Bladder neck tailoring has been marked

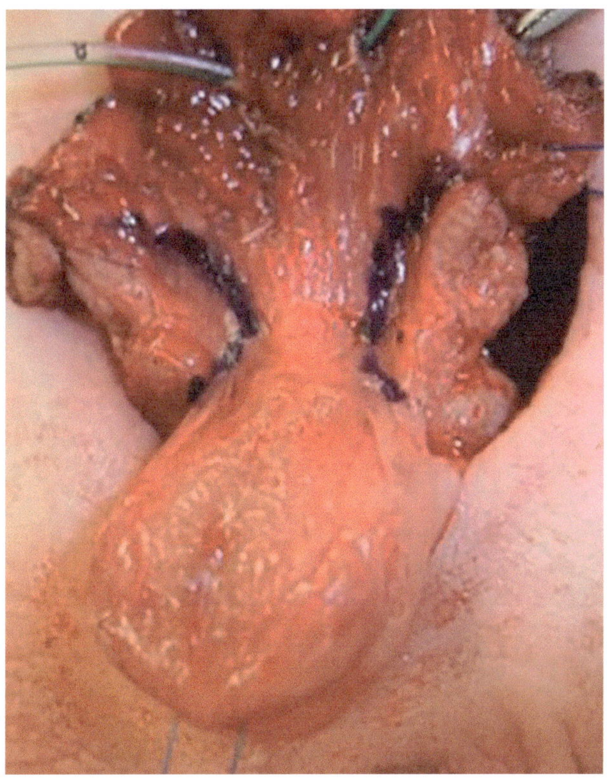

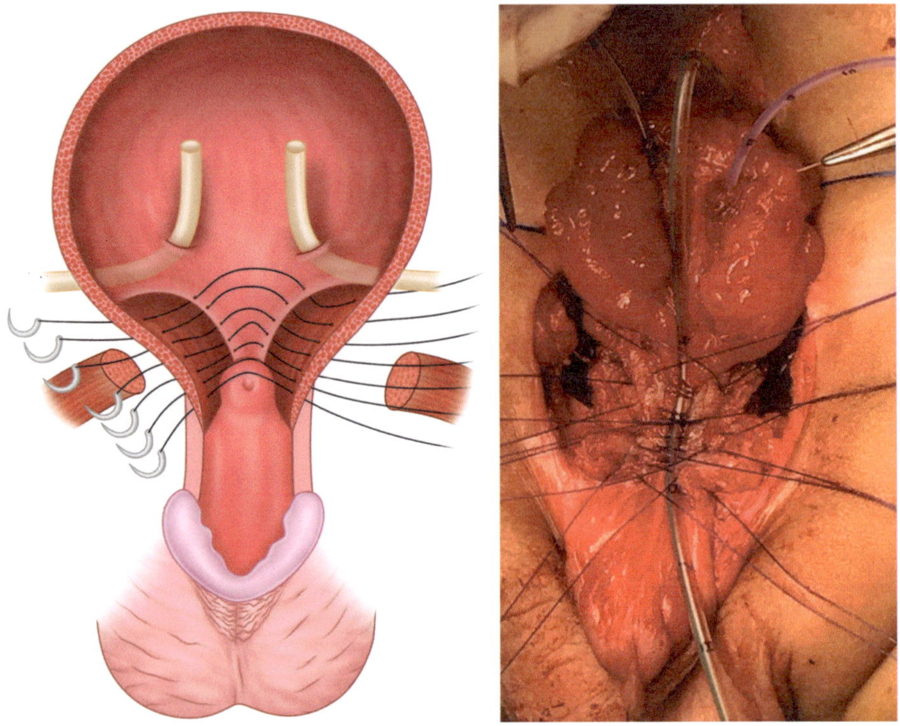

Fig. 10.5 Diagram and intraoperative picture of the bladder neck repair

to cover and reinforce the tailored bladder neck as a second layer (Fig. 10.6 and Video 10.2).

After a suprapubic catheter is inserted, the bladder is closed with interrupted absorbable sutures (Fig. 10.7). During the first surgery, a neo-umbilicoplasty is also performed using a rhomboid skin flap. Bilateral inguinal hernia repairs are routinely performed in boys by undermining the subcutaneous tissue of the original exstrophy incision.

Pelvic Osteotomy

Pelvic osteotomies are performed routinely to bring the pubic bones together in the midline, allowing for deep placement of the bladder in the pelvis and tension-free closure of the abdominal wall. We prefer to utilize bilateral anterior oblique osteotomies as originally described by Salter and modified by Wedge [23]. Infants are kept on modified Bryant's (gallows) traction for 2–3 weeks postoperatively to allow for the osteotomies to heal (Fig. 10.8).

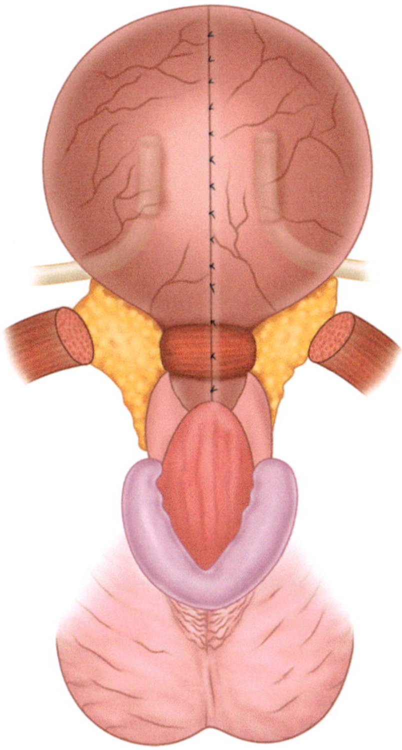

Fig. 10.6 Diagram of the reconstructed bladder neck in two layers and closed bladder

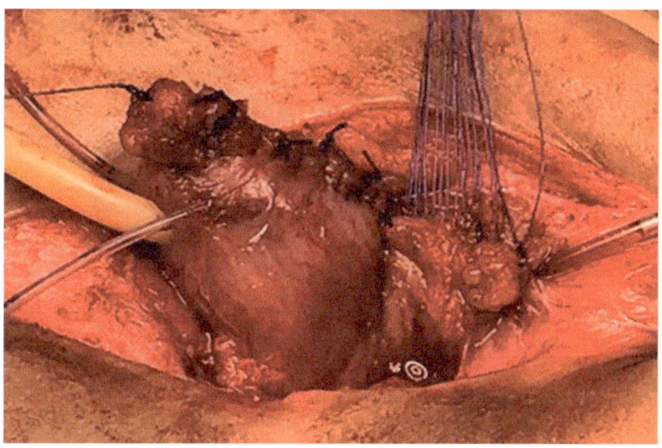

Fig. 10.7 Final aspect of the closed bladder and repaired bladder neck with catheters in place

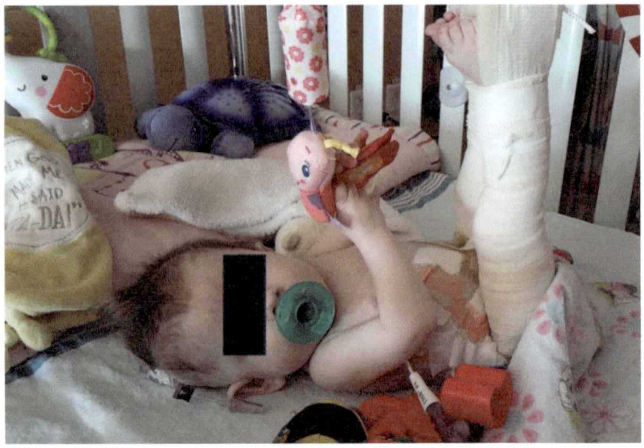

Fig. 10.8 Modified Bryant's traction in a 5-month-old child following classic exstrophy closure

Second Stage Repair: Epispadias Repair and Penile Reconstruction

Preoperative Testosterone Administration

Epispadias and penile reconstruction take place after 9–12 months. Intramuscular injection of testosterone, 2 mg/kg per dose, is administered at 90, 60, and 30 days prior to the epispadias repair.

Epispadias Repair

The repair of epispadias is aimed at correcting the urethral opening and dorsal chordee to achieve a more typical urethral meatus location and a straight penis following bladder closure. The penis is carefully degloved, and initial dissection of the urethra is performed ventrally, separating it entirely from both corpora and allowing it to achieve a ventral position. Both corpora should be dissected until entirely free from the urethra, allowing for natural external rotation when the penis is pulled in a downward direction [35] (Video 10.3). After external rotation, a double layer of interrupted non-absorbable sutures is used to approximate and keep the externally rotated corpora in the midline, both dorsally and ventrally.

The urethroplasty is completed with interrupted absorbable sutures, intended to avoid an accordion effect and allow tissue stretching for the neourethra repair. In most cases, the urethra will reach the tip of the glans or at least a subcoronal location. In some situations where the urethra is too short, it may be necessary to leave it as a hypospadias, which will require further reconstruction. We do not excise the ventral preputial skin when this is anticipated, leaving it available for future staged hypospadias repair.

Penile Skin Reconstruction

Penile skin reconstruction is important, both from functional and cosmetic standpoints. We favor the use of a rotational penile skin flap from the ventral aspect of the penis; this usually provides adequate coverage of the penile shaft (Fig. 10.9). It avoids a dorsal midline scar and ensures a natural appearance with a well-defined

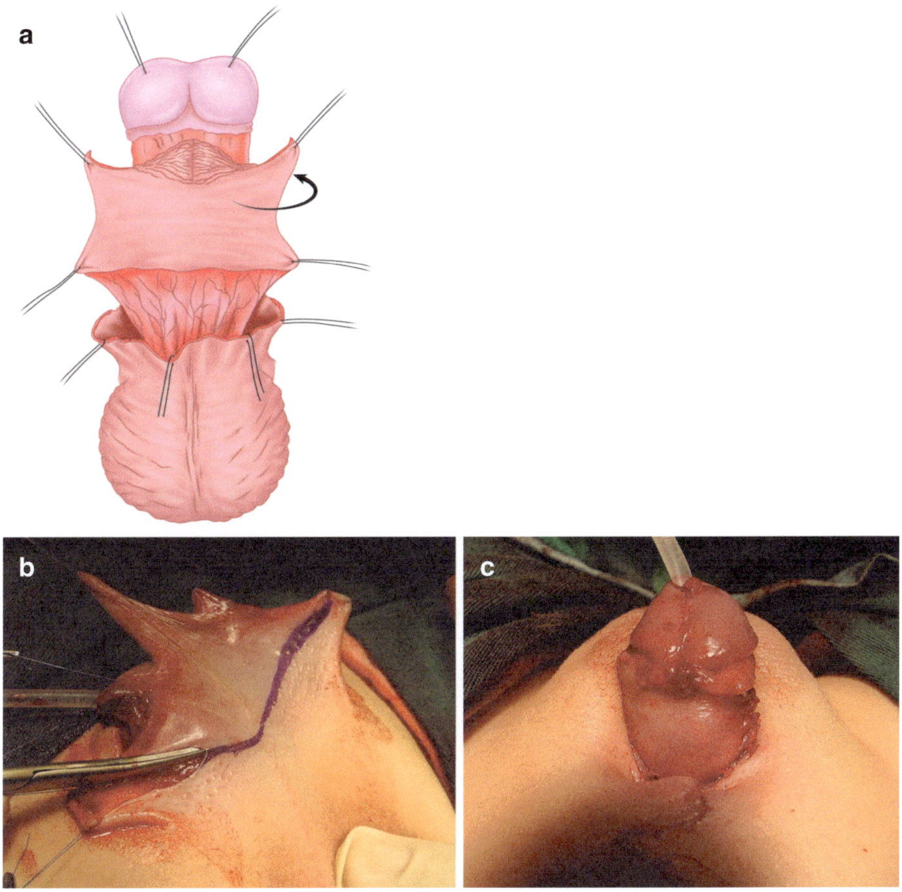

Fig. 10.9 Skin closure after epispadias repair. (**a**) Diagram of the ventral rotational skin flap. (**b**) Harvesting of the skin flap. (**c**) Final aspect of the repair. Note absence of dorsal midline scar

penopubic angle [26]. However, as emphasized above, if the urethra is left as a hypospadias, the ventral prepuce can be left intact for a future staged urethroplasty.

Girls born with exstrophy follow the same principles described for boys except for the genitalia, requiring a feminizing genitoplasty (clitoroplasty—usually approximation of both hemi-clitoris); introitoplasty, Y-V vaginoplasty and monsplasty as described by Pippi Salle [11].

Further Stages: Continence Procedures and Final Touches

Continence Enhancement

Additional procedures may be considered for patients who do not achieve urinary continence following the bladder neck repair. In cases where the bladder neck is not wide open, it is reasonable to attempt its coaptation using bulking materials. Such attempts are more successful when a reasonable bladder capacity is present. We always give the bladder time to develop capacity and, ultimately, continence/dryness with or without intermittent catheterization. Bladder augmentation and neck closure are the last resources that, unfortunately, will be necessary in a proportion of patients [37].

Cosmetic and Functional Refinements

The final stage may also involve cosmetic and functional refinements to the genitalia and bladder, tailored to the individual patient's outcomes from previous surgeries. It is important to achieve an adequate cosmetic appearance of the external genitalia. In many surveys, females resent having a scarred suprapubic area and an abnormal labial appearance [5]. They also care about having a reconstructed umbilicus and a normal mons venus, elements often neglected in the past. This stage is critical for addressing any residual issues and enhancing overall quality of life [11].

Single Institution Experience with the Toronto Approach

Aware of the increased bladder capacities achieved when using the CPRE, we decided to make the modifications described above, aiming to safely maintain these advantages. In 2019, a comparative study was performed at The Hospital for Sick Children (SickKids), aimed at evaluating the outcomes of a single (CPRE) versus a staged (Toronto approach) repair of bladder exstrophy [10]. It is important to note that all patients undergoing CPRE in this series also underwent BUR and bladder neck tailoring, similar to what is performed in the Toronto approach staged repair. A total of 21 patients were analyzed, with 10 undergoing CPRE-BUR and 11 undergoing the Toronto approach.

In terms of intra-operative complications, the CPRE-BUR group experienced two cases (20%) of penile ischemic injury, one of which led to significant tissue loss. In addition, all patients remained with hypospadias, requiring staged oral mucosa urethroplasty later. Penile ischemia was not observed in the Toronto approach group, highlighting its safety profile in preserving penile integrity during surgery. The two groups had similar complications, such as fistulae, strictures, stones, and UTIs.

The study also reported on long-term surgical outcomes and the need for additional procedures. For the CPRE group, 7 out of 10 patients (70%) required further surgical interventions, whereas in the staged Toronto approach group, 6 out of 11 patients (54.5%) underwent additional surgeries. This data suggests a slightly lower, although not statistically significant, rate of additional surgeries in the staged repair group compared to the CPRE group.

The subjective assessment indicated better penile length and cosmetic outcomes in the Toronto approach group, suggesting an advantage in postoperative appearance and patient satisfaction. This finding aligns with the surgical aim to address functional issues and consider the cosmetic outcomes important for the patient's psychological well-being.

In summary, the study presents the Toronto approach as a safer alternative to CPRE-BUR, especially in minimizing the risk of severe intra-operative complications like penile ischemic injury. While long-term outcomes regarding the urinary system's functionality and health appeared comparable between the two groups, the Toronto approach demonstrated potentially better cosmetic results and a slightly reduced need for additional surgeries. Figure 10.5 illustrates the long-term outcomes of genitalia operated with the Toronto approach (Fig. 10.5).

Finally, it is noteworthy that the 1st stage of the Toronto approach had a significantly shorter duration compared to CPRE (median 580 vs. 367 minutes). The authors postulate that this impacts the surgeon's stamina and accuracy when two advanced reconstructive procedures are performed back-to-back (bladder closure and epispadias repair) in the case of CPRE. When the duration of both procedures was added up in patients undergoing the Toronto approach, there was no substantial difference compared to CPRE. However, admittedly, patients undergo two general anesthetics from the outset [10].

Addressing Challenges and Limitations

While the Toronto approach represents a significant advancement in the surgical management of bladder exstrophy, it is not devoid of challenges. The staged repair introduces the potential for increased scarring at the proximal urethra, which may create additional difficulties during the epispadias surgery. However, as the bladder neck was previously addressed, most cases do not require much dissection in that area.

Conclusion

The surgical management of male bladder exstrophy via the Toronto approach is characterized by a nuanced and staged application of various surgical techniques, each meticulously designed to address the distinct phases of treatment required for this complex condition. The approach leverages a deep understanding of bladder exstrophy's anatomical and functional aspects, aiming to restore normal anatomy, preserve renal function, achieve urinary continence, and improve cosmetic outcomes. It is paramount to maintain strict follow-up protocols for patients treated for bladder exstrophy regardless of the technique used for primary closure. Aspects like lower and upper urinary tract function, cosmesis, transition into adulthood, sexuality, and fertility need to be taken into account for the life continuum of children born with this challenging congenital malformation.

References

1. Ahn JJ, Shnorhavorian M, Katz C, Goldin AB, Merguerian PA. Early versus delayed closure of bladder exstrophy: a national surgical quality improvement program pediatric analysis. J Pediatr Urol. 2018;14(1):27.e21–5. https://doi.org/10.1016/j.jpurol.2017.11.008.
2. Baird A, Mathews R, Gearhart J. The use of combined bladder and epispadias repair in boys with classic bladder exstrophy: outcomes, complications, and consequences. J Urol. 2005;174(4 Part 1):1421–4.
3. Baka-Jakubiak M. Combined bladder neck, urethral and penile reconstruction in boys with the exstrophy-epispadias complex. BJU Int. 2000;86(4):513–8.
4. Bar-Yosef Y, Savin Z, Ekstein M, Ben-David R, Dekalo S, Bar-Yaakov N, Sofer M, Ben-Chaim J. Preoperative bladder capacity predicts social continence following bladder neck reconstruction in children born with exstrophy-epispadias complex. Eur J Pediatr Surg. 2023;33(6):510–4. https://doi.org/10.1055/a-2003-1823.
5. Braga LH, Lorenzo AJ, Jrearz R, Bagli DJ, Farhat WA, Salle JLP, Khoury AE. Gender-based outcome analysis after complete primary repair of bladder exstrophy (CPRE). J Urol. 2008;179(4S):95.
6. Braga LH, Lorenzo AJ, Jrearz R, Bagli DJ, Salle JLP. Bilateral ureteral reimplantation at primary bladder exstrophy closure. J Urol. 2010;183(6):2337–41.
7. Canning DA, Gearhart JP, Peppas DS, Jeffs RD. The cephalotrigonal reimplant in bladder neck reconstruction for patients with exstrophy or epispadias. J Urol. 1993;150(1):156–8.
8. Cendron J. Bladder reconstruction. Method derived from that of Trendelenbourg. Ann Chir Infant. 1971;12(6):371–81. (La reconstruction vésicale. Méthode dérivée de celle de Trendelenbourg.)
9. Cervellione RM, Husmann DA, Bivalacqua TJ, Sponseller PD, Gearhart JP. Penile ischemic injury in the exstrophy/epispadias spectrum: new insights and possible mechanisms. J Pediatr Urol. 2010;6(5):450–6.
10. Chua M, Ming J, Fernandez N, Varghese A, Farhat W, Bagli D, Lorenzo A, Salle JP. Modified staged repair of bladder exstrophy: a strategy to prevent penile ischemia while maintaining advantage of the complete primary repair of bladder exstrophy. J Pediatr Urol. 2019;15(1):63.e61–7.
11. Cook AJ, Farhat WA, Cartwright LM, Khoury AE, Pippi Salle JL. Simplified mons plasty: a new technique to improve cosmesis in females with the exstrophy-epispadias complex. J Urol. 2005;173(6):2117–20. https://doi.org/10.1097/01.ju.0000157687.37406.d8.
12. Ellison JS, Ahn J, Shnorhavorian M, Grady R, Merguerian PA. Long-term fate of the upper tracts following complete primary repair of bladder exstrophy. J Pediatr Urol. 2017;13(4):394.e391–6.
13. Grady RW, Mitchell ME. Complete primary repair of exstrophy. J Urol. 1999;162(4):1415–20.
14. Gupta AD, Goel SK, Woodhouse CR, Wood D. Examining long-term outcomes of bladder exstrophy: a 20-year follow-up. BJU Int. 2014;113(1):137–41.
15. Hammouda HM, Kotb H. Complete primary repair of bladder exstrophy: initial experience with 33 cases. J Urol. 2004;172(4):1441–4.
16. Jarosz SL, Weaver JK, Weiss DA, Borer JG, Kryger JV, Canning DA, Groth TW, Lee T, Shukla AR, Mitchell ME, Roth EB. Bilateral ureteral reimplantation at complete primary repair of exstrophy: postoperative outcomes. J Pediatr Urol. 2022;18(1):37.e31–5. https://doi.org/10.1016/j.jpurol.2021.10.012.
17. Jeffs R. Management of the exstrophy-epispadias complex and urachal anomalies. In: Campbell's urology. 5th ed. Philadelphia: WB Saunders; 1986. p. 1882–921.
18. Joshi RS, Eftekharzadeh S, Shukla AR, Ramji J, Hingorani SR, Canning DA, Pippi-Salle JL, Merguerian P, DeFoor WR Jr, Frazier JR. Kidney function outcomes in patients after complete primary repair of bladder exstrophy and penopubic epispadias: results from the international bladder exstrophy consortium. J Pediatr Urol. 2023;19(1):34.e31–9.

19. Khandge P, Morrill CC, Wu WJ, Harris KT, Haffar A, Maruf M, Patel HD, Di Carlo HN, Gearhart JP. Achieving goal capacity for continence surgery: a cumulative event analysis of bladder exstrophy patients. J Pediatr Urol. 2023;19(5):563.e561–8.
20. Lee T, Borer J. Exstrophy-epispadias complex. Urol Clin North Am. 2023;50(3):403–14. https://doi.org/10.1016/j.ucl.2023.04.004.
21. Mathews R, Hubbard JS, Gearhart JP. Ureteral reimplantation before bladder neck plasty in the reconstruction of bladder exstrophy: indications and outcomes. Urology. 2003;61(4):820–4.
22. Mathews R, Gosling JA, Gearhart JP. Ultrastructure of the bladder in classic exstrophy: correlation with development of continence. J Urol. 2004;172(4, Part 1):1446–9. https://doi.org/10.1097/01.ju.0000138248.43831.27.
23. McKenna PH, Khoury AE, McLorie GA, Churchill BM, Babyn PB, Wedge JH. Iliac osteotomy: a model to compare the options in bladder and cloacal exstrophy reconstruction. J Urol. 1994;151(1):182–6. https://doi.org/10.1016/S0022-5347(17)34912-1.
24. Pathak P, Ring JD, Delfino KR, Dynda DI, Mathews RI. Complete primary repair of bladder exstrophy: a systematic review. J Pediatr Urol. 2020;16(2):149–53.
25. Pippi Salle J. Complications of epispadias repair. In: Third international bladder exstrophy symposium. 13–15 Oct 2009.
26. Pippi Salle J, Jednak R, Capolicchio J, França I, Labbie A, Gosalbez R. A ventral rotational skin flap to improve cosmesis and avoid chordee recurrence in epispadias repair. BJU Int. 2002;90(9):918–23.
27. Pippi-Salle JL, Chan P. One stage bladder exstrophy and epispadias repair in newborn male. Can J Urol. 1999;6(2):757–60.
28. Puri A, Mishra K, Sikdar S, Unni KE, Jain AK. Vesical preservation in patients with late bladder exstrophy referral: histological insights into functional outcome. J Urol. 2014;192(4):1208–14. https://doi.org/10.1016/j.juro.2014.04.095.
29. Purves JT, Baird AD, Gearhart JP. The modern staged repair of bladder exstrophy in the female: a contemporary series. J Pediatr Urol. 2008;4(2):150–3.
30. Ramji J, Weiss D, Romao R, Eftekharzadeh S, Shah J, Frazier J, Reddy P, Merguerian P, Salle JP, Canning D. Impact of bilateral ureteral reimplantation at the time of complete primary repair of bladder exstrophy on reflux rates, renogram abnormalities and bladder capacity. J Pediatr Urol. 2021;17(3):393.e391–7.
31. Salle JP. Commentary to “Penile ischemic injury in the exstrophy/epispadias spectrum: new insights and possible mechanisms”. J Pediatr Urol. 2010;6(5):457–8.
32. Shaw MB, Rink RC, Kaefer M, Cain MP, Casale AJ. Continence and classic bladder exstrophy treated with staged repair. J Urol. 2004;172(4):1450–3.
33. Shnorhavorian M, Grady RW, Andersen A, Joyner BD, Mitchell ME. Long-term follow-up of complete primary repair of exstrophy: the Seattle experience. J Urol. 2008;180(4S):1615–20.
34. Shoukry A, Ziada A, Morsi H, Habib E, Aref A, Badawy H, Eissa M, Daw M. Outcome of complete primary bladder exstrophy repair: single-center experience. J Pediatr Urol. 2009;5(6):496–9.
35. Surer I, Baker LA, Jeffs RD, Gearhart JP. The modified Cantwell-Ransley repair for exstrophy and epispadias: 10-year experience. J Urol. 2000;164(3 Part 2):1040–3.
36. Wu WJ, Maruf M, Harris KT, Manyevitch R, Patel HD, Di Carlo HN, Gearhart JP. Delaying reclosure of bladder exstrophy leads to gradual decline in bladder capacity. J Pediatr Urol. 2020;16(3):355.e351–5. https://doi.org/10.1016/j.jpurol.2020.03.019.
37. Yerkes EB, Adams MC, Rink RC, Pope JC, Brock JW. How well do patients with exstrophy actually void? J Urol. 2000;164(3 Part 2):1044–7.

Modified Perineal Approach in the Management of Female Epispadias

11

Joao Luiz Pippi Salle, Rodrigo L. P. Romao, and Michael Chua

Introduction

Isolated female epispadias (IFE) is a rare congenital anomaly, considered the mildest form of the female exstrophy/epispadias complex, with an occurrence of 1 in 480,000 newborn girls [1]. Factors such as Caucasian race, advanced parental age, and in-vitro fertilization have been associated with it [9, 16].

Inheritance patterns in familial cases suggest a complex genetic trait, occurring in less than 1% of cases [9, 16]. The prior study identified three severity levels of IFE: mild (bifid clitoris and patulous meatus) (Fig. 11.1a, b), intermediate (dorsal urethral split, patulous and opened bladder neck) (Fig. 11.2a, b), and severe (complete urethral cleft involving the sphincter, wide diastasis and opened bladder neck, leading to constant incontinence; prolapse in some cases simulating bladder exstrophy) [16] (Fig. 11.3a, b). Treatment aims to achieve good cosmesis, preserve the upper urinary tract, and ensure full urinary continence [5].

Supplementary Information The online version contains supplementary material available at https://doi.org/10.1007/978-3-031-91238-2_11.

J. L. P. Salle
Division of Urology, SickKids Hospital and Co-Director of the Center for Pelvic Reconstruction, Toronto, Canada
e-mail: pippi.salle@sickkisd.ca

R. L. P. Romao (✉)
Division of Pediatric Urology, Division of Pediatric General and Thoracic Surgery, Hospital for Sick Children, University of Toronto, Toronto, ON, Canada
e-mail: rodrigo.romao@sickkids.ca

M. Chua
Division of Pediatric Urology, Hospital for Sick Children, University of Toronto, Toronto, ON, Canada

A. R. Shukla, R. S. Joshi (eds.), *Bladder Exstrophy and Epispadias*, https://doi.org/10.1007/978-3-031-91238-2_11

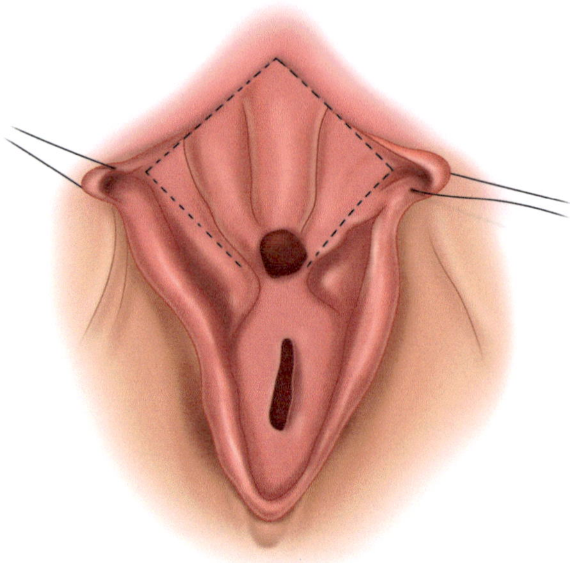

Fig. 11.1 The mucosal strip between the two hemi-clitoris is marked to be further incised

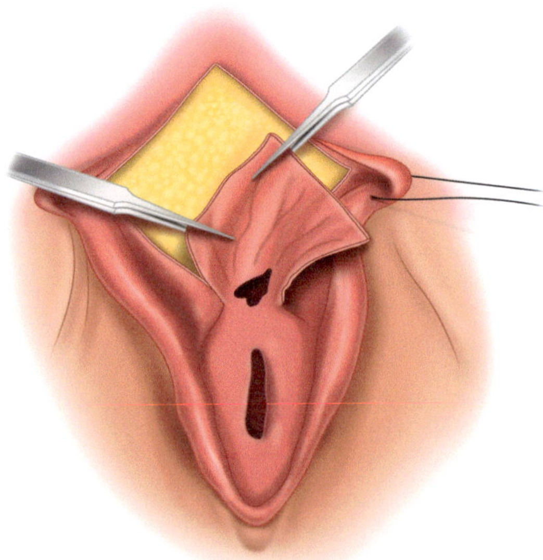

Fig. 11.2 Dissection of the mucosal strip which is used as a handle to retract and expose the BN

Typically, the upper genitourinary tract in IFE patients is normal. Common associated anomalies include a bifid clitoris, an open and patulous urethra, and pubic diastasis; some cases also present with vesicoureteral reflux (VUR). The defect extends to the bladder neck, which is usually incompetent, leading to urinary

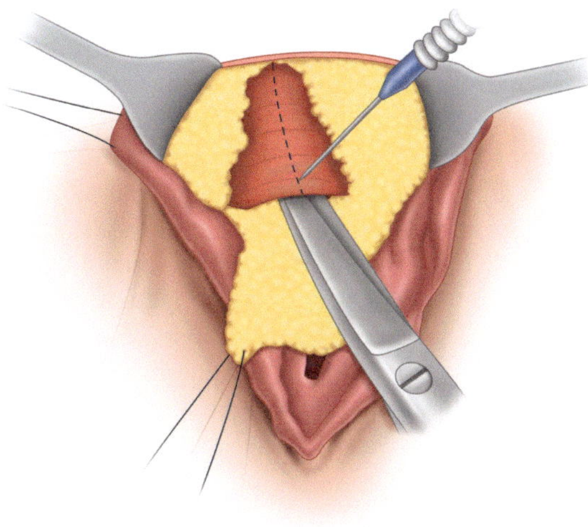

Fig. 11.3 Incision of the intersymphyseal bands to optimize exposure of the BN and anterior bladder wall

incontinence [4]. Diagnosis is generally straightforward, but some cases may be subtle, despite a noticeable bifid clitoris. Misdiagnosis with ambiguous genitalia can occur, and some girls present later with persistent urinary incontinence [1].

Background

The traditional treatment involves urethral and genital reconstruction within the first year, followed by bladder neck reconstruction Young-Dees-Leadbetter cervicoplasty (YDL) when the child reaches the age of social continence [14]. In 2009, Manzoni and Ransley proposed a single-stage technique for repairing the urethra, bladder neck, and clitoris through a perineal approach, without tailoring the bladder neck to enhance outlet resistance [12]. This technique was later modified to include bladder neck tailoring (BNT) via the perineal approach, with studies confirming its feasibility and favorable outcomes [3, 5, 11]. Benefits of this method include earlier surgery, improved continence, reduced morbidity, and potentially fewer additional surgeries.

Modified Perineal Approach Surgical Technique

All patients receive prophylactic antibiotics prior to the procedure. Initially, a cystoscopy is conducted to evaluate the bladder neck and ureteric orifices. The procedure begins with the placement of fine holding stitches into the prepuce of each hemi-clitoris to retract and expose the mucosal strip between them. The mucosal strip between both hemi-clitorises is marked, incised, and dissected from the pubic attachments (Fig. 11.1). Once free, this strip serves as a handle for retracting and exposing the anterior bladder wall (Fig. 11.2). It will eventually be excised along with the approximation of the edges of the hemi-clitoris during the final steps of the genitoplasty. The symphyseal pubic band is exposed and fully incised to enhance the visualization of the bladder neck (BN) and anterior bladder wall (Fig. 11.3). A retro-pubic dissection extending approximately 5 cm is performed to expose the BN and anterior bladder wall. The mucosal strip is further divided in the midline all the way through the BN and extended to approximately 5 cm into the anterior bladder wall (Fig. 11.4). Two longitudinal incisions, 1.5 cm apart, are made in the urethral plate (Fig. 11.5), which is then tubularized over an 8-Fr catheter with interrupted absorbable sutures (after demucolization of its lateral excess) (Fig. 11.6). The demucolized urethral plate is wrapped around the neourethra to reinforce it and to prevent fistulas (Fig. 11.7). The anterior bladder wall and BN are incised, tailored, and sutured to create a funneling configuration. Similarly, the lateral excess of the BN and anterior bladder wall are de-epithelialized, separated from the pubic

Fig. 11.4 The mucosal strip is further divided in the midline all the way through the BN and extended to approximately 5 cm into the anterior bladder wall, allowing wide exposure of the bladder neck and the lateral walls of the bladder which will be funneled

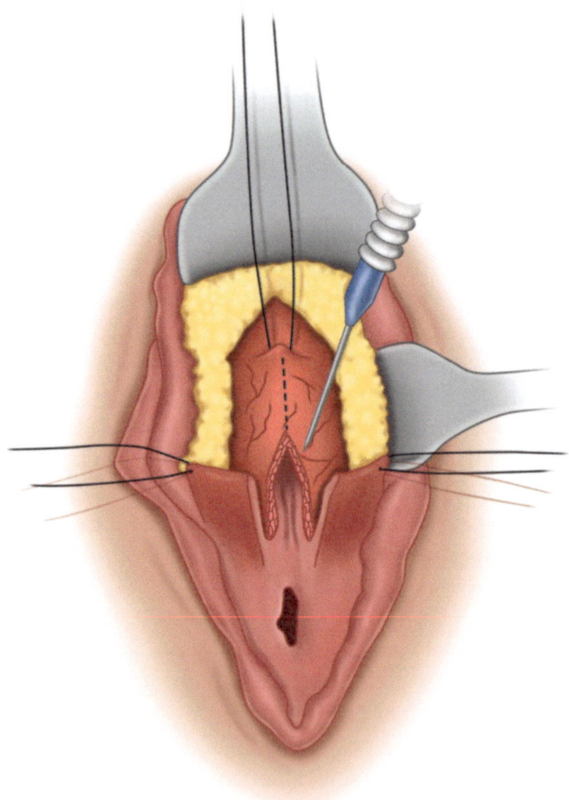

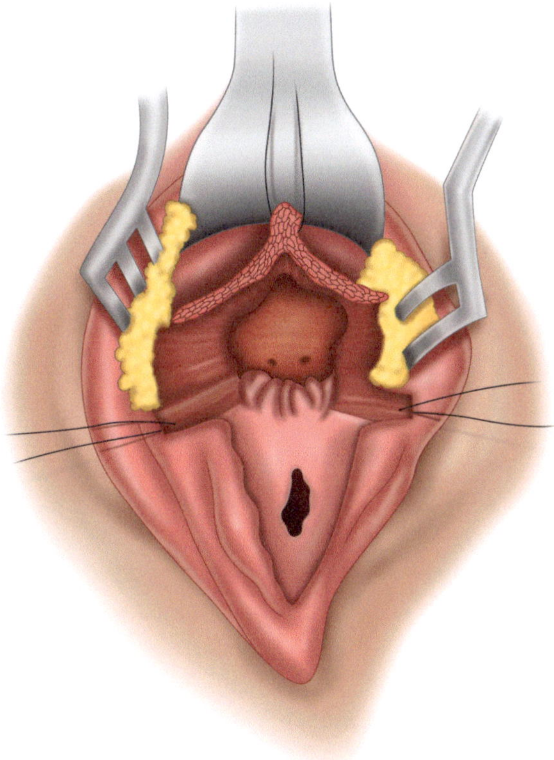

Fig. 11.5 The anterior bladder wall and neck retracted, providing excellent exposure

attachments, and their muscle is wrapped around to reinforce the funneled bladder outlet. The symphyseal pubic bands are approximated, and the suprapubic area is closed in layers with absorbable sutures. Genitoplasty and monsplasty are carried out by lateral mobilization of the suprapubic fat, allowing medial rotation of the diverted labia majora and reconstructing the mons pubis. This mobilization allows both hemi-clitorises to be brought together at the midline, as we previously described [6]. In most cases, a Foley catheter is left in place for 7 days, but in some cases, a suprapubic tube is left for 2–3 weeks when it is clamped and urination is observed. If urination is adequate, it can be removed [15].

The following link depicts the surgical technique and important technical details to perform this procedure:

https://www.dropbox.com/scl/fi/6jigdqamlmn511lj5m3cl/Perineal-Urethrocervicoplasty-for-Female-Epispadias-with-audio-and-credits.mp4?rlkey=kmwvtcj07ylk7r5wf49aghz59&st=ubgrxi3t&dl=0

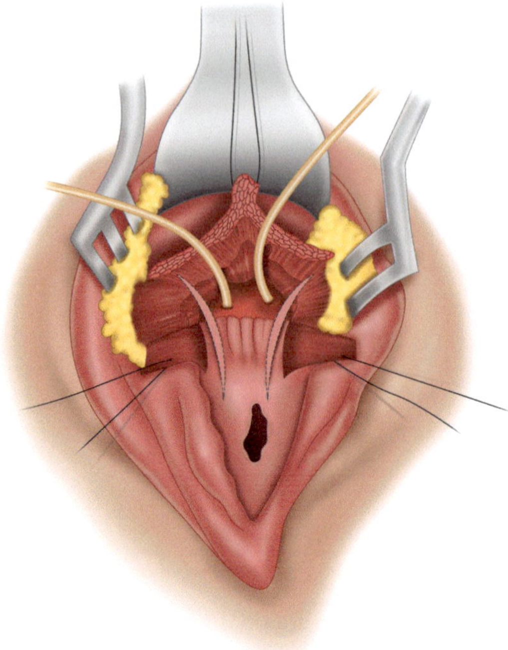

Fig. 11.6 Marking of the mucosa of the urethra (1.5 cm apart), BN, and lateral walls of the bladder which will be funneled and tailored

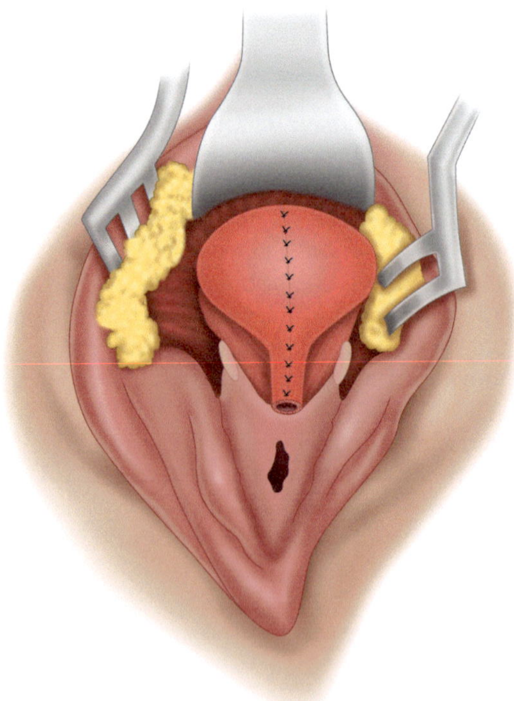

Fig. 11.7 The lateral aspects of the funneled bladder, BN, and urethra are demucosalized. The bladder and urethra are closed with interrupted stitches

Institutional Data on Modified Perineal Technique

A total of nine cases of IFE underwent a modified perineal cervicoplasty and were included in our initial study and compared to three patients historically treated with the classic YDL procedure. Seven of the nine patients (77.8%) were diagnosed at birth, while two were identified later during investigations for refractory urinary incontinence, including one teenage girl. All cases presented with bifid clitoris on the initial examination, and pubic diastasis was noted in every patient. Associated anomalies included three cases with vesicoureteral reflux (VUR), one case of spina bifida occulta, and one anorectal malformation. The mean age at the time of surgery was 4.3 years (range: 1–17 years).

No bladder augmentations or osteotomies were performed in this group. In contrast, all patients who underwent YDL needed augmentation cystoplasty. Ureteric reimplantation was also not performed in the group undergoing perineal cervicoplasty who had an uneventful postoperative course. The mean follow-up duration was 6 years (range: 1–10 years).

Outcomes for urinary continence revealed that four out of seven children (57%), who were old enough for evaluation, achieved continence following the initial procedure. Three incontinent patients received postoperative injections of dextranomer/hyaluronic acid as a bulking agent (Deflux, Q-Med AB, Sweden), resulting in continence for two of them, while one continued to experience stress incontinence. Interestingly, two of these three patients were initially dry but later developed progressive stress incontinence, requiring endoscopic injection of bulking material at the BN to improve outlet resistance [10].

Most patients (7 out of 9) demonstrated volitional voiding, though two were still too young for toilet training assessment but showed signs of cycling their bladders with dry intervals between diaper changes. Subjectively, the cosmetic results were deemed satisfactory from both the surgeon's and parents' perspectives. Sexual function could not be assessed in these patients.

Preliminary findings suggest that the perineal approach is effective for all IFE cases and compares favorably with the traditional YDL technique, supporting previous reports [5]. Our approach, with modified BNT and reinforcement of the bladder neck, achieved continence with voluntary voiding in most patients, eliminating the need for bladder augmentation and ureteral reimplantation [2]. For the perineal approach, complete incision of the inter-symphyseal pubic bands is crucial to facilitate tapering of the anterior bladder wall and bladder neck reinforcement (BNR). Unlike the YDL technique, which can be overly retentive, the modified approach creates a funnel-shaped BN, allowing voluntary voiding. None of the patients required construction of a catheterizable channel. BN reinforcement with bladder tissue, after removing mucosa and urethral, likely enhances outlet resistance, improving continence as demonstrated in this series. Notably, two patients experienced incontinence recurrence years later, highlighting the need for long-term follow-up. Both were successfully treated with BN injections.

One case was diagnosed late in puberty after years of attending voiding dysfunction clinics and unsuccessful pharmacological treatments. This underscores the importance of genital and back examinations in incontinent patients to avoid prolonged suffering and social consequences. Most cases in this series were diagnosed at birth, which could improve psychosocial outcomes and allow earlier treatment.

Achieving adequate cosmesis is important for girls with epispadias and exstrophy. Unfortunately, many women with prior repairs have unsatisfactory genital appearance, persistent bifid clitoris, absent mons, and severe midline scarring. The present technique aimed to improve cosmesis through effective monsplasty and clitoroplasty, receiving positive feedback from parents and the medical team.

Discussion

VUR affects 30–75% of IFE cases [7, 16]. In this series, ureteric reimplantation was not performed during the perineal approach, and no complications related to VUR were observed at long-term follow-up. Patients did not develop recurrent febrile UTIs and were not routinely given antibiotic prophylaxis. If reimplantation is needed, the perineal approach may need to be reconsidered due to inadequate exposure for such a procedure [3].

Bladder capacity in IFE patients is typically low, likely due to poor outlet resistance [11]. Thus, early modified BNT is recommended to increase outlet resistance, allowing the bladder to develop capacity and reducing the need for future augmentation cystoplasty [4, 13, 16].

In this small series, initial YDL approach results were poor, necessitating significant redo surgeries, including augmentation, to achieve dryness. This may be attributed to the retentive nature of the YDL technique and the surgeons' experience with it.

Due to the rarity of cases, data comparing perineal versus classical YDL procedures is limited. The only other study, by Cheikhelard et al., also found favorable results for the perineal approach in achieving continence without the need for augmentation in most patients.

Interestingly, some incontinent IFE patients post-perineal approach could be rendered continent after BN injections. This suggests that injections into a reduced BN can achieve adequate coaptation of its walls, unlike in non-operated patients with a wide-open BN. Similar experiences have been reported by others [8].

Acknowledgement: We acknowledge the work of Dr. Elaine Reck Sangalli, who did the illustrations for our chapter.

References

1. Allen L, Rodjani A, Kelly J, et al. Female epispadias: are we missing the diagnosis? BJU Int. 2004;94:613–5.
2. Alyami F, Fernandez N, Lee L, Metcalfe P, Lorenzo A, Pippi Salle JL. Long-term follow-up after traditional versus modified perineal approach in the management of female epispadias. J Pediatr Urol. 2017;13:497.e1–5.

3. Bhat AL, Bhat M, Sharma R, et al. Single-stage perineal urethroplasty for continence in female epispadias: a preliminary report. Urology. 2008;72:300–3.
4. Caione P, Zavaglia D, Capozza N. Pelvic floor reconstruction in female exstrophic complex patients: different results from males? Eur Urol. 2007;52:1777–83.
5. Cheikhelard A, Aigrain Y, Lottmann H, et al. Female epispadias management: perineal urethrocervicoplasty versus classical young-dees procedure. J Urol. 2009;182:1807–12.
6. Cook AJ, Farhat WA, Cartwright LM, et al. Simplified mons plasty: a new technique to improve cosmesis in females with the exstrophy-epispadias complex. J Urol. 2005;173:2117–20.
7. Gearhart J, Peppas D, Jeffs R. Complete genitourinary reconstruction in female epispadias. J Urol. 1993;149:1110–3.
8. Gundeti M, Large M. Reconstruction of urogenital defects: congenital. In: Neligan P, editor. Plastic surgery E-book, vol. 3. London: Elsevier; 2013. p. 906–14.
9. Kajbafzadeh AM, Tajik P, Payabvash S, et al. Bladder exstrophy and epispadias complex in sibling: case report and review of literature. Pediatr Surg Int. 2006;22:767–70.
10. Kitchens DM, Minevich E, DeFoor WR, et al. Incontinence Following Bladder Neck Reconstruction—Is There a Role for Endoscopic Management? Journal of Urology. 2007;177(1):302-306. https://doi.org/10.1016/j.juro.2006.09.012.
11. Lazarus J, Van Den Heever A, Kortekaas B, et al. Female epispadias managed by bladder neck plication via a perineal approach. J Pediatr Urol. 2012;8:244–8.
12. Manzoni G, Ransley P. Primary surgical intervention for female epispadias. J Pediatr Urol. 2007;3:S73.
13. Mollard P, Basset T, Mure PY. Female epispadias. J Urol. 1997;158:1543–6.
14. Peters C, Gearhart JP, Jeffs R. Epispadias and incontinence: the challenge of the small bladder. J Urol. 1988;140:1199–201.
15. Salle JLP, Fraga JCS, Amarante A, et al. Urethral lengthening with anterior bladder wall flap for urinary incontinence – a new approach. J Urol. 1994;152:803–6.
16. Tantibhedhyangkul J, Copland SD, Haqq AM, et al. A case of female epispadias. Fertil Steril. 2008;90:2017–9.

Osteotomies for Bladder Exstrophy

12

B. David Horn, Soroush Baghdadi,
Piyush Sudamalal Mittal, Vinod Gautam,
and Stefano Cardin

Introduction

Bladder exstrophy-epispadias complex (BE) is a complex congenital anomaly occurring with an incidence of approximately 1 in 50,000 live births [20, 24]. BE is considered a spectrum of disorders, ranging from the milder epispadias to the more severe cloacal exstrophy (OIES syndrome). BE also affects multiple organ systems, including the musculoskeletal, genitourinary, and gastrointestinal systems [24, 26]. Historically, BE resulted in significant morbidity and mortality, although

Supplementary Information The online version contains supplementary material available at https://doi.org/10.1007/978-3-031-91238-2_12.

B. D. Horn (✉)
Department of Orthopedic Surgery, The Children's Hospital of Philadelphia, Philadelphia, PA, USA
e-mail: hornd@chop.edu

S. Baghdadi
Department of Orthopedic Surgery, UCLA, Los Angeles, CA, USA
e-mail: sbaghdadi@mednet.ucla.edu

P. S. Mittal
Department of Orthopaedic, Civil Hospital, B.J. Medical College & Government Spine Institute, Ahmedabad, Gujarat, India

V. Gautam
Department of Orthopedics, Government Medical Collage, Gujarat, India

S. Cardin
Division of Pediatric Orthopaedics, Orlando Health – Arnold Palmer Hospital for Children, Orlando, FL, USA
e-mail: stefano.cardin@orlandohealth.com

A. R. Shukla, R. S. Joshi (eds.), *Bladder Exstrophy and Epispadias*,
https://doi.org/10.1007/978-3-031-91238-2_12

advancements in treatment have improved life expectancy as well as the quality of life for individuals with BE. Despite these advances, however, individuals with BE continue to face challenges related to urinary continence, fertility, and social stigma [6, 24].

BE is a diverse condition influenced by various genetic pathways [26]. BE's embryological pathogenesis is intricate, but an understanding of this helps shed light on anatomical distinctions crucial for orthopedic interventions.

During embryonic development, the cloacal membrane forms through the fusion of ectodermal and endodermal layers in the fourth week of gestation. The subsequent growth of the mesodermal layer, responsible for the musculoskeletal system, forms the urorectal septum, dividing the cloacal membrane into urogenital and anal membranes. Anomalies in this process are believed to stem from deficient mesodermal growth as well as from disruption in the formation of the cloacal membrane [24, 26]. The failure of separation of the urogenital and rectal membranes leads to the complex anomalies observed in BE. These include failure of closure of pubic diastasis (closure normally occurs by the eighth week) as well as the presence of an exstrophied bladder [21, 23, 26].

From an orthopedic perspective, it's also important to recognize that while the pelvic floor muscles exist, they have an atypical orientation. These muscles function to support pelvic organs, but in BE they function as a hammock that pushes organs outward through the exstrophy. This altered role is important in managing BE, particularly during diastasis closure [22, 25, 27].

Earlier treatment approaches primarily focused on covering or closing the exstrophy, yielding high recurrence rates and complications such as wound and bladder dehiscence. Only in the latter half of the twentieth century did surgeons understand the importance of pelvic osteotomy to help decrease the pubic diastasis, prompting the involvement of orthopedic surgeons in the multidisciplinary management of BE [23, 24].

Patho-anatomy of the Pelvis in Bladder Exstrophy

The most obvious osseous feature of BE is the presence of pubic diastasis. While orthopedic surgeons are more accustomed to encountering traumatic causes of pubic diastasis, such as open book pelvic fractures, it's essential to recognize that the anatomical distinctions in BE extend beyond this characteristic finding [20, 23].

In BE, the pelvis exhibits anterior deficiency and external rotation across all of its segments. Detailed analysis of pelvic CT scans in patients with BE revealed an average 30-degree external rotation of each hemipelvis, with the posterior segment (the iliac wing) contributing approximately 12° and the anterior segment around 18° to this rotation. In more severe cases, particularly in cases of OEIS syndrome, the posterior segment showed an average of 25° and the anterior segment 24° of external rotation, respectively, compared to healthy controls. Additionally, the pubic rami in BE are found to be, on average, 30% shorter than in patients of the same age without BE. There is a mean of 4.2 cm of diastasis at birth in BE and 7.2 cm in

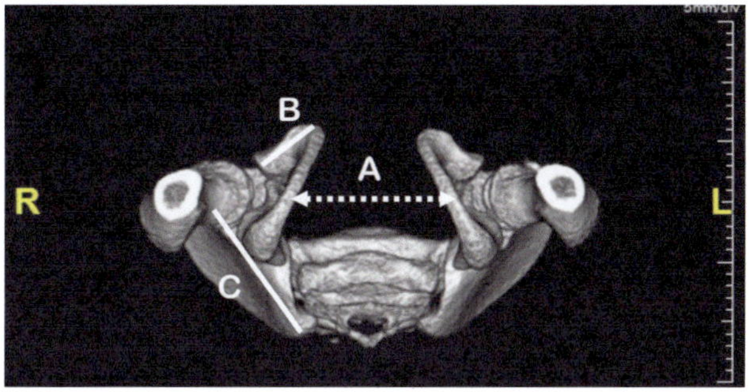

Fig. 12.1 Bony changes seen in exstrophy, including (A) increased inter-triradiate distance, (B) shortened pubic rami, and (C) external rotation of anterior and posterior pelvis

OEIS, which progressively increases with age, reaching a mean of 14.2 cm in adulthood (Fig. 12.1) [20, 22, 26].

Another characteristic feature observed in BE is acetabular retroversion, typically measuring an average of 13° compared to healthy controls, with potential increases into adulthood. This acetabular retroversion, coupled with decreased internal rotation of the hip, contributes to a foot progression angle that may exceed 20° of external rotation [20, 28]. Additional deformities noted in BE patients include increased inter-triradiate distance, rotation and deformity of the sacroiliac joints, and sacral dysmorphism. In summary, the average BE pelvis is characterized by a posterior segment of normal size, a shortened anterior segment, and external rotation across all segments [14, 24].

Summary of key pelvic anomalies in CBE (Fig. 12.1):

- Posterior segment externally malrotated by 12°
- Anterior segment externally malrotated by 18°
- Retroverted acetabula by 15°
- Pubis foreshortened by 30%
- Increased intra-pelvic volume by 30–40%
- Pubis diastasis of 4.2 cm at birth and 14.2 cm in adulthood

Osteotomies in BE Reconstruction

As previously discussed, the complex patho-anatomy of BE coupled with its rarity and variability in severity make soft tissue correction alone challenging. It wasn't until the 1960s that the benefits of osteotomies and reapproximating the pubic diastasis became apparent. Over time, closure of the pelvic ring at the time of urological repair has been shown to have multiple benefits. These include decreased rates of bladder dehiscence, decreased tension on the wound, increased continence rates since the urethra and bladder neck can be placed within the bony pelvis, improved genital reconstruction because of decreased tension on the hemi corpi, and decreased rates of late uterine prolapse. Other theoretical advantages include improved gait, decreased rates of sacroiliac joint arthritis, and decreased rates of hip arthrosis [14, 23, 24, 26]. Shultz, in 1958, reported on the first use of pelvic osteotomies in BE reconstruction [19]. The initial reports described posterior osteotomies, including Lloyd Roberts in 1959 and O'Phelan in 1963 [10, 16]. The anterior approach was first described in 1989 with superior pubic rami osteotomies [4, 17]. This technique gained traction in the 1990s in Europe and was typically performed concomitantly with urologic reconstruction by urologists. This procedure involves cutting the pubis medial to the iliopectineal eminence, within the obturator foramen, and closure with sutures. However, a drawback of this technique is its failure to address external rotation of the pelvis. Overall, the low complication rates and improved outcomes associated with the use of osteotomies have made pelvic osteotomies integral to the care of patients with BE [24, 26].

In general, pelvic osteotomies should be strongly considered in all infants and children more than 72 hours old and in newborn infants with a large pubic diastasis [14, 24]. Osteotomies can be performed either anteriorly or posteriorly. Currently, all of the osteotomies, whether posterior or anterior, have the disadvantage of decreasing intra-pelvic volume [9]. This can make placement of the reconstructed bladder and bladder neck into the pelvis challenging, potentially leading to ischemia of the reconstructed bladder and genitalia.

Posterior osteotomies involve bilateral vertical bony cuts just lateral to the sacroiliac joints. This approach requires prone positioning, so the patient must be repositioned after the osteotomies are performed to allow for the urological reconstruction. Advantages include potential improvement in the acetabular retroversion, although there are concerns that correction may be limited by the soft tissue surrounding the osteotomized segments.

Various anterior iliac osteotomies have been described, including bilateral Salter-type osteotomies extending from just above the anterior inferior iliac spine (AIIS) to the sciatic notch [14, 21], as well as a more oblique osteotomy propagating diagonally from just posterior to the anterior superior iliac spine (ASIS) to the sciatic notch [5, 8, 11]. These are all shown to be successful. In addition, double pelvic osteotomies have been described [14] (Fig. 12.2). These osteotomies will be described in greater detail later in the chapter.

Regardless of the exact technique performed, there are several common preoperative considerations that need to be considered before performing pelvic osteotomies for BE reconstruction. There is approximately a 5% rate of hip dysplasia associated with BE. Patients should be screened for this with a hip ultrasound 4–6 weeks post gestational age [13]. In addition, plain X-rays consisting of an AP pelvis should be obtained to aid in surgical planning. In more complex cases, such as cloacal exstrophy (OEIS) or revision surgery, axial imaging like CT or MRI scans may be helpful to further evaluate pelvic anatomy and search for associated pathologies such as SI joint dysplasia. Close coordination with the urological team is also vital to optimize surgical flow and minimize operative time. Finally, patient factors should be optimized prior to surgery. Patients with cloacal exstrophy, for example, may have nutritional issues that should be addressed prior to undertaking a complex reconstruction.

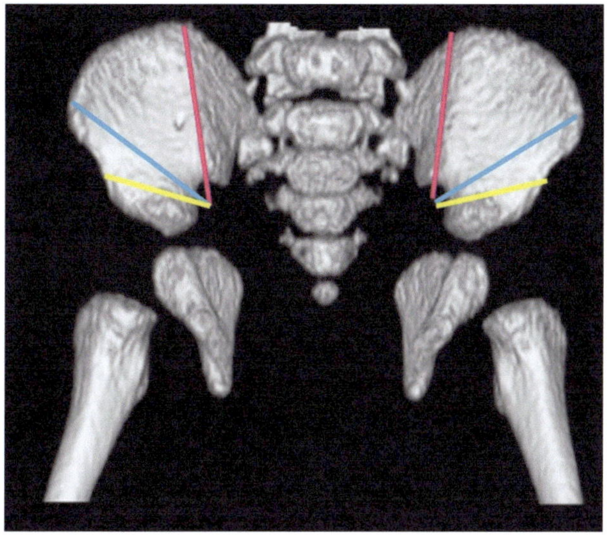

Fig. 12.2 Location of commonly performed pelvic osteotomies. Red—posterior, Blue—oblique, Yellow—anterior and Ahmedabad, Red + Yellow—double anterior

Intraoperative pubic reduction fixation and postoperative immobilization should also be considered in the treatment plan. Many different strategies have been described and used with success. Intraoperative fixation to maintain pubic reduction may involve the use of large absorbable sutures, internal fixation, and/or external fixation. Postoperative immobilization may include skin traction, including modified Bryant's traction, spica casting, and bracing [24].

The role of osteotomies in the treatment of BE is to facilitate the urological reconstruction. The primary goals, therefore, are urological in nature: enhanced healing of the bladder and abdominal wall, urinary continence, renal health, and improved genital function and appearance. Many studies demonstrate improved outcomes when pelvic osteotomies are performed in conjunction with repair of BE [1, 6, 24]. From an orthopedic perspective, the pubic diastasis invariably recurs. This is typically accompanied by external rotation of the pelvis and acetabular retroversion. To date, these differences seem to be well tolerated and have not been associated with decreased ambulatory function, activity level, pain, or hip arthrosis [14, 24, 26]. It is important to bear in mind, however, that the longest follow-up is only in individuals in the fourth decade of life, so true long-term data are not available for this population.

Complications may occur regardless of the specific osteotomy performed. There seems to be an overall 4–5% complication rate associated with osteotomies themselves. These include wound and pin tract infections, skin complications from traction or casting, and nerve palsy (particularly femoral nerve palsy, which was transient) [15, 18].

Posterior Iliac Osteotomies

- Indications:
  - Patients with classic BE <1 year of age.
- Pre-op Imaging:
  - Hip ultrasound.
  - AP pelvis X-ray (Fig. 12.3).
  - Pelvis CT or MRI as indicated.
- Timing
  - The osteotomies are usually performed prior to the urologic repair.
  - The osteotomies can be performed 3–7 days prior to the urological procedure or at the same time as the urological surgery (the latter requires repositioning the patient supine for the exstrophy repair).
- Positioning:
  - The patient is placed prone on gel rolls with all bony prominences appropriately padded (Fig. 12.4).
- Approach:
  - Two parallel longitudinal skin incisions are made. Each should be 4–5 cm in length and about 1 cm lateral to the PSIS (Fig. 12.5).
  - Dissection is performed through subcutaneous fat until deep fascia is reached.
  - Electrocautery is then used to dissect the muscle fibers of the paralumbar muscles off the posterior iliac crest to expose the iliac apophysis.
  - A 15-blade is then used to split the apophysis (the pelvis orientation is vertical). To split the pelvic apophysis, the knife handle will be almost parallel to the body.
  - A small periosteal elevator is used to subperiosteally dissect the inner and outer iliac tables until the sciatic notch is reached on both sides.

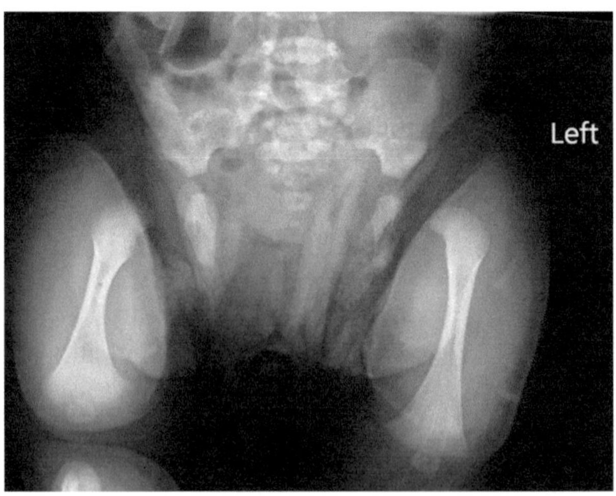

Fig. 12.3 Preoperative radiograph of a 3-month-old girl shows a widened pubic diastasis characteristic of BE

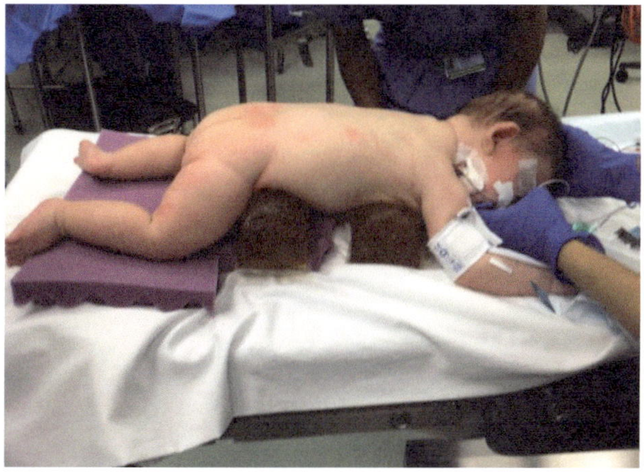

Fig. 12.4 Positioning for posterior iliac osteotomies. The hips should be flexed to improve access to the posterior iliac crests

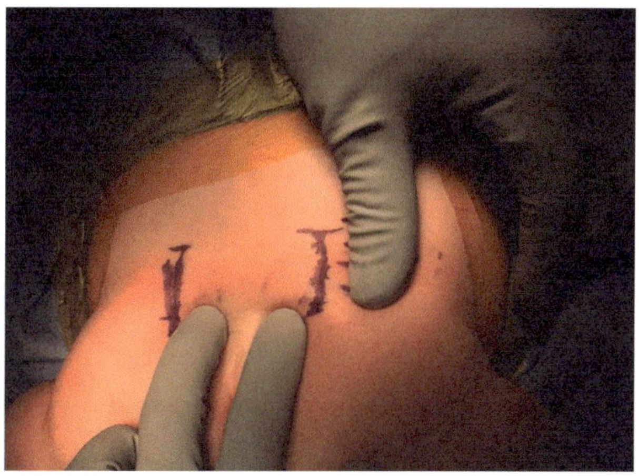

Fig. 12.5 Incisions for posterior osteotomies

    - The surgeon should be aware that the notch tends to be located more medially than expected when dissecting the outer table.
    - In contrast, the notch tends to be located more laterally than expected during the inner table dissection.
  - Once the notch is identified, small Hohmann retractors or periosteal elevators are used to protect its contents.
- Osteotomy:
  - A vertical osteotomy is then performed.
    - This may be created by using small rongeurs, osteotomes, or an oscillating saw.
    - Small osteotomes are used to safely complete the osteotomy.
    - Laminar spreaders may be used to confirm the completion of the osteotomy.
  - Completion of the osteotomy is then verified by hinging the ilium anteriorly, which will result in the osteotomy opening posteriorly.

- Closure is then performed in layers.
- Care should be taken to close the apophysis over the ilium in a separate layer.
  - The overlying fascia is then closed, followed by subcutaneous tissue and skin closure.
- Repeat the surgical technique on the contralateral side.

- Pubic Symphysis Diastasis Reduction:
  - Performed at the time of the urological procedure.
  - The patient is positioned supine once both osteotomies are performed, and the posterior incisions are closed.
  - At the appropriate time in the urology procedure, the pubic symphysis diastasis is typically reduced with manual reduction (a pointed bone reduction clamp may also be used).
    - Pubic diastasis reduction is facilitated by pushing on the greater trochanters of each hip.
  - The reduction is then held by a large, monofilament, absorbable suture between the pubic bones. This helps stabilize the posterior osteotomies.
  - At the conclusion of the procedure, the patient is placed into either a hip spica or a previously made hip spica brace (Fig. 12.6).
- Postoperative immobilization
  - Either a spica cast or a spica brace may be used.
  - Spica brace is the author's preference—two techniques
    - Custom brace fabricated by an orthotist 1–2 weeks prior to surgery (Fig. 12.7)

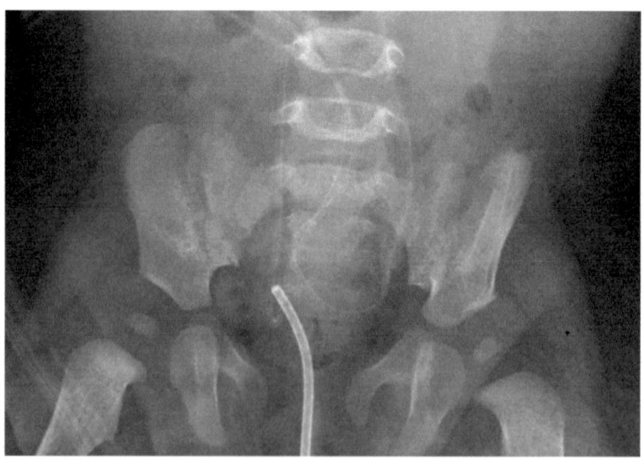

Fig. 12.6 Postoperative radiograph demonstrating posterior osteotomies (dotted lines) and decreased pubic diastasis

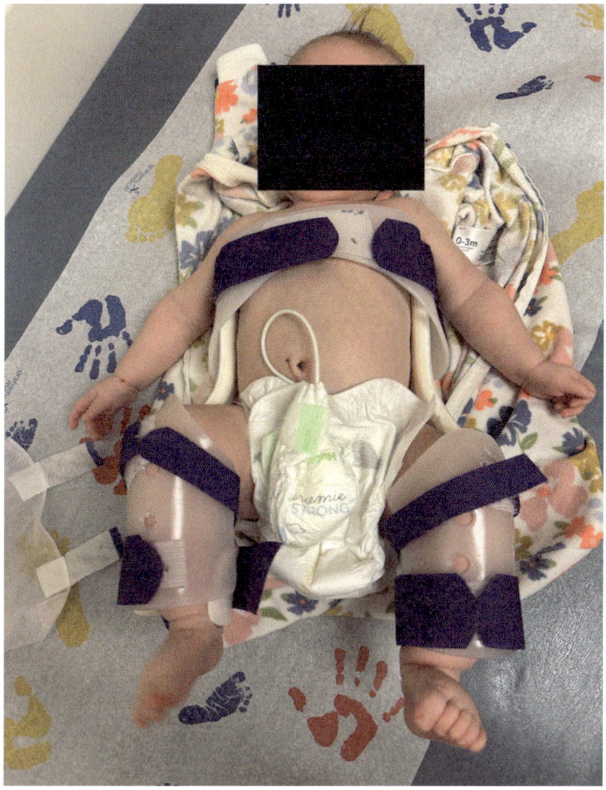

Fig. 12.7 Custom fabricated spica brace

- Bivalved spica cast was placed on the day of surgery
  – The procedure begins with molding for the hip spica brace prior to the beginning of surgical repair.
  – The patient is placed on a spica table, and a double hip spica cast is applied. Care is taken to avoid excessive hip abduction and to keep the hips as adducted as possible. Hip flexion should be 30–60°.
  – The cast is then bivalved and a hip spica brace is then made from the bivalved spica (Fig. 12.8).

- Postoperative Care:
  – Patient remains in spica brace full time for 5 days.
  – The brace may then be removed three times per day for skin checks.
  – The total time of immobilization in a Spica brace is 4–6 weeks (clinical pic at the end of the video).
  – Spica brace allows access for wound care, drains, and hygiene.
  – First postoperative radiographs performed at 4 weeks (postop AP XR pic).

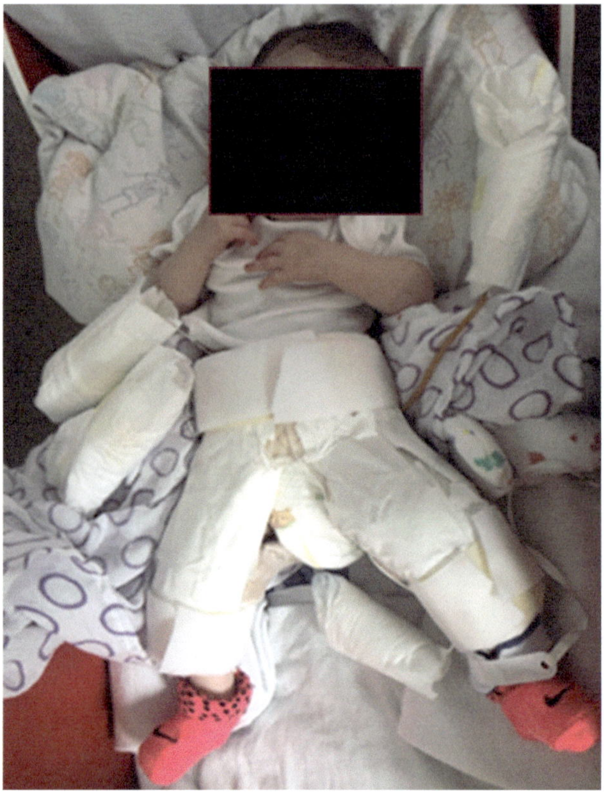

Fig. 12.8 Bivalved spica cast brace

Anterior/Double Iliac Osteotomies [3, 14]

- Indications
  - Single
    - Patients with classic BE <1 year of age.
    - Patients >1 year of age with Cloacal Exstrophy or Epispadius with diastasis <4 cm.
  - Double
    - Substantial diastasis of >4 cm.
    - Late or failed closure of BE in a patient who is >28 days old.
    - Aesthetic purposes for a patient who is >8 years old.
    - Females with BE and accompanying cervical prolapse.
    - Cloacal exstrophy (typically performed when a child is >18 months old).
    - The double osteotomy is usually performed 7–14 days before the urological procedure and stabilized with external fixation.
    - The diastasis is then gradually reduced by adjusting the fixator until the urology surgery.

- Pre-op Imaging:
  - Hip ultrasound.
  - AP pelvis X-ray.
  - Pelvis CT or MRI as indicated.
- Timing:
  - For younger patients (<12 months) or with a diastasis <4 cm, the procedure may be performed in one stage at the time of the urological procedure.
  - For older patients (>12 months) or diastasis >4 cm: Staged Closure.
    - In older children or those with a more severe pubic diastasis, it may not be possible to achieve immediate closure of the pubic symphyseal diastasis.
    - In such cases, closure may need to be done in stages. This involves using an external fixator and gradually adjusting the bar to bring the pubic bones closer together over 7–14 days.
- Positioning:
  - Patient is positioned supine on an operating room table that allows for fluoroscopic visualization of the pelvis.
  - A small (3–4 diameter) gel roll or towel bump is placed midline under the sacrum.
  - The bladder is isolated using a sterile drape.
  - Both legs are placed in sterile stockinette to help keep the patient warm (Fig. 12.9).
  - The pelvis is prepped and draped in a usual sterile fashion.
- Approach:
  - A 5 cm bikini-style incision is performed just below each ASIS along the inguinal crease and beneath the iliac crest.
    - The incision curves proximally to access the iliac crest apophysis.
  - Electrocautery is used to dissect through subcutaneous tissue until external obliques and deep fascia are clearly visualized.

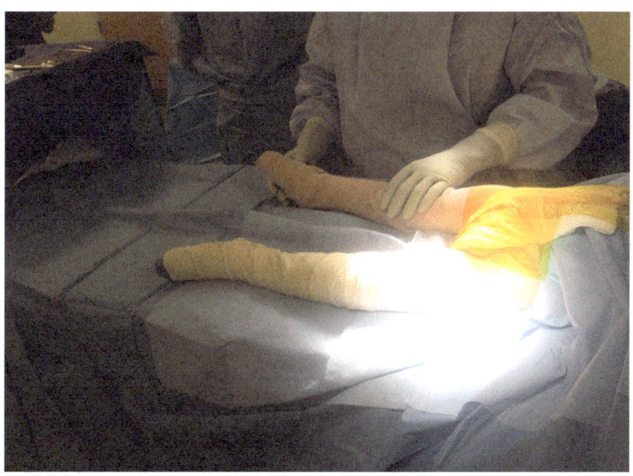

Fig. 12.9 Both legs are wrapped in a sterile stockinette

- The external obliques are gently dissected away from the iliac crest apophysis.
  - Care is taken not to cauterize the cartilage.
- A partial anterior (Smith-Peterson) approach to the hip is used.
  - The interval is between the sartorius and tensor fascia lata (TFL) muscles.
  - The lateral femoral cutaneous nerve (LFCN) is located within this interval.
  - The authors identify the TFL and carefully incise the overlying fascia to protect the LFCN. Blunt dissection is then used to develop the interval between the TFL and Sartorius muscles.
- A 15-blade is then used to split the iliac apophysis midline.
- A subperiosteal elevator is used to expose the inner and outer tables of the pelvis as far as the sciatic notch. Medial dissection on the inner table should stop just short of sacroiliac joint (SIJ) if a double osteotomy is to be performed.

- Osteotomy
  - A 1.1 mm diameter smooth Kirschner wire is placed from the ASIS to the dome of the sciatic notch to serve as a guide for the osteotomy. Fluoroscopy is used to confirm the proper positioning of this wire. Typically the bony cut will be just caudal to this wire (Fig. 12.10).
  - Anterior (Salter-cut) Osteotomy (single):
    - Retractors are carefully placed into the sciatic notch to protect its contents.
    - The osteotomy is then performed from just below the ASIS to the Sciatica notch.
    - An oscillating saw may be used to perform most of the osteotomy (about 4/5 of its length). Osteotomes are then used to complete the last portion of the cut under direct visualization.
    - In older children, a Gigli saw may be used to perform the cut.

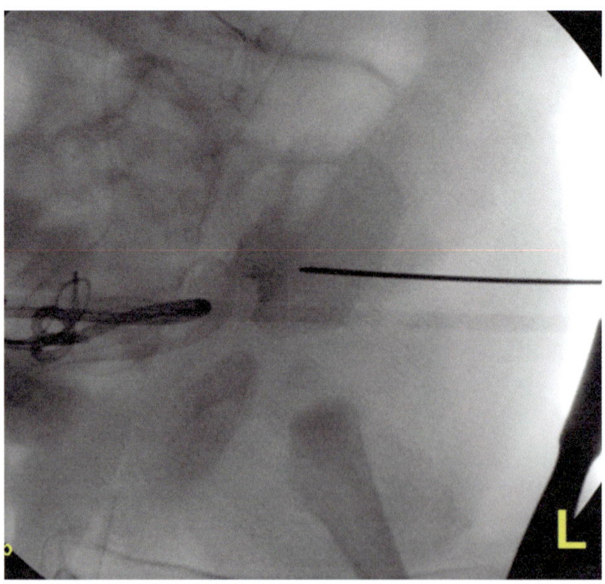

Fig. 12.10 Fluoroscopic image showing the position of guide wire prior to the osteotomy

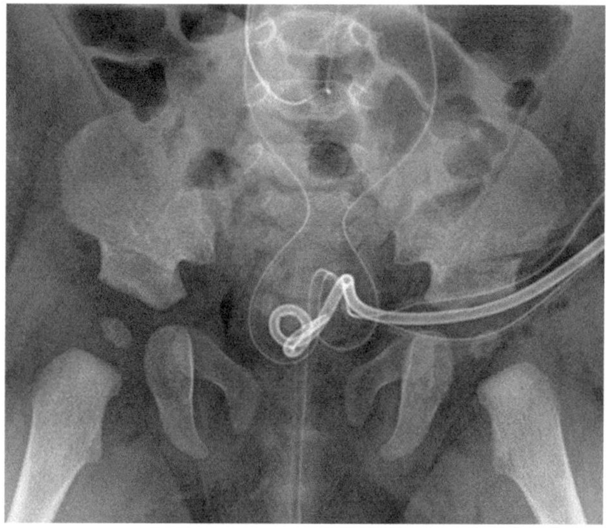

Fig. 12.11 Postoperative pelvis radiograph of a 3-month-old after bilateral anterior osteotomies

    - This osteotomy frees up the distal (acetabular) segment of the pelvis and allows it to internally rotate (Fig. 12.11).
  - Incomplete posterior Iliac Osteotomy (for double osteotomy—performed in conjunction with the anterior (Salter) osteotomy)
    - An incomplete vertical osteotomy is then performed about 1 cm laterally to the SIJ by leaving the posterior cortex intact.
    - This can be made with a burr, rongeur, or oscillating saw.
    - An osteotome can be used distally to free the distal cortical portion of the bone.
    - This creates a "greenstick fracture," which will be used to hinge the iliac wing anteriorly while the hemipelvis continues to be internally rotated (Fig. 12.12).
- Application of external fixator pins
  - Fluoroscopic guidance recommended.
  - Two pins are inserted lateral to medial through the internally rotated distal fragment and parallel to the anterior cut. Bicortical fixation should be obtained with each pin.
  - A third pin is then inserted between the inner and outer tables of the ilium in the iliac wing to stabilize the fragment located between the double osteotomies (Fig. 12.13).
- Pubic Symphysis Diastasis Reduction:
  - Closure of both incisions is then performed in layers.
    - Care is taken to close the apophysis over the ilium in a separate layer.
    - The overlying external oblique fascia is then closed, followed by subcutaneous tissue and skin closure.
  - For younger patients (<12 months) or with a diastasis <4 cm. The reduction is performed in one stage.

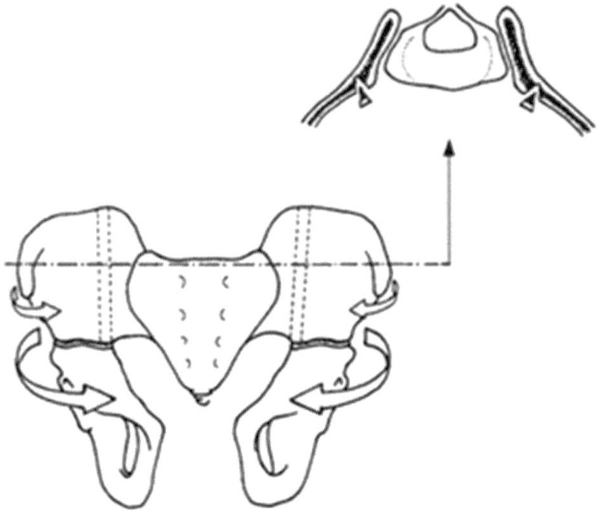

Fig. 12.12 Drawing illustrating anterior iliac wing incomplete osteotomy and correction of deformity. (From de Mattos et al. [3])

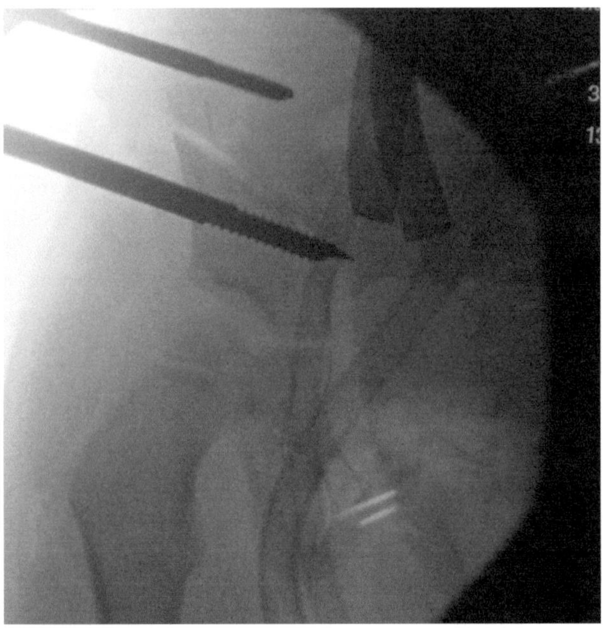

Fig. 12.13 Fluoroscopic image showing external fixator pin position

- The genitourinary repair is then performed by the urology team.
- After the urological procedure, the pubis symphyseal diastasis is reduced.
  - The fixator is adjusted and tightened with the pelvis reduced.
  - A large, monofilament, absorbable suture may also be used to maintain the pubis symphysis reduction.

- For older patients (>12 months) or diastasis >4 cm: Staged Closure
  - In older children or those with a more severe pubic diastasis, it may not be possible to achieve immediate closure of the pubic symphyseal diastasis. In such cases, closure may need to be done in stages. This involves using an external fixator and gradually adjusting the bar to bring the pubic bones closer together over 7–14 days.
  - At the time of the urological procedure, anterior fixation may be performed.
    - Consider anterior fixation in children >2 years and in cloacal exstrophy.
    - An appropriately sized screw (such as a small pedicle screw) may be placed in the canal of the superior pubic ramus.
    - A small plate or rod can then be used to connect these screws to provide anterior stabilization (Figs. 12.14 and 12.15).
- Postoperative immobilization
  - Light skin traction is used (Fig. 12.16).
  - Assess healing after 4–6 weeks.

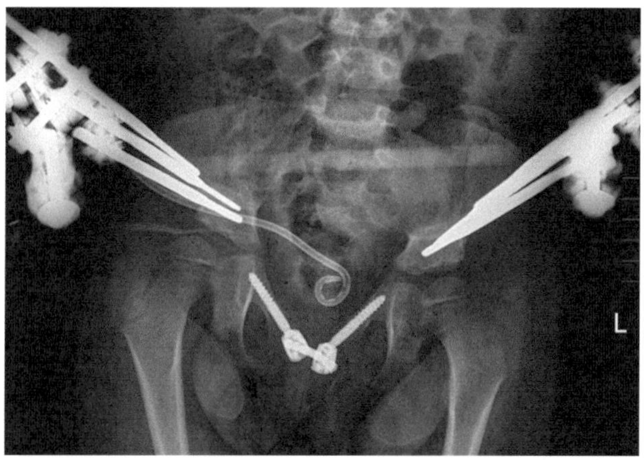

Fig. 12.14 Anterior fixation with pedicle screw within canal of superior pubic ramus in a 4-year-old with cloacal exstrophy before fixator removal

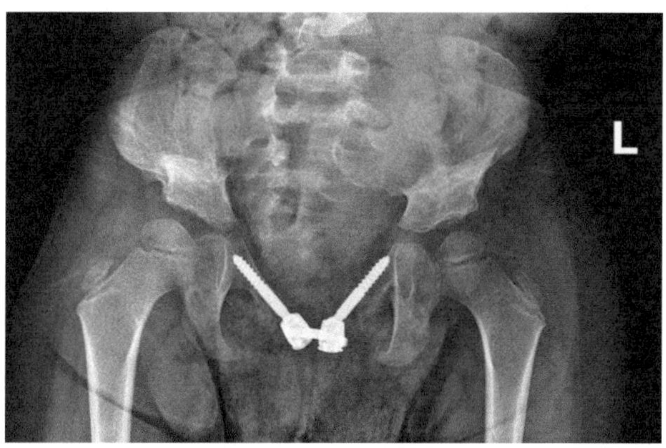

Fig. 12.15 6 months after fixator removal

Fig. 12.16 External fixation and skin traction after double anterior osteotomies

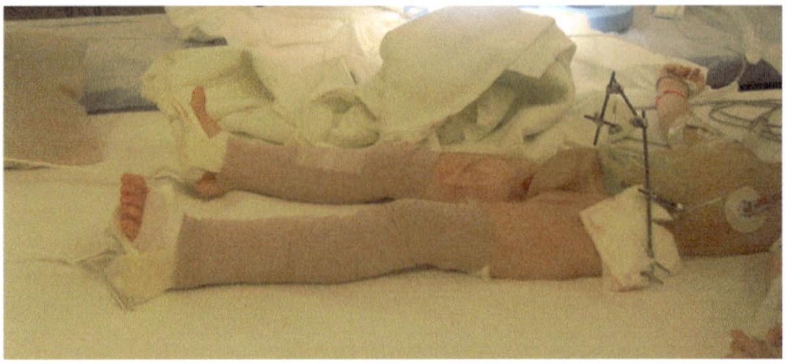

Anterior Oblique Iliac Osteotomies [5, 11]

- Indications
  - Patients with classic BE <1 year of age.
  - Patients >1 year of age with cloacal exstrophy or epispadius with diastasis <4 cm.
- Performed at the time of the urological procedure.
- Positioning:
  - Same as for anterior osteotomy.
- Approach:
  - Same as for anterior osteotomy.
- Osteotomy (Fig. 12.17)
  - The osteotomy procedure is similar to anterior (Salter-cut) osteotomies except that it extends from just posterior to the ASIS to the sciatic notch.
    - For neonates, a bone cutter and osteotome may be used to create the osteotomy.
    - A Gigli saw or oscillating saw may be used in older children.
- Pubic Symphysis Diastasis Reduction is performed as for anterior osteotomies.
- Postoperative fixation/immobilization
  - A spica brace/cast may be used.
  - External fixation along with light skin traction may be used (typically >1 year of age).
  - 4–6 weeks of immobilization is typically required.

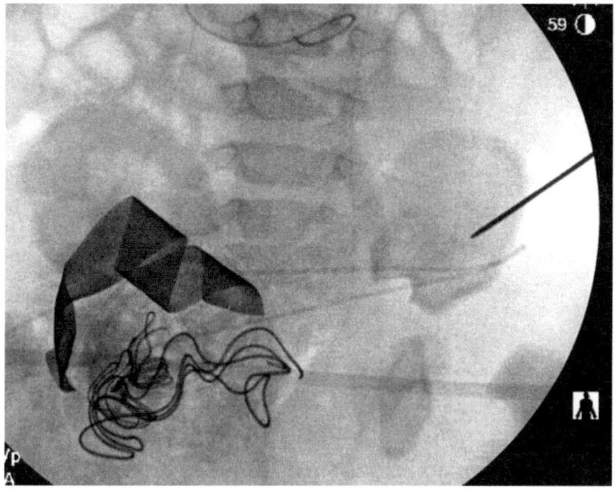

Fig. 12.17 AP fluoroscopic image showing trajectory of an oblique osteotomy

Anterior Bilateral Superior Pubic Rami Osteotomies [4]

- Positioning:
  - The patient is prepared and positioned supine on a flattop table.
  - A rolled towel is placed beneath the patient's buttock to aid in positioning.
- Approach:
  - After urogenital reconstruction is completed, the abdominal skin and its subcutaneous tissues are mobilized through the same incision.
  - The insertion of the rectus femoris on the pubis is identified.
  - The rectus sheath is incised at the lateral border of its insertion where the pubis bone is readily encountered.
  - The origin of the gracilis muscle and adductor longus, magnus, and brevis is identified just medial to the origin of the pectineus muscles.
    - These originate in the same order medially to laterally starting in the pubis symphysis.
  - An intermuscular approach to the superior pubic ramus is made between adductor brevis and pectineus muscle.
    - This will also be just medial to the insertion of the inguinal ligament.
  - The superior pubic ramus periosteum is incised longitudinally along the axis of the bone and circumferentially carefully elevated.
- Osteotomy:
  - Hohmann retractors are placed surrounding the superior pubic ramus deep to the elevated periosteum.
    - This will protect the obturator foramen neurovascular contents.
  - A full-thickness osteotomy is performed with the use of osteotomes or a Gigli saw.

  - The contralateral superior pubic ramus osteotomy is then performed in the same fashion.
- Pubic Symphysis Diastasis Reduction
  - Both osteotomized fragments are freed and tilted toward the midline.
  - An absorbable strong suture is used for approximation of the cartilaginous symphysis with little or no tension.
    - Care must be taken to not entrap the already reconstructed posterior urethra within the approximated symphysis.
  - An external fixator in the form of an A-frame can also be used for further fixation in older patients.
  - The rectus muscles and their sheaths are then closed together in the midline with interrupted suturing.
    - The lateral windows previously made for the approach are then closed in similar fashion.
  - The wound is then meticulously irrigated and closed in multiple layers.

Ahmedabad Osteotomy Technique (P. Mittal, MD and V. Gautam MD, Personal Communication, January 22, 2023)

- Indication
  - May be useful in low-resource environments—can be done without fluoroscopy.
- Positioning:
  - The patient is prepared and positioned supine on a flattop table.
  - A rolled towel is placed beneath the patient's ipsilateral buttock to aid in positioning.
- Approach:
  - The osteotomy is performed after mobilization and reconstruction of the bladder and bladder neck.
  - A 2–4 cm incision is performed centered over ASIS, parallel to the iliac crest.
  - Electrocautery is used to dissect through subcutaneous tissue until external obliques and deep fascia are clearly visualized.
  - The external obliques are gently dissected away from the iliac crest apophysis.
    - Care is taken not to cauterize the cartilage.
  - To access the ASIS, a path is created between the TFL and sartorius muscles, and the lateral cutaneous nerve of the thigh is gently retracted medially.
  - Both sides of the ilium are exposed down to the sciatic notch subperiosteally.
  - Retractors are carefully placed into the sciatic notch to protect its contents.
- We do not recommend dividing the psoas or rectus muscle tendons.

- Pin placement
  - Place 3–3.5 mm diameter half pins in by hand
    - Two on each hemipelvis
      - First pin is superior to ASIS in the iliac crest.
      - Second pin is inferior to ASIS in the supraacetabular region.
    - Pins to be placed at different angles in the axial plane to keep them between the inner and outer tables.
    - Insert by hand and under direct visualization so you can feel when they reach the far cortex.
  - We screen the hip clinically (move each hip through its range of motion while palpating for crepitus or limitation of motion) to ensure there is no joint penetration.
  - We do not normally use fluoroscopy.
- Osteotomy (variation of anterior osteotomy)
  - Perform Salter-type osteotomies with osteotomes and mallet.
  - Avoid levering downward with the osteotome when finishing the cut near the sciatic notch until the osteotomy is complete to prevent propagation of the crack.
  - The wound is then meticulously irrigated and closed in multiple layers.
  - The urological reconstruction is then completed by the urology team.
  - The symphysis is approximated and then held by a large, monofilament, absorbable suture.
- An external fixator is then applied (Figs. 12.18 and 12.19)
  - External fixator stays in place for 4–6 weeks.
  - It is removed when there is satisfactory bone healing.

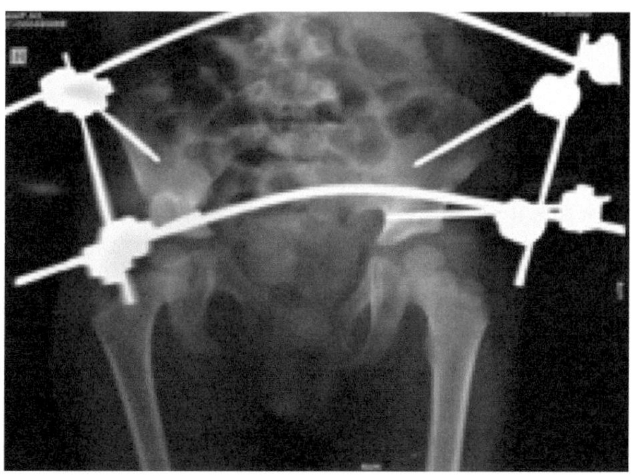

Fig. 12.18 AP Pelvis radiograph showing osteotomy and external fixator

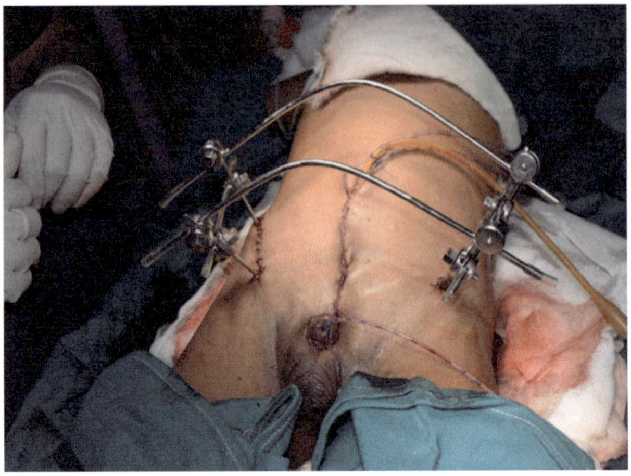

Fig. 12.19 Postoperative appearance of fixator

Postoperative Immobilization

Various immobilization techniques have been explored alongside osteotomies, ranging from elastic bandages and traction to casts, braces, and external fixation. The primary objective of immobilization is to maintain the pelvis in the desired position until osteotomies have healed sufficiently to withstand external rotatory forces. For younger children and smaller diastases, a spica cast or brace with the legs in internal rotation often offers adequate immobilization. However, in more severe cases, especially in repeat osteotomies, some form of rigid fixation may be necessary [12, 18, 24]. As mentioned, external fixation presents an appealing option, facilitating access to the surgical site for urogenital reconstruction and enabling gradual correction [12, 14]. In older patients, internal fixation can be safely employed, including traditional symphyseal plating or pelvic infix, spanning the symphysis [2].

Postoperative immobilization carries inherent risks of complications. Spica casts can lead to pressure sores, and there exists a theoretical risk of compartment syndrome. Internal fixation devices may encounter fixation loss due to the softer bone structure in younger children. Pin tract infections are common with external fixation devices but are typically benign and resolve with proper pin care or pin removal [15].

Complications/Long-Term Outcomes

Long-term outcomes in BE cases are typically contingent upon the severity of anomalies and the success of urologic reconstruction. The anterior abdominal defect closure rate reported in the literature stands at 95%, regardless of whether osteotomies are performed. Notably, the Johns Hopkins group reported the highest closure rate with a comprehensive approach involving osteotomies, external fixation, and Buck's traction [21]. However, attributing the success solely to osteotomies proves challenging due to inherent patient differences between those who receive osteotomies and those who do not. Nonetheless, cases of primary closure failure documented in the literature often lacked osteotomies. Long-term orthopedic outcomes generally lean toward favorability, with most patients achieving normal activity levels and mobility comparable to the general population. However, potential long-term adverse outcomes may include hip dysplasia, osteoarthritis, and excessive external rotation foot progression angle [7].

Complications associated with orthopedic reconstruction are generally rare. According to Okubadejo et al., there is a reported 4% rate of orthopedic complications, excluding pin site problems [15]. Although nerve palsies may occasionally occur following osteotomies, they tend to be transient in nature. Non-union at the osteotomy site is infrequent but may arise with larger corrections. Wound complications, especially those linked with posterior incisions, are not uncommon. Additionally, pressure sores resulting from casts or traction devices require vigilant monitoring and appropriate management, as they represent the most prevalent orthopedic issue [15].

References

1. Baird AD, Sponseller PD, Gearhart JP. The place of pelvic osteotomy in the modern era of bladder exstrophy reconstruction. J Pediatr Urol. 2005;1(1):31–6. https://doi.org/10.1016/j.jpurol.2004.09.001. PMID: 18947531.
2. Cardin S, Herrera-Soto J, Marrero P, Rich M, Swana H, Langford J. Pelvic ring stabilization using anterior subcutaneous internal fixation in bladder exstrophy repair. J Pediatr Orthopaedic Soc North Am. 2020;2(3):132. https://doi.org/10.55275/JPOSNA-2020-132. ISSN 2768-2765.
3. de Mattos CB, Mendes PH, Boechat PR, Júnior JL, da Silva Guimarães L. Bilateral anterior pelvic osteotomy for olosure of bladder exstrophy: description of technique. Rev Bras Ortop. 2015;46(1):107–13. https://doi.org/10.1016/S2255-4971(15)30187-7. PMID: 27026997; PMCID: PMC4799192.
4. Frey P, Cohen SJ. Anterior pelvic osteotomy. A new operative technique facilitating primary bladder exstrophy closure. Br J Urol. 1989;64(6):641–3. https://doi.org/10.1111/j.1464-410x.1989.tb05327.x. PMID: 2627639.
5. Giordano M, Di Lazzaro A, Guzzanti V, Careri S, Bagolan P, Zaccara A, Toniolo R. Oblique pelvic osteotomy in the treatment of bladder exstrophy in neonates. J Pediatr Orthop B. 2019;28(3):207–13. https://doi.org/10.1097/BPB.0000000000000614.
6. Grady RW, Mitchell ME. Complete primary repair of exstrophy. J Urol. 1999;162(4):1415–20. PMID: 10492227.
7. Jani MM, Sponseller PD, Gearhart JP, Barrance PJ, Genda E, Chao EY. The hip in adults with classic bladder exstrophy: a biomechanical analysis. J Pediatr Orthop. 2000;20(3):296–301. PMID: 10823593.
8. Jones D, Parkinson S, Hosalkar HS. Oblique pelvic osteotomy in the exstrophy/epispadias complex. J Bone Joint Surg Br. 2006;88(6):799–806. https://doi.org/10.1302/0301-620X.88B6.17712. PMID: 16720777.
9. Kenawey M, Morakis E, Cervellione R, Keene D, Kelley SP. The true pelvic volume change with various corrective osteotomy techniques for exstrophy-epispadias complex spectrum: the

value of computer-assisted virtual surgery. J Pediatr Orthop B. 2023. https://doi.org/10.1097/BPB.0000000000001145. Epub ahead of print. PMID: 38189741.
10. Lloyd-Roberts GC, Williams DI, Braddock GT. Pelvic osteotomy in the treatment of ectopia vesicae. J Bone Joint Surg Br. 1959;41-B:754–7. https://doi.org/10.1302/0301-620X.41B4.754. PMID: 13853691.
11. McKenna PH, Khoury AE, McLorie GA, Churchill BM, Babyn PB, Wedge JH. Iliac osteotomy: a model to compare the options in bladder and cloacal exstrophy reconstruction. J Urol. 1994;151(1):182–6; discussion 186–7. https://doi.org/10.1016/s0022-5347(17)34912-1. PMID: 8254810.
12. Meldrum KK, Baird AD, Gearhart JP. Pelvic and extremity immobilization after bladder exstrophy closure: complications and impact on success. Urology. 2003;62(6):1109–13. https://doi.org/10.1016/s0090-4295(03)00791-x. PMID: 14665365.
13. Mundy A, Kushare I, Jayanthi VR, Samora WP, Klingele KE. Incidence of hip dysplasia associated with bladder exstrophy. J Pediatr Orthop. 2016;36(8):860–4. https://doi.org/10.1097/BPO.0000000000000571. PMID: 26090968.
14. Nhan DT, Sponseller PD. Bilateral Anterior Innominate Osteotomy for Bladder Exstrophy. JBJS Essent Surg Tech. 2019;9(1):e1. https://doi.org/10.2106/JBJS.ST.18.00018. PMID: 31086719; PMCID: PMC6485763.
15. Okubadejo GO, Sponseller PD, Gearhart JP. Complications in orthopedic management of exstrophy. J Pediatr Orthop. 2003;23(4):522–8. PMID: 12826954.
16. O'Phelan EH. Iliac osteotomy in exstrophy of the bladder. J Bone Joint Surg Am. 1963;45:1409–22. PMID: 14069780.
17. Schmidt AH, Keenen TL, Tank ES, Bird CB, Beals RK. Pelvic osteotomy for bladder exstrophy. J Pediatr Orthop. 1993;13(2):214–9. PMID: 8459014.
18. Shnorhavorian M, Song K, Zamilpa I, Wiater B, Mitchell MM, Grady RW. Spica casting compared to Bryant's traction after complete primary repair of exstrophy: safe and effective in a longitudinal cohort study. J Urol. 2010;184(2):669–73. https://doi.org/10.1016/j.juro.2010.03.057. Epub 2010 Jun 19. PMID: 20639033.
19. Shultz WG. Plastic repair of exstrophy of bladder combined with bilateral osteotomy of ilia. J Urol. 1958;79(3):453–8. https://doi.org/10.1016/S0022-5347(17)66294-3. PMID: 13514903.
20. Sponseller PD, Bisson LJ, Gearhart JP, Jeffs RD, Magid D, Fishman E. The anatomy of the pelvis in the exstrophy complex. J Bone Joint Surg Am. 1995;77(2):177–89. https://doi.org/10.2106/00004623-199502000-00003. PMID: 7844123.
21. Sponseller PD, Jani MM, Jeffs RD, Gearhart JP. Anterior innominate osteotomy in repair of bladder exstrophy. J Bone Joint Surg Am. 2001;83(2):184–93. https://doi.org/10.2106/00004623-200102000-00005. PMID: 11216679.
22. Stec AA, Pannu HK, Tadros YE, Sponseller PD, Fishman EK, Gearhart JP. Pelvic floor anatomy in classic bladder exstrophy using 3-dimensional computerized tomography: initial insights. J Urol. 2001;166(4):1444–9. PMID: 11547108.
23. Suson KD, Sponseller PD, Gearhart JP. Bony abnormalities in classic bladder exstrophy: the urologist's perspective. J Pediatr Urol. 2013;9(2):112–22. https://doi.org/10.1016/j.jpurol.2011.08.007. Epub 2011 Nov 21. PMID: 22105005.
24. Vining NC, Song KM, Grady RW. Classic bladder exstrophy: orthopaedic surgical considerations. J Am Acad Orthop Surg. 2011;19(9):518–26. https://doi.org/10.5435/00124635-201109000-00002. PMID: 21885697.
25. Wakim A, Barbet JP. Connections of the bladder plate and bladder neck with the bony pelvis in a fetus with classic bladder exstrophy. Urology. 2002;60(1):142–6; discussion 146. https://doi.org/10.1016/s0090-4295(02)01715-6. PMID: 12100941.
26. Wild AT, Sponseller PD, Stec AA, Gearhart JP. The role of osteotomy in surgical repair of bladder exstrophy. Semin Pediatr Surg. 2011;20(2):71–8. https://doi.org/10.1053/j.sempedsurg.2010.12.002. PMID: 21453849.

27. Yazici M, Sözübir S, Kilicoglu G, Bernay F, Incesu L, Ariturk E. Three-dimensional anatomy of the pelvis in bladder exstrophy: description of bone pathology by using three-dimensional computed tomography and its clinical relevance. J Pediatr Orthop. 1998;18(1):132–5. PMID: 9449115.
28. Yazici M, Kandemir U, Atilla B, Eryilmaz M. Rotational profile of lower extremities in bladder exstrophy patients with unapproximated pelvis: a clinical and radiologic study in children older than 7 years. J Pediatr Orthop. 1999;19(4):531–5. https://doi.org/10.1097/00004694-199907000-00022. PMID: 10413008.

Common Adjuvant Surgeries in Exstrophy/Epispadias Care

13

Elizabeth Roth, Travis Groth, and John Kryger

Ureteral Reimplantation

Among the many considerations for surgeons at the time of bladder exstrophy repair is whether or not to perform ureteral reimplantation at the time of initial closure. Due to the anterior herniation of the bladder in bladder exstrophy, the ureter inserts posteriorly into the bladder and closer to the bladder neck. There is a significantly shorter intramural tunnel. VUR is present in a large proportion of bladder exstrophy patients after initial bladder closure, with estimates of >75% prevalence postoperatively, Dickson [9]. Recurrent pyelonephritis within this population typically affects 20–50% of patients in the 90-day postoperative period, even with the use of continuous antibiotic prophylaxis, Braga [3], Grady [14]. In certain surgical approaches, such as Young-Dees-Leadbetter bladder neck reconstruction or Kelly radical soft tissue mobilization, ureteral reimplantation may be required to facilitate reconstruction without undue risk of ureteral obstruction, Dickson [9], Tourchi [25]. With complete primary repair of exstrophy (CPRE), there is better bladder urinary cycling due to enhanced sphincter tone at the bladder neck. However, longer periods of urine holding and bladder pressure can also result in worsening VUR. This results in a pressure pop-off mechanism for the bladder and can compromise bladder distension during cycling and can result in worsening hydronephrosis. There may be a theoretical improvement in bladder cycling from bilateral ureteral reimplant (BUR) to facilitate better bladder distension during the dry intervals between voiding. Ureteral reimplant has also reduced hydronephrosis that is secondary to VUR. Lastly, correction of VUR will reduce the incidence of UTI. There is some evidence for larger bladder capacity at age 4 years in children closed with a CPRE-BUR combined approach, Ramji [22].

E. Roth · T. Groth · J. Kryger (✉)
Pediatric Urology, Children's Wisconsin, Medical College of Wisconsin, Milwaukee, WI, USA
e-mail: Eroth@childrenswi.org; Tgroth@childrenswi.org; Jkryger@childrenswi.org

A. R. Shukla, R. S. Joshi (eds.), *Bladder Exstrophy and Epispadias*,
https://doi.org/10.1007/978-3-031-91238-2_13

Cephalo-trigonal or cross-trigonal approaches may be considered and should be driven by the general shape of the bladder plate and which approach will achieve the most optimal tunnel length. With either technique, the procedure starts by identifying each ureteral orifice and cannulating with a small stent or feeding tube (3.5–5 Fr). Each ureteral orifice is circumscribed and dissected free of the intramural tunnel. The trajectory of the ureter will be more medial and caudal than in primary VUR, and there is an increased risk for inadvertent ureteral injury if the altered trajectory is not appreciated. Once the ureter is adequately freed from the intramural tunnel, a new trajectory can be plotted.

Cephalo-trigonal Technique The cephalo-trigonal approach to ureteral reimplantation is a bladder exstrophy-specific surgical technique first described by Canning et al. [4]. It utilizes the known altered trajectory of the ureter in exstrophy patients. There is a posterior insertion of the ureter that enters near the bladder neck. It naturally angles in a cephalad direction. The reimplant is further complicated by a very small bladder. This technique advances the orifice cranially. This allows advancement and elongation of the intramural tunnel while preserving the laterality of the orifice and minimizes risk for extravesical kinking of the ureter that would lead to obstruction.

After dissection of the ureter, a submucosal tunnel is sharply created from the native entry site in a cranial direction on the ipsilateral side of the bladder (Fig. 13.1). As in other ureteral reimplantation techniques, the tunnel length should ideally be 3–5 times the width of the ureter to ensure optimal resolution of VUR postoperatively. Ideal tunnel length may not be possible with a small bladder plate or with a bladder plate with modest craniocaudal dimensions. Care must also be exercised to consider directional shifts of the ureteral trajectory that may occur with corresponding bladder closure. After passing the ureter through the tunnel to the neo-orifice, the ureter is secured to the adjacent mucosa with an absorbable suture in an interrupted fashion. The neo-orifice is then assessed by passing the stent through the reimplanted ureter to ensure a gentle trajectory that passes easily in a retrograde direction. The process is then repeated with the contralateral ureter.

Advantages of a cephalo-trigonal technique include minimization of extravesical ureteral obstruction by taking advantage of the unique trajectory of the ureter in bladder exstrophy and maintaining the laterality of each ureter relative to the midline. Disadvantages include limited tunnel length with a small bladder plate as well as difficulty accessing the ureters cystoscopically through the urethra due to the cranial location and caudal trajectory of the intramural tunnel.

Cross-trigonal Technique (Cohen) First described as a technique for primary VUR, the Cohen cross-trigonal technique is also well suited for use in bladder exstrophy patients, especially in those where the transverse dimensions of the bladder plate exceed the craniocaudal dimensions, Cohen [6]. With this approach, the ureter is mobilized as above, but the submucosal tunnels are created sharply to advance the right ureter across the midline to exit on the left and the left ureter

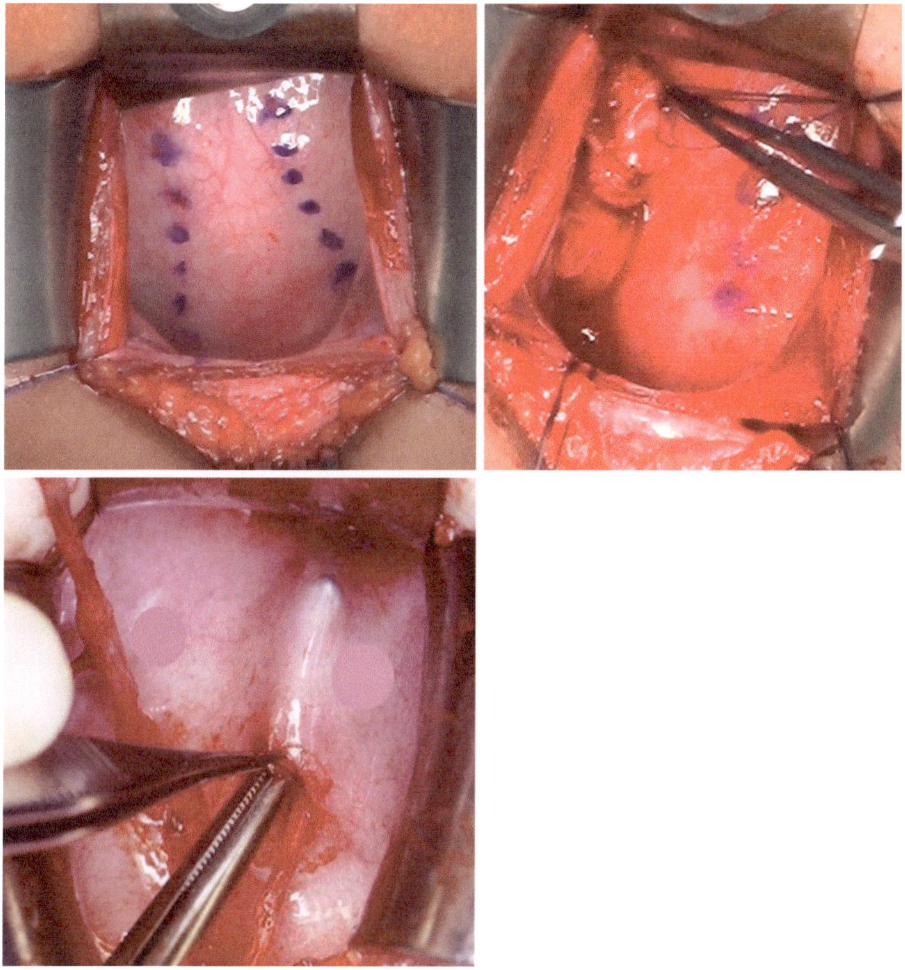

Fig. 13.1 Cephalo-trigonal ureteral reimplant

across the midline to exit on the right (Fig. 13.2). The surgeon will have to choose which ureter to place cranially based on the trajectory and size of the ureters overall. A 1:3–5 ratio of ureteral width to tunnel length is again recommended. The ureteral orifice is secured to the adjacent mucosa at the new site with an absorbable suture. A small-caliber catheter or stent is again placed retrograde to ensure a smooth trajectory of the ureter. Care must be taken to adequately mobilize the ureter to ensure that there is a smooth trajectory for the proposed new ureteral hiatus to avoid issues with extravesical kinking leading to ureteral obstruction. A small segment of the excess ureter may need to be excised to facilitate a smooth trajectory of the reimplanted ureter. Surgeons must also consider how bladder closure may alter ureteral trajectory and avoid advancing the tunnel significantly up the bladder sidewall to avoid obstruction.

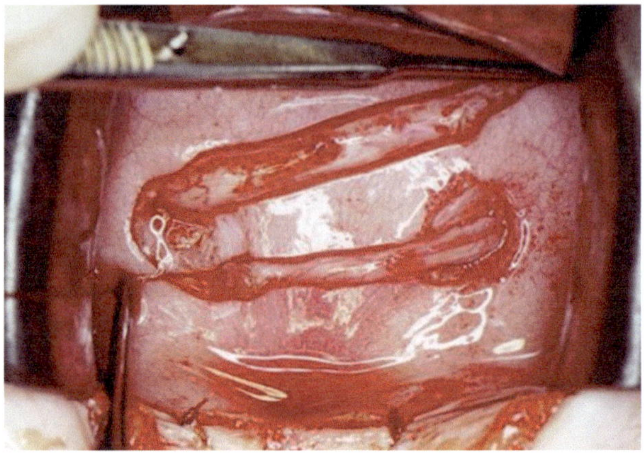

Fig. 13.2 Cross-trigonal ureteral reimplant

Advantages to the Cohen cross-trigonal approach include maximizing tunnel length in patients with limited craniocaudal bladder plate dimensions, better cystoscopic access to the ureters for future urologic surgical needs (but it can still be difficult), and familiarity of the technique to most pediatric urologists and surgeons. Limitations include increased risk for extravesical ureteral obstruction unless familiar with technical modifications for exstrophy and frequent need to resect a portion of distal ureter to ensure an appropriate ureteral trajectory.

Outcomes Multiple surgical groups have published clinical outcomes from bladder exstrophy patients who underwent ureteral reimplantation at the time of initial bladder closure, indicating that it is safe and technically feasible in experienced hands, Dickson [9], Braga [3], Ramji [22], Garat [13], Jarosz [17]. Documented clinical benefits include decreased incidence of febrile UTI, Braga [3], decreased renal scar on nuclear scintigraphy, Dickson [9], and decreased need for subsequent ureteral surgery, Dickson [9], Braga [3], Jarosz [17]. While the rate of VUR is decreased in reported cohorts, the overall rate of postoperative VUR in exstrophy patients is significantly higher than in primary VUR literature (0–40% versus <5%), Dickson [9], Braga [3], Jarosz [17].

Other proposed benefits of early ureteral reimplantation are improved bladder cycling efficiency, potentially leading to the development of greater bladder capacity. The international group based in India noted increased bladder capacity at age 4 years in patients who underwent concurrent BUR at initial closure, though this finding is likely multifactorial, Ramji [22]. In our experience, we have found BUR at the time of initial closure to be helpful in patients with large bladder plates, both male and female.

In carefully selected patients, reimplantation can facilitate improved bladder cycling, protect against recurrent pyelonephritis in the postoperative period, and possibly improve capacity and potential for volitional voiding. However, this must be weighed against the additional operative time, increased tissue handling and mobilization required, and additional surgical complexity added to an already complex surgical problem. Thus treating surgeons must individualize the decision on whether bilateral ureteral reimplantation is warranted on a case-by-case basis.

Inguinal Hernia

It has been well established that classic bladder exstrophy patients have a significantly higher risk of developing inguinal hernias when compared to the general population. Connolly [7] The historically reported incidence of inguinal hernias in classic bladder exstrophy ranges from 56% to 86% in males and 8% to 15% in females. There have been several theories for this, which include innate weakness of the abdominal wall, lack of obliquity of the inguinal canal, along with the increase in intra-abdominal pressure after bladder exstrophy closure, Husmann [16], Muecke [21].

Several studies have assessed risk factors for inguinal hernias in classic bladder exstrophy patients. Male gender is a significant risk factor for developing an inguinal hernia. Most recently in 2021, Lee et al. reported that 64.2% (34 of 53) of males developed inguinal hernias and only 5.3% of (2 of 38) females developed inguinal hernias after CPRE in patients with bladder exstrophy, Lee [19]. It has been previously reported by Lavien et al. that pelvic osteotomy is associated with a decreased incidence of inguinal hernia. In this series, 25% of patients developed an inguinal hernia if an osteotomy was performed versus 46% if an osteotomy was not performed. In their study, both female sex and osteotomies were associated with decreased risk for development of an inguinal hernia along with decreased risk for recurrence. Age at bladder closure was not associated with hernia formation, Lavien [18].

Inguinal hernias in classic bladder exstrophy patients are at risk for incarceration. Lee et al. assessed the timing of inguinal hernias following CPRE. In their study, 17% of patients presented with incarcerated hernias. The greatest risk for inguinal hernia formation was within the first 6 months following CPRE. They also noted decreased rates of development of inguinal hernias after 12 months of age, Lee [19]. Ellison et al. reported that simultaneous hernia closure at the time of CPRE was safe and decreased the risk of future development of inguinal hernias. In their study, 36% (9 of 25) of patients developed inguinal hernias if not repaired at the time of closure versus 11% (2 of 18) who developed inguinal hernias if previously repaired at the time of CPRE, Borenstein [2].

The recurrence rate for inguinal hernias is significantly higher in the bladder exstrophy population than in the general pediatric population. Previous studies have demonstrated a recurrence rate of 17–34% following inguinal hernia repair following bladder exstrophy closure versus a 0.3–1.1% recurrence rate in the general pediatric population, Stringer [23], Lavien [18], Borenstein [2], Ein [10].

Several different approaches for inguinal hernia repairs have been described in bladder exstrophy patients. This includes a pre-peritoneal approach by Connely et al., which is typically performed at the time of bladder closure and standard open inguinal approach, Connolly [7], Ellison [11].

Monsplasty

Another important adjuvant surgical step is the monsplasty. Patients with bladder exstrophy experience significant diastasis of the pubic rami. This results in the separation of the soft tissues above the pubic rami, which is the mons pubis. Even after surgical approximation of the pubic rami, there is separation of the mons pubis in the midline. Often there can be a deep cleft in the pubic midline. This gap can slowly worsen over time as the bony pelvis grows and the pubic diastasis widens.

It has been especially significant in the appearance of the female genitalia that appears more open at the introitus, with a flat or concave mons pubis and bifid clitoris and clitoral hood. Long-term data have shown that women with exstrophy-epispadias complex report dissatisfaction with their genital appearance, Mathews [20], Woodhouse [27]. The appropriate reconstruction of the mons pubis and clitoral structures can greatly enhance the cosmetic appearance of the genital area for girls and boys.

After the approximation of the pubic bones at initial closure, then the monsplasty is undertaken, Cook [8]. This can also be performed in subsequent surgeries at any age. If it is being performed at a later stage of surgery, then the first step is to excise the scar in the midline along its length and excise the non-hair-bearing skin. This will create the natural appearance of the escutcheon at final closure. The lipoma of the mons pubis is then mobilized from each side of the pubis by dissecting the cephalad and lateral and anterior edges until each lipoma can be freely mobilized to the midline. The lipomas are approximated in the midline with layers of 4–0 or 5–0 absorbable interrupted sutures. This creates one central mons above the pubic bones. Sometimes they are sufficiently generous in size to allow them to overlap in the midline and further reduce future separation. The skin edges are excised as much as tension allows to remove non-hair-bearing skin to create the natural appearance of the escutcheon. The skin is approximated cosmetically with absorbable sutures and often Steri-Strips to reduce tension on the skin edges during healing.

Prior to completing the skin closure of the mons, the clitoral hood is reconstructed. The clitoral bodies can be approximated in the midline, and the medial edges of the glans clitoris can be de-epithelialized and approximated with fine absorbable monofilament sutures. But we often do not perform direct approximation of the clitoral bodies on newborn closure to avoid neurovascular injury. Then each clitoral hood can be easily approximated in the midline to enhance the cosmetic natural appearance of the genitalia. The technique described by Grady is a vertical z-plasty, Weiss [26]. Each hemi-clitoral hood is incised along it's medial edge to create two layers. The inferior layers are approximated in the midline with fine absorbable monofilament suture to form the posterior layer of the clitoral hood. Then the superior layers are approximated along their medial edges.

These steps to enhance the mons pubis and clitoral bodies are rather easy steps that add considerable improvement to the pubo-genital appearance.

Umbilicoplasty

Due to the anterior abdominal wall defect in bladder exstrophy, affected children are born with an abnormally low-set umbilical cord at the insertion of the urachus on the exposed bladder dome, rather than the typical location approximately 2/3 of the way between the xiphoid and the pubic symphysis. The umbilicus plays an important aesthetic landmark on the abdomen. The surgical reconstruction of a neoumbilicus should be performed in conjunction with other exstrophy surgeries to create an orthotopic neoumbilicus.

A variety of techniques have been described, Sumfest [24], Cervellione [5], Feyaerts [12], Barroso [1], and Hanna [15]. The site of the neoumbilicus is selected by tracing a line across the anterior abdominal wall between the anterior superior iliac crests. The neoumbilicus is centered on this axis in the midline. Next, a flap or free graft of adjacent skin is selected. The area under the graft or flap is defatted down to the anterior abdominal fascia, and the skin is secured in this location to form an indented neoumbilicus. Three examples of neo-umbilicoplasty (NU) techniques are diagrammed below: Free graft, spiral-flap (S-flap), and rhomboid flap. We conducted an unpublished patient satisfaction survey of our MIBEC patients who were at least 3 years postoperative from umbilicoplasty. The preference was for free graft NU (Figs. 13.3, 13.4, 13.5, 13.6, 13.7, 13.8, and 13.9).

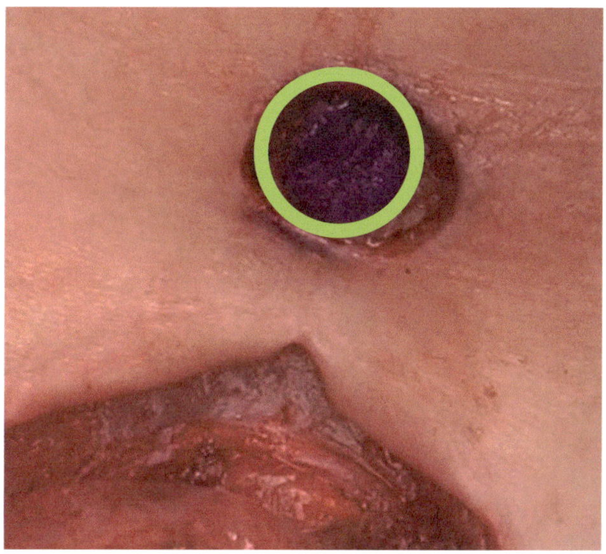

Fig. 13.3 Free Graft NU. A circular graft is harvested from the intended neo-umbilical site which is located at the intersection of the midsagittal line and the level of the iliac crest. After the free graft and underlying fascia have been defatted, the free graft is centrally secured to the exposed fascia with permanent or absorbable monofilament

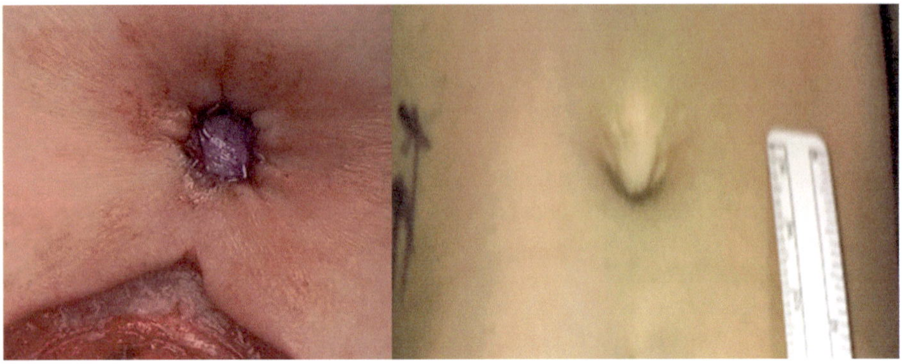

Fig. 13.4 On the left side is the finished Free-Graft NU. Neighboring skin is sutured to the free edges around the circumference of the graft to create a natural indented umbilical appearance. On the right is the long-term appearance of neo-umblilicus

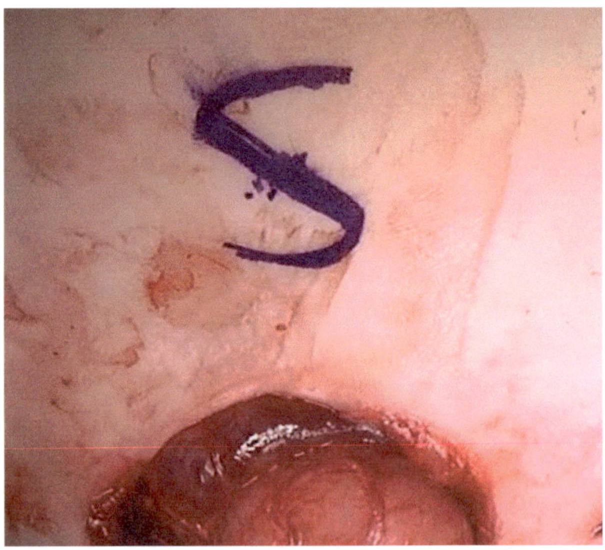

Fig. 13.5 S-Flap NU. Two 2 cm horizontal U-shaped flaps are created by a vertically oriented S-shaped incision centered on the intersection of the midsagittal line and the level of the iliac crest

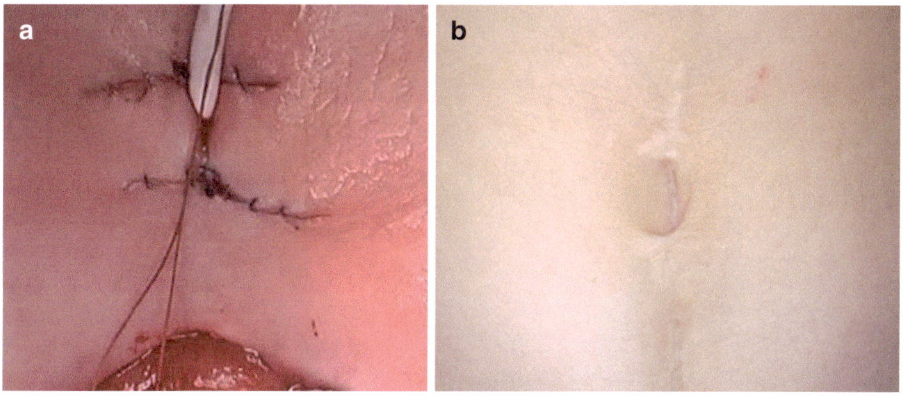

Fig. 13.6 Finished S-Flap NU. (**a**) The U-flaps are opposed to each other after the apex of each flap is anchored to the rectus fascia. The SP tube is located between the two flaps. The flaps are approximated to each other, leaving two horizontal incisions above and below the NU. Once the NU reaches a desired depth, the horizontal incisions are closed with interrupted sutures. (**b**) Long-term appearance of the S-flap

Fig. 13.7 Rhomboid Flap NU. The flap is shifted laterally with its left border running along the midsagittal line. Incisions are made along the green line, preparing the flap for mobilization while also preserving blood supply. A close-up photo showing the incision that outlines the rhomboid flap. There is a malecot catheter exiting the site as a suprapubic tube

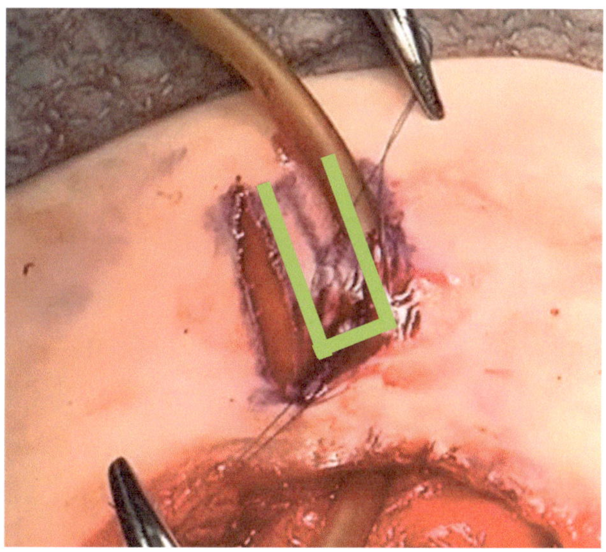

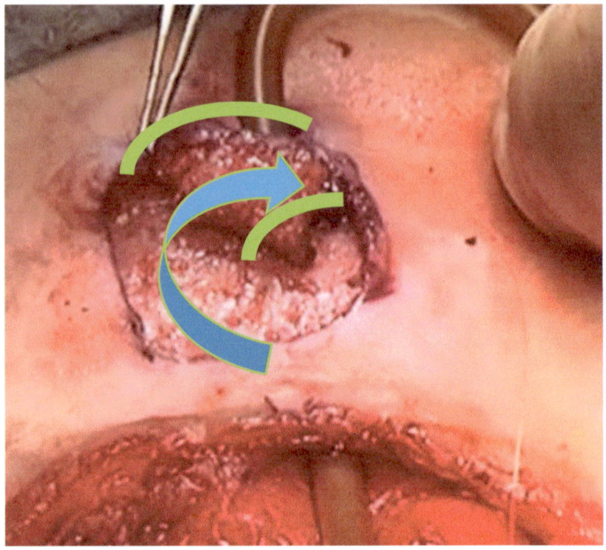

Fig. 13.8 Rotated Rhomboid flap. The rhomboid flap (superior and inferior borders are marked by green lines) is rotated in a counter-clockwise manner (blue arrow) about the SP tube, resulting in the subcutaneous surface of the flap facing outwards, the epidermis centrally oriented towards the SP tube

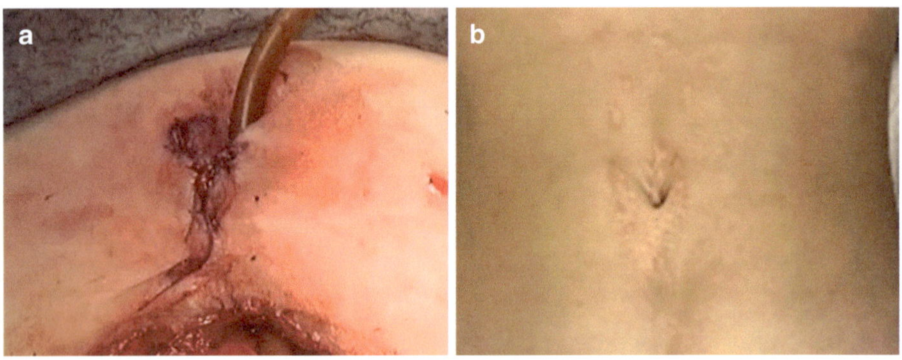

Fig. 13.9 Finished Rhomboid NU. Intra-operative appearance. Long-term appearance

References

1. Barroso U, Jednak R, Barthold JS, Gonzalez R. A technique for constructing an umbilicus and concealed catheterizable stoma. BJU Int. 2001;117:87.
2. Borenstein SH, et al. Effect of subspecialty training and volume on outcome after pediatric inguinal hernia repair. J Pediatr Surg. 2005;40(1):75–80.
3. Braga LHP, Lorenzo AJ, Jrearz R, Bagli DJ, Salle JLP. Bilateral ureteral reimplantation at primary bladder exstrophy closure. J Urol. 2010;183(6):2337–41. https://doi.org/10.1016/j.juro.2010.02.032.
4. Canning DA, Gearhart JP, Peppas DS, Jeffs RD. The cephalotrigonal reimplant in bladder neck reconstruction for patients with exstrophy or epispadias. J Urol. 1993;150(1):156–8. https://doi.org/10.1016/s0022-5347(17)35421-6.

5. Cervellione MR, Kyriazis I, Dickson AP. Construction of a natural looking inverted umbilicus for bladder exstrophy. J Urol. 2008;180:1869–72.
6. Cohen SJ. The Cohen reimplantation technique. Birth Defects Orig Artic Ser. 1977;13:391–5.
7. Connolly JA, et al. Prevalence and repair of inguinal hernias in children with bladder exstrophy. J Urol. 1995;154(5):1900–1.
8. Cook AJ, Farhat WA, Cartwright LM, Khoury AE, Pippi Salle JL. Simplified Mons Plasty: a new technique to improve cosmesis in females with the exstrophy-epispadias complex. J Urol. 2005;173:2117–20.
9. Dickson AP. The management of bladder exstrophy: the Manchester experience. J Pediatr Surg. 2014;49(2):244–50. https://doi.org/10.1016/j.jpedsurg.2013.11.031.
10. Ein SH, Njere I, Ein A. Six thousand three hundredsixty-one pediatric inguinal hernias: a 35-year review. J Pediatr Surg. 2006;41(5):980–6.
11. Ellison JS, et al. Impact of concomitant hernia repair at the time of complete primary repair of bladder exstrophy. J Pediatr Urol. 2016;12(4):211.e1–5.
12. Feyaerts A, Mure PY, Jules JA, Morel-Journel N, Mouriquand P. Umbilical reconstruction in patient with exstrophy: the kangaroo pouch technique. J Urol. 2001;2026:165.
13. Garat JM, de la Peña E, Caffaratti J, Villavicencio H. Prevention of vesicoureteral reflux at the time of complete primary repair of the exstrophy-epispadias complex. Int Urol Nephrol. 2004;36(2):211–2. https://doi.org/10.1023/b:urol.0000034675.34977.b4.
14. Grady RW, Mitchell ME. Complete primary repair of exstrophy. J Urol. 1999;162(4):1415–20. https://doi.org/10.1016/S0022-5347(05)68327-9.
15. Hanna MK. Reconstruction of the umbilicus during functional closure of bladder exstrophy. Urology. 1986;340:27.
16. Husmann DA, et al. Inguinal pathology and its association with classicalbladder exstrophy. J Pediatr Surg. 1990;25(3):332–4.
17. Jarosz SL, Weaver JK, Weiss DA, et al. Bilateral ureteral reimplantation at complete primary repair of exstrophy: post-operative outcomes. J Pediatr Urol. 2022;18(1):37.e1–5. https://doi.org/10.1016/j.jpurol.2021.10.012.
18. Lavien G, et al. Impact of pelvic osteotomy on the incidence of inguinal hernias in classic bladder exstrophy. J Pediatr Surg. 2014;49(10):1496–9.
19. Lee T, et al. Timing of inguinal hernia following complete primary repair of bladder exstrophy. J Pediatr Urol. 2021;17(1):87 e1–6.
20. Mathews RI, Gan M, Gearhart JP. Urogynaecological and obstetric issues in women with exstrophy-epispadas complex. BJU Int. 2003;91:845.
21. Muecke EC. The role of the cloacal membrane in exstrophy: the first successful experimental study. J Urol. 1964;92:659–67.
22. Ramji J, Weiss DA, Romao RLP, et al. Impact of bilateral ureteral reimplantation at the time of complete primary repair of bladder exstrophy on reflux rates, renogram abnormalities and bladder capacity. J Pediatr Urol. 2021;17(3):393.e1–7. https://doi.org/10.1016/j.jpurol.2021.01.020.
23. Stringer MD, Duffy PG, Ransley PG. Inguinal hernias associated with bladder exstrophy. Br J Urol. 1994;73(3):308–9.
24. Sumfest JM, Mitchell ME. Reconstruction of the umbilicus in exstrophy. J Urol. 1994;151(2):453–4.
25. Tourchi A, Di Carlo HN, Inouye BM, et al. Ureteral reimplantation before bladder neck reconstruction in modern staged repair of exstrophy patients: indications and outcomes. Urology. 2015;85(4):905–8. https://doi.org/10.1016/j.urology.2014.12.009.
26. Weiss DA, Steffe E, Borer J, Groth TW, Roth EB, Kryger JV, Shukla AR, Canning DA, Mitchell ME. The Richard Grady Monsplasty: a vertical z-plasty technique. J Pediatr Urol. 2021;17:575–6.
27. Woodhouse CRJ, Hinsch R. The anatomy and reconstruction of the adult female genitalia in classical exstrophy. Br J Urol. 1997;79:618–22.

Continent Anal Urinary Diversions in Bladder Exstrophy

14

Jacqueline P. Morin and V. Rama Jayanthi

Introduction

Despite the evolution of reconstructive procedures over the last several decades, bladder exstrophy continues to present the pediatric urologist with notable challenges. The ultimate goals of exstrophy repair remain to achieve satisfactory cosmetic results, adequate sexual function and fertility, and socially acceptable urinary continence with protection of renal function. The latter has improved over time with the development of novel surgical techniques and high-volume centers, with continence rates boasted as high as 70%; however, contemporary analyses of outcomes continue to demonstrate continence rates as low as 16.7% after primary repair [1, 2]. As there is no standard definition of "continence" in the literature, it is likely that a smaller percentage of patients described as dry may be truly continent, i.e., voiding volitionally with periods of dryness >3 hours [2, 3]. In fact, one systematic analysis of the literature found that only 68% of papers define what it means to be "continent," and most papers include those that require clean intermittent catheterization (CIC) within their definition of continence [3]. Therefore, it is difficult to discern the true rate of dry patients who void volitionally.

Most patients required multiple procedures, and many continue to suffer with life-altering urinary leakage despite these efforts [1, 4, 5]. These patients undergo an average of 2.3 surgeries, upwards of 8 operations for some [6]. It is also postulated that multiple reconstructive procedures of the bladder and bladder neck may compromise bladder urodynamics from previously healthy and safe to low capacity and noncompliant [7]. Continence issues have been found to have a negative impact on self-esteem, mental health, and social interaction for these patients [8]. Furthermore, bladder neck reconstruction has been associated with additional risks of bladder

J. P. Morin (✉) · V. R. Jayanthi
Department of Pediatric Urology, Nationwide Children's Hospital, Columbus, OH, USA
e-mail: rama.jayanthi@nationwidechildrens.org

A. R. Shukla, R. S. Joshi (eds.), *Bladder Exstrophy and Epispadias*,
https://doi.org/10.1007/978-3-031-91238-2_14

outlet obstruction, urethral leakage, pyelonephritis, bladder stones, and bladder perforation [9, 10]. Children who have already undergone sphincteroplasty, bladder augmentations, or additional reconstructive surgeries may not be ideal candidates for further reconstruction [11]. As such, it may be prudent to seek alternative options for continence in a manner that minimizes overall risks.

In patients who continue to suffer with urinary leakage despite extensive reconstruction, an option to achieve dryness is the continent anal urinary diversion (CAUD), of which several surgical methods have been developed over the years. Additionally, a CAUD may be an option for primary reconstruction in cases of bladder exstrophy as well, depending on the goals of the family. The objective of this chapter is to explore the CAUD options and outcomes in patients with history of bladder exstrophy who have failed primary continence reconstruction or who may be candidates for a primary CAUD.

Ureterosigmoidostomy

The ureterosigmoidostomy (US) is the original method of CAUD, during which the ureters are tunneled into the sigmoid colon, thus diverting urine into the rectum [12]. If the patient has normal anal tone, they are likely to achieve dryness through this continence structure. This technique was initially introduced in 1852 and was a very popular method of urinary diversion for many years [13]. The US fell out of favor in the 1950s with the development of the ileal conduit, as it proved to be associated with a variety of life-threatening conditions such as pyelonephritis, renal function deterioration, electrolyte imbalances, and malignancy development [12, 13]. Despite this fact, the US does remain an option for the select patient.

There are many attractive aspects of the US. The procedure itself is relatively straightforward with a short operative time [14]. The procedure offers a method of bladder management that does not include a stoma (with its associated complications often obviating surgical revision), require external appliances, bags, or indwelling catheters, and may be aesthetically preferred by patients and families [14]. Continence rates in the US are excellent. Gobet et al. reported complete continence in 82% of patients by age 20 [10]. Stockle et al. reported daytime continence rates of 97.4%, with complete continence rates as high as 92.3% sustained for >10 years with preserved renal function [15]. Patients report improved quality of life (QOL), and many would select the procedure if given the opportunity again, despite managing complications [10, 13].

Risks in the US can be common and serious. It should be noted that as the ureters are implanted into an intact sigmoid, urinary storage pressures may be elevated, which may result in urinary/fecal incontinence and retrograde reflux with potential upper urinary tract deterioration [11]. Some may require revision surgery to another urinary diversion due to urinary stone formation, colorectal anastomotic stricture formation, recurrent UTIs, pelvic organ prolapse, or malignancy development [10, 16]. The majority of patients (60%) will not demonstrate an increase in creatinine; however, mild to moderate renal insufficiency by glomerular filtration rate estimations only is reported in most patients, with some experiencing additional renal deterioration that requires additional surgery to protect the upper tracts [10, 14, 15]. Pyelonephritis has been reported in 16% of patients [17]. Electrolyte aberrations may occur as a result of absorption of urinary components. Hyperchloremic metabolic acidosis is the most common electrolyte abnormality and may lead to hypokalemia and chronic diarrhea [14]. This is more common in patients with baseline renal insufficiency [14]. Severe and untreated metabolic acidosis can lead to osteomalacia [14]. Hyperammonemia due to rectal absorption of urinary ammonia can occur and, in severe cases, lead to encephalopathy/neurotoxicity, which can be life-threatening if not treated in a timely manner [18]. Urolithiasis, urinary/fecal fistulas, proctitis, bowel leaks, and hernias may occur but are rarer complications [14].

Arguably the most sinister risk is that of colonic adenocarcinoma. Patients with US have a 100–550-fold increased risk of developing colonic adenocarcinoma as compared to the general population unless performed prior to age 25, which portends a 7000-fold increased risk [19]. The exact pathogenesis of malignancy development is unclear, but several theories hypothesize this may be due to chronic inflammation and irritation from mixing fecal and urinary composites. In particular, nitrosamines produced by fecal flora may be activated by the urine, leading to carcinogenesis [20, 21]. The latency period for adenocarcinoma development is an average of 20–25 years following US and is often asymptomatic until advanced [19].

Regardless, the US may be a viable first option, with conversion to an alternate diversion several years later. Care must be taken to resect the ureterocolonic anastomoses at the time of conversion, as adenocarcinoma development at the site of ureteral stumps has been documented following diversion revision [19, 22]. Interestingly, patients who have developed malignancies often request a new ureterosigmoid anastomosis as opposed to a different type of diversion, attesting to the QOL that this rectal diversion may offer [23].

The Sigma-Rectum Pouch (Mainz Pouch II)

An alternative colonic diversion known as the sigma-rectum pouch (SRP), or Mainz pouch II, was introduced in the early 1990s by Fisch and Hohenfellner [24]. This procedure was primarily used to manage adults with bladder cancer but also was applied to children with bladder exstrophy. The Mainz group had significant experience with classic ureterosigmoidostomy but developed SRP in an effort to reduce the incidence of high-pressure complications such as pyelonephritis, renal injury, and incontinence. Rather than simply anastomosing the ureters to the sigmoid colon as with the US, the SRP involves detubularizing the rectosigmoid colon to construct a reservoir in which the ureters are tunneled in an anti-refluxing manner [24]. Anti-refluxing anastomoses are created to help prevent episodes of pyelonephritis and upper tract damage. This diversion allows for a low-pressure, high-capacity reservoir to store urine. In theory, this procedure is superior to the US as it allows for longer storage of urine, thereby reducing urinary frequency/urgency.

Like the US, the SRP is a straightforward procedure of relatively short operative duration. Continence rates for patients with SRP far exceed anything ever demonstrated with a traditional bladder neck repair. Pahernik et al. described 100% daytime continence and 92% nighttime control in 38 children, the majority of whom had history of bladder exstrophy [25]. Hanna et al. described 61 patients who had failed initial closure. Sixteen ultimately underwent an SRP, and all were continent [26]. Hussain et al. wrote on 33 adults with exstrophy who underwent SRP, and all were dry during the day, but 2 had some nighttime bedwetting [27].

As with the US, there are some risks/complications of the SRP. Complications include ureterocolonic anastomotic strictures (4–7%), pyelonephritis despite the anti-refluxing anastomoses (8%), and hydronephrosis [28]. Hyperchloremic metabolic acidosis can occur after SRP, with approximately 60% of patients requiring medical management with alkalizing agents [28].

Certainly the biggest concern with SRP is the theoretical risk of colonic malignancy; however, to date, there have been few, if any, reported cases of tumors developing after this form of rectal diversion. This may simply be due to the fact that the procedure has been in existence for only a few decades, but it will be important for long-term studies to be published. Regardless, acknowledging long-term concerns about malignancy, short-term data as above show the children managed with SRP have markedly improved continence rates compared to traditional bladder neck repairs.

The Cologne Pouch

The Cologne Pouch (CP) is another method of urinary diversion that again uses the anal sphincter as the primary continence mechanism, as with the US and SRP; however, it aims to separate the evacuation of urine and feces. This is accomplished by fashioning a U-shaped segment of sigmoid colon, with one end connected to the rectum. The bladder plate is then attached to the proximal vertex of the "U" [29]. The ureters remain attached to the bladder plate, so no ureterocolonic anastomoses are required. This technique eliminates the risk of ureterocolonic anastomotic strictures that can complicate the US and SRP.

Continence rates are excellent in this procedure as well (100%), with separate urinary and fecal evacuation in 81.5% of patients [29]. This allows for reduced urinary and fecal urgency/frequency due to reduced mixing of the two excretory products. There is only a single series published on the CP [29]. In this cohort of patients, only 7.4% complained of voiding frequency [29]. Similar to the US and SRP, metabolic acidosis may ensue, and patients may require bicarbonate supplementation (55.6%) [29]. As there are no separate ureteral anastomoses performed, there is a reduced risk of both VUR and no ureterocolonic stricture formation, and as such, there may be a reduced incidence of UTIs or upper tract damage [29]. Perhaps due to its relatively recent development as a surgical technique, no malignancies have yet been reported in this series of patients who have undergone CP, with a mean follow-up of 8.3 years (range 1.9–17.4 years) [29].

A modification of this technique has been published where the bladder is augmented with small bowel and the augmented portion of the bladder is anastomosed to the sigmoid colon via a small bowel chimney [30]. As with both this technique and the CP, these methods exemplify the concept of a system whereby the urine is diverted to a pouch separate from the sigmoid that functions as a reservoir, allowing safe urinary storage while minimizing coalescence of feces and urine.

Conclusion

In conclusion, rectal diversion is a viable option for continent urinary diversion for patients with bladder exstrophy either as a primary or a salvage procedure. These procedures boast excellent continence rates and encouraging QOL measurements but are not often at the forefront of exstrophy management. While this is likely due to historical data warning of a variety of risks and complications, those negative implications of a rectal diversion may be balanced with improved QOL and more contemporary techniques and data. Indeed, continence outcomes far exceed what is attainable through more traditional means and these patients often require far fewer surgeries than an exstrophy patient who follows the traditional surgical pathways. This fact suggests that it is worthwhile to explore rectal diversions as an option for either primary or salvage surgical repair for patients, depending on the family's level of risk aversion, social situation, and overall QOL goals. Some families may elect for this approach due to greater continence success rates, the ability to avoid intermittent catheterization, and the more "normal" day-to-day lifestyle.

References

1. Morrill CC, Haffar A, Harris TGW, Crigger C, Gearhart JP. Current management of classic bladder exstrophy in the modern era. Afr J Urol. 2023;29(1):27.
2. Weiss DA, Shukla AR, Borer JG, Sack BS, Kryger JV, Roth EB, et al. Evaluation of outcomes following complete primary repair of bladder exstrophy at three individual sites prior to the establishment of a multi-institutional collaborative model. J Pediatr Urol. 2020;16(4):435.e1–6.
3. Lloyd JC, Spano SM, Ross SS, Wiener JS, Routh JC. How dry is dry? A review of definitions of continence in the contemporary exstrophy/epispadias literature. J Urol. 2012;188(5):1900–4.
4. Maruf M, Manyevitch R, Michaud J, Jayman J, Kasprenski M, Zaman MH, et al. Urinary continence outcomes in classic bladder exstrophy: a long-term perspective. J Urol. 2020;203(1):200–5.
5. Gargollo P, Hendren WH, Diamond DA, Pennison M, Grant R, Rosoklija I, et al. Bladder neck reconstruction is often necessary after complete primary repair of exstrophy. J Urol. 2011;185(6 Suppl):2563–71.
6. Hohenfellner R, Stein R. Primary urinary diversion in patients with bladder exstrophy. Urology. 1996;48(6):828–30.
7. Diamond DA, Bauer SB, Dinlenc C, Hendren WH, Peters CA, Atala A, et al. Normal urodynamics in patients with bladder exstrophy: are they achievable? J Urol. 1999;162(3 Pt 1):841–4; discussion 844–845.
8. Baird AD. Exstrophy in the adolescent and young adult population. Semin Pediatr Surg. 2011;20(2):109–12.

9. Hernandez DJ, Purves T, Gearhart JP. Complications of surgical reconstruction of the exstrophy–epispadias complex. J Pediatr Urol. 2008;4(6):460–6.
10. Gobet R, Weber D, Renzulli P, Kellenberger C. Long-term follow up (37–69years) of patients with bladder exstrophy treated with ureterosigmoidostomy: Uro-nephrological outcome. J Pediatr Urol. 2009;5(3):190–6.
11. Mingin GC, Stock JA, Hanna MK. The Mainz II pouch: experience in 5 patients with bladder exstrophy. J Urol. 1999;162(3 Pt 1):846–8.
12. Koo HP, Avolio L, Duckett JWJ. Long-term results of ureterosigmoidostomy in children with bladder exstrophy. J Urol. 1996;156(6):2037–40.
13. Woodhouse CRJ. The place of the augmented rectal pouch in urinary diversion. BJU Int. 2004;94(6):756–8.
14. Przydacz M, Corcos J. Revisiting ureterosigmoidostomy, a useful technique of urinary diversion in functional urology. Urology. 2018;115:14–20.
15. Stöckle M, Becht E, Voges G, Riedmiller H, Hohenfellner R. Ureterosigmoidostomy: an outdated approach to bladder exstrophy? J Urol. 1990;143(4):770–4; discussion 774–775.
16. Miles-Thomas J, Gearhart JP, Gearhart SL. An initial evaluation of pelvic floor function and quality of life of bladder exstrophy patients after ureterosigmoidostomy. J Gastrointest Surg. 2006;10(4):473–7.
17. Tollefson MK, Elliott DS, Zincke H, Frank I. Long-term outcome of ureterosigmoidostomy: an analysis of patients with >10 years of follow-up. BJU Int. 2010;105(6):860–3.
18. Cascino GD, Jensen JM, Nelson LA, Schutta HS. Periodic hyperammonemic encephalopathy associated with a ureterosigmoidostomy. Mayo Clin Proc. 1989;64(6):653–6.
19. Sathyanarayanaprasad M, Bhat S, Paul F. Adenocarcinoma of the sigmoid colon following ureterosigmoidostomy: a rare long term sequela. J Clin Diagn Res. 2018;12:PD09–10.
20. Crissey MM, Steele GD, Gittes RF. Rat model for carcinogenesis in ureterosigmoidostomy. Science. 1980;207(4435):1079–80.
21. Jian PY, Godoy G, Coburn M, Lynch G, Ro JY, Zhai Q "Jim," et al. Adenocarcinoma following urinary diversion. Can Urol Assoc J. 2012;6(2):E77–80.
22. Pettersson L, Tranberg J, Abrahamsson K, Pettersson S, Sillen U, Jonsson O. Half century of followup after ureterosigmoidostomy performed in early childhood. J Urol. 2013;189(5):1870–5.
23. Silverman SH, Woodhouse CR, Strachan JR, Cumming J, Keighley MR. Long-term management of patients who have had urinary diversions into colon. Br J Urol. 1986;58(6):634–9.
24. Fisch M, Hohenfellner R. Sigma-rectum pouch (Mainz pouch II). BJU Int. 2007;99(4):945–60.
25. Pahernik S, Beetz R, Schede J, Stein R, Thüroff JW. Rectosigmoid pouch (Mainz Pouch II) in children. J Urol. 2006;175(1):284–7.
26. Hanna MK, Bassiouny I. Challenges in salvaging urinary continence following failed bladder exstrophy repair in a developing country. J Pediatr Urol. 2017;13(3):270.e1–5.
27. Hussain M, Qamar U, Abidi S, Guzdar T, Ghori QA, Rizvi SAH. Outcomes of cystectomy with MAINZ pouch II and epispadias repair in exstrophy epispadias complex in adults: a single-centre experience from Pakistan. J Coll Physicians Surg Pak. 2021;31(10):1191–5.
28. Djokić JH, Milojević B, Pejčić T, Aćimović M, Stamenković V, Džamić Z. Sigma-rectum pouch (Mainz pouch II). Acta Chir Iugosl. 2014;61(1):29–34.
29. Klein T, Winkler A, Vahdad RM, Ekamp A, Boemers TM. The Cologne pouch procedure for continent anal urinary diversion in children with bladder exstrophy–epispadias complex. J Pediatr Urol. 2018;14(5):431.e1–6.
30. Phillips J. A new kind of rectal diversion in classic bladder exstrophy – pediatrics nationwide [Internet]. 2021 [cited 2023 Nov 1]. Available from: https://pediatricsnationwide.org/2021/04/28/a-new-kind-of-rectal-diversion-in-classic-bladder-exstrophy/.

Cloacal Exstrophy

15

Ted Lee and Joseph Borer

Introduction

Cloacal exstrophy, also referred to as omphalocele-exstrophy-imperforate anus-spinal defects syndrome, is the most severe form of exstrophy-epispadias complex. Although cloacal exstrophy was initially described in 1709, the first case of long-term survival following successful staged reconstruction was reported in 1960 [1, 2]. Historically, high prevalence of malnutrition, sepsis, and renal failure resulted in elevated infant mortality rates. Advances in neonatal management and surgical reconstructive techniques have resulted in improved life expectancy, with survival rates now approaching nearly 100% [3]. Patients with cloacal exstrophy require lifelong individualized care to optimize nutritional status and renal function. There has been a growing emphasis on long-term quality-of-life issues, such as urinary and fecal continence, health related quality of life, and sexual function [4].

Supplementary Information The online version contains supplementary material available at https://doi.org/10.1007/978-3-031-91238-2_15.

T. Lee (✉)
Department of Urology, Boston Children's Hospital, Boston, MA, USA
e-mail: ted.lee@childrens.harvard.edu

J. Borer (✉)
Department of Surgery, Harvard Medical School, Boston, MA, USA
e-mail: joseph.borer@childrens.harvard.edu

A. R. Shukla, R. S. Joshi (eds.), *Bladder Exstrophy and Epispadias*,
https://doi.org/10.1007/978-3-031-91238-2_15

Epidemiology

The prevalence of cloacal exstrophy is estimated to be 0.5–1 per 100,000, but the true incidence may be higher due to the frequency of undiagnosed omphalocele-exstrophy-imperforate anus-spinal defects (OEIS) syndrome in stillbirths [5–7]. In contrast to the clear male predominance witnessed in classic bladder exstrophy and epispadias, there is conflicting information on sex differences in cloacal exstrophy incidence [5, 8, 9]. Higher incidence in conjoined and monozygotic twins and recurrence within families suggest a genetic contribution to cloacal exstrophy development [10–15].

Embryologic Etiology

A number of theories have been proposed to explain the embryologic origins of exstrophy-epispadias complex. The most well-known theory is cloacal membrane overdevelopment that prevents medial migration of the mesoderm. This results in eventual rupture of the cloacal membrane due to absent mesenchymal support. If the rupture of the cloacal membrane occurs early on in gestation before the presence of the urorectal septum, this results in a lateral entero-vesical fistula seen in cloacal exstrophy. Conversely, if the rupture of the cloacal membrane occurs later in development after medial migration of the mesenchyme in the anterior abdominal wall but not the urethra, it results in epispadias [16, 17]. Other theories include abnormal fusion of the genital hillocks caudal to the cloacal membrane, caudal insertion of the body stalk resulting in failure of interposition of the mesenchymal tissue in the midline, and maldevelopment of the bony pelvis [17–19].

Prenatal Findings

Cloacal exstrophy can be diagnosed with ultrasonography or magnetic resonance imaging during the fetal period. Major diagnostic criteria (>50% of cases) are nonvisualization of the bladder, large midline anterior wall defect or cystic anterior wall structure, omphalocele, and lumbosacral anomalies. Minor criteria (<50% of cases) are lower extremity defects, renal anomalies, ascites, widened pubic arches, a narrow thorax, hydrocephalus, and a single umbilical artery [20]. Fetuses affected by cloacal exstrophy may be distinguished from those with classic bladder exstrophy due to concomitant findings involving the gastrointestinal tract and neural tube. Bladder exstrophy and cloacal exstrophy may also be differentiated by the location of the umbilical cord insertion relative to the abdominal wall defect. An inferior insertion is suggestive of cloacal exstrophy [21].

Prenatal diagnosis of cloacal exstrophy is essential for proper preoperative planning and neonatal management given the severity of comorbidities associated with this condition. Prenatal diagnosis also provides an invaluable opportunity for repeated education, counseling, and preparation for families and caregivers [22].

Reported prenatal diagnosis rates of cloacal exstrophy over the past two decades from tertiary hospitals in North America range between 78% and 89%. This is significantly higher than those reported from earlier time periods, which is likely due to the frequency of prenatal ultrasonography, the quality of the ultrasonography utilized, and the level of expertise of the ultrasonography technician and radiologists [23, 24].

Phenotypic Characteristics and Anatomic Anomalies

Cloacal exstrophy is characterized by exstrophy of the urinary bladder and cecal plate through an abdominal wall defect, anal atresia, hypoplasia of the colon, omphalocele, and anomalous genitalia. The bladder plate is divided in half by the cecal (hindgut) plate. The prolapse or intussusception of the terminal ileum from the exstrophied cecal plate is referred to as the "elephant's trunk deformity." The lateral appendiceal appendages are commonly coined as the "tusks on the face of the elephant" (Fig. 15.1) [25, 26].

Urinary

Abnormalities of the kidneys include renal agenesis, renal ectopia, malrotation, collecting system duplication, congenital cysts, ureterovesical junction obstruction, and vesicoureteral reflux. Ureteral atresia and bladder duplication have also been

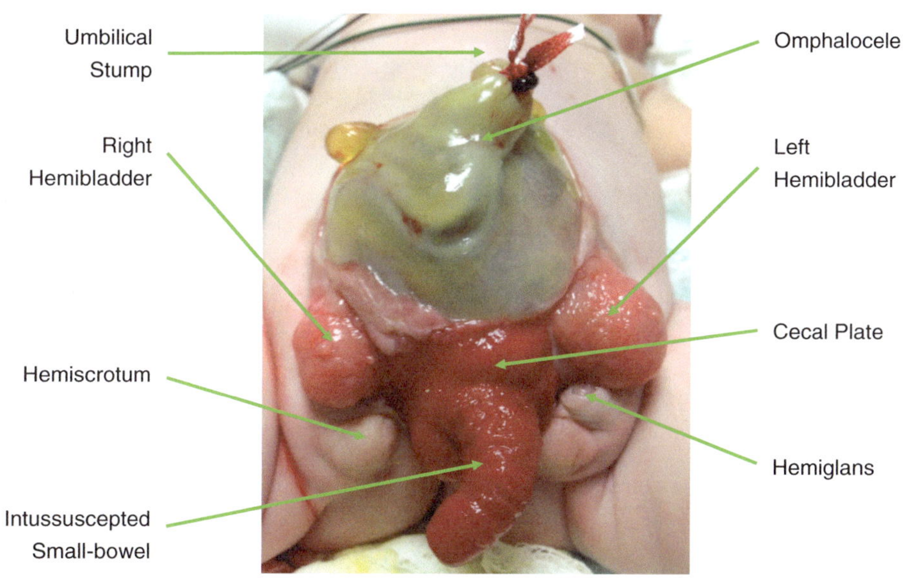

Fig. 15.1 Phenotypic characteristics of cloacal exstrophy

described [27]. In addition to congenital renal anomalies, the upper tracts are at risk of damage from high-pressure bladder dynamics and pyelonephritis. This is evidenced by baseline renal volumes being similar between those with and without cloacal exstrophy [28]. The prevalence of pelvic ectopic kidney ranges from 16% to 30%. Acute renal dysfunction in pelvic ectopic kidneys is of particular concern during bladder closure due to an abrupt increase in abdominal/pelvic pressure following pubic bone approximation during second-stage cloacal exstrophy closure (e.g., compartment syndrome) [29]. Vesicoureteral reflux has been reported in 50–60% following reconstruction and may need to be addressed surgically in the setting of repeated upper tract infections [30].

Gastrointestinal

Congenital short bowel syndrome has been observed in up to 25% of patients. Malabsorption could exist despite sufficient bowel length. This underscores the importance of ileal and colonic preservation, especially at an early age. Other anomalies include intestinal duplications (including of the appendix, ileum, and colon), ectopic perineal anus, malrotation, and duodenal atresia [31–33]. Preservation of the appendix or appendiceal appendages during the initial reconstructive stages is preferred for potential future use as a catheterizable channel. Omphaloceles need to be carefully assessed prior to surgical reconstruction, as rupture requires immediate intervention.

Neurologic

Nearly all cloacal exstrophy patients have underlying spinal dysraphisms, the majority of which are closed. As a result of the closed spinal defect, the prevalence of hydrocephalus is much lower compared to rates within the spina bifida population. The most common defects are spinal lipoma, followed by terminal myelocystoceles. Other defects include myelomeningocele, low-lying conus with tethered cord/fatty filum, diastematomyelia, and meningocele [34, 35]. Intracranial abnormalities, including Chiari malformation, hydrocephalus, and craniosynostosis, may be present [36].

Musculoskeletal

Bony anomalies of the pelvis include externally rotated anterior and posterior pelvis, acetabular retroversion, and diastasis of the pubic symphysis. Pubic diastasis, which is frequently greater than 6 cm, can pose a challenge during surgical reconstruction. Staged approximation may be needed to help approximate the pubic rami gradually, perhaps reducing the risk of pelvic compartment syndrome due to abrupt closure of the pelvic ring [37]. Hip dysplasia is common (16%); therefore, routine physical examinations and plain film X-rays should be performed on newborns [38]. Reported lower limb malformations include clubfoot, equinovarus deformity, and anomalies of the digits. Reported vertebral anomalies include scoliosis, kyphosis, hemivertebrae, sacral anomalies, and duplication [39].

Genital

The penis is often separated into two hemi-phalluses with wide division of the scrotum [40]. Intravesical location of the phallus can be present [41]. Cryptorchidism is common. Absence and duplication of the vas deferens have been described but are not the rule [39, 42].

The clitoral halves are separated with wide division of the labia. Uterus didelphys and other fusion anomalies of the Müllerian duct structures are seen in up to 87% of cloacal exstrophy females. Vaginal agenesis occurs in one-third of cloacal exstrophy females. Vaginal duplication, agenesis, atresia/hypoplasia, and lateral displacement are common. Cervical and ovarian duplication are also reported [42, 43].

Management

Neonatal

In addition to a detailed physical examination, baseline laboratory tests should be obtained (CBC, BMP, blood type). Karyotyping should be considered if sex is not clear on examination. Once stabilized, the umbilical cord should be ligated with a suture instead of an umbilical clamp to prevent abrasion to the bladder or cecal plate. Optimal hydration and nutrition should be established as soon as possible. In addition to breastfeeding and/or enteral feeds, total parenteral nutrition is often necessary to optimize nutritional status. The exposed omphalocele, bladder, and bowel should be covered with occlusive plastic wrap (Tegaderm™) or a hydrated silicone gel dressing (Mepitel®) to keep mucosal surfaces moist [44]. A two-layer dressing may be employed, where the first covering directly on the bladder mucosal surface includes a small hole through which the prolapsed ileum segment is passed. A second superficial dressing covers and protects the prolapsed ileum from diaper abrasion. This second layer of dressing may also be used to help approximate the fascia in the midline and reduce the omphalocele defect. The goal of this dressing technique is to separate the stool from the urine and bladder mucosal surface.

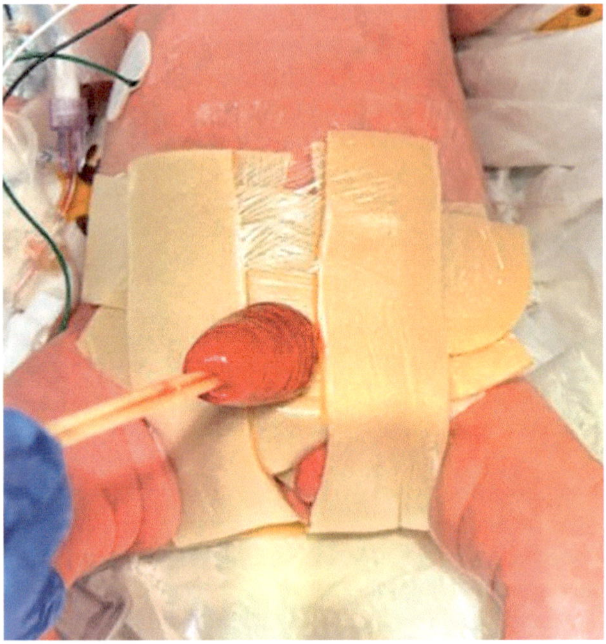

Initial imaging studies include ultrasound of the abdomen and spine as well as abdominal/pelvic plain films. Sonographic examination allows the evaluation of the upper urinary tract, internal genital structures, and spinal cord. Magnetic resonance imaging of the spine is typically performed prior to surgical intervention, and the abdomen/pelvis may be added if anatomy remains unclear following ultrasonography [45].

Surgical Reconstruction

Broad goals of surgical reconstruction include (1) closure of the omphalocele, separation of the cecal plate from the bladder halves, approximation of the posterior bladder halves in the midline, tubularization of the cecum, and incorporation of the hindgut into the gastrointestinal tract via an end colostomy; (2) closure of the exstrophic bladder, approximation of the pubic rami, and genital reconstruction. When patients and families are ready, surgical reconstruction can be performed to achieve social continence. Additional surgical interventions that may be necessary are repair of spinal dysraphism and reconstruction of Müllerian organs prior to menarche.

Most centers have moved from a single-stage reconstruction (closure of the bladder at the time of initial reconstruction) to a staged approach. A staged approach appears to increase the chances of successful primary bladder closure compared to the single-stage approach. Under optimal conditions, a one-stage closure may be considered [47].

Stage 1: Omphalocele Repair, Cecal Plate Tubularization, Hindgut Terminal Colostomy, Reapproximation of Bladder Halves

The timing of initial surgical intervention is dependent on a multitude of factors, including medical stability, nutritional status, and infant size. Important anatomic factors contribute to this decision, including size and status of the omphalocele (e.g., rupture), size of the cecal and bladder plates, and open or closed spinal dysraphism.

Historically, surgery was performed within 72 h of life to minimize the risk of omphalocele rupture, urinary tract infection, and metabolic issues secondary to colonic mucosa being exposed to urine. However, the ventral abdominal closure and genitourinary/gastrointestinal reconstruction can be safely delayed if stool and urine can be separated from the bladder surface and bowel surface, respectively. The omphalocele should also be carefully monitored given the risk of rupture. Attempts may be made to passively reduce the ventral wall fascial defect using dressings prior to initial reconstruction as demonstrated above. This may help prevent worsening of ventral abdominal defect, which may increase the risk of abdominal compartment syndrome at the time of closure. Delay of reconstruction may allow for growth, improvement of nutritional status, and closure of an open neural tube defect [46].

Following careful exam under anesthesia, ureteral catheters are positioned in the ureteral orifices and secured prior to dissection. The omphalocele dissection begins superiorly, and the omphalocele membrane is frequently removed. Following ligation of the umbilical vessels, the bladder plates are separated from the adjacent skin. The medial cecal plate is separated from the two lateral bladder plates to be utilized in the gastrointestinal tract. The bladder halves are approximated in the midline. Inguinal hernias should be repaired if found. The exstrophied cecal plate is then tubularized and placed in continuity with the terminal blind-ending hindgut. The most distal portion of the hindgut is then exteriorized and matured as an end colostomy. Another option may be to retain the cecal plate with the bladder plates at the time of initial surgical reconstruction to maintain the congenital enterocystoplasty or "auto-augment" [48]. However, there are concerns that not incorporating the cecal plate within the gastrointestinal tract during this initial period may result in shortened bowel length and compromised water resorption. Efforts must be made to preserve bowel segments and appendiceal appendages, which can be useful for future bowel, bladder, or vaginal reconstruction.

Creation of an end ileostomy is no longer recommended due to the increased risk of malnutrition and gastrointestinal complications [49]. Leaving the hindgut in continuity with the urinary tract within the pelvis results in complications such as hyperchloremic acidosis, urinary tract infections, failure to thrive, sepsis, dehydration, and TPN dependence. The separation of the hindgut from the urinary tract, dissection of the entire hindgut from the pelvis, creation of gastrointestinal continuity, closure of ileostomy, and creation of colostomy at a later date in patients initially managed this way can improve upon these morbidities. This surgery is referred to as "hindgut rescue" [50].

The omphalocele is ideally completely repaired. However, very large omphaloceles may be left intact due to lack of intra-abdominal domain that can result in abdominal compartment syndrome. In such cases, staged repair of the omphalocele with a silo may be necessary. A biosynthetic patch may be utilized to bridge the "gap" between the two lateral leaflets of the fascia, although this results in a large ventral diastasis postoperatively [44, 45].

Stage 2: Bladder Closure, Reconstruction of the External Genitalia, Pubic Rami Approximation with Osteotomies

The patient is now left with a single exstrophied bladder plate. The exposed mucosa must be protected as previously described. The timing of the second-stage repair is typically between 6 and 24 months of age but ultimately dependent on the overall nutritional status and growth of the patient. Prior to repair, the pubic diastasis must be carefully evaluated. The pubic rami need to be reapproximated at the time of bladder closure to reduce tension off the anterior abdominal soft tissue and reconstructed bladder. To gain pelvic bone mobility for adequate reapproximation, osteotomies are typically required. Osteotomies decrease the risk of wound dehiscence and abdominal wall hernias [51]. If the degree of diastasis is too large (>6 cm), staged osteotomies and gradual approximation of the bones may be necessary to enable pubic rami approximation without an abrupt increase in abdominal and pelvic pressures [37]. An abrupt increase in abdominal and pelvic pressures following lower abdominal wall closure may result in decreased lung volumes, reduced chest wall compliance, compromised renal function, glans ischemia, and prolonged ileus [26]. Pelvic kidneys in particular may experience an increase in renal pelvis pressure, peak systolic velocity, and resistive index compared to orthotopic kidneys at the time of pubic rami approximation. Those with solitary pelvic kidneys may benefit from real-time monitoring during the perioperative period [52].

Genital reconstruction may be pursued during this stage. In males, wide pubic diastasis and rotational deformities of the pelvic skeletal structures contribute to the short, pendular penis often accompanied by dorsal curvature. Radical soft tissue mobilization or the "Kelly repair" has been performed to dissect the corporal bodies off the pubic rami, which enables medial approximation of the corporal bodies. The urethral meatus is typically matured in a hypospadiac location [53]. Glans ischemia, urethrocutaneous fistula, vesicocutaneous fistula, bladder outlet obstruction, and bladder and fascial dehiscence are some of the potential complications that can occur at this stage [26].

It is imperative to avoid urinary obstruction at the bladder outlet level. This can result in urinary stasis and a higher risk of urinary tract infection. Underlying vesicoureteral reflux, which is present in the majority of patients with cloacal exstrophy, may be addressed at this time. However, performing ureteroneocystostomy may place the patient at higher risk of iatrogenic obstruction at the level of the ureterovesical junction [30].

Secondary Procedures

Volitional voiding is typically not an option in those with compromised pelvic innervation associated with spinal dysraphism. In our experience, urinary continence typically becomes a priority when patients reach school age. Other factors include skin breakdown in the perineum from chronic urinary leakage. Prior to any intervention, urodynamics and fluoroscopic studies should be performed to assess bladder compliance and capacity. Cystoscopy and examination under anesthesia may be necessary. Upper tract imaging should be performed. If there is any concern for nephron loss secondary to congenital dysplasia, obstruction, or infection, a nuclear renal scan can be useful to understand baseline split renal function.

Many will require enterocystoplasty using ileum or hindgut due to a small-capacity bladder with low compliance. Prior to the operating room, it is useful to have an understanding of colonic length and degree of dilation through contrast enema via the colostomy. Ideally, dilated portions of the distal hindgut can be utilized as a bowel segment for enterocystoplasty to avoid a bowel anastomosis.

The bladder outlet can be addressed through bladder neck reconstruction or closure. Extensive preoperative counseling is necessary to ensure patients and caregivers are socially ready for urinary reconstruction. Nonadherence to a strict catheterization schedule, especially when the bladder neck is closed, can place the patient at high risk of upper tract damage and bladder perforation. If there is concern for noncompliance, a narrow bladder neck reconstruction may be preferred than a complete bladder neck closure, even if this places the patient at higher risk of stress or overflow incontinence.

It is preferable to utilize the appendix or appendiceal appendage for the creation of an appendicovescistostomy or Mitrofanoff catheterizable channel, since it is a naturally tubularized structure. If an appendix or appendiceal appendage cannot be found, distal hindgut or ileum may be utilized as a segment of bowel to create a Monti catheterizable channel [54].

Fecal continence is also not feasible in majority of cloacal exstrophy patients. Some patients may be candidates for posterior sagittal anorectoplasty and/or colonic pull-through. Children with good colonic length, anocutaneous fistula, and preserved pelvic innervation may be the best candidates for future pull-through [55]. A Malone antegrade colonic enema can be considered in those undergoing pull-through to assist with fecal continence.

Prior to estrogen stimulation, it is challenging to properly assess the anatomy of Müllerian structures due to underdevelopment. It may be beneficial to wait until the beginning stages of puberty to further delineate the anatomy of Müllerian structures. A magnetic resonance imaging study of the abdomen and pelvis is the study of choice to assess the Müllerian structures. Dilation can potentially aid in reconstruction. In the setting of pain associated with an obstructed Müllerian structure, ovarian suppression may relieve pain and allow optimal timing of reconstruction. Abdominal pain related to hematometrocolpos is often mistaken for pyelonephritis, as most of these patients have chronic bacteriuria. Obstructed Müllerian structures may be temporarily drained through a percutaneous approach in the setting of infection or intolerable pain, although this is dependent upon a safe "window" for percutaneous access. Müllerian remnants should be reconstructed or removed based on appearance and shared decision-making with the patient/caregivers. If there is a preexisting channel, vaginoscopy can be useful to assess for an intact cervix. An intact cervix may decrease future infection risk, so its presence may aid in surgical decision-making [43].

Neovaginal reconstruction may be necessary to bridge the gap. Small and large bowel segments may be considered for use for reconstruction with the understanding that there is high risk of side effects of malodorous, mucous build up. If there is a vaginal orifice at the perineal surface, augmentation vaginoplasty with buccal mucosa may be an option [56]. Vaginal stenosis will occur without regular postoperative vaginal dilation. However, vaginal dilation should not be rushed in young patients, as this may cause significant anxiety and psychological trauma. Providers should assess patient/caregiver readiness for vaginal dilation [57]. If not ready, vaginal stenosis can be addressed at an older age.

Outcomes

Urinary Continence

As mentioned above, vast majority of patients will not achieve voluntary urinary control. Achieving urinary continence through surgical reconstruction requires full commitment from patients/caregivers. Multiple surgeries are involved, as surgical reconstruction typically requires revision surgeries. Significant time, effort, and financial resources are utilized to achieve continence even after surgery [58]. Most importantly, it is imperative to counsel patients and caregivers on the risk of upper tract damage from what is essentially the creation of a controlled obstruction of the lower urinary tract.

In a study reporting long-term continence outcomes in 63 cloacal exstrophy patients, 71.4% had a catheterizable channel, 88.9% of whom were continent between catheterizations. Incontinent urinary diversion was present in 9.5%, and 4.8% were catheterized per urethra [3]. A recent multi-institutional study of 160 cloacal exstrophy patients reported that, among young children, 42% were incontinent and 32% were on clean intermittent catheterization. Among older children and adults, 73% were catheterizing, and 88% had a history of enterocystoplasty and creation of a catheterizable channel. In this case series, 28% of adults had incontinent urinary diversions [60].

Renal

Patients with cloacal exstrophy or OEIS are at particularly high risk for chronic kidney disease. Anatomic anomalies of the upper tracts are present in 41–66% [27]. Following urinary reconstruction, the upper tracts are at risk of damage from high-pressure bladder dynamics, pyelonephritis, vesicoureteral reflux, and stone formation from chronic urinary stasis. A single-institutional study reported a quarter of cloacal exstrophy patients having at least stage 1 chronic kidney disease [3].

Fecal Continence

A recent study reported nearly 80% of patients with intestinal diversion. Twenty percent of remaining patients underwent pull-through, half with a concomitant Malone antegrade colonic enema. However, there is significant institutional variability in rates of intestinal diversion [60]. Another single-institutional study with long-term follow-up reported more than a 90% rate of intestinal diversion, with 8% of patients undergoing pull-through [3]. There is wide variability of reported rates of fecal continence despite pull-through (30–85%) [58, 60].

Sexual Function and Fertility

Sexual function in individuals affected by cloacal exstrophy depends on the extent of genital and Müllerian anomalies, which can vary significantly in severity. Testicular histology, architecture of rete testis, epididymis, and vas deferens are typically preserved in genetic males, although natural paternity has not been reported [40, 61]. A recent systematic review of four studies reported that 18% of females were sexually active [61]. Successful pregnancy to term is reported, although uterine prolapse, preterm birth, loss of pregnancy, and cesarean births are also reported [3, 43, 62–65].

Gender Rearing

Historically, genetically male patients with diminutive phallus not suitable for reconstruction often underwent early orchiectomy and were raised as females. However, cloacal exstrophy males typically have normal functioning testicles, thus, normal androgen imprinting in utero. Many genetic males initially assigned female gender have reconverted to male gender roles in adolescence and adulthood [33]. Currently, most pediatric urologists favor gender assignment according to genetic karyotype [66].

Nutrition

There is a high prevalence of malnutrition and short bowel syndrome due to congenital malformation of the gastrointestinal tract. Cloacal exstrophy patients have lower median height-for-age and weight-for-age z-scores compared to the healthy controls. Short bowel syndrome and enterocystoplasty are associated with lower z-scores [67].

Mobility

Many patients with cloacal exstrophy are able to ambulate. Among 63 patients, 37% were ambulated without aids, 13% ambulated with abnormal gait, and 14% ambulated with leg braces or a walker adjunct. Thirty-five percent were wheelchair dependent, and 2% were bedbound [3].

Psychosocial Outcomes

More attention and care should be given to psychosocial outcomes among patients with cloacal exstrophy. A single-institutional study reported anxiety and/or depression in two-thirds of their patients and chronic pain in more than one-fourth of patients. In the same study, 80% of adults attended college and were employed [3].

Conclusion

Cloacal exstrophy, also known as OEIS, involves an anterior abdominal wall defect and a spectrum of urinary, gastrointestinal, skeletal, spinal, and genital anomalies. The initial goal of genitourinary reconstruction is to bring the two hemibladder plates together by excising the omphalocele and separating the cecal plate from the bladder halves. The cecal plate is tubularized and placed in continuity with the blind-ending hindgut, which is exteriorized and matured as an end colostomy. The second surgical step is similar to reconstruction of classic bladder exstrophy, with steps including bladder closure, reconstruction of external genitalia, and approximation of pubic rami with the aid of osteotomies. Given the high prevalence of spinal defects in the cloacal exstrophy population, volitional voiding is typically not an option. When patients and parents/caregivers are socially ready and properly counseled, bladder neck closure/reconstruction and continent catheterizable channels may be created with or without enterocystoplasty in order to achieve urinary continence. There is high prevalence of Müllerian abnormalities, which are typically able to be properly assessed and reconstructed around the time of adolescence. Modern medical management and refined surgical techniques have enabled longer life expectancies for patients with cloacal exstrophy, with reduced rates of malnutrition, sepsis, and renal failure. As patients are surviving childhood and living to adulthood, continual efforts must be made to improve long-term outcomes and quality of life.

References

1. Littre A. Diverse Observations Anatomique. Mem Acad R Sci. 1709;4:9.
2. Rickham PP. Vesico-Intestinal Fissure. Arch Dis Child. 1960;35:97–102. https://doi.org/10.1136/adc.35.179.97.

3. Haney NM, Morrill CC, Haffar A, Crigger C, Gabrielson AT, Galansky L, Gearhart JP. Long-term management of problems in cloacal Exstrophy: A single-institution review. J Pediatr Surg. 2024;59:26–30. https://doi.org/10.1016/j.jpedsurg.2023.09.013.
4. Woo LL, Thomas JC, Brock JW. Cloacal exstrophy: a comprehensive review of an uncommon problem. J Pediatr Urol. 2010;6(2):102–11.
5. Caton AR, Bloom A, Druschel CM, Kirby RS. Epidemiology of bladder and cloacal exstrophies in New York State, 1983–1999. Birth Defects Res A Clin Mol Teratol. 2007;79:781–7.
6. Moore CA, Weaver DD. Exstrophy of cloaca sequence. In: Buyse ML, Dover MA, editors. Birth defects encyclopedia. Centers for Birth defects Information Services, Inc; 1990. p. 648–9.
7. Feldkamp ML, Botto LD, Amar E, Bakker MK, Bermejo-Sánchez E, Bianca S, Canfield MA, Castilla EE, Clementi M, Csaky-Szunyogh M, et al. Cloacal exstrophy: an epidemiologic study from the international clearinghouse for birth defects surveillance and research. Am J Med Genet C Semin Med Genet. 2011;157C:333–43. https://doi.org/10.1002/ajmg.c.30317.
8. Boyadjiev SA, Dodson JL, Radford CL, Ashrafi GH, Beaty TH, Mathews RI, Broman KW, Gearhart JP. Clinical and molecular characterization of the bladder exstrophy-epispadias complex: analysis of 232 families. BJU Int. 2004;94:1337–43.
9. Gambhir L, Höller T, Müller M, Schott G, Vogt H, Detlefsen B, Ebert A-K, Fisch M, Beaudoin S, Stein R, et al. Epidemiological survey of 214 families with bladder Exstrophy-Epispadias complex. J Urol. 2008;179:1539–43. https://doi.org/10.1016/j.juro.2007.11.092.
10. Fullerton BS, Sparks EA, Hall AM, Velazco CS, Modi BP, Lund DP, Jaksic T, Hendren WH. High prevalence of same-sex twins in patients with cloacal Exstrophy: support for embryological association with monozygotic twinning. J Pediatr Surg. 2017;52:807–9. https://doi.org/10.1016/j.jpedsurg.2017.01.043.
11. Lee DH, Cottrell JR, Sanders RC, Meyers CM, Wulfsberg EA, Sun CC. OEIS complex (Omphalocele-Exstrophy-imperforate anus-spinal defects) in monozygotic twins. Am J Med Genet. 1999;84:29–33.
12. Casale P, Grady RW, Waldhausen JHT, Joyner BD, Wright J, Mitchell ME. Cloacal exstrophy variants. Can blighted conjoined twinning play a role? J Urol. 2004;172:1103–6., discussion 1106-1107. https://doi.org/10.1097/01.ju.0000142108.62457.81.
13. Siebert JR, Rutledge JC, Kapur RP. Association of Cloacal Anomalies, caudal duplication, and twinning. Pediatr Dev Pathol. 2005;8:339–54. https://doi.org/10.1007/s10024-005-1157-6.
14. Smith NM, Chambers HM, Furness ME, Haan EA. The OEIS complex (Omphalocele-Exstrophy-imperforate anus-spinal defects): recurrence in sibs. J Med Genet. 1992;29:730–2. https://doi.org/10.1136/jmg.29.10.730.
15. Reutter H, Keppler-Noreuil K, Keegan CE, Thiele H, Yamada G, Ludwig M. Genetics of bladder-Exstrophy-Epispadias complex (BEEC): systematic elucidation of Mendelian and multifactorial phenotypes. Curr Genomics. 2016;17:4–13. https://doi.org/10.2174/1389202916666151014221806.
16. Van der Putte SC. Normal and abnormal development of the anorectum. J Pediatr Surg. 1986;21:434–40.
17. Beaudoin S, Simon L, Bargy F. Anatomical basis of the common embryological origin for epispadias and bladder or cloacal exstrophy. Surg Radiol Anat. 1997;19:11–6.
18. Ambrose SS, O'Brien DP. Surgical embryology of the exstrophy-epispadias complex. Surg Clin North Am. 1974;54:1379.
19. Mildenberger H, Lkuth D, Dziuba M. Embryology of bladder exstrophy. J Pediatr Surg. 1988;23:116.
20. Austin PF, Homsy YL, Gearhart JP, Porter K, Guidi C, Madsen K, Maizels M. The prenatal diagnosis of cloacal exstrophy. J Urol. 1998;160:1179–81. https://doi.org/10.1097/00005392-199809020-00061.
21. Weiss DA, Oliver ER, Borer JG, Kryger JV, Roth EB, Groth TW, Shukla AR, Mitchell ME, Canning DA, Victoria T. Key anatomic findings on fetal ultrasound and MRI in the prenatal diagnosis of bladder and cloacal Exstrophy. J Pediatr Urol. 2020;16:665–71. https://doi.org/10.1016/j.jpurol.2020.07.024.

22. Cacciari A, et al. Prenatal diagnosis of bladder exstrophy: what counseling? J Urol. 1999;161(1):259–61. discussion 262
23. Lee T, Weiss D, Roth E, Bortnick E, Jarosz S, Eftekharzadeh S, Groth T, Shukla A, Kryger JV, Lee RS, et al. Prenatal diagnosis of bladder Exstrophy and OEIS over 20 years. Urology. 2023;172:174–7. https://doi.org/10.1016/j.urology.2022.11.020.
24. Morrill CC, Haffar A, Crigger C, Black M, Jelin A, Nasr I, Gearhart JP. A single-institutional experience with prenatal diagnosis of cloacal exstrophy: room for improvement. J Pediatr Surg. 2023;58:1949–53. https://doi.org/10.1016/j.jpedsurg.2023.04.012.
25. Hurwitz RS, Manzoni GA, Ransley PG, Stephens FD. Cloacal exstrophy: a report of 34 cases. J Urol. 1987;138:1060–4.
26. Lee T, Borer J. Exstrophy-epispadias complex. Urol Clin North Am. 2023;50:403–14. https://doi.org/10.1016/j.ucl.2023.04.004.
27. Suson KD, Inouye B, Carl A, Gearhart JP. Congenital renal anomalies in cloacal Exstrophy: is there a difference? J Pediatr Urol. 2016;12:207.e1-5. https://doi.org/10.1016/j.jpurol.2016.04.008.
28. Rehfuss A, Bourgeois T, Thompson B, Sebastião YV, Wood RJ, Jayanthi VR, Fuchs ME. Baseline renal volumes in children born with cloacal anomalies. Urology. 2021;148:250–3. https://doi.org/10.1016/j.urology.2020.08.010.
29. Lee T, Roth E, Shukla A, Gupta N, Lee R, Kryger J, et al. Pelvic ectopic kidney prevalence and pressure changes during cloacal Exstrophy (Omphalocele-Exstrophy-imperforate anus-spinal defects syndrome) Closure. Urology. 2023;181:124–7.
30. Stolar CH, Randolph JG, Flanigan LP. Cloacal exstrophy: individualized management through a staged surgical approach. J Pediatr Surg. 1990;25(5):505e7.
31. McHoney M, Ransley PG, Duffy P, Wilcox DT, Spitz L. Cloacal Exstrophy: morbidity associated with abnormalities of the gastrointestinal tract and spine. J Pediatr Surg. 2004;39:1209–13. https://doi.org/10.1016/j.jpedsurg.2004.04.019.
32. Davidoff AM, Hebra A, Balmer D, Templeton JM, Schnaufer L. Management of the gastrointestinal tract and nutrition in patients with cloacal Exstrophy. J Pediatr Surg. 1996;31:771–3. https://doi.org/10.1016/s0022-3468(96)90129-3.
33. Sawaya D, Goldstein S, Seetharamaiah R, Suson K, Nabaweesi R, Colombani P, Gearhart J. Gastrointestinal ramifications of the cloacal Exstrophy complex: A 44-year experience. J Pediatr Surg. 2010;45:171–175; discussion 175-176. https://doi.org/10.1016/j.jpedsurg.2009.10.030.
34. Judy BF, Materi J, Lee RP, Tracz JA, Patel J, Weber-Levine C, Crigger C, Mistry P, Gearhart JP, Jackson EM. Spinal Dysraphism in Exstrophy: A single-center study of a 39-year prospective database. J Neurosurg Pediatr. 2023;32:98–105. https://doi.org/10.3171/2023.3.PEDS22447.
35. Kumar N, Chatur C, Balani A, Bisharat M, Tahir Z, Johal N, Sudhakar S, Cuckow P, Thompson DNP, Mankad K. Patterns of spinal cord malformation in cloacal Exstrophy. J Neurosurg Pediatr. 2021;28:1–8. https://doi.org/10.3171/2021.1.PEDS20648.
36. Suson KD, Colombani PM, Jallo GI, Gearhart JP. Intracranial anomalies and cloacal exstrophy–is there a role for screening? J Pediatr Surg. 2013;48:2256–60. https://doi.org/10.1016/j.jpedsurg.2013.06.025.
37. Haffar A, Hirsch AM, Crigger CB, Harris TGW, Haney NM, Galansky LB, Nasr IW, Sponseller PD, Gearhart JP. Multi-staged vs single-staged pelvic osteotomy in the modern treatment of cloacal Exstrophy: bridging the gap. J Pediatr Surg. 2023;58:2308–12. https://doi.org/10.1016/j.jpedsurg.2023.09.003.
38. Mundy A, Kushare I, Jayanthi VR, Samora WP, Klingele KE. Incidence of hip dysplasia associated with bladder Exstrophy. J Pediatr Orthop. 2016;36:860–4. https://doi.org/10.1097/BPO.0000000000000571.
39. Wilcox D, Bischoff A, Ziegler MM. Cloacal exstrophy. In: Pediatric surgery diagnosis and management. Cham: Springer; 2023.
40. Mathews RI, Perlman E, Marsh DW, Gearhart JP. Gonadal morphology in cloacal Exstrophy: implications in gender assignment. BJU Int. 1999;84:99–100. https://doi.org/10.1046/j.1464-410x.1999.00148.x.

41. Benz K, Maruf M, Hatheway C, Kasprenski M, Jayman J, Docimo S, Schneck F, Gearhart J. The Intravesical phallus in patients with cloacal Exstrophy: an embryologic conundrum. J Pediatr Urol. 2018;14(428):e1–428.e5. https://doi.org/10.1016/j.jpurol.2018.05.001.
42. Phillips TM. Spectrum of cloacal Exstrophy. Semin Pediatr Surg. 2011;20:113–8. https://doi.org/10.1053/j.sempedsurg.2010.12.007.
43. Suson KD, Preece J, Di Carlo HN, Baradaran N, Gearhart JP. Complexities of Müllerian anatomy in 46XX cloacal Exstrophy patients. J Pediatr Adolesc Gynecol. 2016;29:424–8. https://doi.org/10.1016/j.jpag.2016.01.124.
44. Holcomb G, Murphy JP, St Peter S. Holcomb and Ashcraft's pediatric surgery, seventh edition. 7th ed; 2019.
45. Weiss DA, Borer JG, Lee RS, Kryger JV, Roth EB, Groth TW, Shukla AR, Mitchell ME, Canning DA. Bladder and cloacal exstrophy. In: Mattei P, editor. Fundamentals of pediatric surgery. Cham: Springer International Publishing; 2022. p. 969–78. ISBN 978-3-031-07524-7.
46. Tirrell TF, Demehri FR, Henry OS, Cullen L, Lillehei CW, Warf BC, Gates RL, Borer JG, Dickie BH. Safety of delayed surgical repair of Omphalocele-Exstrophy-imperforate anus-spinal defects (OEIS) complex in infants with significant comorbidities. Pediatr Surg Int. 2021;37:93–9. https://doi.org/10.1007/s00383-020-04779-w.
47. Jayman J, Tourchi A, Feng Z, Trock BJ, Maruf M, Benz K, Kasprenski M, Baumgartner T, Friedlander D, Sponseller P, et al. Predictors of a successful primary bladder closure in cloacal Exstrophy: A multivariable analysis. J Pediatr Surg. 2019;54:491–4. https://doi.org/10.1016/j.jpedsurg.2018.06.030.
48. Smith CA, Avansino JR, Merguerian P, Lane V, Levitt M. A novel surgical approach for the management of cloacal exstrophy with a giant omphalocele. European J Pediatr Surg Rep. 2021;9(01):e41–5.
49. Husmann DA, McLorie GA, Churchill BM, Ein SH. Management of the Hindgut in cloacal Exstrophy: terminal ileostomy versus colostomy. J Pediatr Surg. 1988;23:1107–13. https://doi.org/10.1016/s0022-3468(88)80324-5.
50. Bischoff A, Brisighelli G, Levitt MA, Peña A. The "Rescue Operation" for patients with cloacal exstrophy and its variants. Pediatr Surg Int. 2014;30:723–7. https://doi.org/10.1007/s00383-014-3512-z.
51. Ben-Chaim J, et al. Applications of osteotomy in the cloacal exstrophy patient. J Urol. 1995;154(2 Pt 2):865–7.
52. Lee T, Roth E, Shukla A, Gupta N, Lee R, Kryger J, Groth T, Canning D, Mitchell M, Weiss D, et al. Pelvic ectopic kidney prevalence and pressure changes during cloacal Exstrophy (Omphalocele-Exstrophy-imperforate anus-spinal defects syndrome) closure. Urology. 2023;181:124–7. https://doi.org/10.1016/j.urology.2023.07.037.
53. Leclair MD, Faraj S, Sultan S, Audry G, Héloury Y, Kelly JH, Ransley PG. One-stage combined delayed bladder closure with Kelly radical soft-tissue mobilization in bladder exstrophy: preliminary results. J Pediatr Urol. 2018;14(6):558–64.
54. Szymanski KM, Whittam B, Misseri R, Flack CK, Hubert KC, Kaefer M, et al. Long-term outcomes of catheterizable continent urinary channels: what do you use, where you put it, and does it matter? J Pediatr Urol. 2015;11(4):210–e1.
55. Srinivas S, Knaus ME, Avansino JR, Badillo A, Calkins CM, Dickie BH, et al. Outcomes from colonic pull-through for cloacal Exstrophy differ by colon length: A multi-institutional study. J Pediatr Surg. 2024;59(2):225–9.
56. Learner HI, Creighton SM, Wood D. Augmentation vaginoplasty with buccal mucosa for the surgical revision of postreconstructive vaginal stenosis: a case series. J Pediatr Urol. 2019;15(4):402–e1.
57. Oelschlager AMA, Debiec K. Vaginal dilator therapy: a guide for providers for assessing readiness and supporting patients through the process successfully. J Pediatr Adolesc Gynecol. 2019;32(4):354–8.
58. Maruf M, Kasprenski M, Jayman J, Goldstein SD, Benz K, Baumgartner T, Gearhart JP. Achieving urinary continence in cloacal Exstrophy: the surgical cost. J Pediatr Surg. 2018;53:1937–41. https://doi.org/10.1016/j.jpedsurg.2018.02.055.

59. Phillips TM, Salmasi AH, Stec A, Novak TE, Gearhart JP, Mathews RI. Urological outcomes in the omphalocele exstrophy imperforate anus spinal defects (OEIS) complex: experience with 80 patients. J Pediatr Urol. 2013;9(3):353–8.
60. Fuchs ME, Ahmed M, Dajusta DG, Gargollo P, Kennedy UK, Rosoklija I, Strine AC, Whittam B, Yerkes E, Szymanski KM, et al. Urinary and bowel Management in Cloacal Exstrophy: a long-term multi-institutional cross-sectional study. J Pediatr Urol. 2023;19(35):e1–35.e6. https://doi.org/10.1016/j.jpurol.2022.10.003.
61. Musleh L, Privitera L, Paraboschi I, Polymeropoulos A, Mushtaq I, Giuliani S. Long-term active problems in patients with cloacal Exstrophy: a systematic review. J Pediatr Surg. 2022;57:339–47. https://doi.org/10.1016/j.jpedsurg.2021.08.020.
62. Gezer A, Guralp O, Yesilbas C, Madazli R. Spontaneous pregnancy and birth with corrected cloacal Exstrophy. Acta Obstet Gynecol Scand. 2011;90:413–4. https://doi.org/10.1111/j.1600-0412.2011.01076.x.
63. Reppucci ML, Alaniz VI, Wehrli LA, de Torre LL, Wood D, Wilcox DT, Appiah LC, Peña A, Bischoff A. Reproductive and family building considerations for female patients with anorectal and urogenital malformations. J Pediatr Surg. 2023;58:1450–7. https://doi.org/10.1016/j.jpedsurg.2022.09.004.
64. Dy GW, Willihnganz-Lawson KH, Shnorhavorian M, Delaney SS, Amies Oelschlager A-M, Merguerian PA, Grady R, Miller JL, Cheng EY. Successful pregnancy in patients with Exstrophy-Epispadias complex: A University of Washington experience. J Pediatr Urol. 2015;11(213):e1–6. https://doi.org/10.1016/j.jpurol.2015.04.019.
65. Seat M, Boxwalla M, Hough A, Goodwin G. A case of congenital cloacal Exstrophy/Omphalocele-Exstrophy-imperforate anus-spinal defects syndrome and a successful pregnancy. Clin Exp Reprod Med. 2022;49:215–8. https://doi.org/10.5653/cerm.2021.05148.
66. Diamond DA, Burns JP, Huang L, Rosoklija I, Retik AB. Gender assignment for newborns with 46XY cloacal Exstrophy: a 6-year Followup survey of pediatric urologists. J Urol. 2011;186:1642–8. https://doi.org/10.1016/j.juro.2011.03.101.
67. Fullerton BS, Sparks EA, Hall AM, Chan Y-M, Duggan C, Lund DP, Modi BP, Jaksic T, Hendren WH. Growth morbidity in patients with cloacal Exstrophy: a 42 year experience. J Pediatr Surg. 2016;51:1017–21. https://doi.org/10.1016/j.jpedsurg.2016.02.075.

Male Epispadias

16

Paul A. Merguerian

Embryology

The embryological theories of epispadias have been explained in a previous chapter. It is believed that abnormalities of the cloacal membrane may be responsible for its occurrence. A large cloacal membrane prevents the normal migration of mesenchymal tissue but is prone to rupture leading to the spectrum of anomalies. In epispadias, the rupture causes nonunion of the distal portion of the urinary tract.

Anatomic Features

The defect involves an absence of the dorsal aspect of the urethra and overlying skin.

Classification of the defect based on the location of the urethral meatus alone is simplistic. It does not take into account other anatomic and functional features such as appearance of the bladder neck, presence or absence of pubic diastasis, and presence of vesicoureteral reflux. The classic assumption is that patients with glandular and penile epispadias are continent in most cases. However, the BN may be abnormal even in distal cases and may affect their ability to achieve continence [3]. In Table 16.1, Cendron et al. have shown that patients with penile epispadias may have an abnormal bladder neck and continence is achieved only in 63% of these patients.

The most common form of this anomaly is *penopubic epispadias* with the defect affecting the bladder neck and the entire urethra. These patients are incontinent of urine and will require a bladder neck reconstruction. The more distal the urethral defect, the less likely that the bladder neck is involved and the continence rate is higher.

P. A. Merguerian (✉)
Seattle Children's Hospital, University of Washington, Seattle, WA, USA
e-mail: paul.merguerian@seattlechildrens.org

A. R. Shukla, R. S. Joshi (eds.), *Bladder Exstrophy and Epispadias*,
https://doi.org/10.1007/978-3-031-91238-2_16

Table 16.1 Cendron et al. series showing that an abnormal bladder neck can be found also in penile epispadias and continence is achieved in only 63% of patients with penile epispadias

Epispadias type	n	Abnormal pubic diastasis	VUR	Abnormal bladder neck	Continence procedures	Continent	Age > 5 years at follow-up
Glandular	4	1(25%)	2(50%)	0	0	3(75%)	3(75%)
Penile	8	3(38%)	1(38%)	3(38%)	0	5(63%)	5(63%)
Penopubic	14	12(86%)	5(29%)	7(50%)	7(50%)	9(64%)	11(79%)
Total	26	16(62%)	8(31%)	10(38%)	7(27%)	17(65%)	19(73%)

All patients with epispadias have a variable degree of dorsal curvature. In its most severe presentation, the penis is directed against the abdominal wall making sexual function difficult. The dorsal curvature is due to an intrinsic deformity of the corporal bodies and not due to tethering of the corpora by the urethral plate [4].

The proximal defects are also associated with diastasis of the symphysis pubis. It was previously thought that the individual corpora cavernosa were of normal caliber but appeared shorter because of the wide separation of the crural attachments, the prominent dorsal chordee, and the shortened urethral groove. However, magnetic resonance imaging (MRI) in adult men with bladder exstrophy compared to age- and race-matched controls showed that the anterior corporeal length of male patients with bladder exstrophy was almost 50% shorter than that of normal controls. The posterior length of the corporeal body was the same as in age-matched controls. The diameter of the anterior corporeal segment was 30% greater than normal. Therefore, the penis appears short not only because of the diastasis of the pubic symphysis but also because of marked congenital deficiency of anterior corporeal tissue [5].

The verumontanum is exposed on the urethral plate. The vas deferens and ejaculatory ducts are not affected. The prostate is also incompletely formed in proximal epispadias [6].

In the epispadias phallus, the neurovascular bundle's course is altered. Rather than being dorsal and close to the midline, the neurovascular bundle lies ventrolateral which is consistent with a medial-to-lateral rotational deformity [7]. At the level of the symphysis, the neurovascular bundles are slightly lateral to the midline at the 11 and 1 o'clock positions. As the nerves course along the phallus distally, they become more ventral and at the distal end are at the 8 and 4 o'clock positions.

The glans has a flattened configuration with excess irregular glans epithelium adjacent to the urethral plate.

The ureterovesical junction may be affected in complete epispadias, and the incidence of reflux has been reported to be between 30% and 40% [8, 9] and in some series up to 80% [10]. In male patients, this has not been shown to be clinically significant.

Epispadias Repair

Male epispadias is one of the most challenging problems that pediatric urologists encounter. The ideal outcome is to render the genitourinary anatomy to its normal location and configuration. The goals of repair include the following:

1. Correction of dorsal curvature
2. Creation of a straight urethra
3. Adequate skin coverage
4. Satisfactory cosmetic outcome
5. Maintenance of erectile function
6. Urinary continence

History of Surgical Repair of Epispadias [11]

In 1845, Dieffenbach freshened the lateral tissue edges and placed approximating sutures, and in 1869, Thiersch rotated local skin flaps to cover the urethral defect. It was not until 1895 that Cantwell performed the first true urethroplasty for complete epispadias. Cantwell completely mobilized the dorsal urethral plate from the corpora cavernosa and transplanted the tubularized urethra below the corpora cavernosa which were then rotated dorsally and approximated in the midline (Fig. 16.1).

In 1918, Young in an attempt to prevent devascularization injury to the urethral plate described a modification of the Cantwell approach. The urethra was detached from the right corpus cavernosum, but it was left attached to the left corpus cavernosum and simply rotated ventrally beneath the corpora.

In 1984, Lepor et al. reported a modified Young urethroplasty in which the urethra remained dorsal to the corpora and was tubularized in continuity in a Thiersch-Duplay fashion from the prostate to the glans penis. Also in 1984 Thmalla and in 1987 Monfort applied the Duckett transverse island flap to male epispadias repair.

Koff and Eakins recognized that rotation of the corporal bodies could correct dorsal curvature. Their techniques involved dissection of the corpora from the urethra and inferior pubic ramus and medial-to-lateral rotation of the corporal bodies in opposite directions with ventral fixation. The urethra remained dorsally located.

To correct the intrinsic nature of the dorsal curvature, Woodhouse and Kellett preferred a fascial release of the tunica albuginea dorsally. This extensive dissection required full mobilization of the urethral plate and preserving the neurovascular bundle.

The combination of the Woodhouse and Kellett concept with the Cantwell repair resulted in the modern-age repair of epispadias as the modified Cantwell procedure which had 3 components: (1) corporal rotation dorsally with cavernocavernostomy, (2) urethral mobilization, and (3) improved glanuloplasty and dorsal skin coverage [12].

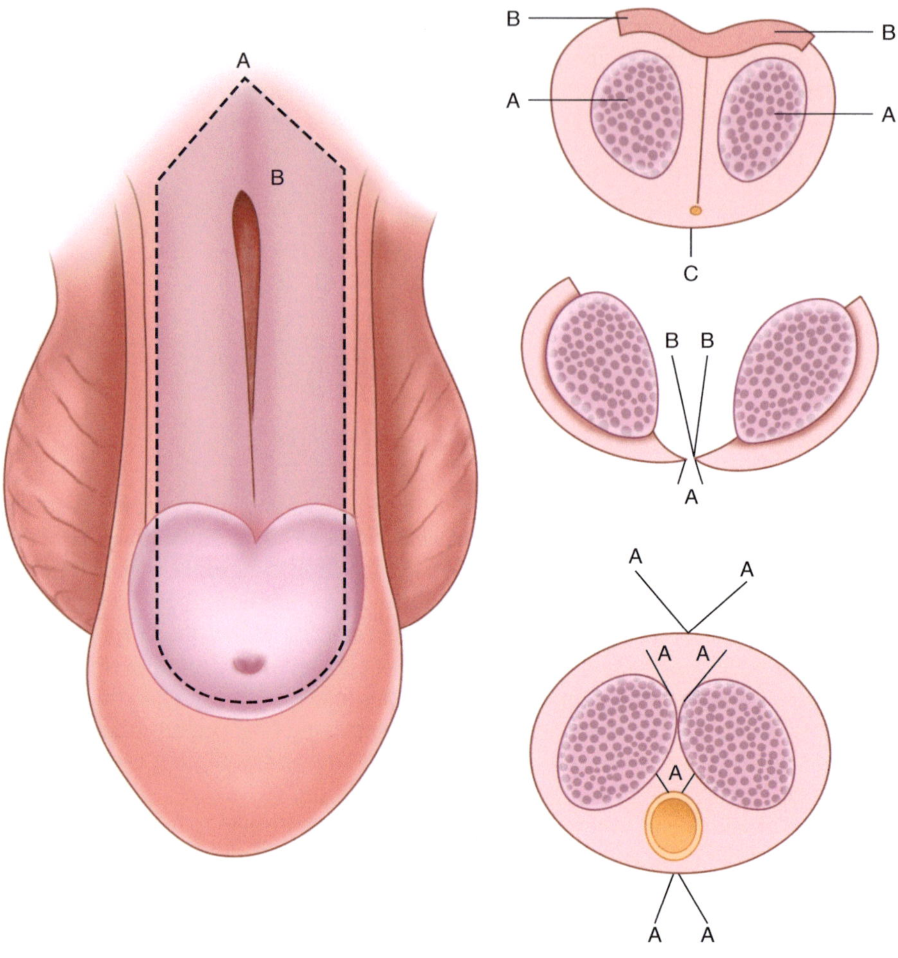

Fig. 16.1 Cantwell epispadias repair. Dorsal urethral plate (**b**) mobilized from corpora, tubularized and positioned ventral to the corpora. Corpora cavernosa rotated dorsal to urethra and approximated

Current Approaches to Male Epispadias Repair

From the various techniques described in the previous section, two reconstructive procedures are currently mostly utilized: the modified Cantwell-Ransley repair and the Mitchell repair [13, 14].

Repair of isolated epispadias is performed at around 6–9 months of age.

Parenteral injection of testosterone preoperatively with two injections (5 weeks prior and 2 weeks prior) of 2 mg/kg of testosterone enanthate has been shown to increase penile length by a mean of 2.7 cm and increase penile circumference by a mean of 2.3 cm without any short-term side effects. The increased length and girth with increased vascularity have the potential to improve outcomes and decrease vascular injury to the urethral plate and skin [15].

Makedonsky described the use of intramuscular HCG administered to patients with epispadias, bladder exstrophy combined with cryptorchidism. HCG was administered intramuscularly at 250–500 IU twice a week for 3 weeks prior to reconstruction. Compared to controls, mean penile length was seen to increase by a mean of 1.8 cm and penile circumference by a mean of 1.2 cm. Epidermal growth factor (EGF) and human epidermal growth factor receptor (Her2/neu),were found to be decreased in exstrophy/epispadias compared to controls, and both EGF and Her2/neu increased by 10% after administration of HCG [16].

Pelvic Osteotomy

Pelvic osteotomy is recommended for proximal epispadias involving the bladder neck as this allows for decreased tension on the tissues of the bladder neck and proximal urethra decreasing complications such as dehiscence and fistulae [17].

Techniques of osteotomy are described in another section of this book.

Modified Cantwell-Ransley Repair

This repair entails three components: (1) corporal rotation dorsally with caverno-cavernostomy, (2) urethral mobilization and reconstruction, and (3) improved glanuloplasty and dorsal skin coverage [18] (Fig. 16.2).

Corporeal Rotation and Cavernocavernostomy

The corporeal bodies are freed completely from the urethra except the distal part of the corpora and hemiglans leaving the mucosa attached to the glans distally therefore assuring improved blood supply and preventing shortening of the urethra.

The corporeal bodies are rotated dorsally (medially) with cavernocavernostomy to secure the corpora and to transpose the urethra ventrally.

In order to avoid damage to the neurovascular bundle, they are mobilized off the corpora. Current modifications avoid the routine mobilization of the neurovascular bundles, since in most of the cases, the incision and the anastomosis of the corporeal bodies can be safely done without their mobilization [19].

Urethral Reconstruction

The urethral plate is dissected to the penile base and distally to the tip of the penile glans with creation of glandular wings. The urethral reconstruction is performed with interrupted absorbable sutures. Dorsal coverage of the urethral suture line by

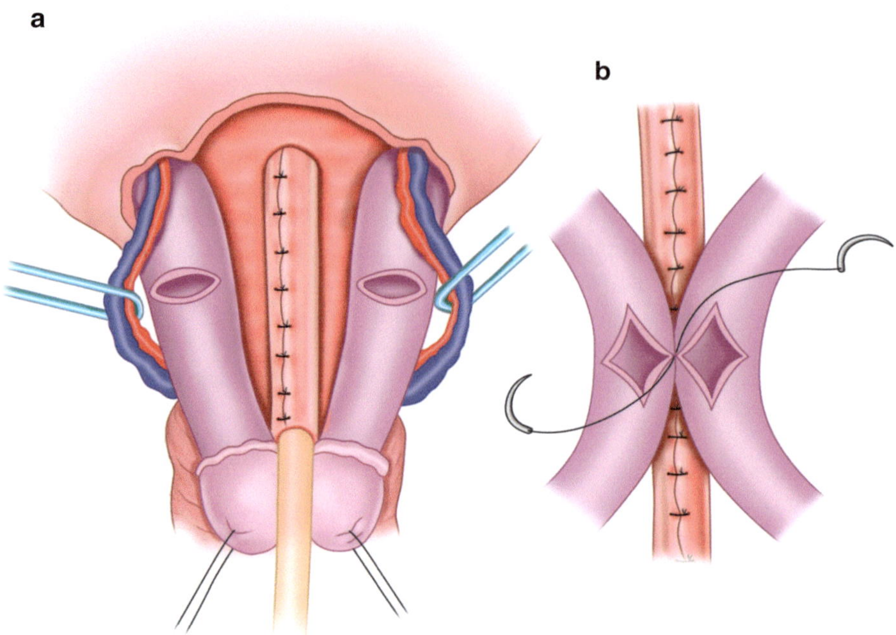

Fig. 16.2 Modified Cantwell-Ransley repair. (**a**) Bilateral transverse corporal incisions are made after complete mobilization of the corpora and neurovascular bundles, and urethral reconstruction. (**b**) Beginning of cavernocavernostomy with corpora overlying reconstructed urethra

the corporal bodies results in a lower fistula rate. The glandular urethra and the meatus are advanced by using a modification of the MAGPI procedure for hypospadias, named IPGAM, which involves a vertical incision in the distal urethral plate and transverse advancement with absorbable sutures.

Glanuloplasty and Skin Coverage

The two main components of the repair that allow normal cosmetic results are the glansplasty and skin coverage.

The epispadias glans wings usually have a bulk of irregular tissue just lateral to the urethral plate. To reconstruct the glans in a conical configuration, this tissue should be aggressively excised and a 2 layer closure of the glans performed with subcuticular absorbable sutures.

Dorsal skin coverage can be difficult, and several methods have been used including a transverse prepucial island flap that is rotated dorsally [11], bilateral rhomboid flaps to aid in proximal dorsal coverage, and Z-plasty brought from the lateral aspect of the midline abdominal incision.

The most common approach is by using reverse Byars flaps and a longitudinal dorsal suture line [20].

Bladder Neck Reconstruction

The majority of patients with penopubic epispadias and a percent of penile epispadias patients will be incontinent and require reconstruction. The two most common bladder neck reconstructions performed today are the Young-Dees-Leadbetter repair and the Mitchell modification.

The bladder neck reconstruction is described elsewhere in this book.

The Mitchell Repair

Bagli and Mitchell first reported results using this technique in 1996 [13]. It was felt that the planes of dissection were such that this technique allows for better access to the bladder neck and to bladder neck reconstruction. Moreover, completely disassembling the urethral plate and the corporal bodies allowed for a more normal appearance of penis and allowed the urethra to be placed ventrally. Because the corporal bodies are completely disassembled, there is no crossed blood supply and the blood supply of each corpus is based on the central artery. The urethral and spongiosal blood supplies come from the proximal urethra. The dorsal nerve complex is not dissected from the corpora cavernosal bodies.

Initial Dissection

The dissection is usually started on the ventral aspect of the penis. The initial plane of dissection occurs just above Buck's fascia. As the dissection progresses medially, the plane will shift from above Buck's fascia to above the tunica albuginea on the ventromedial aspect of each corporal body. The urethral plate with the corpus spongiosum is dissected from the dorsomedial aspect of the corpora cavernosa on the tunica albuginea preserving all of the spongiosal tissue (Fig. 16.3).

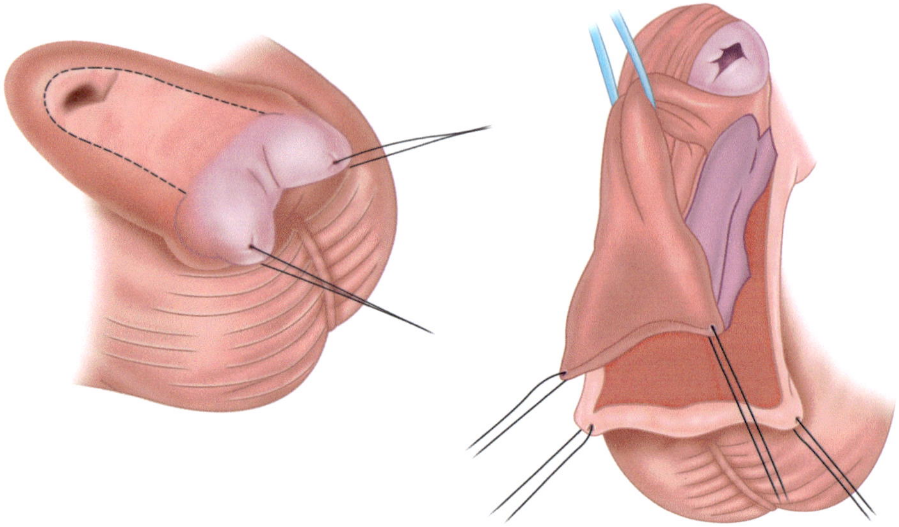

Fig. 16.3 Plane of dissection between the urethral plate and the corpora cavernosa

Careful lateral dissection of the penile shaft skin and dartos fascia from the corporal bodies is performed above Buck's fascia ensuring to keep the neurovascular bundle intact. They are located laterally on the corpora within Buck's fascia.

Penile Disassembly

The penis is disassembled into three components: the right and left corporal bodies with their respective hemiglans and the urethral plate with its underlying corpus spongiosum.

This provides easier access to the proximal urethra and the bladder neck.

The plane of dissection is at the level of the tunica albuginea on the corpora. Once the plane is between the urethral plate/corpus spongiosum and the corporal bodies, the dissection is carried distally to separate the three components from each other. It is important to keep the corpus spongiosum attached to the urethral plate as the blood supply of the urethra is based on the spongiosal tissues. Para-exstrophy flaps cannot be utilized in this technique as this maneuver will devascularize the distal urethra (Fig. 16.4).

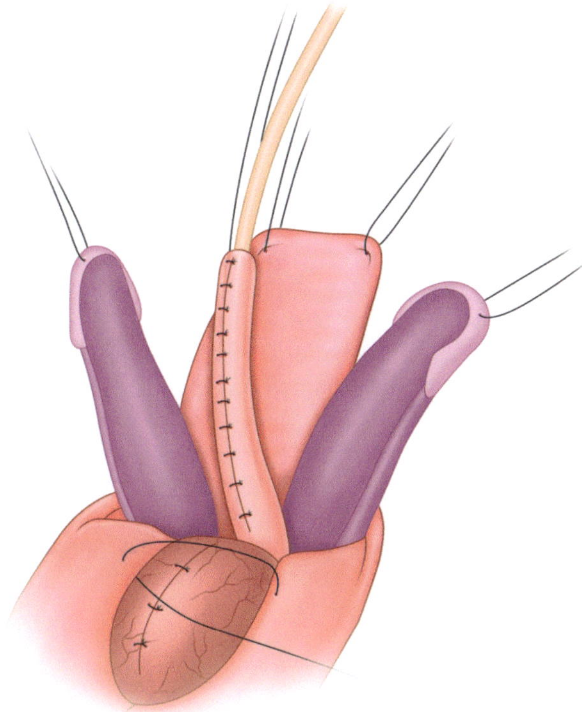

Fig. 16.4 Urethral tubularization in continuity with bladder neck closure

Proximal Dissection

Dissection of the urethral and spongiosum from the corporal bodies is crucial for posterior placement of the bladder neck and proximal urethra. A deep incision of the intersymphyseal ligaments posterior and lateral to the urethral plate is necessary to allow the bladder neck and posterior urethra to be positioned deep in the pelvis.

Bladder Neck Reconstruction

For penopubic epispadias with involvement of the bladder neck, the bladder neck reconstruction is performed next (described in another chapter).

Primary Closure

Once the bladder neck is reconstructed and the corporal bodies and urethral plate with corpus spongiosum are dissected, the closure is started. A suprapubic tube is recommended for the proximal repairs.

The urethra is then tubularized in two layers using monofilament suture in an interrupted fashion so as not to shorten the urethra. The tubularized urethra is then placed ventrally. The corporal bodies are rotated medially. Buck's fascia of each corporal body is then reapproximated in the midline. This medial rotation is important to assist in correcting the dorsal curvature.

If osteotomies were performed, the pubic symphysis is reapproximated using two 0.0 polydioxanone sutures with the knots tied anteriorly to prevent erosion into the bladder neck and proximal urethra (Fig. 16.5).

Dorsally, glans wedges are excised to create a conical appearance of the glans penis. The hemiglans are then reapproximated using subcuticular interrupted monofilament sutures.

The urethra is then brought up to each hemiglans ventrally to create an orthotopic meatus. Occasionally, the urethra may not reach as it is left in a hypospadias location for future reconstruction. The glans is reconfigured ventrally with interrupted monofilament sutures.

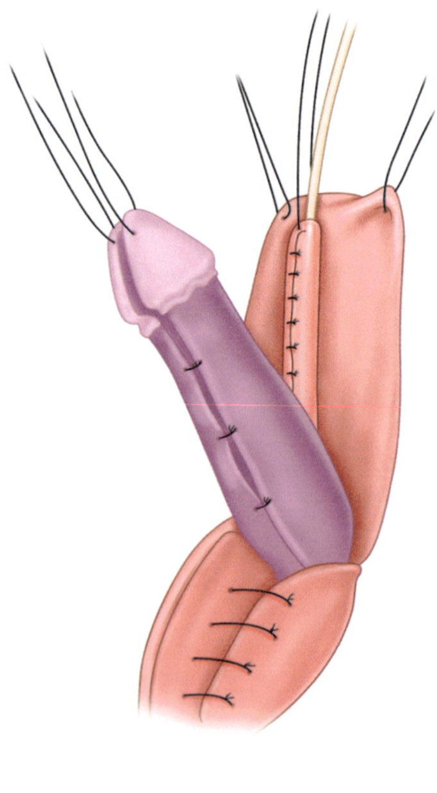

Fig. 16.5 Symphysis pubis is reapproximated after the urethra and bladder neck have moved posteriorly underneath the corporal bodies

Skin Closure

Dorsal skin coverage in epispadias repair can be difficult. Reverse Byars flaps are used to transpose the ventral skin dorsally for coverage.

A transverse island pedicle flap from the ventral prepuce rotated to the dorsum can also be utilized. The remaining ventral prepuce is then used for ventral and lateral coverage. Kramer and Jackson described the use of bilateral rhomboid flaps to aid in proximal dorsal coverage [21].

An alternative approach to proximal shaft coverage has been Z-plasty in which triangular flaps of skin from the lateral aspect of the midline abdominal incision are based distally and reconfigured to close the distal abdominal incision as well as cover the proximal penile shaft.

Modification to the Mitchell-Bagli Epispadias Repair

A modification of the Mitchell-Bagli repair is described in the Video Journal by Pippi Salle et al. [22] (https://doi.org/10.1016/j.urolvj.2022.100127).

It is felt that the most critical aspect of achieving continence is allowing for adequate bladder outlet resistance to allow bladder cycling and increased bladder capacity. Special attention is paid to tailoring the bladder neck so that it has a near-normal funneled configuration.

Another step which is not always achieved with the Mitchell and the Cantwell-Ransley repair is dorsal penile curvature correction and maximizing penile length. This leads to dissatisfaction of cosmetic appearance in adolescence and adulthood. Instead of internally rotating the corporal bodies, external rotation has been shown to achieve a more normal lie of the penile shaft. This requires extensive dissection of the corporal bodies and separation from the urethra [23].

In order to reduce the risk of creating a dimple at the penopubic area, mobilization of fat flaps from the mons pubis on either side to lay on top of the pubic closure at the penopubic angle allows for a flatter penopubic junction.

Finally, the previously described methods of skin closure have the potential of increasing the risk of dorsal curvature recurrence secondary to retraction of the dorsal midline scar. Moreover, redundancy and ventral skin ischemia have been reported after the use of transverse preputial island flaps. The rhomboid flaps have the disadvantage of having hair-bearing skin on the penile shaft.

In an attempt to prevent these complications, Pippi Salle described the use of a ventrally based skin flap that is then rotated to cover the penile shaft with the suture line being on the lateral aspect of the penis, thus preventing the complications related to the abovementioned repairs [24] (Fig. 16.6).

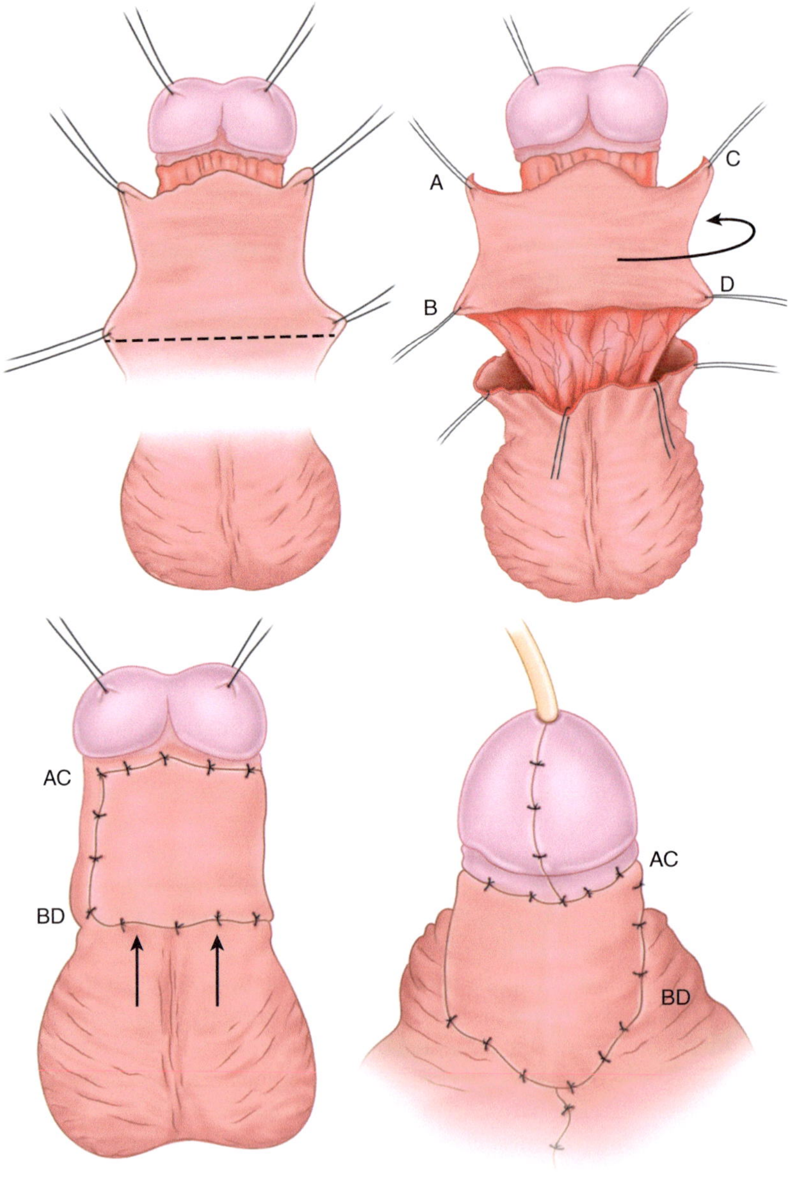

Fig. 16.6 Ventral penoscrotal junction is identified and the incision line demarcated. Dissection of the ventral penile skin flap is directed toward the penoscrotal junction. Mobilization is continued until a flap with sufficient mobility is fashioned to enable dorsal rotation and lateral placement of the longitudinal shaft skin suture line. Rotation of the ventral penile skin flap allows for lateral placement of the suture line

Outcomes

Reported rates of success for epispadias repairs vary. The degree of epispadias, the age of the patient, surgeon experience, and the presence of previously operated tissue all impact the successful outcome of epispadias repair.

Moreover, penile cosmetic result is a subjective measurement. Patient-reported outcomes are lacking, and therefore, cosmetic success of these repairs is difficult to validate and compare.

Fistula Formation

Urethrocutaneous fistula is the most common urethroplasty-related complication. The areas predisposed to fistula formation are the penopubic junction and penoscrotal angle. The rate of urethrocutaneous fistula formation varies from 2.4% to 28% [20, 25, 26].

Gearhart et al. reported a 21% fistula rate in 75 boys who underwent the Cantwell-Ransley epispadias [19].

Thomas et al. [27] in a series of 30 male patients followed for a median of 18.5 years reported a urethrocutaneous fistula rate of 20%.

Braga et al. [28] reported a rate of 24% in 21 patients with penopubic epispadias.

A recent study by Bencic et al. reported a rate of 22.6% in 31 patients with isolated epispadias with a mean age of 17 years. In this study, they also report urethrocutaneous fistula occurring in 2 patients 10 years after closure undermining the importance of long-term follow-up [29].

Urethral Stricture

The incidence of urethral stricture varies between 5% and 10% [27, 29, 30].

Djordjevic described repair of failed epispadias in 23 adult men with complete penile disassembly after failed epispadias repair. The urethra was reconstructed with genital skin or buccal mucosa. In this cohort, the rate of urethral stricture was 43.8% [31].

Residual Curvature

As there is a lack of patient-reported outcomes, the true incidence of residual curvature and especially the incidence of clinically significant residual dorsal curvature are lacking. Moreover, patient-reported outcomes are hard to obtain as shown in the study by Reddy et al. evaluating the long-term sexual outcome of men with epispadias [32]. Out of 74 patients who met inclusion criteria, 15 (20%) agreed to fill out a questionnaire on their sexual function.

Reddy et al. reported on 15 patients of which nine (60%) had persistent curvature of the penis. Moreover, 8 of the 15 patients (53%) underwent chordee repair and penile lengthening during adolescence [32].

Urinary Continence

The true incidence of incontinence after epispadias repair is lacking as the definition of incontinence is not standardized. Also, the types of continence procedure vary from study to study making it difficult to assess outcomes. Moreover, there are no long-term patient-reported outcomes and definition of what is acceptable for patients and their families.

Cendron et al. defined continence as dry intervals of 2 h or more or on clean intermittent catheterization. Of 4 patients with Glandular epispadias, 3 (75%) were continent. Of 8 patients with penile epispadias, 5 (63%) were continent. Of 14 patients with penopubic epispadias, 9 (64%) were continent. In this series, the bladder neck was repaired using the Young-Dees-Leadbetter repair or sling bladder neck suspension [33].

Thomas et al. defined continence as not needing to wear any protection (e.g., incontinence pad for urine leakage) with patient reporting to be dry between voids or catheterizations. Of the 3 distal epispadias, 1 required a continence procedure with a total continence rate of 100%. Of the 3 midshaft epispadias patients, 2 required a continence procedure with the total continence rate of 67% (2/3). Continence surgery included injection of bulking agents (Macroplastique), bladder neck reconstruction (Young-Dees-Leadbetter), bladder neck sling, Kelly procedure, and a combination of above [27].

Braga et al. definition of continence was as follows: continent (dry intervals of at least 4 h), partially continent (2- to 4-h dry intervals), and incontinent (dry intervals of less than 2 h). They also stratified the continence rate based on the procedure performed (Cantwell-Ransley repair versus Mitchell-Bagli repair). Continence was 100% in 3 glandular and 9 penile epispadias patients. Of 17 penopubic epispadias, 11 had undergone the Cantwell-Ransley repair and 6 had undergone the Mitchell-Bagli repair. Of the 11 Cantwell-Ransley repairs, 8 (73%) were continent and 3 (27%) were partially continent. Of the 6 Mitchell-Bagli repairs, 5 (83%) were continent and 1(17%) was partially incontinent [28].

Bencic et al. defined urinary continence as dry for more than 2 h. They reported their results on 31 patients with isolated epispadias. Of the 19 patients with penopubic epispadias, 9 had a single-stage repair, 6 had 2 repairs, and 4 had multiple repairs. Of these, 12 (63%) are continent and 1 (5.3%) is continent on clean intermittent catheterization. Of the 8 patients with penile epispadias, 7 had a single-stage repair and 1 had 2-stage repair. Of these, 7 (87.5%) are continent and 1 (12.5%) is incontinent. All 4 glandular epispadias patients had one repair, and they are all continent [29].

Recently, Weiss et al. reported results from the Multi-Institutional Bladder Exstrophy Consortium (MIBEC). Of 8 patients with glandular epispadias, 5 were continent (dry for 3 h or more), 1 had intermediate continence (dry for 2 h or less), and 1 was incontinent. Of 8 patients with penile epispadias, 6 were continent and 2 had intermediate continence. Of 20 patients with penopubic epispadias, 10 were continent, 2 of whom required clean intermittent catheterization, 5 had intermediate continence with one of them on clean intermittent catheterization, and 5 were wet. This series also showed that the proximal repairs will require a bladder neck reconstruction to achieve continence but that even the more distal defects may have bladder neck incompetence and persistent incontinence [34].

Sexual Function

The cosmetic appearance and sexual function of males undergoing isolated epispadias repair are not robust. Penile length, quality of erections, and ejaculatory function all play a role in sexual function. Reddy et al. reported that 73% of the males with epispadias reported being engaged in sexual activity, yet 67% (10/15)reported having one or more issues related to sexual function [32]. These included abnormal ejaculation, difficult orgasm, decreased sensation, difficulty maintaining erections, penile appearance, and curved erections.

Of Sunil et al. series of patient with male epispadias, only 15 (20%) completed the questionnaire. Although 12 patients (80%) reported overall satisfactory sexual intercourse, 11 (73%) admitted to 1 or more problems with sexual function, including abnormal ejaculation (53%), diminished sensation (20%), and difficulty maintaining an erection (20%) [35].

Of 31 epispadias patients in Bencic et al. series, 7 (22.6%) completed the International Index of Erectile Function (IIEF) questionnaire. The average score was 21.3 (19–26) for the erectile function domain and 8.7 (7–10) for the overall satisfaction domain. Only 2 patients (28.6%) had lower scores in the erectile function domain. Three of the 7 patients had lower scores in the orgasmic domain [29].

Renal Function

Bladder neck reconstruction may place patients with epispadias at risk for renal compromise over time. This risk is lower than in bladder exstrophy as bladder capacity is near-normal in most children with isolated epispadias.

In a series by Joshi et al. from the International Bladder Exstrophy Consortium of 12 patients with isolated epispadias, eGFR was normal in all. Vesicoureteral reflux was present in one patient who also developed renal scarring. This suggests that patients with vesicoureteral reflux are at risk for pyelonephritis and possible renal scarring, and they should be followed closely after repair [36].

Female Epispadias

Primary female epispadias is rare and occurs in an estimated prevalence of 1:160,000 to 1:480,000 live births [37]. Some of these patients present later on in life when they are unable to be toilet-trained.

In this condition, the dorsal aspect of the urethra is absent and the urinary sphincter including the bladder neck is deficient. The clitoris is bifid, the perineal body is broadened, and the vagina is anterior. The mons pubis is absent, and the anterior labia are laterally displaced but are fused in the midline posteriorly. The vagina may be stenotic [1]. The internal genital organs (uterus, fallopian tubes, and ovaries) are usually unaffected.

The goals in managing these patients include the following:

1. Creation of a straight urethra
2. Good cosmetic appearance with reapproximation of the genitalia in the midline
3. Reconstructing the bladder neck for continence
4. Maintaining clitoral function

The traditional surgical approach was a staged reconstruction with the second stage being the bladder neck reconstruction [38]. Manzoni and Ransley presented an alternative single-stage technique in 2009, where the urethra, bladder neck, and clitoris were repaired by a perineal approach, but without tailoring the bladder neck to enhance outlet resistance [39]. This approach was then modified to perform a bladder neck tailoring through a perineal approach with favorable outcomes [40, 41]. The advantages of using this approach include improved continence and reduced morbidity. The radical soft-tissue mobilization described by Kelly has been applied for female primary epispadias [42].

With the complete primary epispadias repair, the bladder neck, urethra, and vagina are mobilized as a unit. Osteotomies may be necessary when the pubic diastasis is wide. The intersymphyseal bands are deeply incised to allow the bladder neck and urethra to move posteriorly. The bladder neck is then reconstructed and the urethra tubularized. The symphysis pubis is reapproximated.

The Richard Grady Monsplasty is then performed. This is a vertical Z-plasty closure to provide a 2-layer closure of the mons that decreases tension and improves cosmetic appearance by recreating a clitoral hood that provides a more normal appearance of the external genitalia for girls with bladder exstrophy. This has been described in the article by Weiss DA et al. that also includes a video of the technique [43].

The perineum is described elsewhere in this book by Pippi Salle et al.

The Kelly repair of female epispadias is described by Leclari MD et al. [42]. Supplementary video related to this article can be found at https://doi.org/10.1016/j.jpurol.2017.08.017.

Through a short transpubic midline incision, the lateral aspect of the bladder is exposed, giving access to the superior aspect of the pelvic floor. The most anterior fibers of the levator ani muscle are incised at the level of their insertion on the internal obturator muscle fascia, providing exposure to the ischiorectal fat and the urogenital diaphragm. Perineal dissection allows adequate exposure to the corpora cavernosa. A muscle stimulator is used to identify the bulbospongiosus, ischiocavernosus, and transverse perineal muscles. The periosteum of the ischiopubic rami is peeled away to allow mobilization of both corpora cavernosa, until the neurovascular pedicle exiting from the Alcock's canal is identified. All striated muscular structures, part of the urogenital diaphragm, linking the urogenital complex to the anterior pelvic ring are detached from the bone. Further dissection, on the medial aspect of the corpora, allows separation of the corpora from the urethral plate, which eventually allows repositioning of the bladder neck deep into the pelvis. Reconstruction included ureteral reimplantation if necessary, bladder neck funneling reconstruction, and urethral reconstruction with tubularization over an 8 or 10F catheter. Muscular fibers detached from the pelvis and fibers of the bulbospongiosus muscle are wrapped around the bladder neck and the upper urethra whenever possible. A corporoplasty is performed by approximating both corpora cavernosa ventrally to the neo-urethra on the midline, and both glans and clitoris are covered by a common clitoral hood.

Outcomes

Alyami et al. reported on the long-term outcomes comparing the traditional Young-Dees-Leadbetter repair versus the modified perineal approach. They had a total of 12 patients with isolated female epispadias, three of whom underwent the traditional repair and 7 underwent the perineal repair. None of the 3 patients who underwent the traditional repair were continent, while 4 of 7(57%) who underwent the perineal approach were continent.

Leclair et al. compared the perineal approach to the Kelly repair [42]. They included 16 patients in their study. Seven females underwent the perineal approach, and of these, 5 of 7 were continent during the day and 4 of 5 were also continent at night. They state that 3 of the 5 required bladder neck injection to achieve continence. Of the 9 patients undergoing the Kelly repair, 8 were evaluable and all achieved diurnal continence and 3 of 8 were fully continent though one required clean intermittent catheterization for obstructive micturition.

There are significant limitations to the above studies including the small number of patients in the surgical group. The comparison groups may also not have been similar as the more severe forms of epispadias most likely required a more radical approach. Because of the rarity of this condition, multi-institutional and longer term studies are required to determine the benefit of the complete primary repair versus the perineal repair versus the Kelly repair.

Conclusion

Epispadias represents one end of the spectrum of the bladder exstrophy-epispadias complex. Repair of epispadias is a challenging operation even in expert hands. The incidence is rare, and repair should be performed in centers of excellence in order to provide the best possible outcome.

As this condition is rare, published long-term outcomes related to continence and sexual function are sparse. Studies show that continence can be achieved in the majority of patients with epispadias but over 80% require multiple procedures to achieve social continence. Erectile and ejaculator functions are satisfactory, yet there is continued dissatisfaction with genital appearance.

References

1. Grady RW, Mitchell ME. Management of epispadias. Urol Clin North Am. 2002;29:349–60.
2. Dees JE. Congenital epispadias with incontinence. J Urol. 1949;62:513.
3. Cendron PS, Cho M, Pennison I, Rosoklija DA, Diamond JG. Borer: Anatomic findings associated with epispadias in boys: Implications for surgical management and urinary continence. J Ped Urol. 2018;14:42–8.
4. Woodhouse CRJ, Kellett MJ. Anatomy of the penis and its deformities in exstrophy and epispadias. J Urol. 1984;132:1122.
5. Silver RI, Yang A, Ben-Chaim J, et al. Penile length in adulthood after exstrophy reconstruction. J Urol. 1997b;158:999.
6. Gearhart JP, Yang A, Leonard MP, et al. Prostate size and configuration in adult patients with bladder exstrophy. J Urol. 1993c;149:308.
7. Hurwitz RS, Woodhouse CRJ, Ransley PG. The anatomical course of the neurovascular bundles in epispadias. J Urol. 1986;136:68.
8. Arap S, Nahas WC, Giron AM, et al. Continent epispadias: surgical treatment of 38 cases. J Urol. 1988;140:577.
9. Kramer SA, Kelalis P. Assessment of urinary continence in epispadias: review of 94 patients. J Urol. 1982a;128:290.
10. Ben-Chaim J, Peppas DS, Jeffs RD, et al. Complete male epispadias: genital reconstruction achieving continence. J Urol. 1995b;153:1665.
11. Diamond D, Ransley PG. Male epispadias. J Urol. 1995;154:2150–5.
12. Gearhart JP, Leonard MP, Burgers JK, Jeffs RD. The Cantwell-Ransley technique for repair of epispadias. J Urol. 1992;148:851–4.
13. Mitchell ME, Bagli DJ. Complete penile disassembly for epispadias repair: the Mitchell technique. J Urol. 1996;155:300–4.
14. Grady RW, Mitchell ME. Management of epispadias. Urol Clin N Am. 2002;29:349–60.
15. Gearhart JP, Jeffs RD. The use of parenteral testosterone therapy in genital reconstructive surgery. J Urol. 1987;138:1077–8.
16. Makedonsky J. The use of Human Chorionic Gonadotropin (HCG) for penile reconstruction in bladder Exstrophy and Total Epispadias. Eur J Ped Surgery. 2006;16:428–31.
17. Suson KD, Sponseller PD, Gearhart JP. Bony abnormalities in classic bladder exstrophy: the urologist's perspective. J Ped Urol. 2013;9:112–22.
18. Diamond DA, Ransley PG. Male epispadias. J Urol. 1995;154:2150–5.
19. Gearhart JP, Sciortino C, Ben-Chaim J, Peppas DS, Jeffs RD. The Cantwell-Ransley epispadias repair in exstrophy and epispadias: lessons learned. Urology. 1995;46:92–5.
20. Bar-Yosef Y, Sofer M, Ekstein MP, Binyamini Y, Ben-Chaim J. Results of Epispadias repair using the modified cantwell-ransley technique. Urology. 2017;99:221–4.

21. Kramer SA, Jackson IT. Bilateral rhomboid flaps for reconstruction of the external genitalia in epispadias-exstrophy. Plast Reconstr Surg. 1986;77:621–31.
22. Pippi Salle JL, Elifranji M, Abbas T, Alhadi A, Elkadhi A, Leslie B, Vallasciani S. Technical details in the primary repair of male epispadias: step by step video. Urol Video J. 2022;13:10027. https://doi.org/10.1016/j.urolvj.2022.100127.
23. Baka-Jakybiak M. Bladder neck, urethral and penile reconstruction in boys with the exstrophy-epispadias complex. BJU Int. 2000;86:513–8.
24. Pippi Salle JL, Jednak R, Capolicchio JP, Franca IMP, Labbie A, Gosalbex R. A ventral rotational skin flap to improve cosmesis and avoid chordee recurrence in epispadias repair. BJU Int. 2002;90:918–23.
25. Kibar Y, Roth C, Frimberger D, Kropp B. Long-term results of penile disassembly technique for correction of epispadias. Urology. 2009;73:510–4.
26. Surer I, Baker LA, Jeffs RD, Gearhart JP. The modified Cantwell-Ransley repair for Exstrophy and Epispadias: a 10-year experience. J Urol. 2000;164:1040–3.
27. Thomas JS, Shenoy M, Mushtaq I, Wood D. Long-term outcomes in primary male epispadias. J Ped Urol. 2020;16(80):e1–6.
28. Braga LH, Lorenzo AJ, Bagli DJ, Khoury AE. Outcome analysis of isolated male epispadias: single center experience with 33 cases. J Urol. 2008;179:1107–12.
29. Bencic M, Bizic M, Joksic I, Stojanovic B, Djordjevic ML. Isolated male Epispadias repair: long-term outcomes. Life. 2024;14:446.
30. Tourchi A, Hoebeke P. Long-term outcome of male genital reconstruction in childhood. J Pediatr Urol. 2013;9:980–9.
31. Djordjevic ML, Bizic MR, Martins F, Kojovic V, Krstic Z. Treatment for failed epispadias repair presenting in adults. J Urol. 2013;190:165–70.
32. Reddy SS, Inouye BM, Anele UA, Abdelwahab B, Le B, Gearhart JP, Rao PK. Sexual health outcomes in adults with complete male epispadias. J Urol. 2015;194:1091–5.
33. Cendron M, Cho PS, Pennison M, Rosoklija I, Diamond DA, Borer JG. Anatomic findings associated with epispadias in boys: Implications for surgical management and urinary continence. J Ped Urol. 2018;14:42–6.
34. Weiss DA, Lee T, Roth EB, Cendron M, Goetz J, Kryger JV, Groth TW, Shukla AR, Mitchell ME, Canning DA, Borer JG. Male epispadias repair: outcomes at three sites prior to the establishment of a multi-institutional collaboration. J Ped Urol. 2024;20:e1-408.e6.
35. Reddy SS, Inouye BM, Anele UA, Abdelwahab M, Le B, Gearhart JP, Rao PK. Sexual health outcomes in adults with complete male Epispadias. J Urol. 2015;194:1091–5.
36. Joshi RS, Eftekharzadeh S, Shukla AR, Ramji J, Hingorani SR, Canning DA, Pippi-Salle JL, Merguerian P, Defoor WR Jr, Frazier J, Weiss DA, Reddy PP. Kidney function outcomes in patients after complete primary repair of bladder exstrophy and penopubic epispadias: results from the international bladder exstrophy consortium. J Ped Urol. 2023;19(34):e1–34, e9.
37. Allen A, Rodjani J, Kelly M, Inoue JM. Hutson: female epispadias: are we missing the diagnosis? BJU Int. 2004;94:613–5.
38. Peters C, Gearhart JP, Jeffs R. Epispadias and incontinence: the challenge of the small bladder. J Urol. 1988;140:1199–201.
39. Manzoni G, Ransley P. Primary surgical intervention for female epispadias. J Pediatr Urol. 2007;3:S73.
40. Cheikhelard A, Aigran Y, Lottmann H, Lortat-Jacob S. Female epispadias management: perineal urethrocervicoplasty versus classical Young-Dees procedure. J Urol. 2009;182(4):1807–11.
41. Bhat AL, Bhat M, Sharma R, Saxena G. Single stage perineal urethroplasty for continence in female epispadias: a preliminary report. Urology. 2008;72(2):300–3.
42. Leclair MD, Faraj S, Villemagne T, Carrouget J, Arnaud A, Heloury Y. Primary female epispadias: perineal approach or Kelly repair? J Pediatr Urol. 2018;14:33–9.
43. Weiss DA, Steffe E, Borer JG, Groth TW, Roth EB, Kryger JV, Shukla AR, Canning DA, Mitchell ME. The Richard Grady Monsplasty: a vertical Z-plasty technique. J Pediatr Urol. 2021;17(4):575–6.

The Failed Exstrophy Repair: Technique and Implications

17

Rakesh S. Joshi and Jaishri Ramji

Introduction

Over the past several decades, there has been a dramatic evolution in the management of bladder exstrophy. Advanced surgical techniques and improved postoperative management have contributed to better results in functional and cosmetic outcomes. Successful primary closure is a key factor for bladder growth and eventually continence. In the modern era, contemporary success rates of exstrophy closure have improved significantly, and the long-term continence rates range around 45–60% depending on the type of repair done [1].

With increasing experience and knowledge of the surgical anatomy, the incidence of complete dehiscence has decreased from 13% to 1% [2]. Yet failures in different forms still occur frequently. A failed exstrophy closure is a devastating setback to subsequent genitourinary reconstruction, urinary continence and long-term impact on the patient and healthcare system.

The occurrence of bladder prolapse, complete dehiscence, vesicocutaneous fistula, outlet obstruction or any combination of factors along with loss of urethra, corpora or glans/clitoris constitutes a failed exstrophy closure. Although repeat closure is often feasible, there are negative implications on the fate of the urinary tract. The chances of achieving continence after failed and multiple closures decrease dramatically. Children with one or more failed closures are ultimately an extremely challenging subset with poorer outcomes.

Supplementary Information The online version contains supplementary material available at https://doi.org/10.1007/978-3-031-91238-2_17.

R. S. Joshi (✉) · J. Ramji
Department of Pediatric Surgery, B. J. Medical College and Civil Hospital, Ahmedabad, Gujarat, India

A. R. Shukla, R. S. Joshi (eds.), *Bladder Exstrophy and Epispadias*,
https://doi.org/10.1007/978-3-031-91238-2_17

In this chapter, we will try to outline the possible reasons for failed closures, the types of outcomes that constitute failure, the early and late management of failed closure, including principles of redo closures, and the outcomes of redo exstrophy closures.

Reasons for Failure of Primary Closure

Regardless of choice of surgery, the objectives of surgery should aim at tension-free closure of bladder, pelvic ring and abdominal wall; protection of the upper tracts by avoiding outlet obstruction and pyelonephritis; and preservation of the genital and urethral soft tissues. Consequently, a failed closure results when any one of these objectives is not accomplished adequately.

Pre-operative, technical or post-operative causes can be the attributable factors for failure, either in isolation, or more commonly, multifactorial.

Pre-operative Factors

Various patient-related factors may contribute to failure of the primary repair; a wide pubic diastasis, an ill or undernourished infant and an unprotected or improperly preserved bladder plate, which delays the primary surgery. Technical precision and the surgeon and institutional experience, along with lack of concomitant osteotomy, are also known to impact the outcomes [3].

Technical Aspects

From a technical point of view, adequate vesicourethral mobilisation is a key factor contributing to successful closure. Experienced surgeons advocate aggressive posterior repositioning of the bladder, bladder neck and the urethra. This is based on the principle that exstrophy represents an anterior bladder herniation. The posterior placement is facilitated by the simultaneous dissection of bladder and urethral plate and division of the intersymphyseal band. Failure to release this band increases the chances of dehiscence [4, 5]. Surer et al. and EL Sherbiny et al. have showed that this principle helps prevent significant complications even in repair of failed closures [4].

The rate of dehiscence may also be correlated with exiting the drainage catheters from the neo- urethra, rather than a suprapubic exit site [6]. This manoeuvre may cause ischaemia, especially if paraexstrophy flaps are used. The flaps can necrose and cause the inter-pubic stitch to erode into the urethra, with resultant infection, dehiscence or urethral stricture. Currently the role of paraexstrophy flaps is limited mostly to staged repairs when there is severe shortening of the urethra [7].

The Role of Osteotomy

Studies have proven the importance of osteotomy in the surgical treatment of bladder exstrophy. The major role of osteotomy is in relaxing the tension on the bladder closure and the abdominal wall closure to allow for tension-free, adequate healing. In the absence of osteotomy, the abnormal separation of the pubic bones and the external rotation of the innominate bones place a significant tension on the soft tissues during reconstruction of the bladder, urethra and the anterior abdominal wall. It has been documented that the use of osteotomy has improved the success rates of soft tissue closure and urinary continence and resolved the gait abnormalities [8].

Some surgeons believe that when the primary repair is done in newborns, ligamental laxity allows the pelvis to be closed without significant tension. Osteotomy becomes mandatory once exstrophy repair is delayed beyond 72 h, in cases of poorly malleable pelvis and when the pubic diastasis is more than 4 cm [9, 10]. A firm anterior pelvic ring resulting from osteotomy supports the urethral suspension and contributes in preventing bladder prolapse or dehiscence [8]. Gearhart has reported in his study of 170 failed repairs that osteotomy had been done in only 29% at the time of the primary repair [11]. The rate of failure of abdominal wall closure and bladder closure has diminished to less than 5% at experienced centres with the incorporation of osteotomy in the repair of bladder exstrophy. Various types of osteotomies have been described, like posterior iliac, anterior osteotomy of the superior pubic rami, anterior diagonal iliac, modified Salter's innominate and vertical iliac ramotomy [8]. The combined transverse innominate and vertical iliac osteotomy have been shown to have lower rates of dehiscence and prolapse compared to other osteotomies [10]. The benefits of osteotomy far outweigh the complication rate of 4% shared collectively by the various osteotomies [8]. At the authors' institute, all primary repairs are done after 3 months of age with osteotomy in all cases. The dehiscence rate has been less than 2%, and there have been very few complications.

On the other hand, certain authors believe that osteotomy is not an essential element of the exstrophy repair. The downsides are the added morbidity, complications and requirement of an expert orthopaedic surgeon. Even after the osteotomy, the pubes eventually drift apart over a period of time; and hence the osteotomy itself may not be a long-term contributor to continence [12]. Bhatnagar et al. and Sudipta et al. have reported good results with the use of rectus flaps to facilitate the closure instead of osteotomy and believe that it is not necessary either for the closure or for the achievement of continence [10, 13].

When talking about failed repairs and redo closures, the pendulum swings greatly in favour of osteotomy. There is ample evidence of osteotomy increasing the success rates of reclosures as reported by various authors [8, 14–16]. The greatest success rates in reclosures have been achieved when the osteotomy was combined with secure post-operative immobilisation with external fixators and modified Buck's traction. Conversely, the outcomes were universally poor regardless of the type of immobilisation, if the osteotomy was not done [15] (Fig. 17.1).

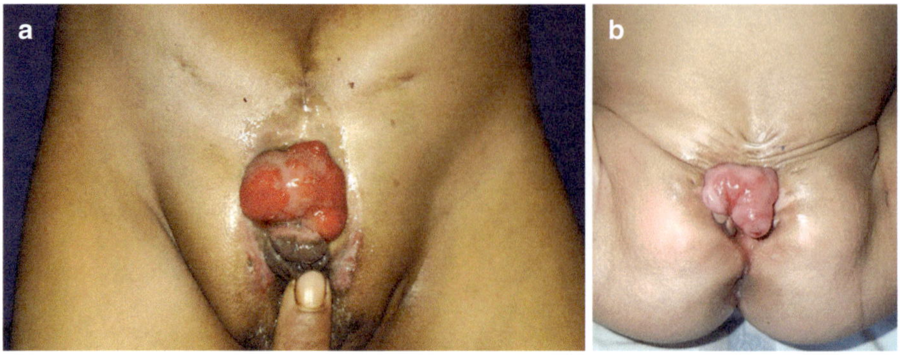

Fig. 17.1 Complete dehiscence within days of closure—no osteotomies done. (**a**) Male. (**b**) Female

Post-Operative Sources of Wound Tension

Successful closure depends as much on reducing the tension on the closure as on maintaining the tension-free closure in the post-operative period. Inadequate analgesia, poor immobilisation, abdominal distension and poor urinary drainage are some of the factors that can increase the wound tension in the post-operative period and lead to a failed repair [14].

In the initial post-operative period, the focus should be on controlling these adverse forces aggressively. Epidural analgesia with hourly pain assessments and adjunctive sedation whenever needed is crucial to keep the child still and comfortable. The nasogastric tube should be removed only when the child is stooling adequately, and abdomen is soft.

Post-operative immobilisation plays a crucial role in successful closure. It allows the tension-free closure enabled by osteotomy to heal adequately. The use of mummy wraps and spica casts has been shown to be rife with complications, with little benefit [15]. Modified Buck's traction or modified Bryant's traction has been advocated with satisfactory outcomes [10, 11]. The best results have been reported with the external fixators along with modified Buck's traction for 6–8 weeks. The leg traction may be the most effective way to control the movement of the legs as well as keep the buttocks and pelvis flat on the bed [15].

Proper management of the outlet of the reconstructed bladder is of prime importance. Early dislodgement of the urinary drainage tubes poses a significant risk for failure [17]. Special attention should be given to securing the tubes and leaving them in for an adequate period. Generally, we leave the ureteric catheters for 14 days, the per-urethral stent for 21 days and the suprapubic tube for 6 weeks. However, there may be institutional variations in the protocol [6, 12, 13]. The closure can also be compromised by wound infection, ultimately leading to dehiscence or a fistula. Hence the importance of broad-spectrum intravenous antibiotics and nutritious diet cannot be overemphasised.

Modes of Failure

Failure of primary exstrophy repair can manifest as dehiscence, prolapse of bladder, vesicocutaneous fistula, urethral stricture or bladder neck obstruction. A complex failure constitutes a combination of one or more of these along with corporal, urethral or glans loss.

Kasprenski et al. have reviewed the outcomes of 170 patients with a failed closure. They documented bladder prolapse and dehiscence as the commonest forms (around 35%) and complex failures comprised another 11% [11].

Modes of primary closure failure	*n*	%
Prolapse	61	35.9
Dehiscence	60	35.3
Vesicocutaneous fistula	05	2.9
Obstruction	06	1.8
Complex	19	11.2
Unknown	15	8.8
Others	07	4.1

Complete dehiscence of the bladder and abdominal wall often occurs early in the post-operative period. The causes for this disastrous occurrence have been described in the previous section. One of the most important causes is the technical failure. Irrespective of the type of repair done, radical mobilisation of the vesicourethral unit for it to be placed deep in the pelvis is the critical step [4, 18]. Gearhart and Jeffs emphasise the need for this radical dissection along with a secure pelvic ring closure in MRSE. A study by Gearhart compared the success rates with and without osteotomy and with different methods of immobilisation. Success rate of 75% was documented with osteotomy and went up to 96% with immobilisation by external fixators or modified Buck's traction. Spica cast and mummy wrapping were found to be far less effective [15].

Complete primary repair of exstrophy (CPRE) as described by Grady and Mitchell also targets at returning the anatomy to more normal location, allowing pelvic diaphragm to assist in continence. The dissection of the intersymphyseal band, the anterior part of the perineal membrane from the pubis, is essential for deep placement of the vesicourethral unit. The bladder, bladder neck and urethra are mobilised and closed as one unit, using penile disassembly and partial bladder neck tailoring [4, 5, 19]. Proponents of CPRE report good early outcomes with low rates of failures in form of dehiscence, fistula and soft tissue loss. The failure rates go up to 58% in cases done without an osteotomy [20, 21].

Another common form of failure is bladder prolapse often not recognised in the early post-operative period as it is less obvious. The abdominal wall is intact as is the bladder closure, but the bladder prolapses inferiorly through a separated pubic diastasis or out the bladder neck. (3) Insufficient dissection of the bladder and urethra from the inferior ramus of the pubis moves the outlet cephalad and increases the chances of bladder prolapse. Similarly, the dissection must be adequate posteriorly and inferiorly upto the levator hiatus with the urogenital fibres lateral to the vesicourethral unit. This is important to prevent the anterior displacement when the pubes are brought together [22]. Gearhart et al. emphasise that during the primary closure, the bladder neck and posterior urethra must be long enough and tight enough to prevent bladder prolapse/ eversion of bladder mucosa, at the same time allowing unimpeded egress of urine [6].

Vesicocutaneous fistulae are technically considered failures, as the management would necessarily imply a redo surgery [23].

Bladder Neck and Outlet

Bladder outlet obstruction is another troublesome form of failed closure. The severe consequences of outlet obstruction on outcomes are main reasons why no formal bladder neck reconstruction is attempted at the primary repair in multi stage repair of exstrophy (MSRE); rather, a bladder outlet is created, which is incontinent, yet provides enough resistance to stimulate bladder growth [14]. In CPRE also, although the epispadias repair is done simultaneously, there is no bladder neck reconstruction. The symphyseal suture may contribute to stricture formation due to erosion into the posterior urethra. Gearhart and associates have reported a high incidence of strictures with the use of long paraexstrophy flaps during bladder closure in MSRE, which are prone to ischaemic necrosis. Ureteric stents exiting from the neourethra may be another culprit, hence the importance of proper placement of tubes and their postoperative management. The neourethra must be calibrated before removing the suprapubic tube [2, 24].

Outlet obstruction has also been observed in CPRE and Kelly's repair, in form of complete obliteration of the urethra. It is unclear whether this is due to technical problems during extensive mobilisation causing ischaemia to the urethra [2].

The possibility of narrowing of the outlet can be suspected if there are episodes of febrile urinary tract infections or development of hydronephrosis on follow-up [6]. Bladder stones, difficult catheterisation, prolonged dry intervals, straining to void with residual urine or recurrent episodes of epididymitis may be some other presentations indicating outlet obstruction [24].

Complications like loss of urethral plate, glans, corporal body and clitoris may happen in isolation or along with major modes of failure, constituting a 'complex failure'. Such soft tissue loss may be because of the radical dissection, more so in CPRE [25]. The penile disassembly technique done incorrectly, accentuated by vagaries in the blood supply of the penis, may contribute to an ischaemic injury to the phallus [22]. Other reasons for the soft tissue injury could be arterial spasm, venous congestion subsequent to compartment syndrome after a tight pubic closure or an abnormal blood supply [25, 26]. Atrophy of one or both clitoral bodies has also been observed, a probable consequence of ischaemic insult [27]. Partial or complete loss of the urethral plate could result from damage to the terminal arteries during dissection. Inadvertent injury to the bulbar artery as it exits from the common penile artery into the corpus spongiosum can lead to complete loss of the urethral plate [25]. In girls, loss of the urethrovaginal septum has been reported secondary to the use of para-exstrophy flaps [26] (Fig. 17.2).

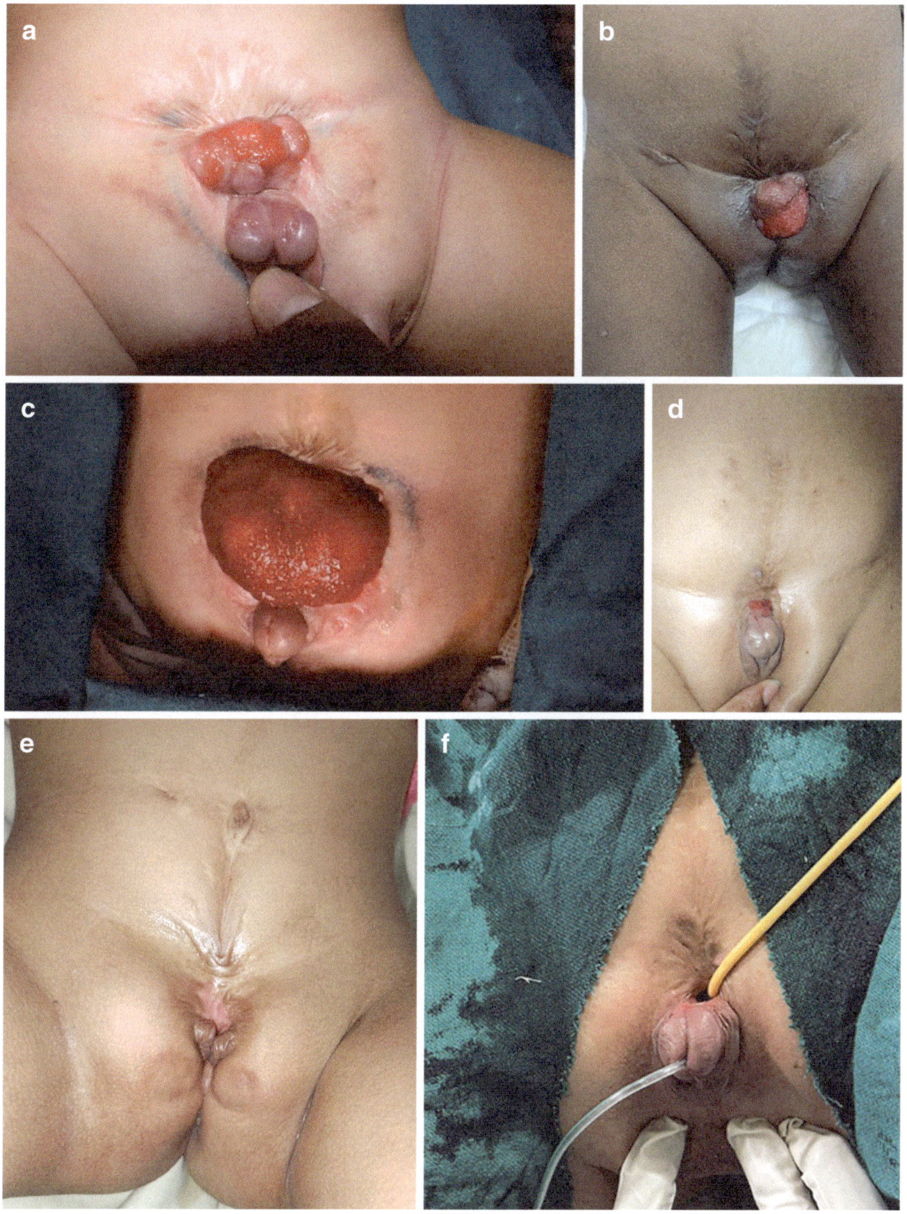

Fig. 17.2 Various modes of failed exstrophy repair. (**a**) Complete dehiscence in a male. (**b**) Complete dehiscence in a female. (**c**) Failed CPRE—bladder dehiscence with intact epispadias repair. (**d**) Bladder prolapse in a male. (**e**) Prolapsing bladder in a female. (**f**) Vesicocutaneous fistula. (**g**) Failed epispadias repair. (**h**) Stenosed hypospadiac meatus after CPRE causing outlet obstruction. (**i**) Complex failure—loss of corpora. (**j**) Complex failure—loss of hemiglans

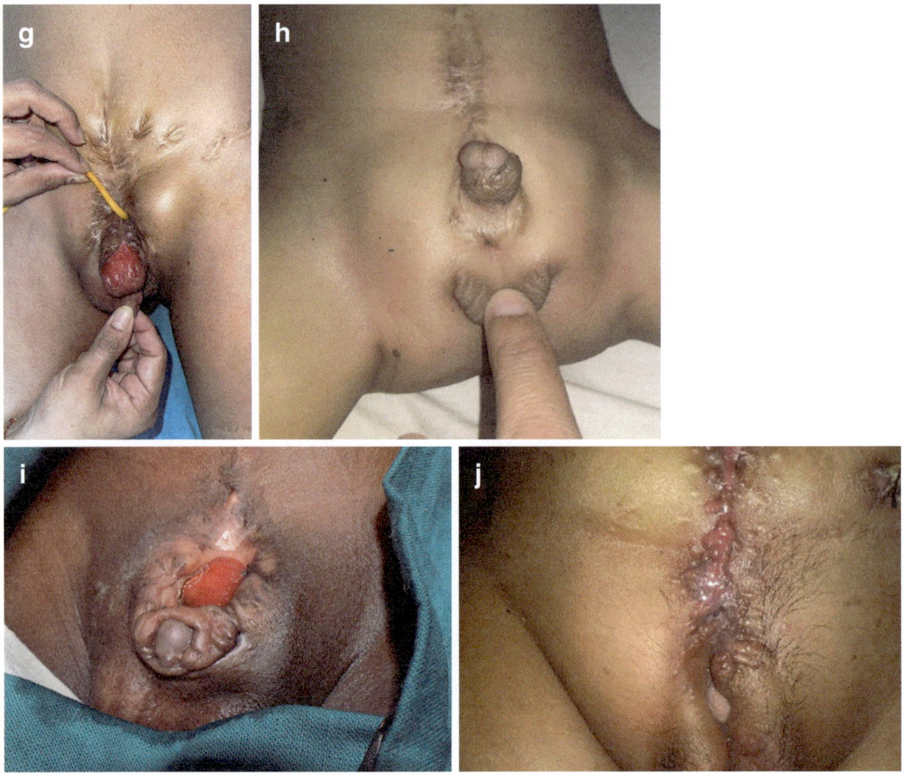

Fig. 17.2 (continued)

Consequences of Failed Repairs

A failed repair has negative long-term impacts on the patient and the healthcare system [11]. The consequences of one or more failed repairs are increased scar formation and collagen deposition, decreased bladder growth, decreased capacity and decreased rates of voided urethral continence [28]. A successful primary bladder closure is the cornerstone to achieve sufficient bladder capacity and eventually continence. Each failed repair decreases the potential to gain adequate bladder capacity [29]. Failure of the primary closure translates as a failure to get adequate bladder capacity in over 50% patients. The MSRE uses the bladder capacity as the main determinant for BNR. Kasprenski M et al. have reported that BNR alone as a continence procedure was successful in only 53.2% of the patients who were eligible for this procedure [11]. Thus, only half of those who acquire reasonable capacity are continent subsequently, suggesting that other factors like bladder compliance also

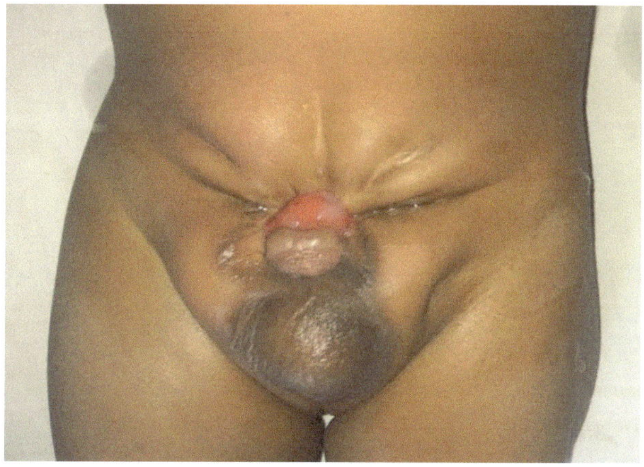

Fig. 17.3 Small capacity bladder with scarred abdominal wall after failed repairs

play an important role [26]. The chances of continence with volitional voiding go down to 30% with two closures and further to 20% with three or more closures [2].

Repeated surgical insults can also lead to fibrosis and contracture of the bladder plate. This leads to a low-volume stiff bladder after reclosure. Peppas et al. have shown the ratio of collagen to smooth muscle to be much higher in bladders that have been subjected to multiple closures. The increased collagen formation decreases the elasticity and compliance of the bladder, preventing the bladder from reaching its full capacity with growth [16]. Hanna MK et al. report changes of cystitis cystica, cystitis glandularis and squamous metaplasia on bladder biopsy in cases of failed repairs [30].

The scarring from previous surgery also increases the difficulty of subsequent repair, particularly the bladder neck reconstruction. It has been suggested by many that 4–6 months should be allowed for the wound to mature. However, waiting for too long a period may aggravate the chronic inflammation of the exposed bladder plate and make it stiff and fibrotic [16] (Fig. 17.3).

Consequences of Stricture and Obstruction Posterior urethral stricture and subsequent outlet obstruction impair the success of any repair significantly. This is a potentially dangerous complication as it poses a serious threat to the upper tracts and slowly leads to deterioration of renal function [2, 22, 24] (Fig. 17.4).

Redo surgeries and other salvage procedure after multiple failures are complicated, requiring longer surgical and post-operative recovery time [31]. The cost to the patient, resource utilisation and burden on healthcare system is compounded significantly when the primary repair fails.

The afore-mentioned clinical and economic consequences of failure have raised the question of centralisation of bladder exstrophy care. Patient outcomes may be better optimised if the surgeries are done exclusively by teams with expertise earned with large volume of cases. The improved outcomes at such high-volume centres of excellence would probably offset the travel obstacles and costs [11, 31]. Long-term

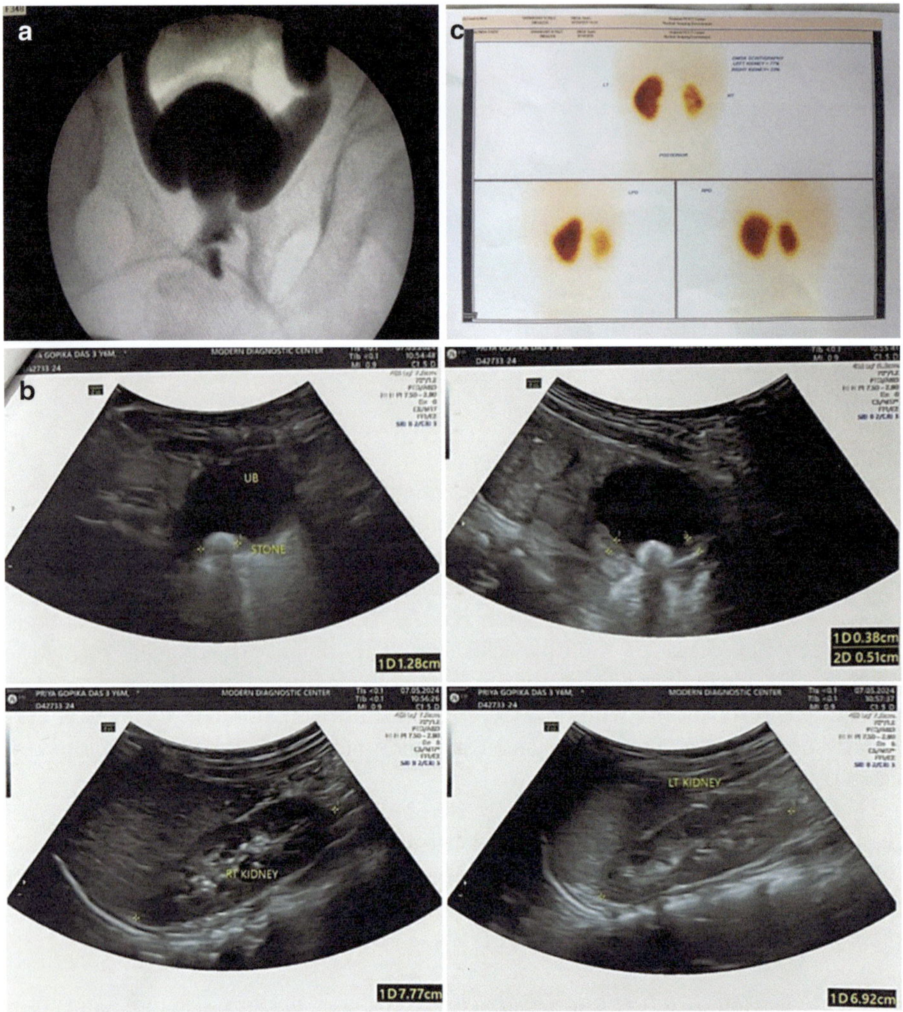

Fig. 17.4 Effects of outlet obstruction. (**a**) High pressure bladder with reflux. (**b**) Stone formation. (**c**) Compromised renal function

multi-institutional collaboratives involving experts from high-income countries combined with local experience at well-equipped dedicated centres in middle- and low-income countries are proving to a feasible model for alleviating the disease burden in these areas [32].

Management

The initial management of a failed repair is conservative with debriding the devitalised tissue, removal of foreign bodies and treating wound infection with culture-appropriate antibiotics. There should be no attempts at immediate repeat closure. A minimum interval of 4–6 months is considered optimal before attempting any surgical procedure [3, 11]. This allows time for the wound to mature and the inflammation to subside.

Before planning any surgical procedure for failure, a complete evaluation is mandatory. This should include examination under anaesthesia, pelvic x-rays, ultrasound and renal scans. Cystograms and cystoscopy are indicated in cases of prolapse, vesicocutaneous fistula or bladder outlet obstruction, while CT scans or MRI is recommended when previous osteotomies have been done.

The options for a surgeon managing a failed exstrophy repair are delayed redo bladder closure, redo bladder closure with epispadias repair, redo bladder closure with concomitant bladder augmentation, excision of the bladder and continent urinary diversion, creating a urinary conduit [6, 33]. The precise management needs to be individualised to correct the factors culpable for the initial failure. It is also necessary to consider the socio-economic circumstances, quality of life, and perception of body image. In adolescents presenting with failure, continent urinary diversion may be planned early [29].

Although a failed repair decreases the chances of a compliant, good capacity and continent bladder, all failed primary repairs should be given a chance for redo repair, if the bladder plate is healthy and genital reconstruction is possible.

Redo Exstrophy repair may be undertaken as a single-stage CPRE or as MSRE. The basic tenets of a redo repair include: (1) radical dissection of the bladder and posterior urethra, (2) deep placement of the bladder, bladder neck and urethra as one unit in the pelvis, (3) osteotomy with external fixators or traction to secure post-operative immobilisation, (4) adequate post-operative sedation, pain relief and control any distracting forces and (5) pre-operative intramuscular testosterone, which by increasing phallic length and girth may reduce likelihood of inadvertent injury [26].

The redo repair outlined below is what the authors follow and is much the same as the complete primary repair described in another chapter in this textbook. The challenge at the outset is to enter the correct surgical planes between the bladder detrusor and rectus fascia circumferentially around the bladder plate. The scarred and fibrous tissue from the previous failed repair will often render these planes difficult to identify, so care must be taken to ensure that the detrusor muscle of the bladder is preserved. Once the planes are identified, the goal is to radically dissect the vesicourethral unit, releasing all the adhesions from the previous surgery. The planes between the detrusor muscle and fascia are often easiest to visualise laterally, where the dissection begins to identify the medial border of the anterior rectus sheath. The idea is to enter the perivesical fat and dissect the bladder superiorly and inferiorly on either side. The superficial ligaments of the bladder are divided, but it is recommended not to continue with the deep pelvic dissection at this point to avoid injury to the corpora cavernosa that may not be fully visualised in this anterior plane.

Rather, the superior dissection at the dome of the bladder is performed, separating the peritoneum and superficial adhesions from the dome. In redo cases, sometimes it is impossible to avoid entering the peritoneum. If this occurs, the peritoneotomy may even facilitate lateral dissection when the planes are especially obliterated from previous surgery.

Once this lateral dissection is completed in an antegrade direction up to the lateral intersymphyseal bands, we proceed to the penile skin dissection. Regardless of whether a previous epispadias repair has been done, the penile skin is degloved, the neurovascular bundles are identified all the way to their course underneath the bone at the corporal insertion into the pubic bone. Often this dissection is particularly difficult as the fibrosis from the previous surgery can cause the bundles to be displaced from their original position. Once the bundles are safeguarded, the deep intersymphyseal bands are accurately identified and divided under vision (Fig. 17.5). The radical division of all the bands in this area between the bladder neck, urethra and the pubis helps to completely free the bladder plate, which can then be easily lifted up or pushed into the pelvis without any restriction. It would be worth bearing in mind that enthusiastic medial dissection at this point could compromise the width of the bladder neck.

Often, a failed repair may also have a failed epispadias repair, or it might be a failure of the first stage of bladder closure in a MSRE, where the epispadias repair had not been undertaken. It is invariably necessary to dissect the urethral plate or the reconstructed tube off the corpora and redo the epispadias repair to adequately mobilise the vesicourethral unit. The modified Cantwell-Ransley technique is applied, separating the urethral plate first ventrally and then dorsally starting at

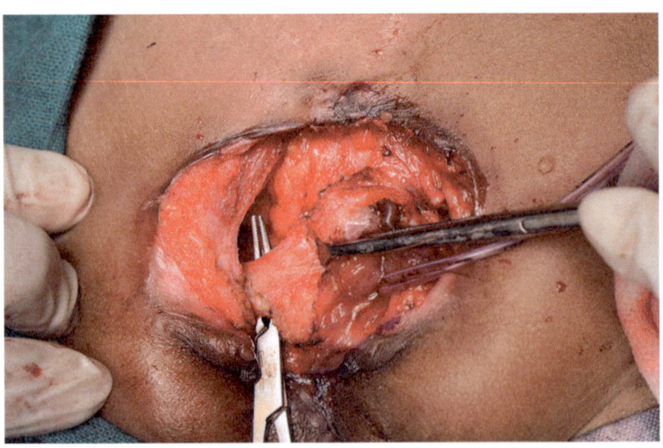

Fig. 17.5 Lateral dissection—identification and division of deep intersymphyseal bands

midshaft and moving proximally and distally. The fibroses from the previous surgery make this dissection tedious. The proximal prostatic and bladder neck dissection is tricky, where the urethra may get thin or narrow. Similarly, the distal dissection from the glans may be troublesome. The tip of the urethral plate is kept connected to the glans. Sometimes, however, the proximal radical mobilisation may shorten the urethra, or the distal plate may not be supple enough, or may have been damaged in the previous surgery. In such cases, it is more advisable to give a hypospadiac meatus, as described by Mitchell and Bagli's modification with a complete disassembly [22]. The pre-operative use of testosterone has been advocated as a means to enhance the growth of the urethral plate, increase its pliability and vascularity and minimise the incidence of hypospadias, especially in redo cases and older children [26, 34]. The authors have also been able to obtain an orthotopic meatus in most cases with the use of pre-operative testosterone enanthate intramuscular injections (2 mg/kg at 5 weeks and 3 weeks before surgery) combined with topical application of testosterone cream.

Concomitant bilateral ureteric reimplantation may be possible in some redo repairs based on the size and quality of the bladder plate. A cephalotrigonal or cross-trigonal method may be used. The safety and efficacy of reimplantation during CPRE has been well established [35].

The closure of the vesico-urethral unit begins at the bladder neck. There is no formal bladder neck reconstruction, but an attempt to funnel the bladder neck area is made to increase the outlet resistance without causing obstruction. This is done by marking an area of approximately 18 to 20 mm width depending on the age and clinical appearance, denuding lateral triangular strips of mucosa for creating a 10 mm length of funnelled wall. Three or four sutures with 4–0 or 5–0 PDS are taken, to be tied later after the bladder closure.

The bladder closure is started after bringing out and securing the ureteric catheters, suprapubic tube and a per-urethral stent. The closure is done in single or double layer with 3-0 PDS, with simple or mattress sutures, as per the quality of the bladder and surgeon's preference. The urethroplasty is done preferably with interrupted sutures, leaving the glansplasty for after pubic bone approximation.

As discussed earlier, osteotomy is imperative for a successful redo closure. An adequate osteotomy will allow the surgeon to place the bladder and posterior urethra in the pelvis while the hip bones are internally rotated to bring the pubes in close approximation to bridge the intersymphyseal gap. Depending on the severity of the diastasis, expertise of the orthopaedic surgeon and whether a previous osteotomy has been done, the osteotomy best suited for the patient can be performed. Sometimes a combination of transverse innominate and vertical iliac osteotomy may be necessary, if the diastasis cannot be overcome by a single osteotomy. The authors have found the modified Salter's osteotomy to be adequate in most cases. Usually, a single strong 1-0 PDS suture securely knotted on the outside is sufficient to keep the approximation in place. Sometimes an additional suture may be necessary. Such a snug approximation can sometimes cause vascular compression and create a penile compartment syndrome. Active bleeding from the glans and any glans congestion should be checked for before being satisfied with the symphyseal

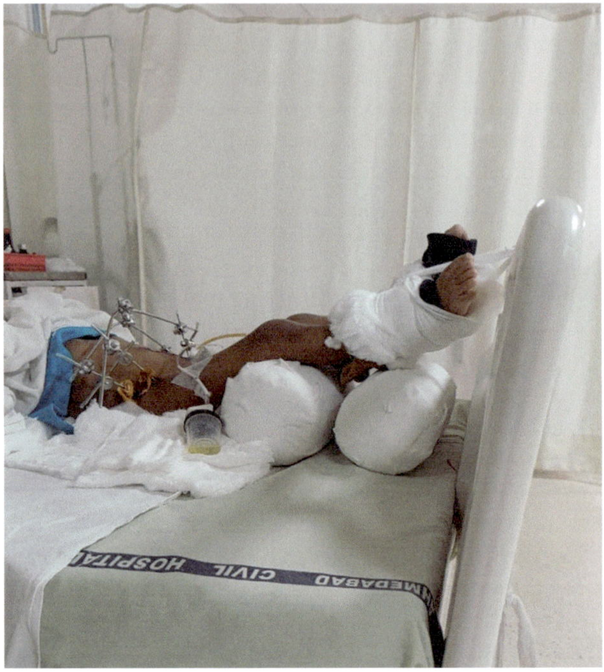

Fig. 17.6 Leg traction and external fixators for secure immobilisation

closure. It may be necessary to release the suture and re-approximate with a small gap between the pubic bones to ensure that there is no vascular compromise.

The glansplasty is now completed; the urethra is shifted ventrally, and the corpora are approximated dorsally in external rotation with 4-5 sutures of 5-0 PDS, as demonstrated by Pippe Salle [36]. Depending on the availability and quality of skin, the penile skin cover can be done by different techniques: a ventral rotational skin flap described by Pippe Salle, dorsal transposition of a ventral flap (reverse Salle technique), a transverse island flap or reverse Byar's flaps. Except for the reverse Byar's, all the others aim at avoiding a dorsal suture line, which improves the cosmesis [37, 38].

The abdominal wall closure can now be done in a tension-free manner. In rare instances, lateral relaxing incisions can be given, to decrease undue tension. It is vital to ensure that the tubes are all securely fixed before the patient is shifted. Our preferred method of immobilisation for stabilising the osteotomy is the use of external fixators for 4 weeks. The addition of leg traction like modified Bryant's may provide extra security (Fig. 17.6).

Post-operative care focuses primarily on immobilisation, adequate pain relief with epidural analgesia, wide spectrum antibiotics and antispasmodics to prevent bladder spasms, along with the prevention of any other causes of raised abdominal pressure such as distension and constipation. Ureteric stents are left in for 2 weeks and suprapubic drainage is maintained for 6 weeks (Fig. 17.7).

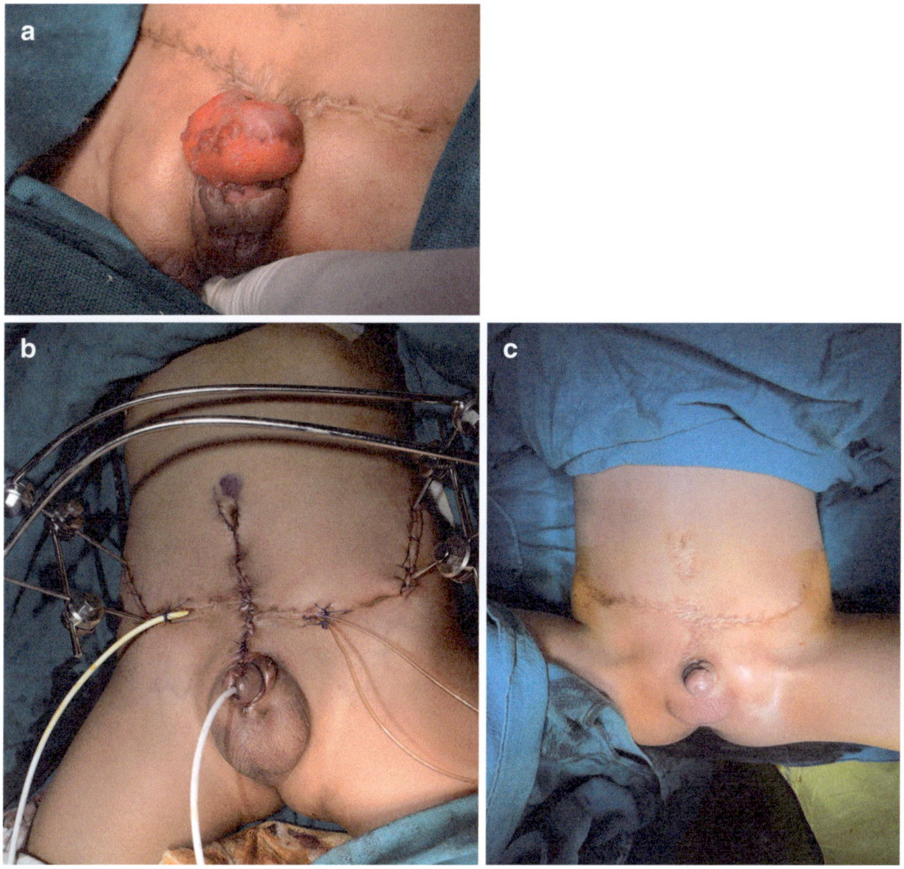

Fig. 17.7 Redo repair in failed exstrophy. (**a**) Failed repair with complete dehiscence. (**b**) Redo CPRE with osteotomies. (**c**) Outcome on 6-month follow-up

Use of Rectus Muscle Flaps

The bladder neck region and intersymphyseal area are the most vulnerable areas for dehiscence or fistula formation. The use of rectus muscle pedicled flaps has been described to reinforce the closure in the inter-pubic gap in redo bladder closures and repair of vesicocutaneous fistulae; as well as in bladder neck closures and bladder augmentation in failed repairs [13, 39, 40] (Fig. 17.8).

We have similarly used the rectus muscle flap in some redo repairs for reinforcing the closure, and sometimes also as an alternative to osteotomy in older patients. The rectus muscle is separated off the anterior and posterior rectus sheaths, taking care not to damage the anterior sheath. The muscle is divided at the upper end of the incision and mobilised till its attachment to the pubic bone and preserving its vascular supply from the inferior epigastric vessels. The muscle flap can now be turned

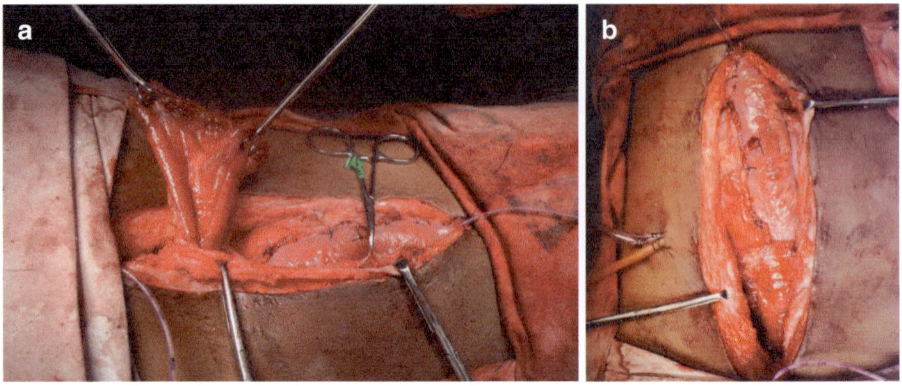

Fig. 17.8 Use of rectus flaps for reinforcement of the bladder augmentation. (**a**) Raising the flap. (**b**) Covering the repair

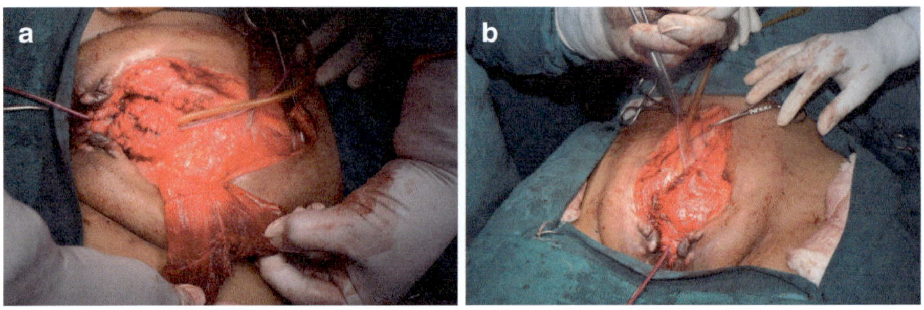

Fig. 17.9 Use of rectus flaps in redo repair. (**a**) Raising the flap. (**b**) Covering the bladder repair

across the inter-pubic gap to cover the bladder repair. The opened rectus sheath is repaired, and both sheaths are anchored to the upper end of the muscle flap, to get a secure abdominal wall closure (Fig. 17.9).

A different technique of using the rectus muscle flap in lieu of osteotomy to close the pelvic brim has also been described. The muscle is detached from the superior pubic ramus on either side, sutured in midline and then pulled caudad and re-anchored at the symphysis to complete the pelvic brim [12].

The possibility of weakness or herniation in the deficit created by transposing the muscle needs to be considered, although there has been no incidence in the short-term follow-up of our cases. Others who have used these flaps have also not reported this consequence [13, 39].

The redo repair in a female patient essentially follows the same principles, with a few noteworthy points to emphasise. A similar radical dissection of the bladder and urethra is done but maintaining the connection to the vagina. The urethrovaginal septum is kept intact to preserve the blood supply. The lateral aspects of the vesico-urethral unit and the lateral vaginal attachments are freed from the pelvic floor. It is

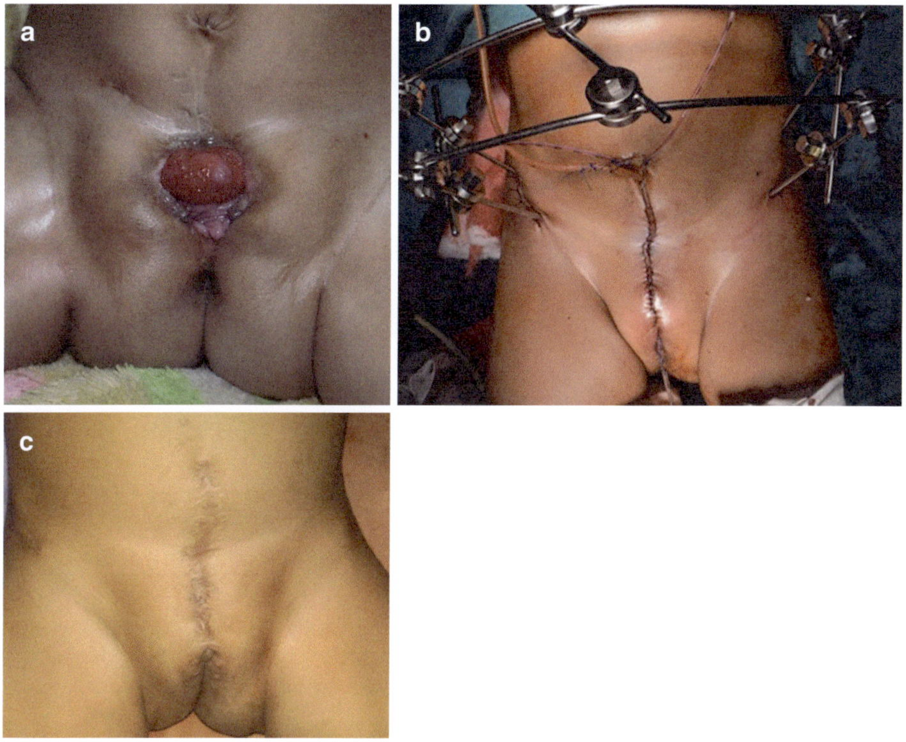

Fig. 17.10 Redo CPRE in a female. (**a**) Failed repair—complete dehiscence. (**b**) Redo CPRE. (**c**) Outcome at 6-month follow-up

important at this point to place a small Hegar's dilator in the vagina to prevent injury to the lateral vaginal wall. The dissection of the vagina goes lateral, posterior and inferior upto the levator hiatus. The genital reconstruction includes a monsplasty and Y-V labioplasty to bring the vaginal introitus out adequately. Rather than suturing the split clitoris (which may disrupt the delicate nerve supply and cause scarring), the clitoral bodies are simply brought together in midline, and anterolateral skin flaps are sutured over them to create the clitoral hood and anterior fourchette [27, 41]. If there is significant scar tissue from the previous surgery, a puboplasty as described by Vanderbrink et al. may be necessary, where a wedge of scar between the clitoral bodies is excised and tissues are approximated to create the anterior fourchette [27] (Fig. 17.10).

A vesicocutaneous fistula, which has not closed spontaneously, often needs to be managed like a complete dehiscence. However, in some cases, the epispadias repair and penile reconstruction may be intact. In such cases, the fistula can be closed by doing a wide local dissection without disturbing the epispadias repair. A rectus abdominus muscle flap can be used to reinforce the fistula repair.

Bladder outlet obstruction due to neourethral stricture is a form of failure that may be quite difficult and prolonged to manage. Initial management begins with identifying the extent of the problem with a cystoscopy and voiding cystourethrogram. Although a few strictures can be managed with dilatations, many require multiple procedures. Serial dilatations, intermittent self-catheterisation, urethrotomy and revision of the urethroplasty with buccal grafts are the options with escalating intensity. Suprapubic diversion or even complete defunctionalisation with a vesicostomy may be necessary with increasing upper tract deterioration. Revision of the outlet wherever possible is preferred over vesicostomy as the latter will result in shrunken bladder unfit for further reconstruction. The need for long-term suprapubic diversion ultimately translates into bladder augmentation with Mitrofannoff [6, 14, 22].

Failed Genital Reconstruction

While a simple urethrocutaneous fistula after the epispadias repair is easily repaired, the management of some of the more complex genital reconstructive failures may prove challenging.

Loss of the entire urethral plate may require staged reconstruction using full thickness skin grafts or buccal mucosal grafts. Tissue expanders with skin grafts may be necessary where there is loss of penile shaft or skin. Neophalloplasty, using complex plastic surgical reconstructive techniques, is an option for patients who have significant loss of glans, corporal bodies and other soft tissues [6, 14, 22]. These are the most challenging situations, where ideal tissue substitutes are not available.

Alternatives to Redo Repair

A failed exstrophy repair may not always be amenable to redo repair. Various factors need to be taken into consideration before deciding the best option for the child, the foremost being the status of the upper tracts. The morbidities of reclosure are also high with redo osteotomies, prolonged immobilisation, epidural analgesia and extended hospital stay. In a child with a poor bladder template, older age or multiple attempts at closure, it might be prudent to provide a urinary diversion.

Ureterosigmoidostomy

The procedure was popular and accepted in the past, being tolerated well and providing continence. However, the long-term morbidities of recurrent pyelonephritis, stone formation, electrolyte imbalance, acidosis and risk of malignancy led to it falling out of favour. Fisch et al. reported the Mainz II, a modification of the classical ureterosigmoidostomy, as an alternative method of internal diversion. By detubularisation and creating submucosal tunnels, the morbidity was reduced, although the risk of malignancy remains the same. Recently, this procedure has again been proposed as a valuable alternative in terms of quality of life for selected patients [22]. A variation of ureterosigmoidostomy using a recto-sigmoid bladder reservoir has been described as an alternative to multiple attempts at redo repair [42]. Sarin et al. have reported encouraging results from Yogesh's cystorectostomy, a modification of Heitz-Boyer-Hovelacque procedure, directly anastomosing the bladder plate to the recto-sigmoid pouch, without mobilising the ureters. Such procedures may have a role in low- and middle-income settings and significantly improve the quality of life, though our preference remains to embark on a redo closure whenever feasible [43].

Augmentation Cystoplasty

The most serious consequence of failed exstrophy repairs—especially after multiple closures—is the effect on the bladder growth. Hollowell and Ransley stated that it was unrealistic to expect the exstrophied bladder to provide compliant continence without augmentation cystoplasty in majority of cases [35]. Thus, in an already abnormal bladder, the chances of attaining good capacity and compliance are reduced drastically after failed repairs. Hence the option of bladder augmentation must be considered depending on the various adverse factors. The need for bladder augmentation in failed exstrophy has been reported to be as high as 73–92% [13]. That said, our initial experience with closure of redo bladders does show similar bladder capacity increase and low risk of upper tract deterioration as compared to primary bladder closures [32, 44]. Therefore, our preference remains to embark on a redo bladder exstrophy closure and observe expectantly for an extended period of time prior to considering bladder augmentation.

The segment used for augmentation can be ileal, ileocaecal, colonic or gastric as reported by various authors. It is often accompanied by bladder neck tightening/closure with provision of a continent catheterisable stoma. A complete discussion of the techniques and outcomes of different modes of augmentation cystoplasty is beyond the scope of this chapter and can be found elsewhere.

Outcomes of Redo Repair

There are some common consensuses about outcomes of reclosure after failed repairs: (1) reclosure with osteotomy has high success rates in terms of the closure; (2) the outcomes in terms of long-term continence are at best around 50%; and (3) multiple re-operative surgeries reduce the chances of attaining a good bladder capacity and consequently continence rates are very low.

Successful repeat closure rates of as high as 95–98% have been reported with redo MSRE as well as redo CPRE, osteotomy being a critical component of this success [6, 11, 14]. Hafez et al. have reported 100% success rates with CPRE for

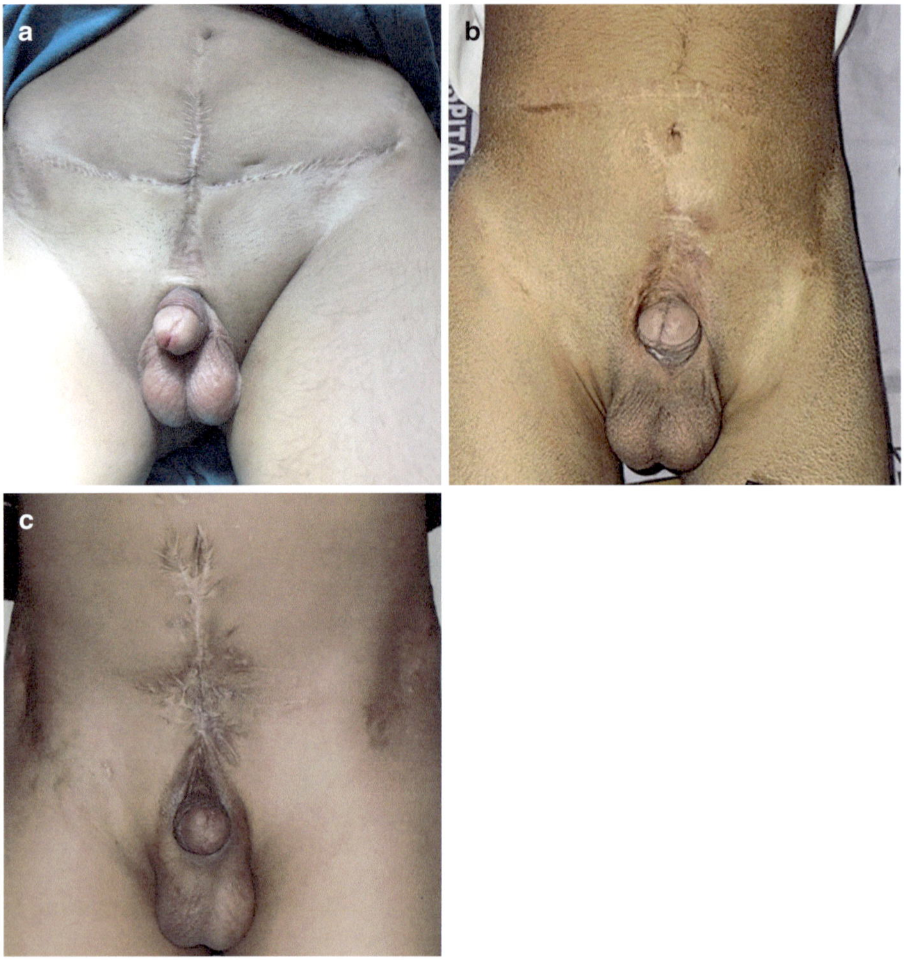

Fig. 17.11 Long-term outcomes of redo CPRE. (**a**) Follow-up at nine years—continent with volitional voiding and with good bladder capacity. (**b**) Follow-up at 4 years—redo CPRE for vesicocutaneous fistula and outlet obstruction done at age 13 years—continent with volitional voiding and with good bladder capacity. (**c**) Follow-up at 5 years—redo CPRE with hypospadiac meatus done at 8 years of age—continent with good bladder capacity

failed repairs, when performed in adjunct with osteotomy and with adequate post-operative immobilisation [14]. In our experience also, we have had encouraging results with redo CPRE and modified Salter's osteotomy with 99.7% successful closures in 32 cases (*unpublished data*). Thus, the experienced surgeon faced with the challenging task of reclosure can find some optimism in these numbers. For the frustrated and anxious parents, counselling regarding this attainable result is imperative [11] (Fig. 17.11).

Another observation with CPRE is the high number of patients (77%) requiring a hypospadiac meatus and further surgeries for correction [14]. The purpose of

CPRE to decrease the number of surgeries is lost with the requirement of staged hypospadias correction. Out of the 32 redo cases in our cohort, ten patients required a hypospadiac meatus. In the past few years, we have been giving the patients pre-operative testosterone. Our observation is that with the use of testosterone along with adequate mobilisation, an orthotopic meatus can be achieved in most patients, save those who have severe chordee and very short urethral length. Methods for urethral plate augmentation at the time of CPRE, like use of a transverse island flap of preputial skin as a tube to achieve an orthotopic meatus, have been reported [45].

Vesicoureteric reflux is almost universal after bladder closure, whether primary or redo. The practice of concomitant ureteric reimplant is still in the evolutionary stage, but preliminary observations are that the incidence of reflux is decreased, and if present, the grades are low [46, 47]. Reimplant at the time of redo closure is also possible in carefully selected cases where the bladder is healthy and pliable. Whether the outcomes in form of reflux and hydroureteronephrosis are similar remains to seen. By preventing or decreasing the grade of reflux, the benefits would probably be improved bladder cycling, enabling the previously compromised bladder to grow better [46]. The detrimental effects of reflux causing urinary tract infections with a high-pressure bladder on the upper tracts may also be neutralised to some extent; however, this can be corroborated only with long-term analysis of larger cohorts subjected to this procedure [47].

With all the importance being given to the role of osteotomy, it is essential to also review the outcomes with respect to redo osteotomy. Many of the failed repairs occur in spite of an osteotomy at the primary surgery, due to the various other factors involved. A redo osteotomy is almost always necessary in these patients. Studies have shown that redo osteotomy is feasible and safe without many complications caused by the repeated disruptions of the bony pelvis [48]. The overall complication rate of osteotomy, including redo osteotomy, is only 4%, which includes neurologic complications (nerve palsies, femoral nerve injury and sciatic nerve injury), bony complications (non-union, malunion) and leg length asymmetry [49]. Novak et al. reported that the gait was normal in 95% cases even with repeat osteotomy [3]. The authors have also found redo osteotomy to be safe and effective with three instances of transient peroneal nerve palsies as the only complication.

While the redo surgery is often successful in experienced hands, the same cannot be said for the bladder growth and continence rates. The repeated surgical stress on the bladder, the fibroses and the pathological changes from a long-exposed bladder mucosa take a severe toll and consequently hinder the growth and chances of being dry. According to a large series of failed exstrophy closures reported from Johns Hopkins, where the patients underwent MSRE and subsequent continence procedures, only 18% of these patients ultimately achieved a good continence outcome per urethra. Of the rest, 90% were dry, but at the expense of ileocystoplasty and lifelong catheterisation. As a matter of fact, only 38% of the patients with successful reclosures were considered suitable for BNR [3].

Similar outcomes have been reported with CPRE done with osteotomy. In the series reported by Hafez et al., only 14% of successful reclosures achieved continence with volitional voiding. The rest required BNR or bladder closure with bladder augmentation [45]. Again, we have adopted an observational approach with early physical therapy for our patients following redo repairs—usually until the children reach puberty, as long as the upper tracts are safe. At that point, if bladder capacity, urodynamic findings and continence history are unlikely to support continence, then further definitive reconstruction such as bladder neck closure with augmentation is considered.

With such low rates of long-term good outcomes, the question that arises is whether to undertake the arduous task of redo surgeries. Although a secure pelvic bone approximation is a requisite for successful reclosure, the low continence rates bring forth the relevance of osteotomy and its morbidities in the setting of a bladder augmentation. Many authors believe that bladder augmentation is the best option for the dehisced exstrophy [13]. Mainz and Stein have advocated abandoning any bladder reconstruction in failed repairs, and instead creating a conduit or rectal reservoir [14]. Many experts believe that this is a viable option in a low-resource setting.

In light of the drastic consequences of a failed repair, it is important that redo surgeries should be undertaken only at high-volume centres, which have the expertise and experience to provide optimal outcomes. As such centres are far and few, the economic burden on the families with respect to prolonged hospital stay and frequent long-distance travel is high. What then is the justification for planning a redo surgery with all the drawbacks rather than bladder augmentation or continent diversion?

Given that our knowledge about the exstrophied bladder is still vastly inadequate, it is impossible to predict which bladders undergoing reclosures will do well in the future. The chance of continence with volitional voiding is less than 30%, yet not negligible. Additional benefits of redo repairs also include correction of rotational pelvis deformity and pelvis support in females, which should be considered. It seems logical to propose that redo repair would be a reasonable option in carefully selected cases with a good bladder template; and when undertaken at a centre with good volume, resources and expertise. The best approach would be to educate and counsel the families thoroughly about different available options and their possible outcomes, understand their expectations as well as their limitations and encourage their participation in charting out a plan which is best suited to the needs of their child.

References

1. Purves JT, Gearhart JP. The bladder exstrophy-epispadias-cloacal exstrophy complex. In: Gearhart J, et al., editors. Pediatric urology. 2nd ed. Amsterdam: Elsevier; 2010. p. 386–415.
2. Elderwy AA, Grady R. The exstrophy epispadias complex. In: Wilcox D, et al., editors. Pediatric urology: surgical complications and management. Blackwell; 2008. p. 83–91.
3. Novak TE, Costello JP, Orosco R, et al. Failed exstrophy closure: management and outcome. J Pediatr Urol. 2010;6:381–4.
4. El-Sherbiny MT, Hafez AT, Ghoneim MA. Complete repair of exstrophy: further experience with neonates and children after failed initial closure. J Urol. 2002;168(4):1692–4.

5. Grady RW, Mitchell ME. Complete primary repair of exstrophy: surgical technique. Urol Clin N Am. 2000;27(3):569–78.
6. Gearhart JP, Peppas DS, Jeffs RD. PAEDIATRIC UROLOGY: the failed Exstrophy closure: strategy for management. Br J Urol. 1993;71(2):217–20.
7. Gearheart JP, Peppas DS, Jeffs RD. Complications of paraexstrophy flaps in the reconstruction of classical bladder exstrophy. J Urol. 1993;150:627–30.
8. Wild AT, Sponseller PD, Stec AA, Gearhart JP. The role of osteotomy in surgical repair of bladder exstrophy. In: Seminars in pediatric surgery, vol. 20, No. 2. WB Saunders; 2011. p. 71–8.
9. Hofmann A, Haider M, Promm M, Neissner C, Badelt G, Rösch WH. Delayed primary closure of bladder exstrophy without osteotomy: 12 year experience in a safe and gentle alternative to neonatal surgery. J Pediatr Surg. 2022;57(10):303–8.
10. Morrill CC, Haffar A, Harris TG, Crigger C, Gearhart JP. Current management of classic bladder exstrophy in the modern era. Afr J Urol. 2023;29(1):27.
11. Kasprenski M, et al. Modern management of the failed bladder exstrophy closure: a 50-yr experience. Eur Urol Focus. 2018;6:383. https://doi.org/10.1016/j.euf.2018.09.008.
12. Bhatnagar V. Bladder exstrophy: an overview of the surgical management. J Indian Assoc Pediatr Surg. 2011;16(3):81–7.
13. Sam CJ, Kurian JJ, Kishore R, Arunachalam P, Sen S. Management and outcome in dehisced exstrophy with a simplified bladder re-closure and further reconstruction. J Pediatr Urol. 2020;16(6):836–e1.
14. Novak TE. Failed exstrophy closure. In: Seminars in pediatric surgery, vol. 20, No. 2. WB Saunders; 2011. p. 97–101.
15. Meldrum KK, Baird AD, Gearhart JP. Pelvic and extremity immobilization after bladder exstrophy closure: complications and impact on success. Urology. 2003;62(6):1109–13.
16. Gearhart JE, Ben-Chaim J, Sciortino C, Jeffs RD. The multiple reoperative bladder exstrophy closure: what affects the potential of the bladder? Urology. 1996;47(2):240–3.
17. Da H. Closure of the exstrophic bladder: an evaluation of the factors leading to its success and its importance on urinary continence. J Urol. 1989;142:522–4.
18. Purves JT. Modern approaches in primary exstrophy closure. In: Seminars in pediatric surgery, vol. 20, No. 2. WB Saunders; 2011. p. 79–84.
19. Grady RW, Mitchell ME. Complete primary repair of exstrophy. J Urol. 1999;162(4):1415–20.
20. Gearhart JP, Baird A, Nelson CP. Results of bladder neck reconstruction after newborn complete primary repair of exstrophy. J Urol. 2007;178(4S):1619–22.
21. Hammouda HM, Kotb H. Complete primary repair of bladder exstrophy: initial experience with 33 cases. J Urol. 2004;172(4):1441–4.
22. Wein AJ, Kavoussi LR, Partin AW, Peters CA. Campbell-Walsh urology E-book: 4-volume set. Elsevier Health Sciences; 2015.
23. Massanyi EZ, Shah B, Schaeffer AJ, DiCarlo HN, Sponseller PD, Gearhart JP. Persistent vesicocutaneous fistula after repair of classic bladder exstrophy: a sign of failure? J Pediatr Urol. 2013;9(6):867–71.
24. Baker LA, Jeffs RD, Gearhart JP. Urethral obstruction after primary exstrophy closure: what is the fate of the genitourinary tract? J Urol. 1999;161(2):618–21.
25. Husmann DA, Gearhart JP. Loss of the penile glans and/or corpora following primary repair of bladder exstrophy using the complete penile disassembly technique. J Urol. 2004;172(4 Part 2):1696–701.
26. Gearhart JP, Baird AD. The failed complete repair of bladder exstrophy: insights and outcomes. J Urol. 2005;174(4):1669–73.
27. VanderBrink BA, Stock JA, Hanna MK. Aesthetic aspects of reconstructive clitoroplasty in females with bladder exstrophy–epispadias complex. J Plast Reconstr Aesthet Surg. 2010;63(12):2141–5.
28. Massanyi EZ, Shah BB, Baradaran N, Gearhart JP. Bladder capacity as a predictor of voided continence after failed exstrophy closure. J Pediatr Urol. 2014;10(1):171–5.
29. Ebert A, Schott G, Hirschfelder H, Rösch WH. Management of failed bladder exstrophy closure in adolescence and adulthood. BJU Int. 2000;86(7):901–4.

30. Hanna MK, Bassiouny I. Challenges in salvaging urinary continence following failed bladder exstrophy repair in a developing country. J Pediatr Urol. 2017;13:270.e1. https://doi.org/10.1016/j.jpurol.2016.12.019.
31. Nelson CP, North AC, Ward MK, Gearhart JP. Economic impact of failed or delayed primary repair of bladder exstrophy: differences in cost of hospitalization. J Urol. 2008;179(2):680–3.
32. Joshi R, Shrivastava D, Ramji J. A model for sustained collaboration to address the unmet global burden of bladder exstrophy-epispadias complex and penopubic epispadias: the International Bladder Exstrophy Consortium (vol 153, pg 618, 2018). JAMA Surg. 2018;153(7):692.
33. Woo LL, Thomas JC, Brock JW. Bladder and cloacal exstrophy. In: Coran A, et al., editors. Pediatric surgery e-book: expert consult-online and print. Elsevier Health Sciences; 2012.
34. Gearhart JP, Mathews R, Taylor S, Jeffs RD. Combined bladder closure and epispadias repair in the reconstruction of bladder exstrophy. J Urol. 1998;160(3 Part 2):1182–5.
35. Bhatnagar V, Dave S, Agarwala S, Mitra DK. Augmentation colocystoplasty in bladder exstrophy. Pediatr Surg Int. 2002;18:43–9.
36. Salle JP, Elifranji M, Abbas T, Alhadi A, Elkadhi A, Leslie B, Vallasciani S. Technical details in the primary repair of male epispadias: step by step video. Urol Video J. 2022;13:100127.
37. Pippi Salle JL, Jednak R, Capolicchio JP, França IM, Labbie A, Gosalbez R. A ventral rotational skin flap to improve cosmesis and avoid chordee recurrence in epispadias repair. BJU Int. 2002;90(9):918–23.
38. Barla RK, Sen S. Skin cover in epispadias repair by dorsal transposition of a ventral Island flap: a modification of the Pippi Salle technique. Pediatr Surg Int. 2015;31:1099–102. https://doi.org/10.1007/s00383-015-3785-x.
39. Friedlander DA, Lue KM, Michaud JE, Gearhart JP, Redett RJ, Di Carlo HN. Repair of vesicocutaneous and urethrocutaneous fistulae with rectus muscle flap in a bladder exstrophy patient. Urol Case Rep. 2017;13:42–4.
40. Michaud JE, Ko JS, Lue K, Di Carlo HN, Redett RJ, Gearhart JP. Use of muscle pedicle flaps for failed bladder neck closure in the exstrophy spectrum. J Pediatr Urol. 2016;12:289.e1. https://doi.org/10.1016/j.jpurol.2016.03.006.
41. Promm M, Roesch WH. Recent trends in the management of bladder exstrophy: the Gordian knot has not yet been cut. Front Pediatr. 2019;7:110.
42. Kanojia RP, Rao KL, Menon P, Agarwal S, Bawa M, Mahajan JK, Samujh R. Recto sigmoid bladder reservoir for patients with exstrophy: three-dimensional evaluation for outcome analysis. J Pediatr Urol. 2014;10(6):1176–80.
43. Sarin YK, Sekhon V. Exstrophy bladder – reconstruction or diversion for the underprivileged. Indian J Pediatr. 2017;84(9):715–20. https://doi.org/10.1007/s12098-017-2419-9. Epub 2017 Jul 18. PMID: 28721463.
44. Joshi RS, Eftekharzadeh S, Shukla AR, Ramji J, Hingorani SR, Canning DA, Pippi-Salle JL, Merguerian P, DeFoor WR Jr, Frazier JR, Weiss D. MP67-04 kidney function outcomes after complete primary repair of exstrophy: results from the international bladder exstrophy consortium. J Urol. 2021;206(Supplement 3):e510.
45. Hafez AT, El-Sherbiny MT, Shorrab AA, El-Mowafi H. Complete primary repair of bladder exstrophy in children presenting late and those with failed initial closure: single centre experience. J Urol. 2005;174(4):1549–52.
46. Ramji J, Weiss DA, Romao RL, Eftekharzadeh S, Shah J, Frazier JR, Reddy PP, Merguerian PA, Salle JP, Canning DA, Joshi RS. Impact of bilateral ureteral reimplantation at the time of complete primary repair of bladder exstrophy on reflux rates, renogram abnormalities and bladder capacity. J Pediatr Urol. 2021;17(3):393–e1.
47. Braga LH, Lorenzo AJ, Jrearz R, Bagli DJ, Salle JL. Bilateral ureteral reimplantation at primary bladder exstrophy closure. J Urol. 2010;183(6):2337–41.
48. Nelson CP, King J, Sponseller PD, et al. Repeat pelvic osteotomy in patients with failed closure of bladder exstrophy: applications and outcomes. J Pediatr Surg. 2006;41:1109–12.
49. Okubadejo GO, Sponseller PD, Gearhart JP. Complications in orthopedic management of exstrophy. J Pediatr Orthop. 2003;23(4):522–8.

Perioperative Management of Bladder Exstrophy

18

Anjana Kundu, Arvid Yung, and Rita Agarwal

Background

Bladder exstrophy is a rare congenital malformation of the genitourinary tract affecting approximately 1 in 50,000 live births, more commonly among males [1, 2] and with a preponderance in low- and middle-income countries (LMICs) [3, 4]. The bladder exstrophy-epispadias complex (BEEC) refers to a malformation including a severe midline abdominal wall defect, wide separation of the pubic symphysis, and an anteriorly positioned open bladder and urethra. Epispadias and classical bladder exstrophy may occur in isolation, but cloacal exstrophy often carries with it various other malformations of the gastrointestinal tract, skeletal system, and neurological system [5]. The bladder remains open on the abdominal wall in both classical bladder exstrophy and cloacal exstrophy.

A surgical repair involves complex and extensive reconstruction of the bladder and its adjacent structures to restore satisfactory functional and cosmetic anatomical integrity, with the goal of achieving urinary continence and a high quality of life. The surgical techniques have been described in detail in the earlier chapters and consist of several different techniques. The most common surgical repair techniques include either a single-staged closure of the bladder and genitalia, i.e., complete primary repair (CPRE) [4, 6] or a planned modern staged repair (MSRE) [7, 8]. Although the majority of surgical repair in high-income countries (HICs) occurs within days of birth, in LMICs, these defects may either go unrepaired well into

A. Kundu (✉) · A. Yung
Department of Anesthesiology and Perioperative Medicine, Golisano Children's Hospital and University of Rochester, Rochester, NY, USA
e-mail: Anjana_Kundu@URMC.Rochester.edu

R. Agarwal
Department of Anesthesiology, Lucille Packard Children's Hospital, Stanford University, Palo Alto, CA, USA

A. R. Shukla, R. S. Joshi (eds.), *Bladder Exstrophy and Epispadias*,
https://doi.org/10.1007/978-3-031-91238-2_18

teenage years or may have been the subject of an improper and poor surgical technique due to lack of access to skilled medical and surgical care [4]. Most patients with this disorder will undergo multiple corrective surgical procedures in their lifetime to achieve functionally and cosmetically acceptable results [9].

Regardless of the surgical approach, approximation of the pelvis, either through manual approximation of a still malleable pelvis among neonates or through pelvic osteotomies for older children, is essential for abdominal closure and for the likelihood of achieving continence [10]. There is a need for extended immobilization postoperatively to promote healing and to maintain pelvic ring integrity. This in turn requires adequate pain management, nutritional support, meticulous nursing care for osteotomy sites, surgical drains and stents, and skin integrity.

Optimal outcomes from such a complex surgery with a prolonged postoperative course involving neonates, young children, or adolescents requires a close interdisciplinary perioperative collaboration between surgeons, anesthesiologists, intensivists, pediatricians, experienced nursing staff, and physical therapists. The surgical correction requires extensive reconstructive procedures to restore anatomical integrity, and the functional outcomes depend significantly on meticulous perioperative management, including adequate pain management, minimizing complications, and optimizing recovery.

In this chapter, we provide an overview of the interdisciplinary perioperative management for the BEEC.

Perioperative Management of Bladder Exstrophy

Preoperative

Preoperative evaluation is crucial in determining the overall health status of the patient and identifying any comorbidities that may impact the perioperative management. The surgical candidates most commonly fall into one of three categories: neonates, older children, and children with previously failed surgeries or complications related to previous surgery.

Typically, these neonates and children do not have any other congenital anomalies or underlying cardiorespiratory derangements. A hemogram to ensure adequate hemoglobin levels and a type and crossmatch for blood transfusion due to a high likelihood of a significant blood loss associated with pelvic osteotomies and staged or repeat surgeries may be the only necessary investigations unless the patient's history and physical exam indicate otherwise. In a patient with cloacal anomaly, a lumbosacral radiograph is useful in identifying any sacrococcygeal or spinal anomalies.

These neonates and children routinely get hemograms and blood chemistry performed as a part of their surgical preoperative workup, along with plain radiographs of the abdomen and pelvis and an abdominal ultrasound KUB to rule out associated anomalies of the upper urinary tract. Upper tract damage and abnormal renal function before bladder plate closure and even after the repair are uncommon despite some risk of postoperative kidney scarring in the intermediate-term follow-up. However, it does not correlate with altered renal function [11].

For older children, preoperative assessment by an anesthesiologist should also include assessment of preoperative anxiety, stress, and fear, as it has been demonstrated to have detrimental effects on intraoperative analgesic and anesthetic use, postoperative pain scores, analgesic requirements, as well as behavioral and sleep disturbance [4, 12, 13]. Management of preoperative anxiety may include age- and development-appropriate behavioral modalities such as preoperative preparation programs providing orientation tours and narrative information, coping and self-management skills such as relaxation and distraction techniques, therapeutic play, toys, art, music, games, and visual aids such as videos, books, and virtual reality [14]. Acupuncture and acupressure have also been shown to reduce preoperative anxiety [15, 16]. The administration of anxiolytics in the United States varies based on the age of the patient and geographical location. The most commonly used anxiolytic medications include midazolam (85% of patients), fentanyl, ketamine, clonidine, or dexmedetomidine, especially when analgesia is also desired or midazolam is contraindicated [14]. The premedication is usually administered orally, but intranasal, intravenous, and intramuscular routes can also be utilized.

Monitoring

Standard American Society of Anesthesiologists (ASA) monitoring (pulse oximeter, electrocardiography (ECG), noninvasive blood pressure, temperature, end-tidal carbon dioxide ($ETCO_2$), inspired oxygen concentration), and neuromuscular blockade are essential. Often in HICs, invasive intra-arterial blood pressure (IABP) monitoring is routinely done, especially for neonates. Obtaining adequate vascular access with two large-bore peripheral intravenous catheters is essential for rapid volume replacement.

Intraoperative Management

The goals of intraoperative anesthetic management include ensuring hemodynamic stability, maintaining adequate renal perfusion, and optimizing surgical conditions for optimal repair.

Surgical repair of BEEC is typically long and requires neuromuscular blockade to facilitate maximal approximation of tissues for optimal surgical repair. It's also associated with significant intraoperative fluid shifts, changes in the vascular volumes due to high insensible losses, third space losses, and blood loss associated with osteotomies. General anesthesia with endotracheal intubation along with regional anesthesia for intraoperative and postoperative analgesia is the most appropriate approach [17].

In patients for whom there is no contraindication, regional anesthesia has proven to be a safe and effective option for intraoperative and postoperative analgesia in neonates, infants, and children [18]. In neonates and infants, the use of epidural analgesia has contributed to limiting postoperative opioid-related adverse effects, facilitating earlier tracheal extubation, and quickening the resumption of normal gastrointestinal function [19, 20].

Induction of general anesthesia may be achieved using either an inhalational or intravenous route. After induction of general anesthesia and endotracheal intubation, an epidural catheter is placed that should cover the low thoracic to sacral dermatomes, thus requiring a relatively large spread of local anesthetic. Catheters can be inserted in the sacral, caudal, or lumbar region. Caudal insertion requires advancement of the catheter tip to the lumbar region [17, 21]. In young infants, blind advancement of the catheter can be achieved in two-thirds of the patients [21]. Correct positioning can be confirmed by epidurogram, which involves injecting a small amount of contrast through the catheter during either fluoroscopy or x-ray, or by using ultrasound to approximate the spread of the local anesthetic. Although not FDA approved for use in the USA, special catheters for placement at the desired location are available, such as the Tsui stimulating or electrocardiography catheter [22, 23].

The caudal insertion site is preferred by many anesthesiologists in neonates and young infants due to a potentially greater safety profile. The spinal cord in young children has a more caudate termination, which could increase the risk of spinal cord injury when a lumbar site is chosen. Unfortunately, compared to the lumbar site, the caudal insertion site is associated with an increased risk of catheter colonization after 3 days [24]. Tunneling the catheter can reduce this risk and should be considered even at the lumbar site, particularly if there is a plan to maintain the catheter for a prolonged period of time as deemed appropriate by the surgical and anesthesiology teams for adequate postoperative analgesia and optimal functional repair. A recent poll by the Society for Pediatric Pain Medicine of the common practices among pediatric anesthesiologists revealed a significant variation in practice around the management and duration of an epidural catheter for bladder exstrophy patients [25].

In our practice (AK and AY), an epidural catheter is initially inserted in the midline via a caudal or lumbar approach through a Touhy epidural needle using the loss of resistance to saline technique to locate the epidural space, and the catheter is advanced to the desired position. To tunnel the epidural catheter, then using the Touhy needle, we identify a trajectory and distance for the tunneled portion of the epidural catheter starting from the exit site of the epidural catheter in the midline and extending it in a lateral and cephalad direction to where the desired exit location of the tunneled part of the catheter is. Then the Touhy needle along with its stylet is inserted at the identified tunneled exit point and advanced under the skin in a caudate and medial direction such that it should exit adjacent to the epidural catheter without damaging it. The stylet is removed, and the epidural catheter is now fed through the epidural needle, ensuring that the catheter does not kink or knot. Finally, the Tuohy needle is withdrawn, and the length of the catheter is gently pulled at its exit site, usually below the iliac crest, until it lies flat under the skin at the initial insertion site. Preferably, a transparent adhesive dressing is applied to the initial insertion site and the catheter exit site, which facilitates an easy inspection for signs of infection. Prior to the application of this transparent dressing, the catheter may be secured at its exit site using different techniques like topical skin adhesives such as Dermabond (Ethicon, Warsaw, IN, USA) or Steri-Strips® (3M Health Care, Saint Paul, MN, USA) to prevent dislodgement and minimize leakage of epidural infusate. The catheter is then injected with a local anesthetic. The dressing at the exit site should be changed every 5 days or if soiled. The dressing at the initial insertion site can be safely removed within a few days, as skin typically seals over the catheter.

After an initial bolus dose, a continuous infusion of local anesthetic with or without opioids or other adjuvants, such as low-dose alpha-2 agonists (clonidine or dexmedetomidine), can be infused intraoperatively through the epidural catheter and continued postoperatively. In neonates, administration of bupivacaine or ropivacaine (1 mg/kg) or chloroprocaine (30 mg/kg) as a bolus can be followed by an infusion rate no higher than 0.4 mg/kg/h for ropivacaine or bupivacaine and 10 mg/kg/h for chloroprocaine [18, 20, 26]. While epidural infusions of 0.2 mg/kg/h of bupivacaine were associated with rising serum levels after 2 days of epidural infusions [27, 28], this is not true of ropivacaine [29]. Therefore, either chloroprocaine or ropivacaine infusions are the safest options for neonates and infants under 180 days of age [26, 29–32]. In older patients, either bupivacaine or ropivacaine can be infused safely at a rate of up to 0.6 mg/kg/h [7, 17, 19].

For synergistic effects and improved analgesia, additives can be combined with local anesthetics during epidural infusion [26, 33–35]. Opioids, such as fentanyl or hydromorphone, and alpha-2 agonists, such as clonidine or dexmedetomidine, are most commonly used. Active toddlers benefit from the addition of clonidine or dexmedetomidine, as it is associated with sedation and anxiolysis, certainly desired effects in this population [33–35]. Dexmedetomidine has limited evidence for its use in the epidural space, perhaps owing to its more recent availability and its pharmacokinetic similarity to clonidine, which has been deemed safe for epidural use.

In patients where an epidural may be contraindicated, or if the family refuses it, a serious consideration should be made for abdominal plane blocks such as transversus abdominis plane (TAP), quadratus lumborum (QL), and erector spinae plane (ESP) blocks with or without catheter placement. Although these blocks would likely only provide incomplete analgesia in these patients missing the visceral components and the pelvic osteotomy-related pain, their utility as part of a multimodal analgesic regimen for abdominal and urological surgeries has been demonstrated [36]. Use of parenteral opioids along with acetaminophen or paracetamol, nonsteroidal anti-inflammatory drugs (NSAIDs) such as ibuprofen, ketorolac, diclofenac, ketoprofen, and other adjuvant medications such as alpha-2 agonists (dexmedetomidine, clonidine), low-dose ketamine, or lidocaine may be required for optimal analgesia [36–45].

Given the prolonged nature of the surgery, special attention must be paid to appropriate positioning and padding of these children to minimize the chances of pressure- and positioning-related injuries [46]. Their head must be cushioned and will require a regular change of position to prevent pressure alopecia [47]. Maintaining normothermia and euvolemia are critical. The exposure of the patient's abdominal cavity for a large portion of the surgery can contribute to heat loss. Monitoring the patient's temperature, active heating using a forced air warmer, warm fluids for irrigation, and IV infusion can preserve normothermia. Replacement of intraoperative fluids and blood loss should be monitored closely [48].

At the conclusion of the surgery, the goal should be to extubate these children after the reversal of the neuromuscular blocking agents. Due to the prolonged use of neuromuscular blocking agents intraoperatively, quantitative monitoring of the neuromuscular blockade and reversal is ideal for minimizing chances of postoperative residual neuromuscular blockade and respiratory insufficiency [49, 50].

Postoperative Management

Postoperative management of the child with bladder exstrophy is extremely crucial, and anesthesiologists play a critical role in ensuring optimal analgesia and a smooth postoperative course. Adequate postoperative analgesia is a key driver in the maintenance of proper immobilization in the postoperative period, reducing surgical stress response and minimizing postoperative complications. Epidural analgesia may also affect immunomodulation in the postoperative period by boosting the body's defense mechanisms, including cellular immunity, natural killer (NK) cell function, and humoral responses [51, 52]. Care must be taken to maintain the immobilization of the lower extremities. Whether an osteotomy is performed or not, immobilization of the lower extremities is generally preferred by most of the pediatric surgeons. For osteotomy, a 4–6 week period of external fixation is generally recommended [10, 53].

The immediate postoperative pain for BEEC patients is primarily managed by epidural analgesia. However, in case of a contraindication or refusal by family of an epidural, a multimodal analgesic regimen consisting of enteral and parenteral medications may be required for optimal analgesia, anxiolysis, or sedation. These medications may include opioids, acetaminophen or paracetamol, NSAIDs, benzodiazepines, alpha-2 agonists, diphenhydramine, and sometimes even barbiturates. Some of these medications may be associated with tolerance and withdrawal effects after prolonged use and may require a gradual weaning. Lidocaine and/or low-dose ketamine infusions, if used intraoperatively, may be continued for postoperative analgesia. Gradual weaning of medications, especially sedatives and anxiolytics, is advised after usage for more than 7–10 days.

In addition to pelvic immobilization, the bladder and kidneys are drained with a suprapubic catheter and ureteral stents for the duration of immobilization to prevent bladder distention, urinary obstruction, or spillage onto the wound. The wound can also be kept dry with the use of a suction drain. Vigilance around infection prevention and control, proper function of various drains, and adequate nutrition would ensure a decrease in the likelihood of postoperative complications and failure of closure [4, 54–56]. Adequate antimicrobial prophylaxis is important for all patients following primary closure. In addition to a higher rate of vesicoureteral reflux associated with the exstrophy-epispadias complex, various tubes, stents, and drains from the urinary tract and osteotomy fixator pins all represent routes and niduses for potential infections of the urine, bone, or wound. This can lead to potential pyelonephritis or wound dehiscence, which would likely necessitate further surgical intervention. Thus, it is imperative that the surgical wound remains dry and free from tension.

Enteral feeds can be started as soon as the child is fully awake and their bowel function returns. Often a nasogastric tube may be placed to decompress the bowel to promote rest, decrease tension on the wound, and facilitate rapid return of normal gastrointestinal function. In patients with cloacal exstrophy, bowel function may not return for 2 weeks. In case of delayed use of the enteral route, total parenteral nutrition may be implemented to maintain proper caloric intake [57]. Epidural analgesia has been shown to promote gastrointestinal motility and an earlier return of bowel function postoperatively [58].

Postoperative introduction of anticholinergic medications to maintain the relaxed state of the detrusor and to avoid detrusor spasms might help. Finally, care must be taken to maintain the indwelling drains and catheter to ensure optimal outcomes.

Following discharge, the majority of the follow-up relates to regular follow-up investigations to ensure the health of the upper and lower urinary tract.

The incidence of persistent or recurrent pain in these patients is currently unknown. However, with multiple risk factors like dysuria, especially after open bladder surgeries, bladder spasms, wound infection, urethral obstruction, stones, strictures, urethral obstruction, urinary tract infections, urethrocutaneous fistula, osteotomy complications, exposure to multiple surgical procedures, and significant psychosocial burden related to their condition, they are at risk for the development of chronic or recurrent pain. Future investigation should be directed toward exploring the true incidence or prevalence of pain among these patients.

Factors Influencing Postoperative Outcomes and Role of Integrated Team Approach

Attainment of a cosmetic primary closure with long-term bladder growth and voided continence is the ideal desired outcome by both the surgeons and the patients. The single most important predictor of that desired outcome is a successful primary closure of the bladder [13, 59–63]. Baradaran et al. found that failure of primary closure of bladder exstrophy during the immediate postoperative period may result from one of the following events: wound dehiscence, bladder prolapse, bladder outlet obstruction, or vesicocutaneous fistula [4, 13, 59–63]. This further demonstrates the importance of excellent pain control and a calm and restful postoperative course to facilitate proper immobilization of the pelvis and the key role anesthesiologists and pain physicians play. Neonates are especially vulnerable, and poor perioperative pain management is associated with increased morbidity and mortality. The use of opioids, which are the most commonly used analgesics for moderate-to-severe pain in patients of all ages, is often limited in newborns because of the fear of inducing respiratory depression. Epidural anesthesia with local anesthetics can provide profound intra- and postoperative analgesia without impairing respiratory drive and may even facilitate earlier recovery [58].

The nursing teams play an integral part in ensuring meticulous care of all the drains, wound care, infection prevention, and maintenance of skin integrity. Physical and occupational therapists play a major role in the postoperative recovery of these patients after the immobilization period, assisting with proper range of motion, strengthening and stretching of the lower body, and bolstering pelvic as well as core strength. The engagement of a dietician to ensure adequate nutritional status also plays a critical role in the improved outcomes among the BEEC patients.

Finally, the psychological, social, and economic burden of this condition cannot be underestimated and requires a multidisciplinary biopsychosocial approach to care of these patients and families [13].

A rare, complex, and chronic condition like this requires pooling of resources, skills, infrastructure, and commitment in the form of integrated multidisciplinary teams and multi-institutional collaborations [4, 13, 54].

Conclusion

Over the past few decades, management of bladder exstrophy has significantly improved with a significant increase in the number of complete primary repairs of the bladder, pelvic osteotomies—except for the youngest patients—postoperative immobilization, infection control, management of severe postoperative pain (sometimes sedation for a prolonged period), nutritional management, and advanced pediatric nursing care, all of which govern the chances for the best functional and cosmetic result. Perioperative management of bladder exstrophy surgery warrants a coordinated multidisciplinary approach for the achievement of optimal outcomes. Diligence in preoperative assessment and intra- and postoperative management are essential to minimize complications and to ensure optimal surgical repair along with improved function and quality of life for these patients and families.

References

1. Nelson CP, Dunn RL, Wei JT. Contemporary epidemiology of bladder exstrophy in the United States. J Urol. 2005;173(5):1728–31.
2. Siffel C, Correa A, Amar E, Bakker MK, et al. Bladder exstrophy: an epidemiologic study from the International Clearinghouse for Birth Defects Surveillance and Research, and an overview of the literature. Am J Med Genet C Semin Med Genet. 2011;157C(4):321–32.
3. World Health Organization. Congenital anomalies: 2012 fact sheet no. 370. Geneva: WHO. http://www.who.int/mediacentre/factsheets/fs370/en/. Accessed 26 June 2024.
4. Joshi RS, Grady R, Kundu A, Shukla AR, et al. A model for sustained collaboration to address the unmet global burden of bladder exstrophy-epispadias complex and penopubic epispadias: the International Bladder Exstrophy Consortium. JAMA Surg. 2018;153(7):618–24.
5. Diamond DA, Jeffs RD. Cloacal exstrophy: a 22-year experience. J Urol. 1985;133(5):779–82. https://doi.org/10.1016/s0022-5347(17)49224-x. PMID: 3989916.
6. Grady RW, Mitchell ME. Complete primary repair of exstrophy. J Urol. 1999;162(4):1415–20.

7. Massanyi EZ, Gearhart JP, Kost-Byerly S. Perioperative management of classic bladder exstrophy. Res Rep Urol. 2013;5:67–75.
8. Nelson CP, Dunn RL, Wei JT, Gearhart JP. Surgical repair of bladder exstrophy in the modern era: contemporary practice patterns and the role of hospital case volume. J Urol. 2005;174(3):1099–102.
9. Ellison JS, Shnorhavorian M, Willihnganz-Lawson K, Grady RW, Merguerian PA. A critical appraisal of continence in bladder exstrophy: long-term outcomes of the complete primary repair. J Pediatr Urol. 2016;12(4):205.e1–7.
10. Meldrum KK, Baird AD, Gearhart JP. Pelvic and extremity immobilization after bladder exstrophy closure: complications and impact on success. Urology. 2003;62(6):1109–13.
11. Joshi RS, Eftekharzadeh S, Shukla AR, Ramji J, et al. Kidney function outcomes in patients after complete primary repair of bladder exstrophy and penopubic epispadias: results from the international bladder exstrophy consortium. J Pediatr Urol. 2023;19(1):34.e1–9.
12. Kain ZN, Mayes LC, Caldwell-Andrews AA, Karas DE, McClain BC. Preoperative anxiety, postoperative pain, and behavioral recovery in young children undergoing surgery. Pediatrics. 2006;118(2):651–8.
13. Spencer KA, Ramji J, Kundu A, Weiss DA, Shukla AR, Joshi R, Frazier JR, et al. Caregiver distress: a mixed methods evaluation of the mental health burden of caring for children with bladder exstrophy. Front Pediatr. 2022;10:948490.
14. McCann MEMD, Kain ZN. The management of preoperative anxiety in children: an update. Anesth Analg. 2001;93(1):98–105.
15. Borji M, Pouy S, Yaghobi Y, Nabi BN. Effectiveness of acupressure on anxiety of children undergoing anesthesia. Int J Adolesc Med Health. 2019;33(4). https://doi.org/10.1515/ijamh-2018-0177.
16. Wang SM, Escalera S, Lin EC, Maranets I, Kain ZN. Extra-1 acupressure for children undergoing anesthesia. Anesth Analg. 2008;107(3):811–6.
17. Kost-Byerly S, Jackson EV, Yaster M, Kozlowski LJ, Mathews RI, Gearhart JP. Perioperative anesthetic and analgesic management of newborn bladder exstrophy repair. J Pediatr Urol. 2008;4(4):280–5.
18. Maitra S, Baidya DK, Pawar DK, Arora MK, Khanna P. Epidural anesthesia and analgesia in the neonate: a review of current evidences. J Anesth. 2014;28(5):768–79.
19. Ecoffey C, Dubousset AM, Samii K. Lumbar and thoracic epidural anesthesia for urologic and upper abdominal surgery in infants and children. Anesthesiology. 1986;65(1):87–90.
20. Muhly WT, Gurnaney HG, Kraemer FW, Ganesh A, Maxwell LG. A retrospective comparison of ropivacaine and 2-chloroprocaine continuous thoracic epidural analgesia for management of postthoracotomy pain in infants. Paediatr Anaesth. 2015;25(11):1162–7.
21. Valairucha S, Seefelder C, Houck CS. Thoracic epidural catheter placed by the caudal route in infants: the importance of radiographic confirmation. Paediatr Anaesth. 2002;12(5):424–8.
22. Tsui BC, Seal R, Koller J, Entwistle L, Haugen R, Kearney R. Thoracic epidural analgesia via the caudal approach in pediatric patients undergoing fundoplication using nerve stimulation guidance. Anesth Analg. 2001;93(5):1152–5.
23. Tsui BC, Seal R, Koller J. Thoracic epidural catheter placement via the caudal approach in infants by using electrocardiographic guidance. Anesth Analg. 2002;95(2):326–30.
24. Kost-Byerly S, Tobin JR, Greenberg RS, Billett C, Zahurak M, Yaster M. Bacterial colonization and infection rates of continuous epidural catheters in children. Anesth Analg. 1998;86(4):712–6.
25. Society for Pediatric Pain Medicine Poll of the Month. January 2024. https://pedspainmedicine.org/poll-of-the-month-archives/.
26. Gibbs A, Kim SS, Heydinger G, Veneziano G, Tobias J. Postoperative analgesia in neonates and infants using epidural chloroprocaine and clonidine. J Pain Res. 2020;13:2749–55.
27. Mevorach DL, Perkins FM, Isaacson SA. Bupivacaine toxicity secondary to continuous caudal epidural infusion in children. Anesth Analg. 1993;77(6):1305–6.
28. Larsson BA, Lönnquist PA, Olsson GL. Plasma concentrations of bupivacaine in neonates after continuous epidural infusions. Anesth Analg. 1997;84(3):501–5.

29. Bösenberg AT, Thomas J, Cronje L, Lopez T, et al. Pharmacokinetics and efficacy of ropivacaine for continuous epidural infusion in neonates and infants. Paediatr Anaesth. 2005;15(9):739–49.
30. Berde CB, Yaster M, Meretoja O, McCann ME, et al. Stable plasma concentrations of unbound ropivacaine during postoperative epidural infusion for 24–72 hours in children. Eur J Anaesthesiol. 2008;25(5):410–7.
31. Rapp HJ, Molnár V, Austin S, Krohn S, Gädeke V, Motsch J, Boos K, Williams DG, Gustafsson U, Huledal G, Larsson LE. Ropivacaine in neonates and infants: a population pharmacokinetic evaluation following single caudal block. Paediatr Anaesth. 2004;14(9):724–32.
32. Farid IS, Kendrick EJ, Adamczyk MJ, Lukas NR, Massanyi EZ. Perioperative analgesic management of newborn bladder exstrophy repair using a directly placed tunneled epidural catheter with 0.1% ropivacaine. A A Case Rep. 2015;5(7):112–4.
33. Klamt JG, Garcia LV, Stocche RM, Meinberg AC. Epidural infusion of clonidine or clonidine plus ropivacaine for postoperative analgesia in children undergoing major abdominal surgery. J Clin Anesth. 2003;15(7):510–4.
34. Haque MM, Banik D, Akhtaruzzaman AK, Bhowmick DK, Kader MA, Reza R, et al. Dexmedetomidine as an adjuvant to bupivacaine in caudal analgesia in children undergoing infra-umbilical surgery. Mymensingh Med J. 2023;32(3):833–40.
35. Fan M, Li J, Cao R, Hu L, Lu S. Efficacy and safety of dexmedetomidine-ropivacaine versus sufentanil-ropivacaine for epidural labor analgesia: a randomized controlled trial. Ann Palliat Med. 2022;11(4):1410–20.
36. Ardon A, Hernandez N. The use of peripheral nerve blockade in laparoscopic and robotic surgery: is there a benefit? Curr Pain Headache Rep. 2022;26(1):25–31.
37. Olkkola KT, Hamunen K, Maunuksela EL. Clinical pharmacokinetics and pharmacodynamics of opioid analgesics in infants and children. Clin Pharmacokinet. 1995;28(5):385–404.
38. Thigpen JC, Odle BL, Harirforoosh S. Opioids: a review of pharmacokinetics and pharmacodynamics in neonates, infants, and children. Eur J Drug Metab Pharmacokinet. 2019;44(5):591–609.
39. Ceelie I, de Wildt SN, van Dijk M, van den Berg MM, van den Bosch GE, Duivenvoorden HJ, de Leeuw TG, Mathôt R, Knibbe CA, Tibboel D. Effect of intravenous paracetamol on postoperative morphine requirements in neonates and infants undergoing major noncardiac surgery: a randomized controlled trial. JAMA. 2013;309(2):149–54.
40. Baarslag MA, Allegaert K, Van Den Anker JN, Knibbe CA, Van Dijk M, Simons SH, Tibboel D. Paracetamol and morphine for infant and neonatal pain; still a long way to go? Expert Rev Clin Pharmacol. 2017;10(1):111–26.
41. Wong I, St John-Green C, Walker SM. Opioid-sparing effects of perioperative paracetamol and nonsteroidal anti-inflammatory drugs (NSAIDs) in children. Paediatr Anaesth. 2013;23(6):475–95.
42. Ziesenitz VC, Welzel T, van Dyk M, Saur P, Gorenflo M, van den Anker JN. Efficacy and safety of NSAIDs in infants: a comprehensive review of the literature of the past 20 years. Paediatr Drugs. 2022;24(6):603–55.
43. Stone SB. Ketorolac in postoperative neonates and infants: a systematic review. J Pediatr Pharmacol Ther. 2021;26(3):240–7.
44. Schwenk ES, Viscusi ER, Buvanendran A, Hurley RW, Wasan AD, Narouze S, Bhatia A, Davis FN, Hooten WM, Cohen SP. Consensus guidelines on the use of intravenous ketamine infusions for acute pain management from the American Society of Regional Anesthesia and Pain Medicine, the American Academy of Pain Medicine, and the American Society of Anesthesiologists. Reg Anesth Pain Med. 2018;43(5):456–66.
45. Dunn LK, Durieux ME. Perioperative use of intravenous lidocaine. Anesthesiology. 2017;126:729–37.
46. Patterson H, Eady J, Sommerfield A, Sommerfield D, Hauser N, von Ungern-Sternberg BS. Patient positioning and its impact on perioperative outcomes in children: a narrative review. Pediatr Anesth. 2024;34:507–18.

47. Khokhar RS, Baaj J, Alhazmi HH, Dammas FA, Aldalati AM. Pressure-induced alopecia in pediatric patients following prolonged urological surgeries: the case reports and a review of literature. Anesth Essays Res. 2015;9(3):430–2.
48. Maruf M, Jayman J, Kasprenski M, Benz K, Feng Z, Friedlander D, Baumgartner T, Trock BJ, Di Carlo H, Sponseller PD, Gearhart JP. Predictors and outcomes of perioperative blood transfusions in classic bladder exstrophy repair: a single institution study. J Pediatr Urol. 2018;14(5):430.e1–6.
49. Faulk DJ, Karlik JB, Strupp KM, Tran SM, Twite M, et al. The incidence of residual neuromuscular block in pediatrics: a prospective, pragmatic, multi-institutional cohort study. Cureus. 2024;16(3):e56408.
50. Thilen SR, Weigel WA, Todd MM, Domino KB, et al. 2023 American Society of Anesthesiologists practice guidelines for monitoring and antagonism of neuromuscular blockade: a report by the American Society of Anesthesiologists Task Force on Neuromuscular Blockade. Anesthesiology. 2023;138(1):13–41.
51. Koltun WA, Bloomer MM, Tilberg AF, Seaton JF, Ilahi O, Rung G, Gifford RM, Kauffman GL Jr. Awake epidural anesthesia is associated with improved natural killer cell cytotoxicity and a reduced stress response. Am J Surg. 1996;171(1):68–72; discussion 72–3.
52. Wang L, Liang S, Chen H, Xu Y, Wang Y. The effects of epidural anaesthesia and analgesia on T lymphocytes differentiation markers and cytokines in patients after gastric cancer resection. BMC Anesthesiol. 2019;19(1):102.
53. Anand S, Lotfollahzadeh S. Bladder exstrophy. [Updated 2023 Jun 3]. In: StatPearls [Internet]. Treasure Island (FL): StatPearls Publishing; 2024. Available from: https://www.ncbi.nlm.nih.gov/books/NBK563156/.
54. Weiss DA, Groth TW, Abdulfattah SA, Eftekharzadeh S, Lee T, Lee R, Canning DA, Kryger JV, Shukla AR, Roth EB, Mitchell ME, Borer JG. Multi-institutional bladder exstrophy consortium after 8 years: the short- and intermediate-term outcomes. J Urol. 2024;212(1):177–84.
55. Shnorhavorian M, Grady RW, Andersen A, Joyner BD, Mitchell ME. Long-term followup of complete primary repair of exstrophy: the Seattle experience. J Urol. 2008;180(Suppl 4):1615–9. discussion 1619–1620.
56. Schaeffer AJ, Stec AA, Purves JT, Cervellione RM, Nelson CP, Gearhart JP. Complete primary repair of bladder exstrophy: a single institution referral experience. J Urol. 2011;186(3):1041–6.
57. Davidoff AM, Hebra A, Balmer D, Templeton JM Jr, Schnaufer L. Management of the gastrointestinal tract and nutrition in patients with cloacal exstrophy. J Pediatr Surg. 1996;31(6):771–3.
58. Guay J, Suresh S, Kopp S, Johnson RL. Postoperative epidural analgesia versus systemic analgesia for thoraco-lumbar spine surgery in children. Cochrane Database Syst Rev. 2019;1(1):CD012819. https://doi.org/10.1002/14651858.CD012819.pub2. PMID: 30650189; PMCID: PMC6360928.
59. Husmann DA, McLorie GA, Churchill BM. Closure of the exstrophic bladder: an evaluation of the factors leading to its success and its importance on urinary continence. J Urol. 1989;142:522.
60. Novak TE. Failed exstrophy closure. Semin Pediatr Surg. 2011;20(2):97–101.
61. Novak TE, Costello JP, Orosco R, Sponseller PD, Mack E, Gearhart JP. Failed exstrophy closure: management and outcome. J Pediatr Urol. 2010;6(4):381–4.
62. Baradaran N, Cervellione RM, Orosco R, Trock BJ, Mathews RI, Gearhart JP. Effect of failed initial closure on bladder growth in children with bladder exstrophy. J Urol. 2011;186(4):1450–4.
63. Alpert SA, Cheng EY, Kaplan WE, Snodgrass WT, Wilcox DT, Kropp BP. Bladder neck fistula after the complete primary repair of exstrophy: a multi-institutional experience. J Urol. 2005;174(4 Pt 2):1687–9. discussion 1689–1690.

Exstrophy as a Global Health Concern: Strategies for Addressing the Burden of Disease

19

Katelyn A. Spencer, Aseem R. Shukla, and Rakesh S. Joshi

Global Health, Global Surgery, and Their Role Within Treating Bladder Exstrophy

The World Health Organization (WHO) has defined health to be "a state of complete physical, mental, and social well-being, and not merely the absence of disease or infirmity" since the advent of the organization in 1948 [1]. This definition pushed health beyond the binary of solely sick versus well and enshrined the idea that health is a state which can be promoted. This opened the door for global health advocates to work to improve the health of people around the world and across defined country borders.

Global health is a concept that has changed in its definition and scope over the years. It is most commonly defined as "an area for study, research, and practice that places a priority on improving health and achieving equity in health for all people worldwide" [2]. Of note, global health is distinctly different from that of public health or international health according to current definitions. Public health has traditionally been constrained by national borders, while global health focuses on issues that transcend borders. Additionally, conversely to international health,

K. A. Spencer · A. R. Shukla
Children's Hospital of Philadelphia, Philadelphia, PA, USA

Perelman School of Medicine, University of Pennsylvania, Philadelphia, PA, USA
e-mail: ShuklaA@chop.edu

R. S. Joshi (✉)
Department of Paediatric Surgery, Ahmedabad Civil Hospital, Ahmedabad, Gujarat, India

A. R. Shukla, R. S. Joshi (eds.), *Bladder Exstrophy and Epispadias*,
https://doi.org/10.1007/978-3-031-91238-2_19

which was initially developed through the lens of colonialism with knowledge, services, and interventions exclusively coming from high-income countries (HICs) to low- and middle-income countries (LMICs), global health attempts to shift the power imbalance. It aims to promote partnership or pooling of expertise between high-, middle-, and low-income countries in addition to reducing health inequity by advocating for social equity. Global health also works to include population-level prevention without neglecting the importance of individual-level clinical care through multidisciplinary strategies that draw on health and social sciences in addition to fields like engineering, urban planning, climate science, and others.

Despite global health being a large field that encompasses many domains, surgery has not always been considered a primary element [3]. As the field has traditionally been defined by specific populations (i.e., mothers, children, etc.) and diagnoses (i.e., HIV), surgery is a hard entity to fund, as it intersects all patient populations and includes a variety of disease pathologies. There has been a more recent push to define global surgery and include it within the umbrella of global health [4]. This includes supporters of the addition such as Jim Kim, the 12th President of the World Bank, who has stated that "surgery is an indivisible, indispensable part of health care and of progress toward universal health coverage" [5]. The addition of surgery within the field is especially important since common surgical procedures are cost-effective and comparable to other widely accepted global health interventions (i.e., antiretroviral therapy) when performed in LMICs [6].

There is a large burden of surgical disease worldwide and a disproportionate allocation of resources currently. Three-fourths of all surgeries take place in the wealthiest third of the world [7]. As a result, there are two billion people who do not have access to surgical care [8]. This is all due to differing levels of resource availability and capacity. For example, HICs have 10 times as many operating rooms [8] and 11 times as many trained surgeons [9] per person as LMICs.

Conversely, the burden of disability-adjusted life-years from surgical conditions is concentrated within LMICs [10]. Approximately 94% of complex congenital anomalies that require surgical intervention occur in LMICs [11]. When specifically examining genitourinary conditions, they are incredibly common [12]. They are five to ten times more likely than cleft lip and/or palate and are the third most common non-chromosomal anomaly behind congenital heart and limb defects. While rare compared to other genitourinary anomalies, bladder exstrophy epispadias complex (BE) occurs in 1 in 50,000 live births [13]. As such, it can account for a significant number of cases, especially in places with higher birthrates. It is a common trend within LMICs to have higher birth rates than HICs, and this can contribute to an increased burden of disease [14]. Global surgery endeavors to treat conditions like BE and should not be viewed as too costly [6] or complex because the burden of disease within these countries is significant. Outside of cost, from a moral standpoint, there is an obligation that exists to provide the highest level of care possible for these children and their families.

Unique Challenges of Bladder Exstrophy in LMICs

Outside of the standard challenges of surgical conditions within LMICs, including lack of access to care, decreased resource availability, etc., BE provides unique challenges to patients and providers designing interventions to treat this population.

Delay in Diagnosis and Closure

BE is primarily diagnosed prenatally via ultrasound in HICs. As a result, parents can be counseled on what to expect, and surgical planning about closure can be done before delivery. However, access to and equity of prenatal care within and between countries impacts early detection of BE [15, 16]. In LMICs there is less access to prenatal ultrasounds, and so, less of these children are diagnosed prior to delivery. This then creates a delay in closure because surgical planning is delayed. Additionally, due to the rare nature of BE, diagnosis can be further delayed as parents are sent through the referral network until they finally reach a physician with knowledge of the condition. Then, there is further time required for parents to reach a physician who can perform the closure operation.

Delayed closure for BE also comes with its own challenges. Closing children with BE at older ages, which is common in LMICs because of all of the reasons listed above, is associated with a higher failure rate [17], greater challenges with continence, and the need for repeat closures and other operations throughout the lifetime of the child [18]. All of these challenges contribute to worsening the sequelae of mental health challenges that come with BE.

Complex Level of Medical and Surgical Care Required for Bladder Exstrophy

Treating BE successfully requires a high degree of technical skill and experience. While the timing and type of closure for BE remain a debated topic among pediatric urologists [19], there is definitive support that well-performed initial closures are more successful for patients than redo closures after a failed initial attempt [18]. In order to achieve this, the initial closure should be performed by well-trained urologists with the assistance of orthopedic surgeons. This creates a challenge in LMICs, where the access to and availability of highly trained surgeons is low in general. There is a high rate of failure when less experienced surgeons attempt to perform the initial closure, and this creates future challenges if the child needs a repeat procedure due to the presence of scar tissue and altered anatomy.

Additionally, these children need dedicated and specific postoperative care and long-term follow-up to facilitate a successful closure and good quality of life. This includes having well-trained nurses postoperatively who are familiar with the unique needs of these children. These children will also need continued follow-up care to monitor their long-term outcomes, including continence, renal function, fertility, and sexual function. All of this is complicated in the LMIC setting, where access to care and medical specialties is limited.

Mental Health Concerns

Children with BE, irrespective of their location, are at a dramatically increased risk of psychosocial adjustment issues, including suicidal ideation and behaviors, depression, and anxiety compared to their anatomically intact peers [20–25]. This is complicated by the fact that children in LMICs have less access to mental health services [26].

The mental health concerns of this population also extend to the caregivers of these children. It has been documented that parents of children with BE have stress levels comparable to the parents of children with other long-term diagnoses such as type one diabetes [27]. Parents, in general, are concerned about the long-term impacts of BE, including helping with hygiene and uncertainty about their child's future [28]. Primarily these parents are concerned about their child's ability to get married, have children, achieve independence, and obtain complete continence, and these worries increase with subsequent surgeries.

Mental health within LMICs for this patient population is uniquely complicated by the cultural traditions and beliefs surrounding religion within those countries. Specifically, in many LMICs around the world, there is an increased rate of multigenerational housing [29], and living within close quarters creates challenges for families with children with BE due to the constant leakage of urine. This can contribute to perceived and experienced stigma from family, school classmates, and community members [28]. All of this is compounded by lower financial resources for disposable diapers, mental health services, etc., While some of these challenges are not unique to the LMIC setting, they can compound to create different challenges for patients and their caregivers that must be understood and addressed within interventions created to address this need.

Strategies to Design a Global Surgery Collaboration

In order for a global surgery collaboration to be successful, it must address the challenges the specific population of interest has holistically and treat all aspects of the disease [4]. The focus cannot just be on creating anatomic integrity and then leaving, as might be seen within many "short-term surgical missions." These programs, which have become common within the field of global surgery, are typically focused on increasing surgical volume over a short timeframe and do not always lead to improved surgical capacity for host institutions [30]. They are not designed to cultivate long-term follow-up for patients and have been known to result in higher complication rates that are outside of the local health system's capacity to address [31]. Furthermore, when volunteer teams are not well integrated with the local hosts, they can burden local providers, stress hospital resources, and create negative opinions of HIC volunteers [32]. While conceived and executed with the best of intentions, these global surgery programs can cause more harm than good for local populations.

In response to these programs, the American Surgical Association Working Group (ASAWG) on Academic Global Surgery created a set of guiding principles for ethical engagement within global surgery. They are as follows [10]:

1. Local priority: The interests of the local partners and patients should take precedence in all decision-making.
2. Resources: Programs should not hinder existing infrastructure, and obtained HIC resources should be focused on the host site and partners.
3. Clinical care: HIC surgeons and staff should create a plan for complication management and long-term follow-up.
4. Capacity building: Training should be applicable to the LMIC setting in which host partners will function, focus on local as opposed to visiting surgeons, and not contribute to out-migration.
5. Research: Research should be mutually collaborative and equitably attribute authorship.
6. General: All HIC partners should practice cultural sensitivity and uphold the standards of care and practice that exist in their HIC.

The Ahmedabad Model of Excellence

Successful global surgery collaborations employ the above strategies and put an emphasis on capacity building. An example of a robust global surgery collaboration, irrespective of disease of interest, is the International Bladder Exstrophy Consortium (IBEC) based in Ahmedabad, Gujarat, India. The program began in 2009 when surgeons from two academic research centers in the United States joined with the Department of Pediatric Surgery at the Civil Hospital and BJ Medical College in Ahmedabad, Gujarat, India, to form a multi-institutional collaboration. Since then, the partnership has grown to include the Children's Hospital of Philadelphia, Cincinnati Children's Hospital, Seattle Children's Hospital, surgeons from the Hospital for Sick Children in Toronto, Canada, and a pediatric anesthesiologist specialized in pediatric pain management. The Civil Hospital, a government-financed public hospital offering free medical care to a primary catchment area of 60 million people, serves as the host institution. The collaboration includes at least one annual visit from the same team of surgeons, during which new patients are evaluated and care plans are made, while all previous patients are recalled for long-term follow-up. Patients undergo yearly urodynamic evaluation, cystogram, ultrasound, DMSA scan, and bloodwork. The collaboration also evolved toward a more holistic approach to care, including mental health screenings, educational sessions with family members, and community-building activities for the entire cohort.

The IBEC is an example of successfully putting the criteria outlined by the ASAWG into practice in order to exact long-term benefits for patients. The following sections will outline the unique benefits of the collaboration and how they have been implemented according to the ASAWG principles.

Local Priority

The IBEC has a conscious focus on maintaining local priority throughout all aspects of the collaboration. The coordinators from both the host and visiting teams frequently discuss the priorities of local partners throughout the planning process. This includes focusing on the host team's goals and adjusting the collaboration so it best serves the local patient cohort. For example, the first few years of the collaboration identified a greater need for patient education, so the collaboration added novel education initiatives that included a doll representative of a BE patient to better explain to patients, their caregivers, and nursing staff what they should expect after surgery [33].

A gap in care and support for the caregivers was also identified, and research endeavors were added to focus on the patients' quality of life and strategies to best support them [28]. Patient- and family-centered educational lectures were strengthened based on the gathered data, and social workers and psychologists were added to the group to offer support. Patients and families who attend the collaboration annually can gain several ancillary psychosocial benefits, including group support through a family-coordinated WhatsApp group, one-on-one counseling, and social resources.

Resources

The collaboration has focused on leveraging the existing infrastructure to provide more care to a greater number of patients as the geographic catchment area of the collaboration has increased [34]. Collaboration funding is prioritized for the host institution's needs, including purchasing necessary resources for the collaboration and providing services to patients. Importantly, funds are not overwhelmingly dedicated to travel for the visiting team.

Clinical Care

The clinical care plan for complication management for the collaboration was devised together with the host and visiting providers and is based on pathways produced over several years [17]. The clinical care aspect of the collaboration is centered on an annual commitment of the primary surgeons from HICs to return for patient follow-up. Additionally, all interval follow-up care is completed by the host team with support from the teams from HIC through regular teleconference communication.

Long-term follow-up is an essential element of the collaboration to create the continuity of care required to treat such a complex condition. Specifically for BE, consistent follow-up is required to ensure that the long-term consequences of even successful BE closures are captured within data and addressed either through medical or surgical management. For many global surgery programs, including short-term surgical missions, there is little data on long-term outcomes because there is not a large emphasis placed on coordinating follow-up [35]. As a result, these programs are hard to evaluate. Previous work has found that the postoperative follow-up for many of these programs typically stops after 6 months. For the small number of programs that do follow patients for longer than 6 months, their follow-up rate is on average 56% with a 22.3% complication rate [35]. Conversely, the IBEC has continued to follow patients years after their original procedure and has a consistent follow-up rate of 76% [17]. This is despite the various challenges within the LMIC setting.

This is a testament to the original inception of the IBEC. It was prospectively constructed to include a long-term commitment between the host and visiting surgeons. The collaboration includes rigorous preoperative counseling and setting expectations of care with patients to ensure that they not only return for follow-up but also undergo a comprehensive examination.

Capacity Building

All aspects of the collaboration are committed to capacity building. All repairs are performed with at least one resident of the host institution participating in the surgery. Emphasis is placed on knowledge sharing between host and visiting stakeholders, with a focus on training local residents and attending physicians to create autonomous surgeons that have the capacity to perform the CPRE with the same outcomes as the teams from the HIC academic research centers. As a result, the host team has increased experience and greater competency in performing a CPRE. Over the last 5 years, almost as many closures have been performed outside of the time of annual collaboration as during the set window, with comparable results. This is the ultimate showcasing of capacity building, as the host institution is now able to independently provide an extremely high level of care for this specific patient population.

Also, essential to capacity building for the IBEC was the selection of the host institution that had the ability to house the collaboration and expand with it as it grew. The IBEC purposefully selected the second-largest hospital in Asia to partner with. Civil Hospital has a pediatric surgery department that oversees 100 beds and performs 2500–3000 surgical procedures per year. When selecting a host institution, Civil Hospital had demonstrated through these parameters that it possessed the capacity to care for postoperative patients with BE.

Research

The collaboration has been focused on research and, as such, has produced several collaborative manuscripts [17, 28, 34, 36–38]. Each of these projects has equitably credited host partners with first, co-first, or corresponding authorship.

General Principles

Cultural sensitivity is of primary importance for the collaboration, so local partners lead all patient interactions, and all visiting partners are educated on cultural sensitivity prior to attending the collaboration.

Equally as important is the commitment to providing care to the IBEC cohort of patients that is equivalent to the standard of care within the visiting surgeons' home institutions. The IBEC has reported outcomes that are comparable with those seen in HICs [17].

Overall, the IBEC offers a model for a sustainable, long-term global surgery collaboration. It has generated positive, long-term benefits for local partners and patients with surgical outcomes on par with HICs. By focusing on surgical capacity over volume, the collaboration's scope has widened to increase the geographic catchment area for patients [34]. But, like all things in the field of global health, there is always more work to be done to address gaps in care. Even well-designed interventions, like the IBEC, are still trying to address the unique challenges of BE to bring earlier referrals, operate on children at younger ages, and provide strategies to make the collaboration even more equitable for individuals of all social classes within the region [34].

Despite the continued work that is ongoing, the IBEC offers a template for global surgery collaboration when focused on addressing the burden of BE. Such projects must embody the principles of the ASAWG and should push the field forward by maintaining its commitment to a sustainable, long-term collaboration. While this specific program deploys a large volume of resources for a rare disease such as BE, it serves as a template for other pathologies. BE, being a global genitourinary deformity, mastery of the procedure enables downstream expertise in other genitourinary reconstructive procedures such as hernia repairs, reimplantation of ureters, hypospadias, bladder neck reconstruction, and more. By using BE and the IBEC as a model for global collaboration, we submit that there are a multitude of benefits for many more children with less rare conditions.

References

1. WHO. Constitution of the World Health Organization. World Health Organization; 1948. p. 1–18.
2. Koplan JP, Bond TC, Merson MH, et al. Towards a common definition of global health. Lancet. 2009;373(9679):1993–5. https://doi.org/10.1016/S0140-6736(09)60332-9.

3. Farmer PE, Kim JY. Surgery and global health: a view from beyond the OR. World J Surg. 2008;32(4):533–6. https://doi.org/10.1007/s00268-008-9525-9.
4. Dare AJ, Grimes CE, Gillies R, et al. Global surgery: defining an emerging global health field. Lancet. 2014;384(9961):2245–7. https://doi.org/10.1016/S0140-6736(14)60237-3.
5. Jim Kim, President of the World Bank, Addresses the Inaugural Meeting of the Lancet Commission on Global Surgery in Boston, MA, USA on January 17 2014. 2014. Accessed 7 July 2023. https://www.lancetglobalsurgery.org/january-videos.
6. Grimes CE, Henry JA, Maraka J, Mkandawire NC, Cotton M. Cost-effectiveness of surgery in low- and middle-income countries: a systematic review. World J Surg. 2014;38(1):252–63. https://doi.org/10.1007/s00268-013-2243-y.
7. Weiser TG, Regenbogen SE, Thompson KD, et al. An estimation of the global volume of surgery: a modelling strategy based on available data. Lancet. 2008;372(9633):139–44. https://doi.org/10.1016/S0140-6736(08)60878-8.
8. Funk LM, Weiser TG, Berry WR, et al. Global operating theatre distribution and pulse oximetry supply: an estimation from reported data. Lancet. 2010;376(9746):1055–61. https://doi.org/10.1016/S0140-6736(10)60392-3.
9. Hoyler M, Finlayson SRG, McClain CD, Meara JG, Hagander L. Shortage of doctors, shortage of data: a review of the global surgery, obstetrics, and anesthesia workforce literature. World J Surg. 2014;38(2):269–80. https://doi.org/10.1007/s00268-013-2324-y.
10. Debas H, Alatise OI, Balch CM, et al. Academic partnerships in global surgery: an overview American Surgical Association Working Group on Academic Global Surgery. Ann Surg. 2020;271(3):460–9. https://doi.org/10.1097/SLA.0000000000003640.
11. Congenital anomalies. Accessed 28 Nov 2021. https://www.who.int/news-room/fact-sheets/detail/congenital-anomalies.
12. Data & Statistics on Birth Defects | CDC. Centers for Disease Control and Prevention. Published June 28, 2023. Accessed 18 July 2023. https://www.cdc.gov/ncbddd/birthdefects/data.html.
13. Siffel C, Correa A, Amar E, et al. Bladder exstrophy: an epidemiologic study from the International Clearinghouse for Birth Defects Surveillance and Research, and an overview of the literature. Am J Med Genet C: Semin Med Genet. 2011;157(4):321–32. https://doi.org/10.1002/ajmg.c.30316.
14. Pezzulo C, Nilsen K, Carioli A, et al. Geographical distribution of fertility rates in 70 low-income, lower-middle-income, and upper-middle-income countries, 2010–16: a subnational analysis of cross-sectional surveys. Lancet Glob Health. 2021;9(6):e802–12. https://doi.org/10.1016/S2214-109X(21)00082-6.
15. Arroyave L, Saad GE, Victora CG, Barros AJD. Inequalities in antenatal care coverage and quality: an analysis from 63 low and middle-income countries using the ANCq content-qualified coverage indicator. Int J Equity Health. 2021;20(1):102. https://doi.org/10.1186/s12939-021-01440-3.
16. Arsenault C, Jordan K, Lee D, et al. Equity in antenatal care quality: an analysis of 91 national household surveys. Lancet Glob Health. 2018;6(11):e1186–95. https://doi.org/10.1016/S2214-109X(18)30389-9.
17. Joshi RS, Shrivastava D, Grady R, et al. A model for sustained collaboration to address the unmet global burden of bladder exstrophy-epispadias complex and penopubic epispadias: the International Bladder Exstrophy Consortium. JAMA Surg. 2018;153(7):618–24. https://doi.org/10.1001/jamasurg.2018.0067.
18. Gearhart JP, Ben-Chaim J, Sciortino C, Sponseller PD, Jeffs RD. The multiple reoperative bladder exstrophy closure: what affects the potential of the bladder? Urology. 1996;47(2):240–3. https://doi.org/10.1016/s0090-4295(99)80424-5.
19. Promm M, Roesch WH. Recent trends in the management of bladder exstrophy: the Gordian knot has not yet been cut. Front Pediatr. 2019;7:110. https://doi.org/10.3389/fped.2019.00110.
20. Reiner WG, Gearhart JP, Kropp B. Suicide and suicidal ideation in classic exstrophy. J Urol. 2008;180(4 Suppl):1661–3; discussion 1663–1664. https://doi.org/10.1016/j.juro.2008.03.115.

21. Immelt S. Psychological adjustment in young children with chronic medical conditions. J Pediatr Nurs. 2006;21(5):362–77. https://doi.org/10.1016/j.pedn.2006.02.006.
22. Bujons A, Lopategui DM, Rodríguez N, Centeno C, Caffaratti J, Villavicencio H. Quality of life in female patients with bladder exstrophy-epispadias complex: long-term follow-up. J Pediatr Urol. 2016;12(4):210.e1–6. https://doi.org/10.1016/j.jpurol.2016.05.005.
23. Dellenmark-Blom M, Sjöström S, Abrahamsson K, Holmdahl G. Health-related quality of life among children, adolescents, and adults with bladder exstrophy–epispadias complex: a systematic review of the literature and recommendations for future research. Qual Life Res. 2019;28(6):1389–412. https://doi.org/10.1007/s11136-019-02119-7.
24. Pennison MC, Mednick L, Rosoklija I, et al. Health related quality of life in patients with bladder exstrophy: a call for targeted interventions. J Urol. 2014;191(5S):1553–7. https://doi.org/10.1016/j.juro.2013.09.089.
25. Hankinson JC, Eldridge MA, Ostrander R, et al. Emotional and behavioral functioning in children with bladder exstrophy-epispadias complex: a developmental perspective. J Pediatr Urol. 2014;10(1):136–41. https://doi.org/10.1016/j.jpurol.2013.07.013.
26. Kieling C, Baker-Henningham H, Belfer M, et al. Child and adolescent mental health worldwide: evidence for action. Lancet. 2011;378(9801):1515–25. https://doi.org/10.1016/S0140-6736(11)60827-1.
27. Earnshaw VA, Quinn DM, Park CL. Anticipated stigma and quality of life among people living with chronic illnesses. Chronic Illn. 2012;8(2):79–88. https://doi.org/10.1177/1742395311429393.
28. Spencer KA, Ramji J, Unadkat P, et al. Caregiver distress: a mixed methods evaluation of the mental health burden of caring for children with bladder exstrophy. Front Pediatr. 2022;10. Accessed 2 Nov 2022. https://www.frontiersin.org/articles/10.3389/fped.2022.948490.
29. Samanta T, Chen F, Vanneman R. Living arrangements and health of older adults in India. J Gerontol B. 2015;70(6):937–47. https://doi.org/10.1093/geronb/gbu164.
30. Botman M, Hendriks TCC, Keetelaar AJ, et al. From short-term surgical missions towards sustainable partnerships. A survey among members of foreign teams. Int J Surg Open. 2021;28:63–9. https://doi.org/10.1016/j.ijso.2020.12.006.
31. Hendriks TCC, Botman M, Rahmee CNS, et al. Impact of short-term reconstructive surgical missions: a systematic review. BMJ Glob Health. 2019;4(2):e001176. https://doi.org/10.1136/bmjgh-2018-001176.
32. Chaus M. The dark side of doing good: a qualitative study to explore perceptions of local healthcare providers regarding short-term surgical missions in Port-au-Prince, Haiti. J Glob Health Rep. 2020;4:e2020002. https://doi.org/10.29392/001c.11876.
33. Families in India learn post-surgical care for bladder exstrophy. Association for the Bladder Exstrophy Community. Published January 14, 2017. Accessed 24 Feb 2022. https://www.bladderexstrophy.com/families-learning-post-surgical-bladder-care-bladder-exstrophy-support-recovery/.
34. Spencer K, Joshi R, Ramji J, et al. Global surgical collaboration to treat bladder exstrophy-epispadias in India led to a larger geographical catchment area. J Glob Health Rep. 2023;7:e2023007. https://doi.org/10.29392/001c.74378.
35. Luan A, Mghase AE, Meyers N, Chang J. Are we curing by cutting? A call for long-term follow up and outcomes research in global surgery interventions – perspective. Int J Surg. 2021;87:105885. https://doi.org/10.1016/j.ijsu.2021.01.011.
36. Joshi RS, Eftekharzadeh S, Shukla AR, et al. Kidney function outcomes after complete primary repair of exstrophy: results from the International Bladder Exstrophy Consortium. J Urol. 2021;206:E510.
37. Ramji J, Weiss DA, Romao RLP, et al. Impact of bilateral ureteral reimplantation at the time of complete primary repair of bladder exstrophy on reflux rates, renogram abnormalities and bladder capacity. J Pediatr Urol. 2021;17(3). https://doi.org/10.1016/j.jpurol.2021.01.020.
38. Ramji J, Eftekharzadeh S, Fischer KM, et al. Variant of bladder exstrophy with an intact penis: surgical options and approach. Urology. 2021;149:E15–7. https://doi.org/10.1016/j.urology.2020.11.046.

Incontinence in Exstrophy-Epispadias: Should We Change Our Thinking?

20

Dana A. Weiss

Introduction

When a child is born with the bladder outside the body, an open bladder neck, and an open urethra, with a short phallus or bifid clitoris, there are multiple goals for the future. These goals focus initially on restoring normal anatomy with an internalized bladder and reconstructing a more normal appearance for the genitalia. Next, the focus shifts to urinary function, optimizing the bladder to hold urine at safe storage pressures and to empty at low pressures to prevent urinary tract infections and to preserve renal function. The next phase naturally aims to achieve dryness, again while ensuring protected renal function. Finally, as a child shifts into adulthood, the focus shifts to optimizing sexual function and fertility.

While these aims can be approached separately, each is interrelated. Closure of the bladder and bladder neck must be achieved with just the right amount of resistance. If the resistance is too low, the kidneys might remain safe, as there will be no urine stasis or elevated bladder pressures, but gross incontinence may mean that the bladder will not grow and cycle. If the bladder outlet resistance is too high, the bladder will overwork, become hypertrophic, and transmit elevated pressures to the kidneys, leading to chronic kidney disease or even renal failure. Next, if a bladder neck reconstruction is done with the goal of dryness through intermittent catheterization, and especially if the bladder is augmented, then the child and later the teen and adult are committed to a consistent and regimented catheterization schedule with attendant risks of infections, bladder stones, damage to the kidneys, and even more catastrophic events, such as perforation of the augment and death. Thus, it is critical to gauge interest and buy-in both from a family wishing their child to be "normal" and

D. A. Weiss (✉)
Children's Hospital of Philadelphia, Philadelphia, PA, USA

Perelman School of Medicine at the University of Pennsylvania, Philadelphia, PA, USA
e-mail: Weissd1@chop.edu

A. R. Shukla, R. S. Joshi (eds.), *Bladder Exstrophy and Epispadias*,
https://doi.org/10.1007/978-3-031-91238-2_20

from the child, who needs to want to engage in these practices not just for the present, but also throughout the teenage years, when often there is resistance to participating in any fixed routine.

Other chapters in this book are focused on how to achieve continence with a surgical approach. This chapter is intended to bring focus to the questions of what, when, and why to achieve continence.

Defining Continence

Since continence is one of the key outcome measures in exstrophy, one would think that there would be a clear definition. However, one of the challenges in interpreting results across time and institutions is the lack of a consistent definition. Moreover, as there are some general themes that are shared among the various definitions, the question then arises as to where these came from. Did patients participate in the assessment and creation of these definitions, or are they physician-made?

Continence versus Dryness

Most studies and outcomes distinguish continence with the ability to void from continence with the need to catheterize. One way to clarify these disparate outcomes is perhaps in the wording: the word continence means the ability to hold urine and volitionally empty the bladder via the urethra, while the word dryness would indicate the ability to hold urine but with the requirement of a catheter to empty the bladder or the use of a drainage bag. Going forward in this chapter, the words continence and dryness will be used to differentiate between these two groups.

Dry Interval: How Long Is Long Enough?

The next variation in outcomes reported is the time interval required to be considered continent, or dry. The most commonly accepted interval is 3 hours. A review of the literature by Lloyd et al. in 2012 determined that out of 87 studies from 2000 to 2012, the most common definition used to assess continence was "dry with voiding/catheterization every 3 hours" [1]. This is important because the most common definition did not separate voiding vs. catheterization; however, the time interval was the same.

The time interval for defining continence or dryness in patients with exstrophy has not been uniform. In 1978, the definition used for continence for exstrophy was "being completely dry for a minimum of 2 hours while the patient was awake without pharmacological or mechanical aids" [2]. That 2-hour interval was used in the setting of patients undergoing a combined Young-Dees urethroplasty and Marshall-Marchetti-Krantz bladder neck suspension, with assessment of outcomes at an average age of 14 years (range 7.5–24.5 years).

In a follow-up of 207 patients from 1945 to 1985 treated at Columbia, which was then a major exstrophy center, continence was defined as "excellent" if the criteria were met that "the patient maintained a daytime dry interval of at least 3 hours with rare episodes of nighttime wetting and stress incontinence" [3]. This study also included an intermediate continence marker, which is helpful for those who may be quite satisfied with voiding a little more frequently: "A good result was defined as a postoperative daytime dry interval of 1–3 hours…" Finally, "a poor result was a dry interval of less than 1 hour" [3].

Dry Intervals: What Is Meaningful

While 3 hours seems to have become the gold standard for being considered "continent" or "dry," there have not been enough studies on what these dry intervals mean for the patient. How different is it for a child—or adult—to have to void every 2 hours compared to every 3 hours? And should the timing be different if they have to catheterize vs. if they can void? And at what price is it worth it?

In the adult literature, there has been an increasing number of investigations concerned with the degree of and bother of incontinence in both males after prostate surgery and females with stress urinary incontinence. For some men, who have spent a lifetime not having to think about their bladders, even a drop of urine, or the need for the use of a pad, is a significant burden, while healthy women may be much more prone to having 1–2 leaks per 24-hour period, ranging from small to larger volumes, even at a young age [4].

A challenge in reviewing the literature regarding the importance or significance of specific dry intervals concerns the condition being evaluated. The literature on patients with spina bifida and patients with dysfunctional voiding who are otherwise anatomically normal tend to focus on incontinence episodes rather than dry intervals. This is difficult to correlate to BEEC, since for most children with BEEC the question is how long they can stay dry between voiding. Even in the spina bifida literature, the definition of continence has changed over time. For example, initially continence was defined by the survey question of "dry, with or without interventions, during the day." This definition shifted to a question stating "Quantify frequency of bladder incontinence during the day over the last month (when not having a UTI)," and for this question, the answers of "Never" or "Less than once per month" fit the classification of "continent" [5].

Diversion Versus Continence

In the age of incontinent diversion, there was a different balance to consider, as the child would be destined for either a stoma bag or leakage per urethra. Each camp had its advocates—one placing emphasis on dryness of the genitalia for later normal sexual activities, despite the presence of a stoma bag, while the other advocated for management of urethral incontinence and living without a stoma bag [6]. Even at that time, Lattimer, a leader in exstrophy care, felt that waiting for continence was better than upfront diversion. In his study, he worked with pediatric psychiatrists to evaluate the long-term (over 20 years) outcomes of patients and concluded, "Our psychological studies have indicated that the wait several years for the possibility of urinary continence does not leave these patients with insurmountable psychological trauma." While the trade-off that he spoke of was closing the bladder and waiting compared to diversion with an abdominal stoma, one could extrapolate that he may take this trade-off even for complex continent diversions and all the complications associated with those procedures.

Timing and Cost of Continence

Timing

The next question, that follows after assessing the interval of dryness needed to define continence or dryness, is the timing at which dryness or continence can or should be achieved. While on average children toilet train between 2 and 3 years of age [7], there are some children that remain wet through their fourth year, and a pediatric urology clinic sees children through school age and into high school with urgency, frequency, and even wetting; some manage with voiding every 2 hours to avoid leaks. So, should a child who is born with an open bladder that never has had the normal developmental chance to cycle and grow be expected to achieve the same bladder capacity and develop continence at the same age as a child with a normal bladder? If we allow for children to void every 2 hours in our dysfunctional voiding clinic, why should voiding every 2 hours for a child with exstrophy be considered not good enough? Children with exstrophy are often very well adjusted to their lives and many times do not have significant bother by being in a pull-up even into school-age years. The distress usually comes from external influences, such as parent and teacher concerns. We see this often in the setting of nocturnal enuresis, where the child, even until 10–12 years of age, does not mind being wet at night, but the wetness—and often more than the wetness, the lack of distress from the child—causes the greatest distress to the parent. To this end, encouraging a 5- or 6-year-old to take on the challenges of continence, to demand timed voiding or catheterization on a set schedule when they would much rather be carefree and time-free, perhaps adds undue stress to the otherwise happy child.

In children with BEEC, studies have indeed found that continence develops later in life, often developing after puberty [8]. Development of continence requires a combination of factors: enlarging growth of the bladder to provide a large enough reservoir to hold the urine and adequate bladder outlet resistance in the form of a competent bladder neck and external sphincter complex. Even for patients who undergo a formalized bladder neck reconstruction in the setting of a staged repair, bladder capacity greater than 100 cc has been found to be a predictor of the development of continence [9–12]. Khandage et al. recently demonstrated that there was a 50% chance of reaching this goal of 100 cc by 5.7 years of age. However, they also showed that bladder capacity continues to increase over time, and up to 80% of patients had achieved 100 cc capacity by 8 years of age [11]. While the focus of these studies is to demonstrate that 50% would have an adequate bladder capacity for BNR by age 5–6, the data also indirectly supports the concept that over time, the bladder grows in the setting of gentle outlet resistance, and with continued bladder growth, there is continued potential to develop longer dry intervals. Perhaps in another 20 years, as trends shift from proceeding with reconstruction at 5–6 years of age to 8–9 and even older past puberty, we will finally know the real numbers who have the potential to achieve continence over time.

While the data are still immature, we have anecdotally seen children develop gradually increasing dry intervals over time. In children who were closed as a newborn, we have seen continence increase by 20–30 minute intervals year after year. In some children who had the bladder closed at a later age, sometimes 10–11 years, as part of our international surgical collaboration, we have even found that they achieve 2–3 hour dry intervals within a year. Thus, by looking at trends and gradual changes for each child, physicians can provide personalized expectations and treatment plans.

Cost of Continence

The next question in the calculus of achieving dryness or continence is to what lengths a child and family want to go to achieve dryness vs. how long they are willing to wait to see if continence will develop with time. This varies significantly between families but also varies significantly based on external influences and discussions with surgeons and care givers. In centers where the routine is to give time to gradually develop growth of the bladder and improve sphincteric control, families are more likely to tolerate and manage the wet child and to give time for the achievement of continence, gaining motivation from each gradual increase in dry interval. On the other hand, in centers where from the start, the plan is to progress to dryness, either through bladder neck reconstruction or bladder neck closure, the family will be gearing up from birth for that day when dryness is achieved, and for some, that time cannot come soon enough.

The goal for early dryness comes from the motivation to normalize children among their peers and to get them out of diapers and pull-ups as soon as they are willing to participate in a catheterization regimen. This early dryness comes with the cost of further surgeries, the need to catheterize on a strict regimen, and the risk, especially in the setting of an augmentation or bladder neck closure, of significant complications. These costs are multiplied over a lifetime. Lastly, the promise of dryness even with a bladder neck reconstruction is not a guarantee after just one surgery. From one of the largest experiences in BNR, almost 41% of children progressed to other procedures after an initial BNR, and even nearly 28% of those who underwent BNR with augmentation and/or catheterizable channel went on to further surgeries [13]. Moreover, families must know that even a bladder neck closure is not a 100% guarantee for continence, as 9/124 patients in this large series remained incontinent even after BNC and continent diversion [13]. Probably with enough surgery, these all can become dry, but again, when the question is what is the cost of dryness, each surgery adds up.

The flip side of the argument is that while childhood dominates the present and the desire to be dry is real, ultimately childhood—including the teenage years—is only a small fraction of a lifetime. If there is the potential to achieve voiding with continence during the 50+ years of adulthood, is it worth being wet, to some degree, for the first 10–20 years of life?

Physical Therapy for Continence

To follow along with the question of "At what cost dry?", we must also look at what it takes to be continent. We don't presume that the majority will be magically dry when they hit their 13th birthday. The thought is that over time, with gradual development of the external sphincteric muscles in parallel with the gradual growth of the bladder, a child will be able to hold more and more urine. As detailed in another chapter, the role of pelvic floor physical therapy is coming to the forefront in all areas of urinary health, and none more so than in the management of bladder exstrophy. Much of this therapy involves intensive work by the child and the family. This starts with bladder training to really focus on the bladder, spending a concentrated effort, both at home and during therapy sessions, on feeling and responding to the bladder, voiding on a strict timed schedule, and tracking improvements. In addition, at times, the improvements will be directly related to the intensity of the training: at times of rigorous training, the person may be dry, but when they lessen their intensity, wetness recurs. This can be frustrating.

Challenging Dogma

The goal of this chapter is to challenge dogma. If we don't do that, we will never advance the care of our patients. So the questions I propose are: What is magical about 3 hours? Why is the drive to be dry at 5 years, or to be dry by kindergarten, driving our medical care? Where does freedom and independence without worrying about the bladder play a role?

Many studies use an all-or-nothing approach to dry intervals; more than or less than 3 hours without the use of any pads. Others offer an "intermediate" success outcome: a dry interval of 2 hours. But what if a child is happy and functional being continent if they void every 1.5–2 hours, then that should count for something—and that child should be considered continent. If a child or young adult can wear a pad or liner for minor leaks and peace of mind, they may still be considered "wet," but they may be functionally happy. So, some children and families might decide that the benefit of becoming completely dry is not worth the cost.

While each management decision needs to be based on a discussion between the patient/family and the physician, there are now outside influences that are much more prevalent than 15 years ago. Social media has allowed for ongoing discussions and conversations at best, or passive observations at worst, that tell a parent what they should be doing, how they should be thinking, and what choices they should make for their child. Some may be pressured to seek dryness by age 5–6 and may consider anything later than that as a failure. But what if the child doesn't care?

We have made patience the hallmark of our approach to continence in bladder exstrophy. We lay the foundation for this from the earliest meeting—be it prenatally or in the first visit in clinic. Our goal is to keep each child safe and healthy and allow the best chance for them to void normally. While we hope that with newer techniques of closure we will see increasing numbers of children who achieve continence with voiding after only a single surgery, even the prospect that 20% will be able to be continent with voiding is enough to keep families working toward the goal. Even some older children who have not achieved continence are now minimally bothered by the wetting that even when offered a procedure, they decline.

References

1. Lloyd JC, Spano SM, Ross SS, Wiener JS, Routh JC. How dry is dry? A review of definitions of continence in the contemporary exstrophy/epispadias literature. J Urol. 2012;188:1900–4. https://doi.org/10.1016/j.juro.2012.07.017.
2. Toguri AG, Churchill BM, Schillinger JF, Jeffs RD. Continence in cases of bladder exstrophy. J Urol. 1978;119:538–40. https://doi.org/10.1016/S0022-5347(17)57541-2.
3. Connor JP, Hensle TW, Lattimer JK, Burbige KA. Long-term followup of 207 patients with bladder exstrophy: an evolution in treatment. J Urol. 1989;142:793–5. https://doi.org/10.1016/S0022-5347(17)38890-0.
4. Lukacz ES, Falke C, Geynisman-Tan J, Wyman JF, Mueller ER, Markland AD, et al. Healthy bladder storage and emptying functions in community-dwelling women measured by a 2-day bladder health diary. Neurourol Urodyn. 2023;42:725–35. https://doi.org/10.1002/nau.25169.
5. Wiener JS, Suson KD, Castillo J, Routh JC, Tanaka ST, Liu T, Ward EA, Thibadeau JK, Joseph DB; National Spina Bifida Patient Registry. Bladder management and continence outcomes in adults with spina bifida: results from the national spina bifida patient registry, 2009 to 2015. J Urol. 2018;200(1):187–94. https://doi.org/10.1016/j.juro.2018.02.3101. Epub 2018 Mar 26. PMID: 29588216; PMCID: PMC6919313.
6. Lattimer JK, Beck L, Yeaw S, Puchner PJ, Macfarlane MT, Krisiloff M. Long-term followup after exstrophy closure: late improvement and good quality of life. J Urol. 1978;119:664–6. https://doi.org/10.1016/S0022-5347(17)57583-7.
7. Vermandel A, Van Kampen M, Van Gorp C, Wyndaele J. How to toilet train healthy children? A review of the literature. Neurourol Urodyn. 2008;27:162–6. https://doi.org/10.1002/nau.20490.
8. Taskinen S, Suominen J, Mäkelä E. Development of late continence in bladder exstrophy and epispadias patients. Urology. 2020:S0090429520307937. https://doi.org/10.1016/j.urology.2020.06.034.
9. Bar-Yosef Y, Savin Z, Ekstein M, Ben-David R, Dekalo S, Bar-Yaakov N, et al. Preoperative bladder capacity predicts social continence following bladder neck reconstruction in children born with exstrophy–epispadias complex. Eur J Pediatr Surg. 2023;33:510–4. https://doi.org/10.1055/a-2003-1823.

10. Chan DY, Jeffs RD, Gearhart JP. Determinants of continence in the bladder exstrophy population: predictors of success? Urology. 2001;57:774–7. https://doi.org/10.1016/S0090-4295(00)01102-X.
11. Khandge P, Morrill CC, Wu WJ, Harris KT, Haffar A, Maruf M, et al. Achieving goal capacity for continence surgery: a cumulative event analysis of bladder exstrophy patients. J Pediatr Urol. 2023;19:563.e1–8. https://doi.org/10.1016/j.jpurol.2023.04.039.
12. Massanyi EZ, Shah BB, Baradaran N, Gearhart JP. Bladder capacity as a predictor of voided continence after failed exstrophy closure. J Pediatr Urol. 2014;10:171–5. https://doi.org/10.1016/j.jpurol.2013.08.003.
13. Maruf M, Manyevitch R, Michaud J, Jayman J, Kasprenski M, Zaman MH, et al. Urinary continence outcomes in classic bladder exstrophy: a long-term perspective. J Urol. 2020;203:200–5. https://doi.org/10.1097/JU.0000000000000505.

21 Surgical Options for Refractory Urinary Incontinence in Classic Bladder Exstrophy

Brian A. VanderBrink

Introduction

The congenital defect in classic bladder exstrophy (CBE) results in significant aberrations in typical urinary tract anatomy. Despite a successful primary repair, regardless of the technique employed, there is frequent urinary incontinence in this patient population [1–4]. The urinary symptoms contribute to a decreased patient-reported quality of life [5, 6]. Therefore, interventions aimed at improving the urinary symptoms are pursued, each with their own varying degrees of effectiveness and invasiveness.

The social consequences of urinary incontinence begin to manifest as the child approaches primary school age when most of their peers are toilet trained and not using protective undergarments. The timing of active interventions for urinary incontinence differs amongst patients and their families and may be dependent upon their respective psychosocial circumstances and physician biases. Many nonsurgical methods have been recommended in the form of surveillance and psychosocial support, pelvic floor therapy, pharmacotherapy, and clean intermittent catheterization (CIC) via urethra prior to additional surgery undertaken for purposes of achieving continence. This chapter is aimed at discussing and reviewing the surgical options for refractory urinary incontinence in CBE patients following primary surgery.

B. A. VanderBrink (✉)
Division of Pediatric Urology, Cincinnati Children's Hospital Medical Center, Cincinnati, OH, USA
e-mail: Brian.vanderbrink@cchmc.org

A. R. Shukla, R. S. Joshi (eds.), *Bladder Exstrophy and Epispadias*,
https://doi.org/10.1007/978-3-031-91238-2_21

Preoperative Counseling

It is extremely helpful to set realistic expectations for the CBE patients and their family about observed urinary continence outcomes after primary bladder surgery in the surgeon's personal experience, as well as published series. In the author's opinion, this message can never be communicated too early nor too often to CBE patients and their families/care providers. They should be informed that the prospect of volitional voiding accompanied by urinary continence both day and night is the exception rather than the norm in CBE population based upon existing literature. Large retrospective reviews in single and multiple institutions have seen this "holy grail" outcome in CBE patients of urinary continence while voiding, with or without additional bladder neck surgery, and not catheterizing in only 20–25% of patients [3, 7, 8]. Therefore to achieve social continence, the majority of CBE patients will likely require additional lower urinary tract reconstructive surgery following primary bladder closure.

An emphasis on proper patient selection for any of the continent reconstruction surgeries discussed in this chapter cannot be understated. Assessment of the degree of bother from the urinary continence will undoubtedly influence the intensity of and desire for further intervention. Bother can be quantified with patient-reported outcomes utilizing validated quality of life (QOL) questionnaires or also more simply by asking the patient or parent during the clinical encounter [9]. But it must be underlined that parent-reported (or proxy-reported) responses as to their child's QOL is an observers' impression of a child's internal experience: it is not interchangeable with the child/patient-reported QOL. Parents, healthcare providers, and other proxies typically underestimate patents' QOL [10]. Therefore, a single visit and response may not be adequate prior to complex urologic reconstruction for incontinence to discover or understand these nuances of patient/family preferences or social determinants of health.

Due to the frequent need for additional procedures following and complications associated with a complex lower urinary tract reconstruction discussed in this chapter [11], it is this author's practice pattern to not schedule surgery upon first meeting the patient or family despite obvious indications/presence of bothersome urinary incontinence. The Johns Hopkins team has advocated for an intense pre–bladder neck repair program conducted by a senior urology nurse practitioner, senior clinical nurses, and a child psychologist well versed in voiding issues prior to bladder reconstruction [12]. These sessions are begun for both child and parents at least 6 months before the proposed bladder outlet procedure with successful completion of the program required before surgery is scheduled. Bladder capacity has been observed to be a predictor of continence after bladder neck reconstruction (BNR) alone. [13, 14] However, additional nonphysiological considerations such as emotional maturity of the patient, adherence to lifestyle modifications, and adequate family support may have an impact on urinary continence [3]. As such, patient selection, which represents a collective consideration of all of these factors, likely remains the most important tool for achieving continence after reconstructive surgery.

The social problem of urinary incontinence must not be converted to a medical problem secondary to the continence procedure. An incompletely emptied bladder places the upper tracts at risk that is amplified following procedures such as BNR/closure or continent urinary diversion. Reconstructive strategies that are predicated on CIC at regular intervals may overwhelm continence mechanisms leading to leakage via continent catheterizable channel (CCC) or bladder/reservoir perforation [11]. It is important to consider the patient's cultural background, socioeconomic situation, and access to medical supplies when determining the surgical treatment plan. Reliable and uninterrupted access to catheter supplies to perform CIC is another fundamental part of surgical decision-making. In some circumstances due to either socioeconomic status, cultural norms, or other factors, the use of catheter-independent procedures such as urostomy or ureterosigmoidostomy may be considered superior to reconstructions reliant upon CIC such as augmentation cystoplasty (AC) or continent diversion.

The reconstructive surgeries performed in the CBE patients are either aimed at incompetent bladder outlets and/or insufficient bladder reservoirs. This chapter will begin with a review of procedures performed to increase bladder outlet resistance. Surgical procedures to enhance bladder outlet resistance may be done by three basic surgical categories: procedures with either injection of material under the mucosa or an external compression device; procedures to reconfigure the bladder outlet into a more efficient continence valve and closure of the bladder outlet.

Compression of the Lumen of Bladder Outlet

Bladder Neck Bulking Agent Injection

When surgery is pursued, the least surgically invasive method to improve urinary continence secondary to an incompetent bladder outlet is endoscopic bulking agent urethral or bladder neck injection (BNI). The allure of BNI is its simplicity, relatively low risk to the patient compared to open procedure, an opportunity for repetition in the event of failure, and yet not exclude more complex treatment options that might be needed in the future. BNI can serve as both primary therapy and an adjunct to reconstructive surgery for achieving urinary continence. Various bulking agents have been utilized with varying characteristics and success rates. Most studies have demonstrated that BNI as primary treatment for incontinence in children is often ineffective and not cost-effective to other surgical treatments

The BNI technique involves cystoscopic visualization of the urethra and bladder neck in either a retrograde or in combination with an antegrade manner via suprapubic cystotomy or CCC [15]. An injection needle is placed through the working channel of the cystoscope and multiple injections are performed. (Fig. 21.1) The needle is directed submucosally and a bleb is raised under direct visualization while injecting the material until submucosal accumulation occurs. The goal would be material injected until full coaptation is achieved by cystoscopic inspection.

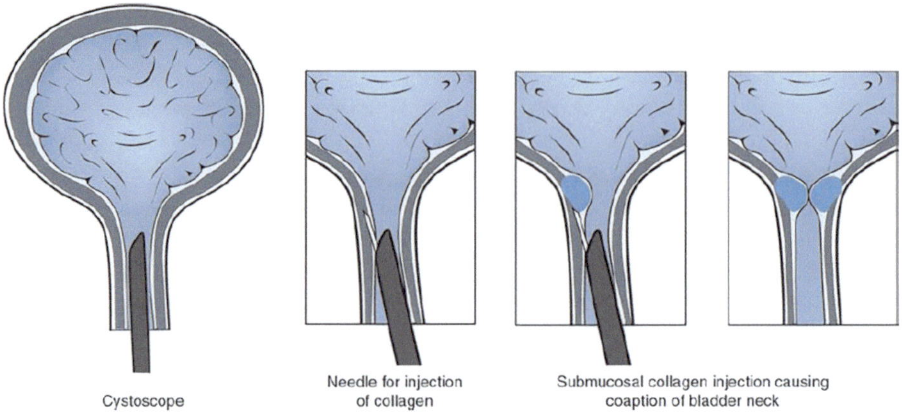

Fig. 21.1 Injection of the bladder neck with various materials is accomplished by passing the needle through the cystoscope. The material is injected submucosally either retrograde through the urethra or antegrade from suprapubic approach. The material provides passive pressure to help occlude the bladder outlet. (Used with Permission from Taylor and Francis- Kelalis-King-Belman Textbook Clinical Pediatric Urology 5E)

The original material used for BNI was polytetrafluoroethylene (Polytef®/Teflon®) and showed promising results with its first description in pediatric population in 1985 by Vorstman et al. [16] Dyer et al. reported their experience with Teflon® BNI as primary therapy in 13 CBE patients with 0% success rate of producing continence [17] . The controversy and observations regarding Teflon® particle migration to nonurologic body sites have truncated further use of this agent [18]. Cross-linked glutaraldehyde bovine collagen (Contigen®) was the next promoted BNI agent and multiple reports of its use in children [19–22]. Unfortunately, Contigen® was not immune to adverse effects and is associated with allergic reactions, thus, requiring pre-injection skin testing for a hypersensitivity reaction. The positive effects of Contigen® BNI observed were largely temporary in durability and putatively secondary to degradation of the material due to its biodegradability. Burki et al. described their experience with yet another BNI material, polydimethylsiloxane (Macroplastique®), in a CBE/epispadias population [23]. They reported its use in 52 patients with success in 9 patients (17%) defined as being dry without pads/diapers while another 17 (33%) significantly improved. Those patients with a positive outcome comprised just 4/34 (12%) patients with a diagnosis of CBE. Macroplastique®'s continued use in pediatrics has been tempered by fear of reports of migration and non-biodegradability [24].

Dextranomer hyaluronic acid (Deflux®) has been utilized for BNI and has not been implicated in particle migration [17, 25–28, 30–32]. It has been described as primary therapy by Dyer et al. in a CBE population and the authors described, as they observed with their using Teflon® uniformly no improvement in continence or bladder capacity following Deflux® BNI [17]. Several other authors have described Deflux® BNI in either primary or adjunct following BNR in CBE pediatric patients

[25–28]. The characteristics of Deflux® show that the implant volume decreases in size due to a reduction in the aqueous volume of the implant and/or displacement of the implant from its injection site before its consolidation by endogenous collagen [29]. This property of Deflux® can result in some patients following BNI showing improvement in urinary continence followed by a rapid deterioration in continence parameters depending on when they were assessed. Caione et al. showed that after the first 3 months continence results remained relatively stable and they advocated that it may be difficult to judge Deflux® BNI success within the first 3 months and repeat BNI should be reserved until after 3 months [25].

The Paris, France group has published the most on Deflux® BNI in peer-reviewed literature [26, 30–32]. Fiorenza et al. reported their experience in 22 patients with CBE (18 males, 4 females) using Deflux® BNI [30]. Modern staged reconstruction was performed in all patients except one. Previous BNR had been performed in the majority of patients, but not in all patients with five patients who had undergone previous AC. Dryness was observed in 7 patients (32%), improvement was observed in 3 patients (14%), and no change was observed in 12 patients (55%) with CBE. Patients with previous BNR tended to have longer failure-free survival. The authors concluded that BE patients are unlikely to benefit from Deflux® BNI without previous BNR. This same institution shared its observations with outcome of further continence procedures after failure of Deflux® BNI [31]. In their series, 24 patients had a subsequent bladder neck procedure: artificial urinary sphincter (AUS, 7—all dry), bladder neck plasty (9–7 dry, 1 improved, and 1 still incontinent), bladder neck closure (BNC, 1—dry), and fascial sling (3–2 dry and 1 improved). At the time of surgery, the authors state that the Deflux® paste was easily identified with minimal surrounding tissue inflammatory reaction. This group from Paris, France, has advocated that even if the success rate is limited in the long term, due to its relative simplicity Deflux® BNI should be proposed to manage major incontinence in children as a primary procedure or as a salvage procedure with a failed bladder neck procedure [32]. The authors advocate information that is not over-optimistic should be provided to the patient and parents regarding the expected success rate of Deflux® BNI.

Artificial Urinary Sphincter

One of the benefits of BNI is the high likelihood of maintenance of the ability for continued volitional voiding; however as previously described, one drawback is the relatively low success rate in achieving urinary dryness in CBE patients. The AUS is another surgical intervention where spontaneous bladder emptying with voiding can be preserved but confers a much higher continence rate compared to a single BNI. The AUS is a hydraulic device that is composed of three parts: an inflatable cuff that surrounds and compresses the bladder neck or bulbous urethra; a pressure-generating balloon; and a pump control module. (Fig. 21.2) The AUS gives the patient the ability to deflate the cuff and reduce the compression of the bladder neck at will. The pressure exerted on the urethra is regulated by the balloon/reservoir. The

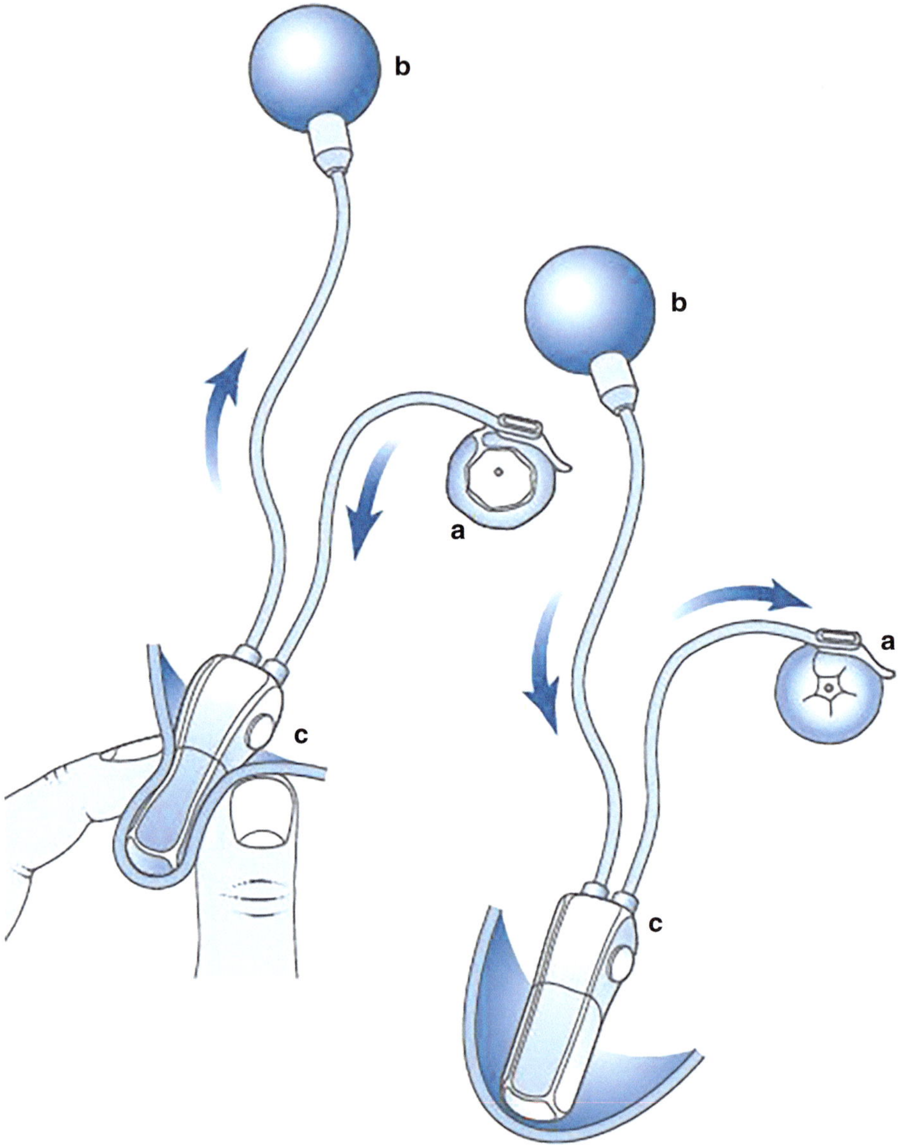

Fig. 21.2 The artificial urinary sphincter is a mechanical device composed of three components: (**a**) an inflatable cuff, (**b**) a pressure-regulating reservoir balloon, and (**c**) a control pump. It functions by using hydraulic pressure to inflate the cuff, which compresses the urethra and provides continence. By squeezing the pump (implanted in the scrotum or labia), the patient can manually deflate the cuff and allow voiding or catheterization through the urethra. The pressure in the balloon then restores pressure throughout the system and reinflates the cuff in 3 minutes. (Used with Permission from Taylor and Francis- Kelalis-King-Belman Textbook Clinical Pediatric Urology 5E)

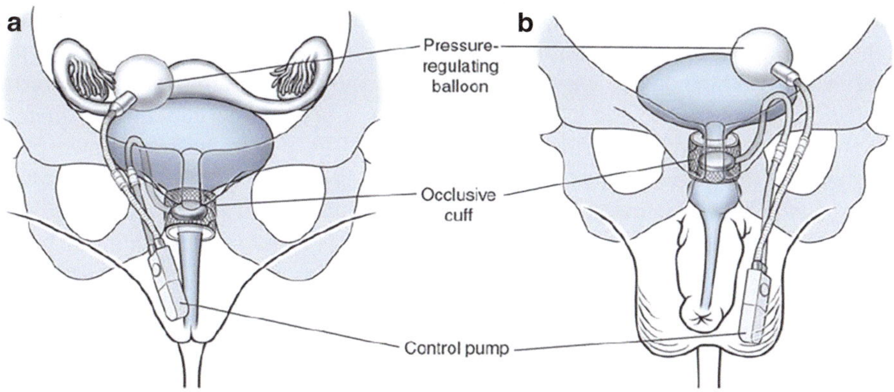

Fig. 21.3 (**a**) Artificial urinary sphincter components in a female with the pump implanted in the labia. (**b**) Artificial urinary sphincter components in a male with the pump implanted in the scrotum. Both examples demonstrate the cuff implanted around the bladder neck. (Used with Permission from Taylor and Francis- Kelalis-King-Belman Textbook Clinical Pediatric Urology 5E)

bladder neck is the preferred site of placement of inflatable cuff in children (Fig. 21.3). The pump is placed in the scrotum or labia, and the entire device is contained within the body.

The AUS was originally only placed in patients who could void as there were concerns that performing CIC through the implanted sphincter could cause damage to the tissue compressed by the cuff and lead to erosion. However, as previously mentioned, the use of CIC is frequently seen in children with CBE [3, 8]. Barrett and Furlow reported a series of children who could not void after AUS implantation and found that CIC could be performed safely if the cuff was deflated prior to passage of the catheter [33]. Continence was good and no patients suffered erosion due to catheterization. The AUS device is not activated immediately after implantation, as cuff pressure immediately after surgery may cause erosion of the cuff into the bladder. The sphincter may be activated after 6–8 weeks with less risk of erosion. Eventually, all AUS will wear out and fail, requiring replacement, but if complications can be avoided the mean survival of the new devices in children well over 10+ years.

Light and Scott, as pioneers of the AUS implantation procedure, published the first series of CBE patients with AUS in 1983 [34]. Surgical implantation with the AS792 model of AUS in 10 CBE patients resulted in a reported continence in 90%. Removal of the device occurred in one patient secondary to bladder neck obstruction and resulting upper tract dilation, which resolved after explanation. Concerns over the placement of the cuff around the previously operated bladder neck were not observed in this original case series; however, as experience grew with the AUS device erosion of the cuff was observed. Decter et al. reported their experience with the AMS 800 device in 11 patients with CBE and 5 patients with epispadias [35]. A total of 13 patients had failed prior BNR. Of these 16 patients, 10 currently have an active device in place and 9/10 continent. To accomplish these results, however, these 10 patients required 10 additional procedures, including 6 revisions and 4 other operations for complications associated with the procedure. Three patients had erosion and the device was removed (1 underwent successful reimplantation).

Ruiz et al. described the use of AUS in 23 non-neurogenic patients (19 males) where 12 had extrophy epipspadias complex (EEC) with mean follow-up of 80 months [36]. Three sphincters in patients with exstrophy were removed because of erosion and/or infection at 5, 49, and 60 months after initial surgery. CBE patients and those with previous bladder procedures were exposed to more complications such as erosion compared with patients with epispadias or anorectal malformation. Hafez et al. reported their experience with AUS in five CBE patients as a small subset of larger pediatric cohort (n = 89) patients [37]. The authors noted that a history of CBE was the only significant factor with detrimental effect on AUS survival as four of the five patients (80%) had their AUS removed secondary to erosion relative to a total of 12/84 (14%) erosions in the remaining cohort. Castera et al. reported in a small series of seven patients with EEC that five patients were continent, with two of the five patients had epispadias only and two CBE patients underwent concomitant AC [38]. AUS cuff erosion developed 2 years later in one of these two CBE patients and the device was removed. These authors argued that patients who undergo bladder neck or urethral surgical procedures before AUS placement may benefit from the lowest balloon pressures (51–60 cm. water) capable of maintaining closure of the bladder neck to minimize further ischemia to the compromised bladder neck substrate.

Others have not reported as high a rate of erosion in the CBE population. Bosco et al. and Levesque et al. reported the Boston children's 5- and 10-years of experience, respectively, with AUS in children with varying causes of incompetent bladder outlet with the majority being from neurogenic causes [39, 40]. In Levesque's study, **32** of **39 (82%)** of the patients with sphincters in place were dry [39]. The authors demonstrated that the AUS was a viable and successful option for the incontinence associated with CBE in a very small sample size ($n = 4$). Bosco et al. demonstrated that the risk of cuff erosion in girls and boys was similar if they have not had prior bladder surgery [40]. Herndon et al. and the Indiana group had 20+ years of experience published with over 100 children with AUS implantation and 10 had CBE within the 21 patients having EEC [41]. Risk factors for erosion were evaluated but in their series placement of the AUS directly on the segment of bowel used to create the neourethra was the only significant clinical factor, while previous bladder neck repair or use of CIC in this large series did not significantly increase the erosion rate. Patients in whom the latest model of AUS (AMS 800) was implanted had a much lower revision rate than those with a previous model and almost 60% had no mechanical complications.

Increasing the outlet resistance with the AUS, as with any bladder outlet procedure, can potentially alter the bladder storage dynamics in a manner deleterious to the upper urinary tracts. This delayed clinical phenomenon after AUS implantation has been reported by several authors [42–45]. This deterioration has been hypothesized to be secondary to two factors: a failure to void efficiently in some patients and the new development of detrusor hypertonicity in others. Deterioration of detrusor function after AUS placement occurs in as many as 20% of patients, and there is currently no reliable method to predict which patients will undergo these changes or the timetable for risk [45]. Because of this threat, it is necessary to closely follow patients with AUS with upper tract imaging and urodynamics, as needed indefinitely after placement of the sphincter.

AC has been performed in a significant number of CBE patients for a variety of indications to create a low-pressure, adequate-volume reservoir [PUMA]. Augmentation may be performed at the same time as AUS placement but has been associated with an increased risk of device infection if the colon and small bowel are the substrates used for the augmentation [46]. At the current time, the use of the AUS in patients who require AC and CIC may offer little advantage over other surgical methods to increase bladder outlet resistance.

Procedures to Surgically Reconfigure the Bladder Outlet into a Continence Valve

Bladder Neck Reconstruction

Due to the congenital exstrophic bladder and bladder outlet in CBE, the primary repair to close the bladder, bladder neck, and urethra may not result in urinary continence. Hugh Hampton Young of Johns Hopkins University in 1922 described a procedure in epispadias to reconstruct the bladder outlet by excising redundant dorsal tissue and then both narrowing and lengthening the bladder outlet to narrow it using "Boomerang Needle Holder" that Young himself created [47]. John Dees of Duke University in 1949 expanded upon Young's procedure by describing a posterior urethral flap to lengthen the neourethra [48]. He removed the mucosa from the muscle on the lateral aspect of this flap and, after closing the central flap of mucosa into a tube, he closed the muscle over the mucosa in a second layer. This provided additional muscle around the neourethra. Guy Leadbetter of Massachusetts General Hospital in 1964 further improved upon the Young–Dees bladder neck repair by moving the ureters to a new location higher along the posterior bladder wall and away from the urethra [49]. This maneuver allowed the posterior bladder strip to be even longer and produce a long neourethra and a much higher bladder neck. This last modification of these prior techniques is currently known as Young-Dees-Leadbetter (YDL) BNR.

The Johns Hopkins team has published extensively on the use of YDL in CBE patients and typically performs BNR when a patient is 5–8 years of age and has a strong desire to be continent [3, 50–52]. As previously mentioned, they advocate that the patient must be mentally prepared to commit to an intense voiding program and, in addition, must have adequate bladder capacity as BNR may result in loss of capacity [12]. The Johns Hopkins group state contraindications to BNR alone include a prior failed exstrophy closure, small bladder capacity, or unfavorable urodynamic parameters such as poor compliance, elevated detrusor pressure, or low contractility that would suggest poor emptying [52].

Reports of urethral continence using the YDL BNR alone have been observed in 25–70% of CBE patients with variable follow-up periods from different institutions [3, 4, 50–57]. However this continence rate post-BNR can be challenging for the reader to discern at first glance for a number of reasons due to variable reporting metrics [58]. Is continence after BNR defined as dry without the use of any incontinence protection? Is continence after BNR defined as dry within 2-h or 3-h or 4-h intervals? Is continence after BNR with spontaneous voiding or via CIC or AC. Bladder capacity has been reported to be a predictor of continence after BNR alone [13, 14]. A minimum bladder capacity of 100 cc has been advocated as a metric to assist in surgical decision-making between BNR or CCC with or without AC [59].

Early series reported continence rates with voiding alone in 80% with modern staged reconstruction with YDL BNR [60, 61]. In the most recent review from Johns Hopkins, 350 CBE patients with continence data known at least 3 months postoperatively and 7 years median follow-up. In those who underwent BNR alone, the continence rate was 91 of 142 (64.1%) with 80 of the 91 voiding spontaneously per urethra and 11 of 91 performing CIC [3]. One of the disadvantages of the YDL BNR includes the loss of bladder capacity that results from the reallocation of bladder wall tissue to the urethral continence mechanism. The neourethra following YDL, as most BNR, may be tortuous and difficult to catheterize. Such extensive bladder neck surgical reconfiguration with YDL BNR, as with all BNR techniques, carries the potential for postoperative neuromuscular dysfunction. Therefore, it may be difficult for CBE patients following YDL BNR to exhibit normal voiding characteristics. Yerkes et al. examined 27 patients with EEC who had undergone YDL without AC with 2 or more years of follow-up [57]. Dry intervals of at least 2 h were achieved by 18 patients and all were considered by parents to void well. Despite near or total subjective continence and "good" voiding, 13 of these 18 patients (72%) had clinical problems related to emptying, which included recurrent urinary tract infections in 10, epididymitis in 2, and bladder calculi in 4. Objective urodynamic parameters confirmed poor voiding in most patients.

Other surgeons have modified the YDL BNR in a quest to improve urethral continence. Mollard in 1980 described his results using a BNR technique in 15 patients with CBE [62]. (Fig. 21.4) On one side, the trigonal muscle is cut in the transverse direction at the level of the new bladder neck. On the other side, the trigone is cut parallel to the urethra, thus leaving a triangle attached to the bladder by its base and tubularized. The muscular triangle, still attached to the urethra, is turned inward and sutured to the other side of the urethra. The muscular triangle on the other side is pulled upward in front of the new bladder neck and the lowest part of the detrusor. This will reconstitute a muscular loop in front of the new bladder neck and a clear urethrovesical angle. A long-term follow-up (mean 11 years) from this center in Lyon, France, using the Mollard BNR technique in 80 CBE patients showed that 36 (45%) patients presented with a dry interval of >3 h with 18 patients using CIC (16 via Mitrofanoff) after one BNR [63]. Twenty-two patients (27%) underwent AC. Fifty-one percent of all patients required an endoscopic procedure within

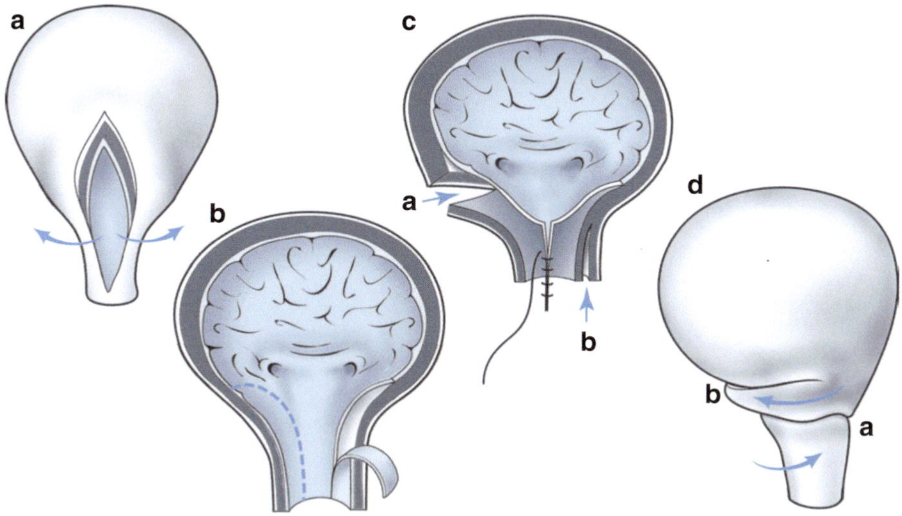

Fig. 21.4 Mollard bladder neck reconstruction. Molalrd's variation of the Young-Dees-Leadbetter procedure is similar in the construction of the neourethra from a long posterior strip of urethra and bladder. It differs in that one of the triangular flaps is incised vertically and parallel to the neourethra. This flap is then rotated horizontally across the midline to create an angle of the anterior bladder neck. (**a**) The bladder is opened in the midline (**b**) The mucosa lateral to the central urethra strip is excised. (**c**) The two lateral muscle flaps are incised, one vertically and one horizontally. (**d**) Flap [A] is wrapped around the neourethra like Young-Dees-Leadbetter operation while Flap [B] is rotated horizontally across the repair to create an anterior bladder neck. (Used with Permission from Taylor and Francis- Kelalis-King-Belman Textbook Clinical Pediatric Urology 5E)

3 months after the BNR either in the form of dilation of BNR for urine retention or BNI (n = 3) for persistent urethral leakage.

Koff's variation on the YDL also differs from the original in its use of the periurethral muscle flaps [64]. His description involves the initial incision on the lateral aspect of the bladder neck, rather than the midline, and this produces a single long muscle flap on one side of the bladder. (Fig. 21.5) After ureteral reimplantation in a cephalotrigonal fashion, the mucosa is stripped from the long muscle flap, leaving a midline strip of urethra and bladder to tubularize for the neourethra. The long muscle flap is then wrapped around the neourethra, producing what Koff termed 'the cinch'. Koff reported results in 10 CBE patients with continence day and night achieved in 6 patients (3 voiding and 3 on CIC) while daytime-only continence was achieved in an additional 2 patients for 80% continence rate. Four patients had underwent AC in this Koff series (3 prior to BNR and 1 concomitantly). Hanna et al. described a variation of the Cinch procedure but instead of an initial transverse incision, the muscular flap was created in longitudinal fashion [65].

Both Mollard's and Koff's BNR techniques use bladder muscle flaps to create more outlet resistance at the expense of making the bladder smaller by reducing the bladder itself. Jones et al. originally described a series of patients using a modification of the YDL which has been the Mitchell BMR after Michael Mitchell [66]. The

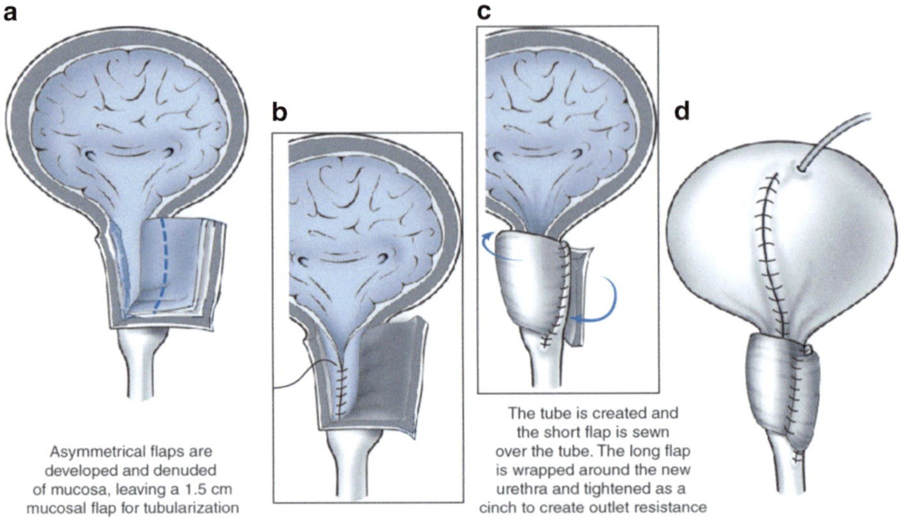

Fig. 21.5 Koff's Cinch bladder neck reconstruction. It is another variation of the Young–Dees–Leadbetter procedure that creates the neourethra from a posterior flap of urethra and bladder and covers it with a flap of demucosalized muscle. The construction of this flap is different to other repairs that rely on two flaps. The technique is predicated on lower transverse lateral incision of the bladder neck instead of opening the anterior midline. This creates a single long flap on one side of the neourethra. The flap is then wrapped around the neourethra and sewn to itself with permanent sutures. It acts as a constant compression of the bladder outlet. (**a**) The bladder outlet is opened on one side. (**b**) A midline mucosal strip is tubularized and the mucosa is dissected from the remaining muscle flap. (**c** and **d**) The muscle flap is then rotated around the bladder outlet. (Used with Permission from Taylor and Francis- Kelalis-King-Belman Textbook Clinical Pediatric Urology 5E)

Mitchell BNR technique returned to Hugh Hampton Young's original concept of a narrowed neourethra without added muscular support. Mitchell's BNR does not decrease bladder capacity as the anterior bladder and urethral flap are incorporated into the bladder. The technique through low transverse incision mobilizes a triangular full-thickness flap of the anterior urethra and bladder neck and then narrows the bladder outlet. The flap is then rotated cephalad and integrated into the bladder. Continence was achieved in 64% of patients who all voided in a mixed group of children including neuropathic bladders and CBE. DeCambre et al. reviewed another modification of Mitchell BNR in a series of four CBE patients using a demucosalized detrusor muscle pedicle to wrap around the bladder neck base [67]. Three of the four CBE patients underwent simultaneous enterocystoplasty and concomitant Mitrofanoff channel. Urinary continence rate, defined as no leaking via bladder neck, was 50% after the first procedure in the CBE patients and 100% after the BNI injection. The authors advocated for the detrusor wraparound in combination with the Mitchell modification of YDL BNR to be most useful in difficult redo operations in which sufficient bladder tissue is available for repair. Burki et al. from Great Ormod Street, London, described the utility of the Mitchell BNR in just that clinical scenario [55]. Burki et al. reported on 30 CBE patients with a history of failed prior BNR. Of the patients, 15 already had undergone AC, 12 had undergone a Mitrofanoff procedure and 12 had been treated with BNI in an attempt to achieve continence. Four patients had undergone more than 1 bladder neck procedure. Postoperatively 28 patients were using CIC to empty the bladder (5 per urethra, 23 via Mitrofanoff). Although redo BNR can render a significant number of patients dry, it was only effective if performed in conjunction with AC. Ashraf Hafez of Mansoura, Egypt, described his experience with the Mitchell BNR and detrusor wraparound flaps in 28 children with CBE [68]. His manuscript was described as mini-trigonal tubularization and bladder neck wraparound with a demucosalized detrusor flap. With a mean follow-up of 2.5 years, all 13 patients with augment on CIC via reconstructed outlets were continent which was significantly higher than the non-augmented cohort. Complete dryness was achieved in 20 (71%) of 28 patients.

The use of non-detrusor muscular flaps as an additional substrate for coaptation/compression of the bladder outlet with or without BNR has been described. The pyramidalis, rectus abdominis, and gracilis muscles have been harvested as wraparound flaps of reconstructed bladder outlet to augment resistance and improve continence [69–71].

Bladder Neck Closure

Persistent incontinence after BNR as described can be challenging to achieve urinary continence. Repeat BNR may denervate the posterior urethra and distal trigone, and ultimately impair any potential for spontaneous voiding. In patients who have undergone multiple surgical procedures involving the bladder neck with intractable urinary incontinence, the muscle quality may be questionable or extensive scarring may exist. This clinical scenario does not lend itself to reconstructive efforts. BNC or transection may be the singular way to achieve urethral continence albeit at the expense of alternative bladder drainage in the form of CIC or urostomy. Patient selection is paramount as with any lower urinary tract reconstruction but may be magnified as BNC is most frequently paired with the creation of a CCC using the Mitrofanoff principle. Compliance with CIC is critical to avoidance of bladder perforation and upper urinary tract preservation.

Standard BNC is accomplished by approximating the anteroposterior bladder neck edges in two layers. The distal urethra may or may not be closed, and omentum or a rectus muscle flap is usually interposed between the closed bladder neck and urethra [72–74]. Despite these measures, BNC is often associated with such complications as leakage or fistula. Khoury et al. described a modification of the standard technique of BNC that involves extensive mobilization of the posterior edge of the bladder neck, elevating it at least 2 cm. off of the vagina or rectum in female and male patients, respectively [72]. This free edge of the posterior bladder neck is rolled anteriorly and, hence, the anastomosis is placed anterior and not directly inferior. When concomitant enterocystoplasty is performed, the anterior suture line is begun in the midline by suturing the edge of the detubularized and reconfigured bowel plate to the anteriorly rolled edge of the bladder base.

Many series of BNC have been reported with success rates of 40–100% [72, 75–81]. Bladder perforation is the most feared complication because of inadequate drainage and excessive pressures but does not seem to occur at higher rates than BNR. Nguyen and Baskin reported high calculus formation and fistula rates (40%) in 20 patients (n = 12 CBE patients) who underwent AC and BNC, largely attributable to poor compliance with CIC [78]. They also found that incomplete division of the bladder neck portended fistula formation. At 3 months after surgery, 40% of the patients were completely dry, 20% had leakage via the stoma and 40% had a urethral fistula. After additional surgeries, 85% of the patients were completely continent 2 years following BNC (15% declined further surgeries or had an ileal conduit). Of the 15 patients with follow-up longer than 3 years, only 40% remained completely dry, and leakage via the stoma developed in 47% after being dry for 1 year. Repeat urodynamic studies did not show any adverse changes in bladder dynamics in the incontinent patients. Stomal stenosis of the CCC occurred in 30% of the patients and bladder stones developed in 40%. Novak et al. described 76 patients (n = 42 CBE patients) who underwent AC with BNC [79]. After a mean follow-up of 44 months, continence was achieved in 98% of patients and there were no reports of bladder perforation. Complications included two bladder neck fistulas and five patients with stomal leakage. Landau et al. described 12 patients (n = 5 CBE patients), who underwent BNC with a 10-year follow-up [80]. Continence was achieved in all patients, and upper tract dilation was noted in the only patient who did not concurrently receive AC. There were no reports of bladder perforation.

Continent Catheterizable Channel: Mitrofanoff Principle

CIC through the reconstructed urethra in the CBE patients either with or without BNR may not allow for easy, reliable performance of it. Therefore, an alternative conduit for CIC can be quite advantageous, and in 1980, Paul Mitrofanoff published his clinical series utilizing the appendix as the conduit for a CCC for CIC [81]. The Mitrofanoff principle is based on the implantation of a supple tube within a submucosal tunnel with seromuscular support. The urinary reservoir pressure will rise during filling and coapts the lumen of the CCC to prevent retrograde leakage through the CCC and provide continence. The seromuscular layers of detrusor in a bladder or gastrointestinal reservoir, when the bladder is absent or insufficient, can be utilized for the site of implantation of the conduit.

Although this Mitrofanoff principle has been applied frequently with the appendix, other substitutes have included transversely tubularized bowel segments (Yang-Monti) or ureteral remnants. Careful patient selection and ensuring a low-pressure urinary reservoir are critical elements to achieving the successful outcome of the CCC with a high rate of channel continence. Failure to regularly catheterize and completely empty the bladder or reservoir can lead to urinary tract infection, hydronephrosis, or reservoir perforation.

When the appendix is utilized for the CCC, assessment of the appendiceal length and its mesenteric vascular anatomy is important. The appendix can be removed with a cuff of cecum to provide length and a wider stoma to help minimize stenosis at the skin level. The mesoappendix should be mobilized until the desired stomal location can be reached without tension. As with ureteral reimplantation, creation of the antireflux mechanism can be accomplished in an intravesical or extravesical fashion. For intravesical technique, the bladder can be opened in the sagittal plane to allow for concomitant reconstructive procedures such as bladder outlet procedure and/or AC as indicated. The distal end of the appendix can be tunneled into the bladder through neohiatus with a minimal submucosal tunnel length of 3 cm [81, 82]. Securement of the appendix to the outer bladder wall at the entry into the neohiatus into the submucosal tunnel with 3-0 absorbable suture assists to minimize channel retraction. Bladder immobilization using abdominal wall hitch stitch minimizes catheterization angulation and false passages. For the extravesical technique, the bladder is distended via the indwelling catheter and a 3 cm incision is made in the detrusor and seromuscular flaps are created on the anterior-lateral bladder wall [83]. The bladder mucosa is not entered during this extravesical dissection. At the distal aspect of the trough, a mucosotomy is made and the bladder mucosa to appendiceal mucosa anastomosis is performed circumferentially using absorbable 4–0 suture. The seromuscular flaps of the trough are brought anterior to the channel and sutured to each other. Incorporating the serosa of the appendix with the suture used for seromuscular flap closure sutures helps maintain the length of the antireflux tunnel as well.

Implantation of the CCC into the detrusor muscle is the desired method however in the CBE patients this may present a unique challenge if the native bladder is too small or otherwise unsuitable for CCC tunneling. In these cases, a "serosal trough" strategy can be used to implant the CCC into a bowel segment used for augmentation [84, 85]. Two parallel incisions through the augmented bowel serosa are created to expose the muscularis mucosa and submucosa. A full-thickness insertion orifice for the channel is made at the distal end of these incisions. The channel is laid into the tunneled serosal "trough" and implanted into the augmented bladder orifice. The serosal flaps of the parallel incisions are used to overlay the tunneled channel segment.

It is important regardless of the implantation technique used, the Mitrofanoff channel is intra-operatively tested on multiple occasions, and each time any operative step is completed, for ease of catheterizability and stomal continence while the bladder is filled. This will permit the surgeon to identify which step introduced any change or difficulty and adjust accordingly. Depending on stomal location, guide the appendiceal base to the umbilicus or through the rectus muscle after creating a cruciate incision in the rectus fascia. Mature the stoma at the skin level by spatulating the proximal end of the appendix and securing a wide-based V- or U-shaped skin flap at the apex of the spatulation. Key technical points are to maintain the shortest channel possible to facilitate ease of catheterization; avoid kinking; and if possible, fixation of the bladder to the undersurface of the abdominal wall.

When the appendix is absent, insufficient in its length, or other factors preclude its use for Mitrofanoff, an alternative substrate is needed for Mitrofanoff. Colon or ileum is most frequently used and the latter is favored due to the more robust blood supply of the small bowel relative to the large bowel. After assessment of mesenteric vascular anatomy, a 2–3 cm segment of ileum is isolated from gastrointestinal continuity on a vascularized pedicle. This segment is opened transversely along the antimesenteric border according to the technique described by Monti [86]. Tubularization of the reconfigured intestinal segment in a longitudinal fashion over a 12- to 14-Fr catheter is performed in two layers using a 5-0 absorbable monofilament suture. Implantation of the reconfigured channel into the bladder and stomal maturation occurs using the aforementioned surgical techniques as with the appendix. Another alternative technique for creation of a CCC is the Macedo technique which mandates concomitant AC due to the technique [87]. The CCC is constructed from the same bowel segment that AC occurs. From 35 cm of ileum, a 3 cm width flap from the anterior and posterior wall of ileum in the mid part of the isolated segment. The continence mechanism of the CCC is based on *angulation* and a serous-lined tunnel created with three to four nonabsorbable seromuscular sutures.

CCC has been utilized frequently in the CBE population due to the aforementioned challenges of CIC through the reconstructed bladder outlet or following BNC. Kasprenski et al. from the Hopkins team described the simultaneous creation of a CCC at the time of BNR in a series of 24 EEC (n = 18 CBE) patients who were felt not to be candidates of BNR by the authors due to their institution's eligibility criteria [53]. The median bladder capacity of these 18 CBE patients was 220 mL and 2 had prior failed bladder closure. For patients with greater than 6 months of follow-up time (n = 17), 12 (71%) had dry intervals greater than 3 h. Of the 10 patients who were completely dry, 7 (58%) achieved volitional voiding per urethra with residual urine emptied through their CS. The remaining 5 (42%) were continent by stomal catheterization alone and did not achieve voiding per urethra. Of the 5 patients, 29% did not achieve continence following a BNR-CCC procedure. Three of the 5 patients (60%) established eventual continence following BNC. In the Maruf series of 350 patients with EEC where continence outcomes were evaluated, a CCC was used in 157 patients as part of BNC and continent diversion with 60 additional patients as part of BNR with (n = 30) or without (n = 30) AC [3]. This series reported that in those patients who underwent BNR with AC with CCC, 61.3% were continent, with all of these patients performing CIC alone without voiding. Of those who underwent BNC and continent diversion, all 133 patients were on CIC via CCC. Ulman et al. reported their experience with six CBE patients who had undergone YDL-BNR with an adjuvant CCC [88]. Four patients had a breakdown of their reconstructed bladder necks due to CIC via urethra. AC was performed in all six patients at the same setting as the creation of the CCC. Szymanski et al. as part of the multicenter study of five North American pediatric centers from 1980 to 2016 examined the use of CIC in 216 CBE patients [8]. At the last follow-up, 67.4% of all patients performed CIC. Among 95 patients with an intact native bladder, 30.5% performed CIC (72.4% via CCC). Among those without BNR or with an AUS, 14.8% performed CIC, compared to 54.8% after BNR and 100% after BNC. Among 107 patients who underwent AC, all performed CIC, typically via CCC (86.9%). Older patients on CIC were more likely to use a CCC, increasing from 61.5% for those younger than 10 years to 88.3% for patients >18 years. Of 76 adults without a diversion, 85.5% performed CIC. The CIC rate was 100% in adults who underwent AC and 31.3% in adults with a native bladder. These clinical series emphasize the use of CIC via CCC as a frequently utilized intervention in the CBE population.

Complications from CCC arise with short-term and extended follow-up. *Stomal stenosis* at the skin level is the most commonly reported problem with a reported incidence between 10% and 40% [89–92]. *False passages* can also occur from repeated erroneous catheterizations or excessive angulation within the channel and can usually be managed with a temporary indwelling catheter [93]. *Stomal incontinence* is infrequent and may be due to a short intravesical tunnel, persistently elevated reservoir pressures, or a fistula between the channel and the bladder. Lowering elevated detrusor pressures either medically or surgically can resolve the stomal incontinence when secondary to abnormal storage pressures. For inadequate continence mechanism due to shortened antireflux tunnel, endoscopic management with Deflux has been reported [94]. A formal subfascial revision with redo implantation to address the inadequate antireflux mechanism of the channel is another surgical intervention performed as well for stomal incontinence.

Augmentation Cystoplasty

The chapter thus far has focused on surgical techniques to address incompetent bladder outlets and alternative bladder emptying conduits in the form of CCC. However, the urinary incontinence in CBE patients may be secondary to impaired bladder capacity with or without abnormal storage characteristics resulting in an insufficient bladder reservoir. Use of pharmacotherapies (i.e. anticholinergics and/or beta-3 agonists) should be used prior to surgical procedures to improve bladder storage characteristics. When medical management is ineffective, AC is a highly effective procedure to simultaneously decrease elevated detrusor end-filling pressures, improve bladder compliance, and increase bladder capacity.

The use of which gastrointestinal segment is utilized for AC varies by patient anatomy and surgeon preference. Gastric, ileal, and colonic segments have all been used in CBE patients [8, 95, 96]. Gastric segments are less utilized for AC compared to other segments due to the typical normal small and large intestine anatomy of CBE patients. Advantages of sigmoid colon for AC are its anatomic proximity to the bladder and the thick muscular taenia of the colon may serve as a more robust substrate for ureteral or CCC implantation than the thinner seromuscular layer of ileum. This author preferentially uses ileum for AC because of its mesenteric mobility, relative abundance compared to sigmoid colon, and tendency to generate less mucous than the colon. Detubularization and reconfiguration of the intestinal segment used for AC into a U- or W-shape provide multiple advantages, including maximization of the volume achieved for any given surface area, blunting of bowel contractions, and improvement of overall capacity and compliance. This augment patch is then sutured to the bladder after making a sagittal incision to provide wide enterovesical anastomosis.

AC has been performed in varying rates of CBE published series. Szymanski et al. in a multicenter study over three decades retrospectively reviewed 212 CBE patients who underwent primary bladder closure where 108 (50.9%) underwent augmentation, 10 (4.7%) diversion (1 with a previous augmentation), and 95 (44.8%) neither [8]. After controlling for follow-up time in this series using survival analysis, the probability of AC was 14.9% by age 5 years, 50.7% by 10 years, and 70.1% by 18 years. After controlling for follow-up time, this probability varied significantly by treatment center; the probability at 10 years ranged between 26.7% and 64.5%, depending on the center. Among 87 children who underwent a bladder outlet procedure without simultaneous AC for persistent urinary incontinence after primary closure, the probability of future AC was 46.4% at 5 years and 60.7% at 10 years after the bladder outlet procedure and did not differ among centers. Maruf et al. published that out of 432 CBE cohorts treated at Johns Hopkins, 76 and 165 patients underwent AC with BNR or BNC, respectively (56%, 241/432) [3]. Cervellione et al. reviewed 32 CBE patients who underwent bladder closure using a staged repair technique that underwent a salvage procedure for continence [97]. AC was performed in 23/32 (72%) and the remaining 9 patients had either neobladder or urinary diversion procedures.

The complete primary repair technique for CBE has been touted to normalize anatomy at the initial repair, thereby allowing early bladder filling and cycling which may influence bladder function, capacity, and possibly the need for AC. In a multicenter study of CBE patients, Weiss et al. showed 54 CBE patients who underwent bladder closure using a complete primary repair technique reviewed at three centers prior to the creation of a clinical consortium between the centers over a 20-year period (1993–2013) [7]. The median age of patients at the last follow-up was 12 years, and they reported AC was performed in 10/54 (19%) with BNR or BNC. Ellison et al. and DiCarlo et al. reported their own single-institution experience with continence outcomes and procedures following complete primary repair technique in 29 and 61 CBE patients, respectively [1, 51]. Ellison et al. reported that 6/29 (20%) underwent AC which was very similar to 12/61 (19%) in the DiCarlo series undergoing AC. No study has been published to date to discern if the CPRE proves to carry a lower risk for AC.

Surgical technique is critical when performing AC to minimize complications. Adequate length of the intestine (20 cm of either the large or small intestine) utilized will minimize the risk of re-augmentation [98]. Benz et al. reviewed a total of 166 patients with CBE who underwent AC and 17 (10%) patients underwent a re-augmentation. The length of the bowel used for AC was predictive of the need for re-augmentation. In the re-augmentation cohort, the mean amount of bowel used during the first AC procedure was 12 cm compared to the mean amount of bowel used for non re-augmentations which was 20.8 cm. There is also a need to widely open the bladder to minimize the risk of postoperative hourglass deformity contributing to poor drainage and persistent abnormal bladder storage characteristics. Bladder perforation is once again the most feared complication of AC and in large series has been reported to occur 5–10% in large clinical series of patients with CBE and other diagnoses [99–101]. Detubularization and retubularization are useful for minimizing the risk of bladder perforation [102]. The most commonly reported need for additional surgery after AC is the presence of bladder calculi and occurs in 15–30% of patients [102–105] There is a high recurrence rate observed in patients with AC that initially developed a stone-acquiring second bladder calculi within a short period of time of their first occurrence. Recurrence of the bladder stone in the AC patient was independent of the method of removal and found to be similar for both open or endoscopic extraction [106, 107].

Continent Urinary Diversion

In the first half of the twentieth century, standard care of the CBE patients was not predicated on bladder preservation as closure and functional use of the exstrophic bladder was met with poor success rates [108, 109]. Urinary diversion, with cystectomy, was near universal and this frequently involved urorectal anastomosis for CBE patients as first described by Simon in 1852 [110]. Coffey in 1930 refined the ureteral anastomosis technique to reduce the risk of reflux and ureterosigmoidostomy was pursued as a standard of care for CBE patients [111]. The ureterosigmoidostomy was accompanied by a high incidence of metabolic acidosis and intestinal dysfunction. This was noted in patients who underwent ureterosigmoidostomy with extended follow-up and improved survival, an increased risk of colorectal carcinoma which dampened the enthusiasm for this technique [112–115]. At the same time as the initial reports describing neoplastic complications following ureterosigmoidostomy became more published, Eugene Bricker popularized the ileal conduit as an incontinent form of urinary diversion—the so-called "Bricker Bladder" [116]

To overcome the disadvantages of the classical ureterosigmoidostomy and reduce the number of postoperative upper urinary tract complications as well as to improve the continence rates, Fisch and Hohenfellner introduced the rectum-sigma pouch (Mainz Pouch II), which transformed the high-pressure segment of the rectosigmoid into a low-pressure reservoir by detubularization and reconfiguration [117]. Fixation of the rectosigmoid junction at the promontory as well as parallel ureteral implantations guarantee a straight ureteral path and prevent kinking and subsequent obstruction. The antimesenteric opening of the bowel creates a low-pressure reservoir, which is expected to be essential for good day and night continence and confers advantages for the upper urinary tract. The group from Mainz described their technique for minimizing the upper tract complications with antireflux ureteral reimplantation whether the ureter was normal caliber or dilated [118]. D'elia et al. utilized the Mainz II pouch in 123 patients over 10 years (n = 26 with EEC) with reported continence rates day and night of 97% and 95%, respectively [119]. 70% of the patients were on alkalinizing oral medications to address subclinical acidosis seen on blood gas to prevent the development of clinical hyperchloremic acidosis. Mingin et al. [17] described five patients with bladder exstrophy who underwent the Mainz pouch II procedure between 1996 and 1998 to create a rectosigmoid pouch, allowing urine to drain into and be eliminated via the rectum [120]. Three patients required oral sodium bicarbonate to correct metabolic acidosis, but upper tracts remained nondilated, all patients were continent during daytime and nighttime, and there were no episodes of pyelonephritis during follow-up, which was between about 1 and 3 years.

Despite the surgical and technical advances for the modern staged reconstruction of the bladder involving the preservation of the bladder early in life, there is a subset of CBE patients where the bladder is not deemed a suitable substrate for reconstruction utilizing many of the lower urinary tract reconstruction previously discussed in this chapter such as BNR, CCC, and AC. Cystectomy of the exstrophic bladder is rarely performed in contemporary practice where the modern staged repair is the preferred surgical philosophy. Ko et al. described the Johns Hopkins experience in 18 patients of whom (n = 15 with CBE), six were performed primarily with diversion and twelve were performed secondarily. Of the patients with primary cystectomy this occurred at age ranges of 1–9 years due to what authors state were "small, fibrotic, noncompliant, polyp-covered bladders" of poor quality unsuitable for immediate closure [121]. Bladder template size and tissue quality were followed in these patients before determining that they were "unsuitable for closure." [121] The authors concluded from this series and their extensive experience that cystectomy should be considered in select CBE patients where the bladder template is of inadequate size or of too poor quality to permit primary closure, patients with low bladder capacity after prior closure either due to inadequate growth or loss of capacity, particularly at the time when a continence procedure is being considered.

When rectal diversion is not pursued an incontinent conduit with ileum or colon into abdominal wall stomal appliance has been employed. The relative simplicity of the procedure compared to continent reconstructive techniques has been offset by the long-term complications from a urostomy stoma (retraction/stenosis) as well as ureterointestinal anastomotic complications. Deterioration of the upper urinary tract and renal function, calculi formation, and stomal stenosis are observed as late complications at rates of 50–86% with ileal conduits in pediatric patients [122, 123]. With ileum, there is typically a refluxing ureteral anastomosis while colon affords the opportunity of non-refluxing ureterocolic anastomosis. The group from Mainz reported on 105 pediatric patients (n = 16 CBE) with colonic conduit with non-refluxing ureteral anastomosis with a mean follow-up of 16 years in 84 patients [124]. Early and late stenosis at the ureterocolic anastomosis and stomal stenosis occurred in 7.6 and 15.5% of the cases, respectively. Eight kidneys without function after recurrent pyelonephritis, calculi, or stenosis at the ureterocolic anastomosis were removed during follow-up. A total of 31 patients had complications during follow-up and 18 underwent conversion to continent urinary diversion.

When the use of closed continent urinary diversion is preferred or selected over a conduit, and the bladder deemed unusable, there are various continent urinary reservoirs (CURs) that have been described in the literature [82, 87, 125–128]. As with AC, the creation of CUR is predicated on detubularized and reconfigured bowel segment with typical nonrefluxing ureteroenteric anastomosis. The CUR relies upon a continent catheterizable efferent limb created from a variety of substrates such as in situ appendix, tapered ileum, or reconfigured bowel. The appendiceal lumen can influence the maximal diameter of the catheter used for drainage.

Wiesner et al. retrospectively compared the intussuscepted ileal nipple and in situ, submucosally embedded appendix as continence mechanisms in 400 patients who underwent cutaneous ileocecal pouch (Mainz pouch I) [129]. Continence mechanisms were nearly equal between the two techniques. 36% of the entire cohort required intervention for a stomal complication with a higher rate of stomal stenosis seen (32% v 17%) in an in situ, submucosally embedded appendix compared to intussuscepted ileal nipple, most likely due to the smaller diameter of the appendix. However, stone complication was seen in 20% of the ileal nipple group compared to 10% in the appendiceal group likely related to the use of metal staples to create the intussuscepted ileal nipple. Continence rates of the two outlets were very good (82% in ileal and 93% for appendix). The complications associated with CUR increase with increased follow-up and are not dissimilar to that of AC; such as reservoir calculi, reservoir perforation, metabolic disturbances, and gastrointestinal [130].

As long-term follow-up of reconstructive procedures in CBE patients such as conduits, AC, or CUR have revealed a considerable complication rate; interest in ureterosigmoidostomy as a simple and appliance-free technique of continent urinary diversion has rekindled. Whether bladder reconstruction techniques performed for continence that preserves the exstrophy bladder, which frequently are dependent on CIC, are superior to the rectal urinary diversion which can be emptied voluntarily via the natural rectal sphincter and is performed at a single operation, will continue to be the subject of much controversy and discussion over time.

References

1. Ellison JS, Shnorhavorian M, Willihnganz-Lawson K, Grady R, Merguerian PA. A critical appraisal of continence in bladder exstrophy: long-term outcomes of the complete primary repair. J Pediatr Urol. 2016;12(4):205.e1–7.
2. Hammouda HM, Shahat AA, Oyoun NA, Safwat AS, Elderwy AA, Elgammal MA. Long term evaluation of continence after complete primary bladder exstrophy repair. J Pediatr Urol. 2023;19(6):696.e1–6.
3. Maruf M, Manyevitch R, Michaud J, Jayman J, Kasprenski M, Zaman MH, Benz K, Eldridge M, Trock B, Harris KT, Wu WJ, Di Carlo HN, Gearhart JP. Urinary continence outcomes in classic bladder Exstrophy: a long-term perspective. J Urol. 2020;203(1):200–5.
4. Shaw MB, Rink RC, Kaefer M, Cain MP, Casale AJ. Continence and classic bladder exstrophy treated with staged repair. J Urol. 2004;172(4 Pt 1):1450–3.
5. Taskinen S, Suominen JS, Mattila AK. Health-related quality of life and mental health in adolescents and adults operated for bladder Exstrophy and Epispadias. Urology. 2015;85(6):1515–9.
6. Diseth TH, Bjordal R, Schultz A, Stange M, Emblem R. Somatic function, mental health and psychosocial functioning in 22 adolescents with bladder exstrophy and epispadias. J Urol. 1998;159(5):1684–90.
7. Weiss DA, Shukla AR, Borer JG, Sack BS, Kryger JV, Roth EB, Groth TW, Frazier JR, Mitchell ME, Canning DA. Evaluation of outcomes following complete primary repair of bladder exstrophy at three individual sites prior to the establishment of a multi-institutional collaborative model. J Pediatr Urol. 2020;16(4):435.e1–6.

8. Szymanski KM, Fuchs M, Mcleod D, Rosoklija I, Strine AC, VanderBrink B, Whittam B, Yerkes E, Gargollo PC, Pediatric Urology Midwest Alliance (PUMA). Probability of bladder augmentation, diversion and clean intermittent catheterization in classic bladder Exstrophy: a 36-year, multi-institutional, retrospective cohort study. J Urol. 2019;202(6):1256–62.
9. Szymanski KM, Kaefer M, Fossum M, Kalfa N, Herbst KW, Braga LH, Cascio S, Garriboli M, Nelson CP, Nieuwhoff-Leppink A, Bagli D, Harper L, ESPU Research Committee. What are validated questionnaires and which ones measure quality of life? J Pediatr Urol. 2023;19(4):469–70.
10. Albrecht GL, Devlieger PJ. The disability paradox: high quality of life against all odds. Soc Sci Med. 1999;48:977–88.
11. Inouye BM, Shah BB, Massanyi EZ, Di Carlo HN, Kern AJ, Tourchi A, Baradaran N, Stewart D, Gearhart JP. Urologic complications of major genitourinary reconstruction in the exstrophy-epispadias complex. J Pediatr Urol. 2014;10(4):680–7.
12. Gearhart JP, Mathews R. Exstrophy-epispadias complex. In: Wein AJ, Kavoussi LR, Partin AW, Peters CA, editors. Campbell-Walsh urology. 11th ed. Philadelphia: Elsevier; 2016. p. 3182–234.
13. Chan DY, Jeffs RD, Gearhart JP. Determinants of continence in the bladder exstrophy population: predictors of success? Urology. 2001;57(4):774–7.
14. Khandge P, Morrill CC, Wu WJ, Harris KT, Haffar A, Maruf M, Patel HD, Di Carlo HN, Gearhart JP. Achieving goal capacity for continence surgery: a cumulative event analysis of bladder exstrophy patients. J Pediatr Urol. 2023;19(5):563.e1–8.
15. Dean GE, Kirsch AJ, Packer MG, Scherz HC, Zaontz MR. Antegrade and retrograde endoscopic dextranomer/hyaluronic Acid bladder neck bulking for pediatric incontinence. J Urol. 2007;178(2):652–5.
16. Vorstman B, Lockhart J, Kaufman MR, Politano V. Polytetrafluoroethylene injection for urinary incontinence in children. J Urol. 1985;133:248–50.
17. Dyer L, Franco I, Firlit CF, Reda EF, Levitt SB, Palmer LS. Endoscopic injection of bulking agents in children with incontinence: dextranomer/hyaluronic acid copolymer versus polytetrafluoroethylene. J Urol. 2007;178(4 Pt 2):1628–31.
18. Malizia AA, Reiman HM, Myers RP, et al. Migration and granulomatous reaction after periurethral injection of Polytef (Teflon). JAMA. 1984;251:3277–81.
19. Capozza N, Caione P, De Gennaro M, Nappo S, Patricolo M. Endoscopic treatment of vesicoureteric reflux and urinary incontinence: technical problems in the paediatric patient. Br J Urol. 1995;75(4):538–42.
20. Caione P, Lais A, de Gennaro M, Capozza N. Glutaraldehyde cross-linked bovine collagen in exstrophy/epispadias complex. J Urol. 1993;150:631–3.
21. Bomalaski MD, Bloom DA, McGuire EJ, Panzl A. Glutaraldehyde cross-linked collagen in the treatment of urinary incontinence in children. J Urol. 1996;155(2):699–702.
22. Ben-Chaim J, Jeffs RD, Peppas DS, Gearhart JP. Submucosal bladder neck injections of glutaraldehyde cross-linked bovine collagen for the treatment of urinary incontinence in patients with the exstrophy/epispadias complex. J Urol. 1995;154(2 Pt 2):862–4.
23. Burki T, Hamid R, Ransley PG, Mushtaq I, Duffy PG. Injectable polydimethylsiloxane for treating incontinence in children with the exstrophy-epispadias complex: long-term results. BJU Int. 2006;98:849–53.
24. Henly DR, Barrett DM, Weiland TL, O'Connor MK, Malizia AA, Wein AJ. Particulate silicone for use in periurethral injections: local tissue effects and search for migration. J Urol. 1995;153(6):2039–43.
25. Caione P, Capozza N. Endoscopic treatment of urinary incontinence in pediatric patients: 2-year experience with dextranomer/hyaluronic acid copolymer. J Urol. 2002;168(4 Pt 2):1868–71.
26. Lottmann HB, Margaryan M, Bernuy M, Rouffet MJ, Bau MO, El-Ghoneimi A, Aigrain Y, Stenberg A, Läckgren G. The effect of endoscopic injections of dextranomer based implants on continence and bladder capacity: a prospective study of 31 patients. J Urol. 2002;168(4 Pt 2):1863–7.

27. Shah BB, Massanyi EZ, Dicarlo H, Shear D, Kern A, Baradaran N, Gearhart JP. Role of urethral bulking agents in epispadias-exstrophy complex patients. J Pediatr Urol. 2014;10(1):176–80.
28. Misseri R, Casale AJ, Cain MP, Rink RC. Alternative uses of dextranomer/hyaluronic acid copolymer: the efficacy of bladder neck injection for urinary incontinence. J Urol. 2005;174(4 Pt 2):1691–3.
29. Stenberg A, Larsson E, Lindholm A, Ronneus B, Stenberg A, Läckgren G. Injectable dextranomer-based implant: histopathology, volume changes and DNA-analysis. Scand J Urol Nephrol. 1999;33(6):355–61.
30. Fiorenza V, Hukkinen M, Alova I, Clermidi P, Broch A, Botto N, Blanc T, Lottmann HB. Dextranomer endoscopic injections for the treatment of urinary incontinence in bladder Exstrophy-epispadias complex. J Urol. 2023;209(3):591–9.
31. Alova I, Margaryan M, Verkarre V, Bernuy M, Lortat Jacob S, Lottmann HB. Outcome of continence procedures after failed endoscopic treatment with dextranomer-based implants (DEFLUX®). J Pediatr Urol. 2012;8(1):40–6.
32. Lottmann HB, Margaryan M, Lortat-Jacob S, Bernuy M, Läckgren G. Long-term effects of dextranomer endoscopic injections for the treatment of urinary incontinence: an update of a prospective study of 61 patients. J Urol. 2006;176(4 Pt 2):1762–6.
33. Barrett D, Furlow W. Incontinence, intermittent self catheterization and the artificial genitourinary sphincter. J Urol. 1984;132:268–9.
34. Light JK, Scott FB. Treatment of the epispadias-exstrophy complex with the AS792 artificial urinary sphincter. J Urol. 1983;129(4):738–40.
35. Decter RM, Roth DR, Fishman IJ, Shabsigh R, Scott FB, Gonzales ET. Use of the AS800 device in exstrophy and epispadias. J Urol. 1988;140:1202–3.
36. Ruiz E, Puigdevall J, Moldes J, Lobos P, Boer M, Ithurralde J, Escalante J, de Badiola F. 14 years of experience with the artificial urinary sphincter in children and adolescents without spina bifida. J Urol. 2006;176(4 Pt 2):1821–5.
37. Hafez AT, McLorie G, Bägli D, Khoury A. A single-centre long-term outcome analysis of artificial urinary sphincter placement in children. BJU Int. 2002;89(1):82–5.
38. Castera R, Podestá ML, Ruarte A, Herrera M, Medel R. 10-Year experience with artificial urinary sphincter in children and adolescents. J Urol. 2001;165(6 Pt 2):2373–6.
39. Levesque PE, Bauer SB, Atala A, Zurakowski D, Colodny A, Peters C, Retik AB. Ten-year experience with the artificial urinary sphincter in children. J Urol. 1996;156(2 Pt 2):625–8.
40. Bosco P, Bauer S, Colodny A, Mandell J, Retik A. The long-term results of artificial sphincters in children. J Urol. 1991;146:396–9.
41. Herndon CD, Rink RC, Shaw MB, Simmons GR, Cain MP, Kaefer M, Casale AJ. The Indiana experience with artificial urinary sphincters in children and young adults. J Urol. 2003;169(2):650–4.
42. Roth D, Vyas P, Kroovand R, Perlmutter A. Urinary tract deterioration associated with the artificial urinary sphincter. J Urol. 1986;135:528–30.
43. Kronner K, Rink R, Simmons G, Kropp BP, Casale AJ, Cain MP. Artificial urinary sphincter in the treatment of urinary incontinence: preoperative urodynamics do not predict the need for future bladder augmentation. J Urol. 1998;160:1093–5.
44. Bauer S, Reda E, Colodny A, Retik A. Detrusor instability: a delayed complication in association with the artificial sphincter. J Urol. 1986;135:1212–5.
45. Light K, Pietro T. Alteration in detrusor behavior and the effect on renal function following insertion of the artificial urinary sphincter. J Urol. 1986;136:632–5.
46. Light J, Lapin S, Vohra S. Combined use of bowel and the artificial urinary sphincter in reconstruction of the lower urinary tract: infectious complications. J Urol. 1995;153:331–3.
47. Young H. An operation for the cure of incontinence associated with epispadias. J Urol. 1922;7:1–32.
48. Dees J. Congenital epispadias with incontinence. J Urol. 1949;62:513–22.
49. Leadbetter G Jr. Surgical correction of total urinary incontinence. J Urol. 1964;91:261–4.
50. Purves T, Novak T, King J, Gearhart JP. Modified Young-Dees-Leadbetter bladder neck reconstruction after exstrophy repair. J Urol. 2009;182(4 Suppl):1813–7.

51. Di Carlo HN, Manyevitch R, Wu WJ, Maruf M, Michaud J, Friedlander D, Gearhart JP. Continence after BNR in the complete repair of bladder exstrophy (CPRE): a single institution expanded experience. J Pediatr Urol. 2020;16(4):433.e1–6.
52. Surer I, Baker LA, Jeffs RD, Gearhart JP. Modified Young-Dees-Leadbetter bladder neck reconstruction in patients with successful primary bladder closure elsewhere: a single institution experience. J Urol. 2001;165(6 Pt 2):2438–40.
53. Kasprenski M, Benz K, Jayman J, Lue K, Maruf M, Baumgartner T, Gearhart JP. Combined bladder neck reconstruction and continent stoma creation as a suitable alternative for continence in bladder Exstrophy: a preliminary report. Urology. 2018;119:133–6.
54. McMahon DR, Cain MP, Husmann DA, Kramer SA. Vesical neck reconstruction in patients with the exstrophy-epispadias complex. J Urol. 1996;155(4):1411–3.
55. Burki T, Hamid R, Duffy P, Ransley P, Wilcox D, Mushtaq I. Long-term followup of patients after redo bladder neck reconstruction for bladder exstrophy complex. J Urol. 2006;176(3):1138–41.
56. Capolicchio G, McLorie GA, Farhat W, Merguerian PA, Bägli DJ, Khoury AE. A population based analysis of continence outcomes and bladder exstrophy. J Urol. 2001;165(6 Pt 2):2418–21.
57. Yerkes EB, Adams MC, Rink RC, Pope JC IV, Brock JW 3rd. How well do patients with exstrophy actually void? J Urol. 2000;164(3 Pt 2):1044–7.
58. Lloyd JC, Spano SM, Ross SS, Wiener JS, Routh JC. How dry is dry? A review of definitions of continence in the contemporary exstrophy/epispadias literature. J Urol. 2012;188(5):1900–4.
59. Di Carlo HN, Maruf M, Jayman J, Benz K, Kasprenski M, Gearhart JP. The inadequate bladder template: its effect on outcomes in classic bladder exstrophy. J Pediatr Urol. 2018;14(5):427.e1e7.
60. Ferrer FA, Tadros YE, Gearhart J. Modified Young-Dees-Leadbetter bladder neck reconstruction: new concept about old ideas. Urology. 2001;58:791–6.
61. Baird AD, Nelson CP, Gearhart JP. Modern staged repair of bladder exstrophy: a contemporary series. J Pediatr Urol. 2007;3:311.
62. Mollard P. Bladder reconstruction in exstrophy. J Urol. 1980;124:525–9.
63. Mouriquand PD, Bubanj T, Feyaerts A, Jandric M, Timsit M, Mollard P, Mure PY, Basset T. Long-term term results of bladder neck reconstruction for incontinence in children with classical bladder exstrophy or incontinent epispadias. BJU Int. 2003;92(9):997–1001.
64. Koff SA. A technique for bladder neck reconstruction in exstrophy: the cinch. J Urol. 1990;144(2 Pt 2):546–9.
65. Hanna MK. Bladder neck sphincteroplasty: the cinch procedure. Atlas Urol Clinics NA. 2001;9(1):31–6.
66. Jones J, Mitchell M, Rink R. Improved results using amodification of the Young–Dees–Leadbetter bladder neck repair. Br J Urol. 1993;71:555–61.
67. DeCambre M, Casale P, Grady R, Swartz M, Mitchell M. Modified bladder neck reconstruction in patients with incontinence after staged exstrophy/epispadias closures. J Urol. 2006;176(1):288–91.
68. Hafez AT. Detrusor wraparound for bladder neck reconstruction in cohort of children with bladder exstrophy. Urology. 2011;78(4):881–5.
69. Gershbaum MD, Stock JA, Hanna MK. Gracilis muscle sling for select incontinent "bladder exstrophy cripples". J Urol. 2001;165(6 Pt 2):2422–4.
70. Mingin GC, Youngren K, Stock JA, Hanna MK. The rectus myofascial wrap in the management of urethral sphincter incompetence. BJU Int. 2002;90(6):550–3.
71. Stoeckel W. Uber die verwendung der Musculi Pyramidalis bei der operativen behandlung der incontinentia urinae. Zentrabl Gynakol. 1917;41:11.
72. Khoury AE, Agarwal SK, Bägli D, Merguerian P, McLorie GA. Concomitant modified bladder neck closure and Mitrofanoff urinary diversion. J Urol. 1999;162(5):1746–8.
73. Michaud JE, Ko JS, Lue K, Di Carlo HN, Redett RJ, Gearhart JP. Use of muscle pedicle flaps for failed bladder neck closure in the exstrophy spectrum. J Pediatr Urol. 2016;12(5):289.e1–5.

74. McGrath JS, SP MD. Use of pedicled rectus abdominis muscle flap to protect against fistula formation after bladder neck closure. BJU Int. 2005;95(3):450.
75. Kavanagh A, Afshar K, Scott H, AE MN. Bladder neck closure in conjunction with enterocystoplasty and Mitrofanoff diversion for complex incontinence: closing the door for good. J Urol. 2012;188(4 Suppl):1561–5.
76. De Troyer B, Van Laecke E, Groen LA, Everaert K, Hoebeke P. A comparative study between continent diversion and bladder neck closure versus continent diversion and bladder neck reconstruction in children. J Pediatr Urol. 2011;7(2):209–12.
77. Macedo A Jr, Ottoni SL, Garrone G, Mattos RM, Leal da Cruz M. The search for continence in bladder exstrophy: bladder neck transection and Macedo catheterizable reservoir to augment the native bladder. J Pediatr Urol. 2020;16(4):506–7.
78. Nguyen HT, Baskin LS. The outcome of bladder neck closure in children with severe urinary incontinence. J Urol. 2003;169(3):1114–6.
79. Novak TE, Salmasi AH, Lakshmanan Y, Mathews RI, Gearhart JP. Bladder neck transection for intractable pediatric urinary incontinence. J Urol. 2009;181(1):310–4.
80. Landau EH, Gofrit ON, Pode D, Jurim O, Shenfeld OZ, Duvdevani M, Gross EM, Merguerian PA, Katz R. Bladder neck closure in children: a decade of followup. J Urol. 2009;182(4 Suppl):1797–801.
81. Mitrofanoff P. Trans- appendicular continent cystostomy in the management of the neurogenic bladder. Chir Pediatr. 1980;21(4):297–305.
82. Duckett JW, Snyder HM 3rd. Use of the Mitrofanoff principle in urinary reconstruction. Urol Clin North Am. 1986;13(2):271–4.
83. VanderBrink BA, Kaefer M, Cain MP, Meldrum KK, Misseri R, Rink RC. Extravesical implantation of a continent catheterizable channel. J Urol. 2011;185(6 Suppl):2572–5.
84. Keating MA, Kropp BP, Adams MC, Patil UB, Rink RC. Seromuscular trough modification in construction of continent urinary stomas. J Urol. 1993;150(2 Pt 2):734–6.
85. Baradaran N, Stec AA, Gupta A, Keating MA, Gearhart JP. Using a serosal trough for fashioning a continent catheterizable stoma: technique and outcomes. BJU Int. 2013;111(5):828–33.
86. Monti PR, Lara RC, Dutra MA, de Carvalho JR. New techniques for construction of efferent conduits based on the Mitrofanoff principle. Urology. 1997;49(1):112–5.
87. Macedo A Jr, Srougi M. A continent catheterizable ileum-based reservoir. BJU Int. 2000;85(1):160–2.
88. Ulman I, Ergün O, Avanoğlu A, Gökdemir A. The place of Mitrofanoff neourethra in the repair of exstrophy-epispadias complex. Eur J Pediatr Surg. 1998;8(6):352–4.
89. Liard A, Séguier-Lipszyc E, Mathiot A, Mitrofanoff P. The Mitrofanoff procedure: 20 years later. J Urol. 2001;165(6 Pt 2):2394–8.
90. Leslie B, Lorenzo AJ, Moore K, Farhat WA, Bägli DJ, Pippi Salle JL. Long-term followup and time to event outcome analysis of continent catheterizable channels. J Urol. 2011;185(6):2298–302.
91. Szymanski KM, Whittam B, Misseri R, Flack CK, Hubert KC, Kaefer M, Rink RC, Cain MP. Long-term outcomes of catheterizable continent urinary channels: what do you use, where you put it, and does it matter? J Pediatr Urol. 2015;11(4):210.e1–7.
92. Jacobson DL, Thomas JC, Pope J 4th, Tanaka ST, Clayton DB, Brock JW 3rd, Adams MC. Update on continent Catheterizable channels and the timing of their complications. J Urol. 2017;197(3 Pt 2):871–6.
93. Casey JT, Zhang M, Chan KH, Szymanski KM, Judge B, Whittam B, Kaefer M, Misseri R, Rink RC, Cain MP. Does endoscopy of difficult to catheterize channels spare some patients from formal open revision? J Pediatr Urol. 2016;12(4):248.e1–6.
94. Roth CC, Donovan BO, Tonkin JB, Klein JC, Frimberger D, Kropp BP. Endoscopic injection of submucosal bulking agents for the management of incontinent catheterizable channels. J Pediatr Urol. 2009;5(4):265–8.
95. Di Benedetto V, Beseghi U, Bagnara V, Monfort G. The use of gastrocystoplasty in patients with bladder exstrophy. Pediatr Surg Int. 1996;11(4):252–5.

96. Gearhart JP, Jeffs RD. Augmentation cystoplasty in the failed exstrophy reconstruction. J Urol. 1988;139(4):790–3.
97. Cervellione RM, Bianchi A, Fishwick J, Gaskell SL, Dickson AP. Salvage procedures to achieve continence after failed bladder exstrophy repair. J Urol. 2008;179(1):304–6.
98. Benz KS, Jayman J, Doersch K, Maruf M, Baumgartner T, Kasprenski M, Gearhart JP. Bladder re-augmentation in classic bladder exstrophy: risk factors and prevention. Urology. 2018;115:157–61.
99. DeFoor W, Tackett L, Minevich E, Wacksman J, Sheldon C. Risk factors for spontaneous bladder perforation after augmentation cystoplasty. Urology. 2003;62(4):737–41.
100. Metcalfe PD, Casale AJ, Kaefer MA, Misseri R, Dussinger AM, Meldrum KK, Cain MP, Rink RC. Spontaneous bladder perforations: a report of 500 augmentations in children and analysis of risk. J Urol. 2006;175(4):1466–70.
101. Elder JS, Snyder HM, Hulbert WC, Duckett JW. Perforation of the augmented bladder in patients undergoing clean intermittent catheterization. J Urol. 1988;140:1159–62.
102. Szymanski KM, Misseri R, Whittam B, Hollowell N, Hardacker RE, Swenson CR, Kaefer M, Rink RC, Cain MP. Additional surgeries after bladder augmentation in patients with Spina bifida in the 21st century. J Urol. 2020;203(6):1207–13.
103. Kaefer M, Hendren WH, Bauer SB, Goldenblatt P, Peters CA, Atala A, Retik AB. Reservoir calculi: a comparison of reservoirs constructed from stomach and other enteric segments. J Urol. 1998;160(6 Pt 1):2187–90.
104. Palmer L, Franco L, Kogan S, Rda E, Gill B, Levitt S. Urolithiasis in children following augmenation cystoplasty. J Urol. 1993;150:726–9.
105. DeFoor W, Minevich E, Reddy P, et al. Bladder calculi after augmentation cystoplasty; risk factors and prevention strategies. J Urol. 2004;172:1964–6.
106. Szymanski K, Misseri R, Whittam B, et al. Cutting for stone in augmented bladders: what is the risk of recurrence and is it impacted by treatment modality. J Urol. 2014;191:1375–80.
107. Roberts W, Gearhart JP. Time to recurrent stone formation in patients with bladder or continent reservoir reconstruction: fragmentation versus intact extraction. J Urol. 2004;172:1706–8.
108. Ladd WE, Lanman TH. Exstrophy of the bladder. N Engl J Med. 1937;216:637.
109. Higgins CC. Exstrophy of the bladder, a review of one hundred and fifty-six cases. JAMA. 1959;171:1922.
110. Simon J. Ectopia vesicae (absence of the anterior walls of the bladder and pubis abdominal parietis); operation for directing the orifices of the ureters into the rectum; temporary success; subsequent death; autopsy. Lancet. 1852;60:568.
111. Coffey RC. Production of aseptic ureteroenterostomy by a suture transfixing the ureteral wall and the intestinal mucosa. JAMA. 1930;94:1748.
112. Clarke BG, Leadbetter WF. Ureterosigmoidostomy: collective review of results in 2897 reported cases. J Urol. 1955;73:999–1008.
113. Jacobs A, Stirling WB. The late results of ureterocolic anastomosis. Br J Urol. 1952;24:259–90.
114. Sooriyaarachchi GS, PP JROC. Neoplasms of the large bowel following ureterosigmoidostomy. Arch Surg. 1977;112:1174.
115. Spence HM, Hoffmann WW, Fosmire GP. Tumours of the colon as a late complication of ureterosigmoidostomy for exstrophy of the bladder. Brit J Urol. 1979;51:446.
116. Bricker EM. Bladder substitution after pelvic evisceration. Surg Clin N Am. 1950;30:1511–20.
117. Fisch M, Wammack R, Muller SC, Hohenfellner R. The Mainz pouch II (sigma rectum pouch). J Urol. 1993;149(2):258–63.
118. Fisch M, Hohenfellner R. Sigma-rectum pouch (Mainz pouch II). BJU Int. 2007;99(4):945–60.
119. D'elia G, Pahernik S, Fisch M, Hohenfellner R, Thüroff JW. Mainz Pouch II technique: 10 years' experience. BJU Int. 2004;93(7):1037–42.
120. Mingin GC, Stock JA, Hanna MK. The Mainz II pouch: experience in 5 patients with bladder exstrophy. J Urol. 1999;162(3 Pt 1):846–8.

121. Ko JS, Lue K, Friedlander D, Baumgartner T, Stuhldreher P, DiCarlo HN, Gearhart JP. Cystectomy in the pediatric exstrophy population: indications and outcomes. Urology. 2018;116:168–71.
122. Shapiro SR, Lebowitz R, Colodny AH. Fate of 90 children with ileal conduit urinary diversion a decade later: analysis of complications, pyelography, renal function and bacteriology. J Urol. 1975;114(2):289–95.
123. Schwarz GR, Jeffs RD. Ileal conduit urinary diversion in children: computer analysis of follow-up from 2 to 16 years. J Urol. 1975;114(2):285–8.
124. Stein R, Fisch M, Stöckle M, Demirkesen O, Hohenfellner R. Colonic conduit in children: protection of the upper urinary tract 16 years later? J Urol. 1996;156(3):1146–50.
125. Rowland RG, Mitchell ME, Bihrle R. The cecoileal continent urinary reservoir. World J Urol. 1985;3:185–90.
126. Bissada NK, Abdallah MM, Aaronson I, Hammouda HM. Continent cutaneous urinary diversion in children: experience with Charleston pouch I. J Urol. 2007;177(1):307–10.
127. Kaefer M, Tobin MS, Hendren WH, Bauer S, Peters CA, Atala A, Colodny AH, Mandell J, Retik AB. Continent urinary diversion: the Children's Hospital experience. J Urol. 1997;157:1394–9.
128. Chowdhary SK, Rao KL, Kandpal DK, Sibal A, Srivastava RN. Indiana pouch in children: a 15-year experience. J Pediatr Urol. 2014;10:911–6.
129. Wiesner C, Stein R, Pahernik S, Hähn K, Melchior SW, Thüroff JW. Long-term followup of the intussuscepted ileal nipple and the in situ, submucosally embedded appendix as continence mechanisms of continent urinary diverision with the cutaneous ileocecal pouch (Mainz pouch I). J Urol. 2006;176(1):155–9.
130. Novak TE, Salmasi AH, Mathews RI, Lakshmanan Y, Gearhart JP. Complications of complex lower urinary tract reconstruction in patients with neurogenic versus nonneurogenic bladder–is there a difference? J Urol. 2008;180(6):2629–34.

22 Urinary Reconstruction for Bladder Exstrophy in the Developing World: Special Consideration and Technique

Sudipta Sen, Pavai Arunachalam, and Ravi Kishore Barla

Abbreviations

BA	Bladder augmentation
BNC	Bladder neck closure
CIC	Clean intermittent catheterization
RAM	Rectus Abdominis Muscle flap
YDL	Young-Dees-Leadbetter bladder neck plasty

Introduction

This article is based on our experience in managing exstrophy over 40 years in two large tertiary care hospitals in India. We do not intend to sum up the published literature on the subject with its wide variation in the methods of management and the results obtained thereby. Results obtained with regard to continent voluntary voiding are stressed in the majority of published literature, including textbook chapters. However, the management of "failed exstrophy" is not given sufficient importance even though these comprise a large proportion of children plagued by dehisced repairs, uncertain continence, urinary infection, upper tract deterioration, calculi,

S. Sen (✉)
Department of Pediatric Surgery, PSG IMS&R, Coimbatore, Tamil Nadu, India

Department of Pediatric Surgery, CMC Hospital, Vellore, Tamil Nadu, India

P. Arunachalam
Department of Pediatric Surgery, PSG IMS&R, Coimbatore, Tamil Nadu, India

R. K. Barla
Department of Pediatric Surgery, CMC Hospital, Vellore, Tamil Nadu, India

A. R. Shukla, R. S. Joshi (eds.), *Bladder Exstrophy and Epispadias*,
https://doi.org/10.1007/978-3-031-91238-2_22

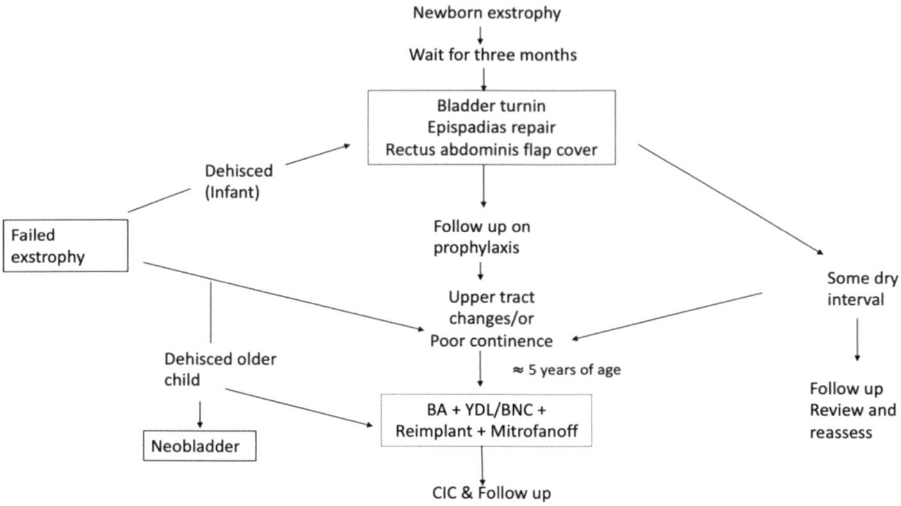

Fig. 22.1 Management protocol for exstrophy

and male sexual inadequacy. Added to this are the financial and psychological burdens of repeated surgery with less-than-optimal results. These issues have forced us to shift the goalpost from "continence and voluntary voiding" to "dryness on clean intermittent catheterization (CIC) with protected upper tracts" as the essential and more realistic goal in exstrophy management. The patients who presented with exstrophy (not including the patients referred after failed surgery) were mangaed in two stages by us. In infancy, exstrophy epispadias repair was completed and around five years of age, they undergo bladder augmention, bladder neck plasty, ureteric reimplant and appendicular Mitrofanoff for intermittent catheterization. We have developed modifications to the standard techniques of the above repairs, which will be described herein (Fig. 22.1).

Operative Technique

Bladder Turn-In and Epispadias Repair with Rectus Abdominis Muscle Flap (RAM) Cover [1]

An incision is made around the bladder plate and then vertically extended cephalad in the midline until the proposed site of the neo umbilicus. Subcutaneous flaps are reflected bilaterally. On the left side, the subcutaneous dissection is continued until the lateral margin of the left rectus sheath is seen. Any associated inguinal hernia is now corrected. The left anterior rectus sheath is vertically opened in the paramedian position along the medial border of the left rectus muscle. The rectus muscle is then separated off the anterior and posterior rectus sheaths, taking care at the fibrous intersections to avoid damage to the anterior rectus sheath. The rectus muscle at the upper end of the incision is divided. The lower half of the left rectus muscle is mobilized by serially dividing the neurovascular supply entering its lateral aspect. The inferior epigastric vessels are carefully preserved. This results in a flap of the lower rectus abdominis retaining its attachment to the pubic bone and being supplied by the inferior epigastric vessels. This muscle flap is turned across the interpubic defect to cover the repaired bladder.

The retropubic space is now developed bilaterally, and the bladder plate is isolated by dividing its lateral attachments to the pubic bone (inter-symphysial band). In the male, the lowermost attachments to the pubis are left undivided until the epispadias are dissected and corporal neurovascular bundles are visualized. The dome of the bladder is now mobilized by dividing the urachus and the umbilical arteries and separating the peritoneum until the ureteral entry into the back of the bladder is visualized.

Dissection for epispadias correction begins at the penile ventrum. Keeping the neurovascular bundles in view, the bladder and urethral plate are completely separated as a single unit from the corporal bodies and the lower pubic attachments, while keeping the glans attachment intact (Cantwell–Ransley technique) [2]. Bladder closure is now done, leaving ureteric and suprapubic catheters, which are brought out through the bladder dome. The urethra is constructed over an 8 Fr feeding tube. Glansplasty is done. Intercorporeal sutures are placed medial to the neurovascular bundle, in the zone from which the urethral plate had been dissected, thus approximating the corporal bodies dorsal to the reconstructed urethra.

The rectus abdominis muscle (RAM) flap is turned medially over the repaired bladder to bridge the gap between the pubic bones. The cut edge of the rectus flap is sutured to the right pubic bone and right rectus sheath, thus providing anterior support to the repaired bladder. These sutures (2–0 polyglactin) should be of the horizontal mattress type and should incorporate the nearest fibrous intersection of the RAM flap to prevent it from cutting through the muscle of the RAM flap. In addition, the lower margin of the muscle flap is utilized to provide a cover to the penopubic angle by a triangular stitch incorporating the two corporal bodies and the lower edge of the muscle flap (Fig. 22.2).

The opened left rectus sheath is now repaired. At the upper edge of the transposed muscle, both rectus sheaths are anchored to the RAM flap to get a secure abdominal closure. The catheters exiting the bladder dome are brought out through the body of the transposed RAM flap, traverse a subcutaneous course, and exit at the proposed neo-umbilical site. Midline skin closure is made possible because of the mobilized skin flaps. The penile skin closure is performed by a modified Pippi Salle method utilizing an island flap from the ventral penile skin [3].

Catheters are left in double diapers. A child is not immobilized and fed after 6 hours if concomitant augmentation is not done. The urethral catheter is removed after a week.

Ureteric and suprapubic catheters are kept for a period of 3 weeks.

This method of doing away with pubic bone approximation (with or without osteotomy) and bridging the musculo-fascio-skeletal defect in the anterior abdominal wall with the mobilized RAM has given us very satisfactory results.

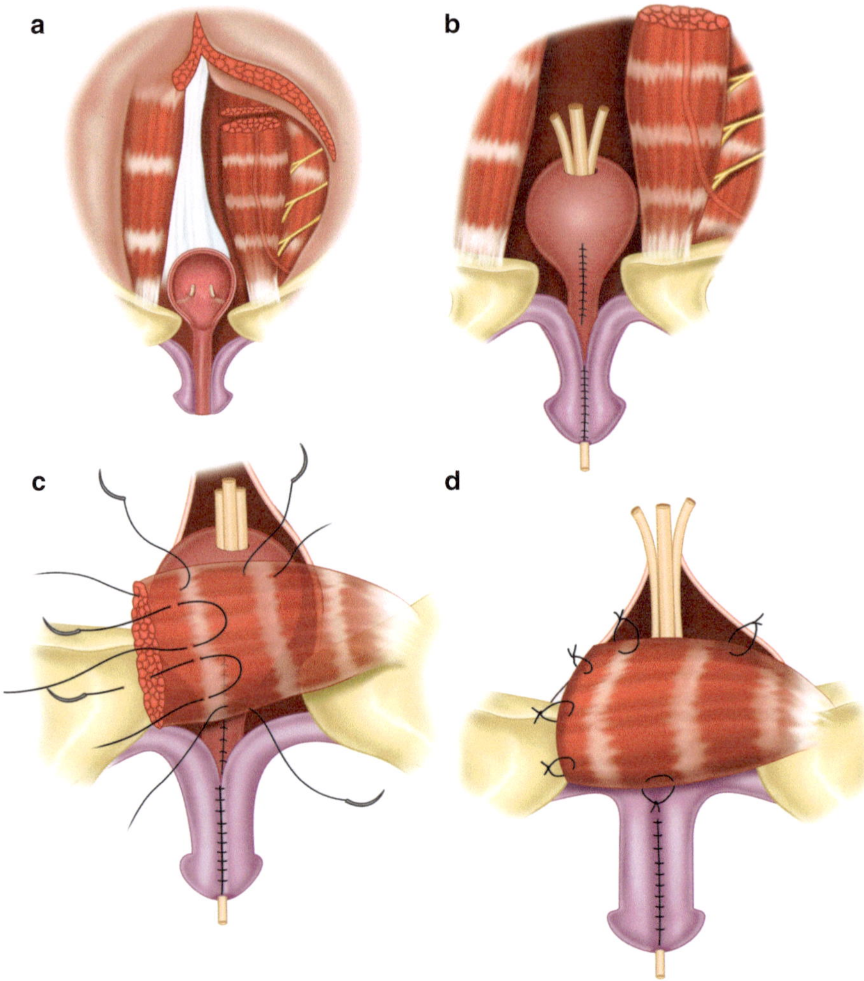

Fig. 22.2 Schematic diagram (**a**–**d**) illustrating repair of exstrophy using RAM flap cover to bridge the inter-pubic gap. The lower half of the left RAM is dissected from within the rectus sheath, dividing the muscle in the mid-abdomen, dividing its lateral neurovascular supply, but retaining its attachment to the pubic bone and supply from the left inferior epigastric vessels. The bladder and urethra are closed as a single unit, and the RAM flap is turned inferior medially to bridge the interpubic gap in front of the repaired bladder. A triangular suture at the lower edge of the RAM flap closes the peno-pubic gap

The operation is simple, with minimal blood loss, free of tension, and does not require any internal or external fixation. We have found it very suitable for a developing country for primary and redo repairs, with concomitant epispadias repair. Bladder augmentation can also be done concomitantly in older children [1] (Fig. 22.3).

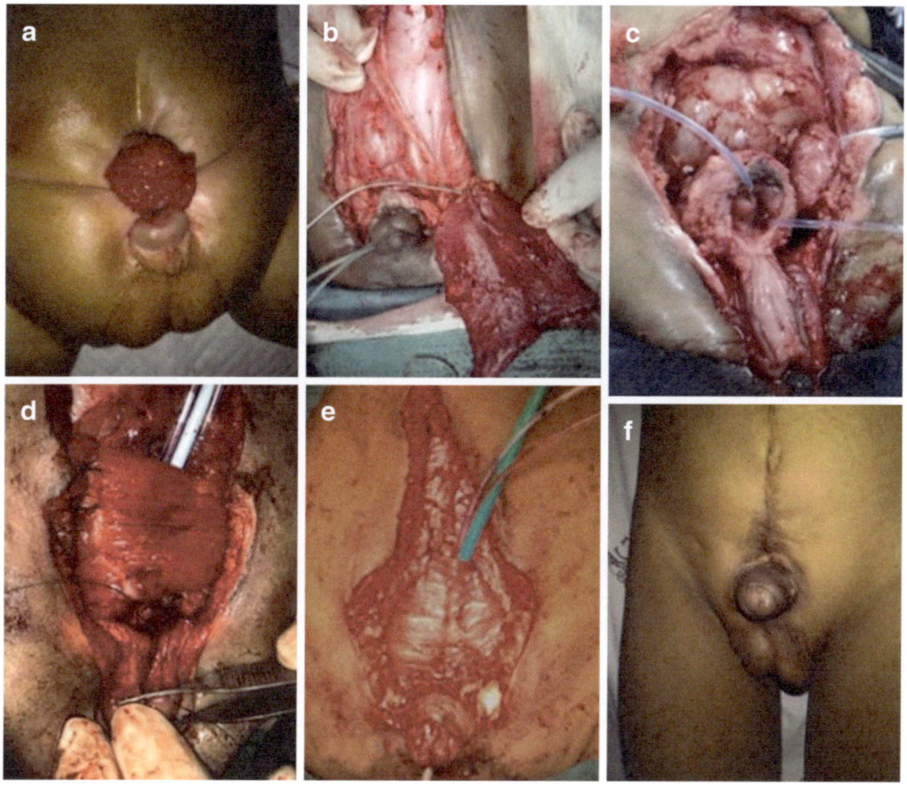

Fig. 22.3 Preoperative (**a**), operative (**b–e**), and follow-up pictures (**f**) of a case of dehisced exstrophy repaired using the RAM flap technique, showing polypoid bladder plate (**a**) lower left rectus abdominis isolated from within the rectus sheath, retaining its pubic attachment and the left inferior epigastric vessels (**b**). The bladder and urethral plate were dissected off their lateral attachments and repaired as a single unit (**c**). The RAM flap is used to bridge the inter-pubic gap, triangular suture buttressing the peno-pubic angle (**d**). Abdominal musculofascial closure completed (**e**)

The Final Reconstruction

The bladder plate in exstrophy, especially after previous failed surgery, is often small and, as such, results in a small-volume bladder. After bladder neck surgery, this small-volume bladder can result in high bladder pressures. This, in addition to the VUR (in exstrophy, VUR is universal), causes renal scarring, HUN, and ultimate renal damage. In addition, dryness is also not achieved. The usual solution to all the above is bladder augmentation. There are, however, several other issues during bladder augmentation for exstrophy. They are as follows:

1. Bladder neck repair is essential to provide dryness. This is usually done as a long YDL plasty. In failed cases with stiff bladder plates, bladder neck closure may be required.

2. Ureters are generally refluxing in the exstrophy-epispadias complex, and ureteric reimplantation will be needed, even if the bladder is being augmented. The safest technique is cephalotrigonal reimplantation, which moves the ureters cephalad, thus avoiding the bladder neck zone.
3. A reliable Mitrofanoff port for easy CIC is essential, as the repaired (even closed) bladder neck is difficult to catheterize. Augmented patients are dependent on CIC.

While ileocystoplasty and colocystoplasty can be used for augmentation in exstrophy, we have devised the ileocecal donut augmentation, which we have found to be very useful in exstrophy. The ileocecal segment has an "in situ" appendix, which is not disconnected for implantation as a Mitrofanoff port, but the reconfigured ileocecal loop as a donut around the appendix provides an effective non-refluxing Mitrofanoff. Thus, appendicular implantation into the already small bladder is not needed. (The small bladder plate has to provide space for YDL and bilateral reimplants.)

The steps of the final reconstruction are detailed under the following headings:

1. YDL bladder neck plasty/bladder neck closure
2. Ureteric reimplantation into the bladder plate/colon segment of the augment
3. Donut bladder augmentation with "in situ" appendicular Mitrofanoff

Young-Dees-Leadbetter Bladder Neck Plasty

The bladder neck area is thoroughly freed from its fibrous attachments to the pelvic bones. This allows the neck to become pliable to enable the YDL plasty. The bladder is opened by a low "smile" incision, which yields the maximum area of the bladder plate for reimplantation and YDL plasty. This is because both the posterior and most of the anterior bladder wall now become the open bladder plate (Fig. 22.4).

The lateral edges of the bladder at the level of the ureteric orifice are cut in a transverse or slightly oblique fashion to meet and encircle the ureteric orifices.

The two parallel vertical incisions are now made only in the mucosa from the level of the ureteric orifice caudal through the trigone into the urethra as far as possible. This outlines a vertical strip of bladder mucosa, which will be tubularized to provide a long urethral channel. The mucosa lateral to the strip is removed to denude the detrusor.

The ureters are mobilized sufficiently via intravesical and extravesical exposure to allow tension-free cephalo-trigonal reimplantation. This moves the ureters away from the bladder outlet. The longitudinal mucosal strip in the trigone and proximal urethra is now tubularized over an 8 Fr catheter. The denuded detrusor on either side is sutured over the tubularized mucosal channel. This completes the YDL bladder neck plasty.

It will be noted that the new bladder neck as well as the bladder plate would have moved cephalad by the above procedure. It is now ready to receive the augmentation (with in-situ Mitrofanoff). The augmentation is sutured onto the bladder plate,

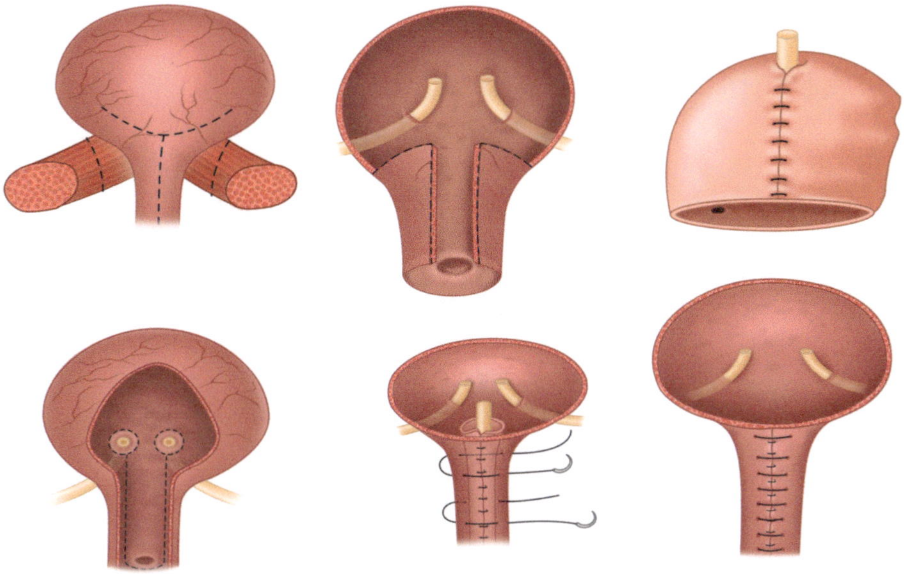

Fig. 22.4 Steps of bladder neck repair (see description below)

which will complete the reconstruction. Herein the donut augmentation is shown. However, ileo- or colocystoplasty with a separately implanted appendix Mitrofanoff is also feasible.

Bladder Neck Closure

Bladder neck closure is done primarily for very small or stiff bladders not suitable for YDL or failed bladder neck plasty.

The bladder is opened by a low "smile" incision, as for YDL. The bladder neck is divided above the verumontanum. Upward traction on the bladder plate during division with electrocautery will expose the correct plane easily. Ureteral reimplantation by the cephalon-trigonal method is required, as in YDL plasty (Fig. 22.5).

The lower edge of the bladder plate is mobilized to expose the posterior wall of the bladder. This increases separation from the divided urethra below and also makes this edge turn anteriorly rather than face downward.

The anteriorly turned lower cut edge of the bladder plate receives the augmentation, which is then sutured to the rest of the bladder plate. A rectus muscle flap is interposed between the divided neck and the urethra to prevent fistulation. If the RAM flap had been used earlier, this can be remobilized from the abdominal wall anterior to the bladder. The author prefers not to close the upper urethral end [4].

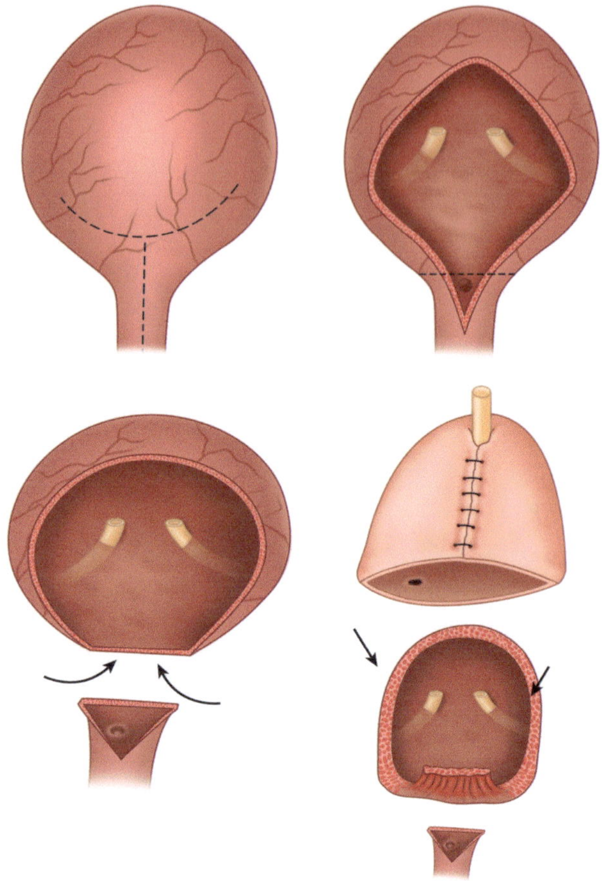

Fig. 22.5 Steps of bladder neck division (closure)—see description below

Operative details

We believe that ureteric reimplantation should always be done at the time of continence surgery, as persistent VUR in a child with an augmented bladder and CIC can result in pyelonephritis, even with a low-pressure urinary reservoir. We prefer to implant the ureters onto the bladder plate.

Ureters are mobilized extravesically and enter the submucosal tunnel from the lateral edge of the bladder plate. The mucosa is lifted off from the detrusor. The submucosal tunnel is made in a cephalotrigonal direction. A neo hiatus of ureteral entry is avoided to prevent obstruction by kinking or fibrosis at the neo hiatus. When

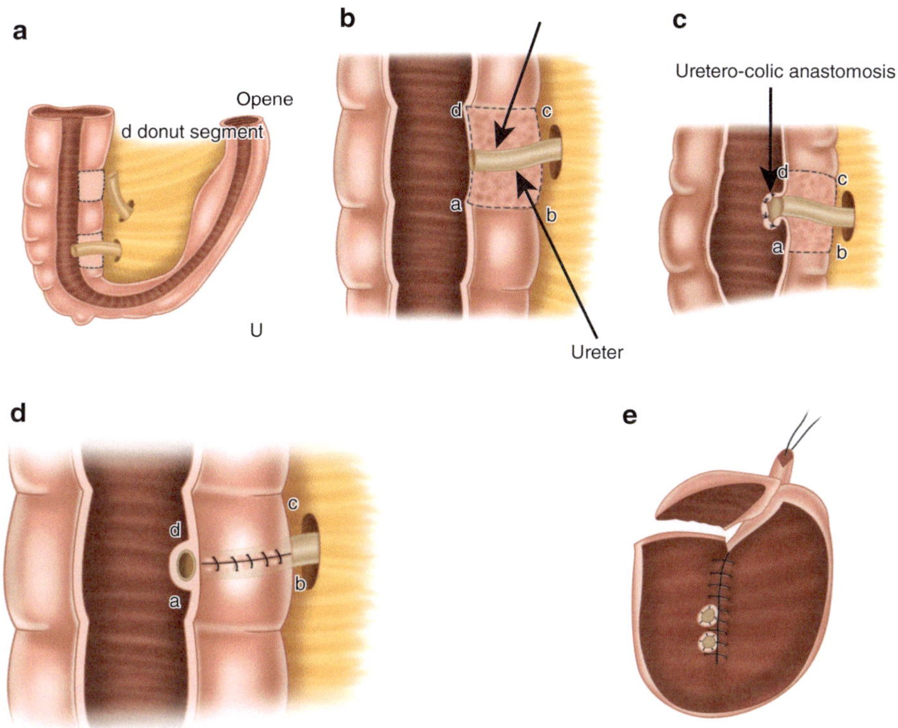

Fig. 22.6 Operative procedure—uretero-colic implantation. (**a**) Ureter brought through colonic mesentery of the detubularized bowel. (**b**) Raw area "abcd" created over the colon by removal of the colonic seromuscular layer, creating a bed for the ureter. (**c**) Ureter laid on the bed "abcd" and uretero-colic anastomosis done between the ureter and mucosal edge "ad". (**d**) Sero-muscular edges "ab" and "dc" sutured over the ureter to complete the submucosal tunnel. The elevated column of colonic mucosa visible from inside the lumen of the colon indicates the ureter lying in the submucosal tunnel. (**e**) Implanted ureters lie between adjacent portions of the reconfigured bowel

the augment patch is sutured onto the bladder plate, care is taken to suture only the bladder mucosa to the augment at the region of ureteral entry to avoid obstruction. Reimplants are stented by 6 Fr feeding tubes for 2 weeks (Fig. 22.6).

When the bladder plate is very unhealthy, our option would be a neobladder, with ureters implanted into the colonic segment of the augmentation by a serosal denudation and colonic wall infolding technique described by us [5].

Ureteric Reimplant into the Colon Segment of the Donut

Operative details are self explanatory.

The Bladder Augmentation by the Donut (Doughnut) Technique [6, 7]

The ileocecal loop is opened on the antimesenteric border, cutting open the ileocecal valve, except in the zone of ileum A A^1, which is behind the appendix. This zone A A^1 will be wrapped around the appendix as it exits the abdomen to form the Mitrofanoff stoma. The opened loop has an inner margin of $ABFCF^1B^1A^1$ and an outer margin of $ADEGG^1E^1D^1A^1$. The inner margins ABFC will be sutured to $A^1B^1F^1C$ to form the posterior wall of the augmentation. Ileal edge DB will be sutured to colonic edge EF. The outer edges of ADEG will be sutured to $A^1D^1E^1G^1$ to form the anterior wall of the augmentation. The portion G to G^1 (now a circular opening) will be left open to fit onto the bladder plate. The cecal opening of the appendix is seen (Figs. 22.7, 22.8, and 22.9).

The bladder plate has been prepared to receive the augmentation (YDL plasty and bilateral cephalo-trigonal reimplantation done). The unopened segment of ileum AA^1 goes around the appendix and is further sutured to provide a fundoplication-like effect around the appendix. (Thus AA^1 is not seen in the figure, being buried by the additional sutures of ileum to ileum around the appendix.) At least one of these sutures also includes the seromuscular layer of the appendix to prevent retraction of the appendix with the augment. The "fundoplication" is also anchored to the anterior abdominal wall to avoid a "dangling" Mitrofanoff port.

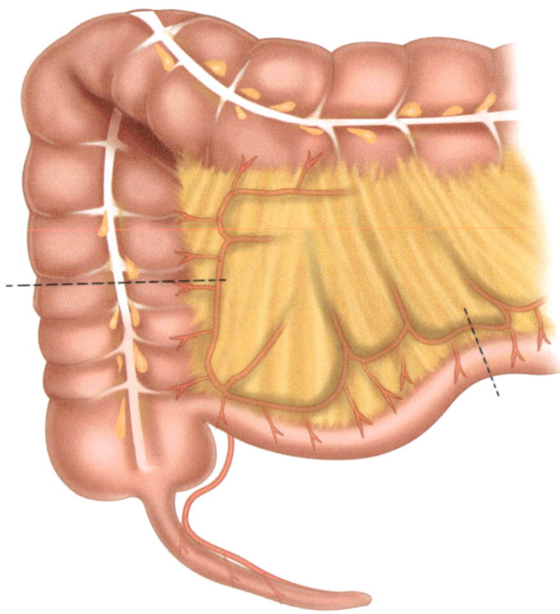

Fig. 22.7 The right colon is mobilized, and the ileocecal loop based on the ileocecal vessels is isolated, including the appendix. The cecum, appendix, half or more (if colon reimplantation is required) of the ascending colon, and about 8 inches of the terminal ileum are included in the isolated segment to be used for the donut augment

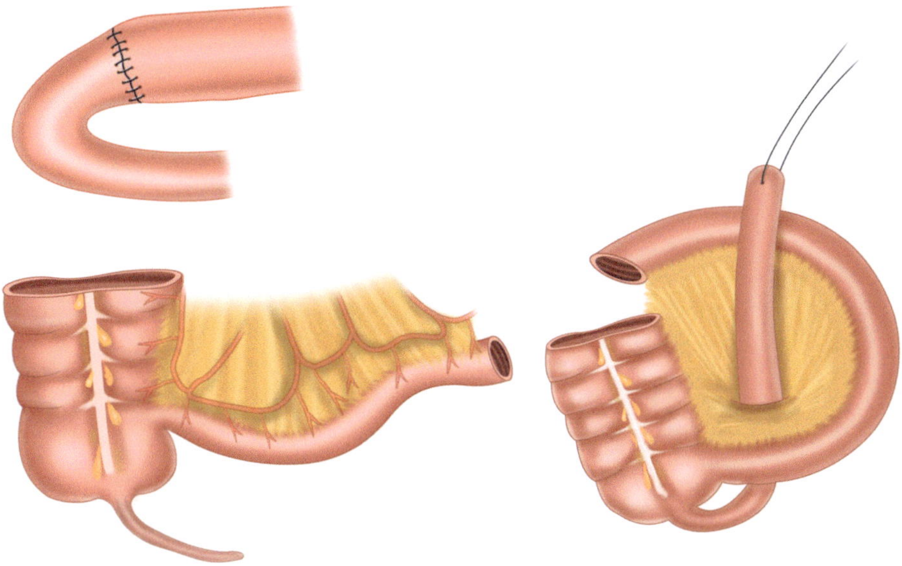

Fig. 22.8 Ileo-transverse colon anastomosis is completed after isolating the ileocecal segment. The ileocecal loop is arranged in the form of a ring (donut) around the appendix. The appendix tip is taken on a stay suture, travels behind the terminal ileum, through an opening made in the mesentery, and is brought cephalad anterior to the ileal loop

Note: A modification of the donut augmentation in young adults—"the inverted" donut.

Occasionally in the older patient, the cecum is higher up in the abdomen and may not directly come down to meet the bladder plate without tension on the ileocecal vessels. In such a situation, the ileocecal segment is "tumbled down" so that the transected ascending colon reaches the bladder plate. A loop of terminal ileum is looped around the appendix and sutured around it to provide the fundoplication effect. (There is no need for the appendix to traverse through the ileal mesentery.) The colon and ileum are opened on the anti-mesenteric aspect and anastomosed to provide a detubularized augmentation around the bladder plate (Fig. 22.10).

This augmentation is also very effective, although a disadvantage compared to the usual method is that the catheter entry into the appendicular port does not reach the most dependent part of the augmentation.

The reconstructed bladder is drained for 3 weeks by two ureteric stents (feeding tubes) and a Malecot's catheter in the augmented bladder. The catheters are brought out via the colonic segment of the augment, which is anchored to the anterior abdominal wall at their point of exit.

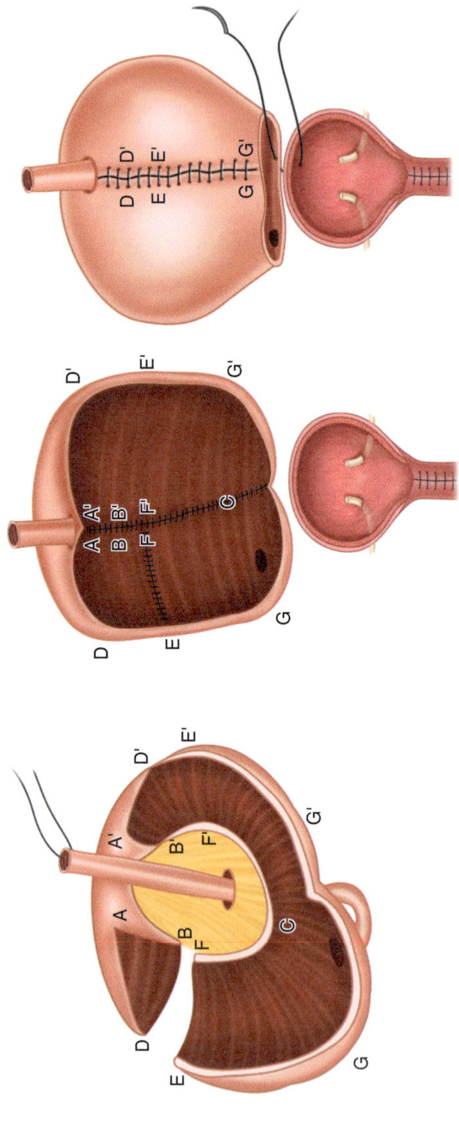

Fig. 22.9 Steps of donut augmentation (see description in text)

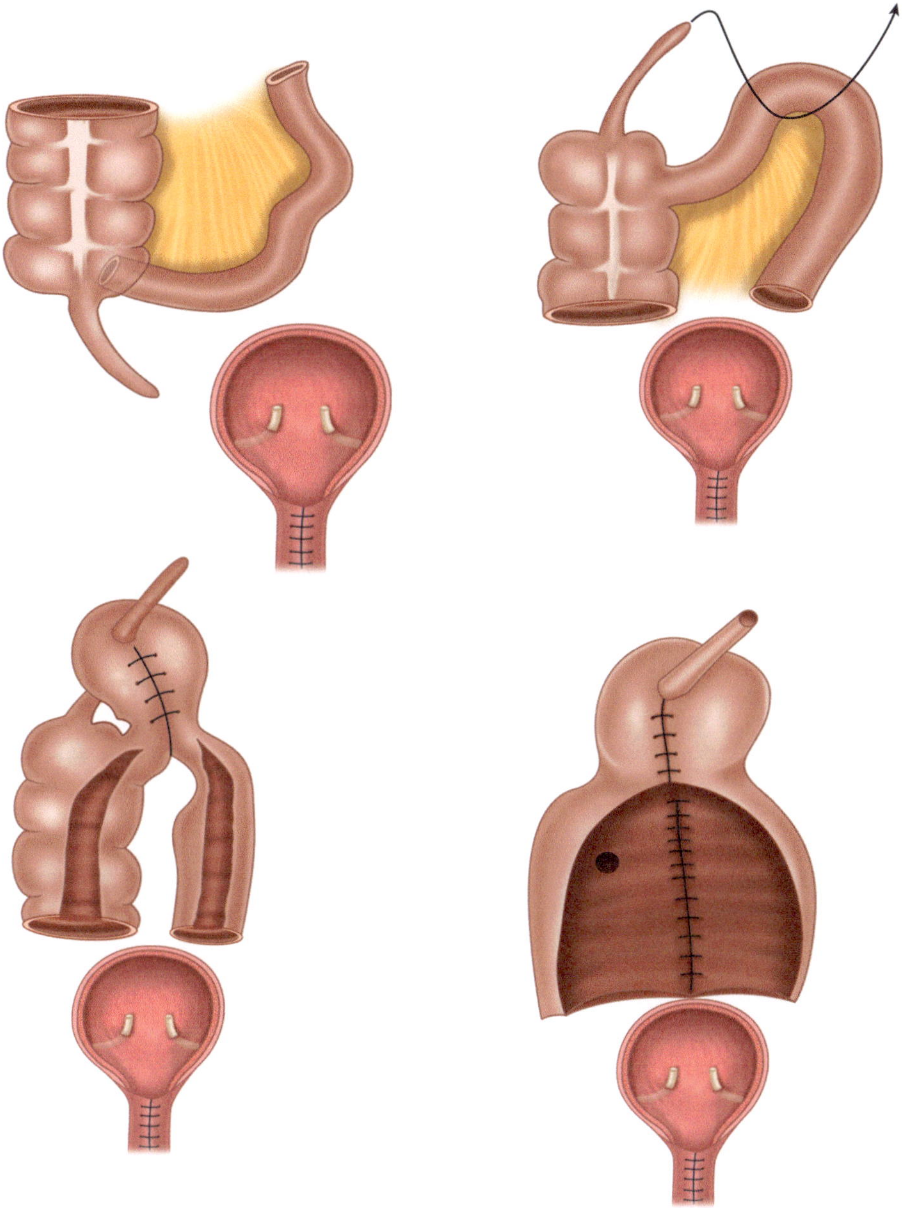

Fig. 22.10 The inverted donut—using the tumbled-down ileocecal segment

Outcome of Reconstruction

The outcome of reconstruction without an augmentation was unsatisfactory, as mentioned earlier. For the past 20 years, we have opted for a policy of BA in most (if not ultimately all) patients.

In the period 2006–2021, 157 children were seen, of whom 125 underwent BA. Of these, 100 underwent ileocecal donut augmentation as described herein, including three with ileocecal neobladders. Since initial bladder turn-in followed by BA using the donut technique has become the standard protocol, we present the outcome in these 100 consecutive children (34 females) with a follow-up of up to 14 years (mean 5 years).

At the time of BA (mean age 6.3 years), 70 of these children had healed bladder turn-in (after multiple attempts in 33), all but two of whom were incontinent. In 30 children, the BA (three neobladder) was done concomitantly with bladder turn-in, mostly in older children [1]. Out of 200 renal units, 48 had HUN, which was gross in 24. Demonstrable VUR was seen in 105 of 140 units (30 bladders were open), with 64 units showing dilating reflux. Dilating VUR and/or HUN were associated with renal scars on DMSA, which were present in 26% of renal units studied. Lower than normal eGFR (<90 ml/min) was seen in 30% of children.

At follow-up, dryness on CIC was achieved in 95 of the 100 children. In the five who remained, wet BN reconstruction had been deferred in three due to pre-existing upper tract changes in a young child, and two had failed YDL. The combination of YDL and BA achieved dryness in 72 of 79 children. BNC, when done primarily (N = 18) or after a previously failed YDL (No = 5), was always successful. The Mitrofanoff port using the "in situ" appendix was trouble-free in 94 children, being easy to catheterize and having no leakage of urine (unless the bladder was excessively full). Two ports had minor urine leakage, which settled with time, and two needed minor skin-level revision. One port was necrosed in the immediate postoperative period and had to be replaced with a gastric tube.

Follow-up ultrasound showed no hydronephrosis in 157 of 200 kidneys. 20 renal units showed new-onset mild pyelectasis, which is being watched. Preoperatively noted HUN (N = 48) showed complete resolution in 25 kidneys and stabilization in the rest.

Evaluation of VUR (available in 194/200) showed no VUR in 165 and persistent VUR in 29. Persistent VUR was seen in 10% of bladder reimplantation, 15% of ureteric implants into the bowel, and 30% of ureters that had not been reimplanted. The eGFR improved from a mean of 116 ml/sq.m/min preoperatively to 139 ml/sq.m/min at follow-up after reconstruction. Preoperatively, 30% of children had an eGFR <90, while at follow-up, only 11% remained below this. In children with preoperative eGFR <90, there was a statistically significant improvement from a mean of 71 to a mean of 106 ($p = 0.036$) (Fig. 22.11).

Cystometry at follow-up showed a large-capacity, compliant, augmented bladder in 90% of 32 studies.

Postoperative complications included adhesive intestinal obstruction (N = 16), minor urinary leak (N = 2), and skin-level wound dehiscence (N = 16). While

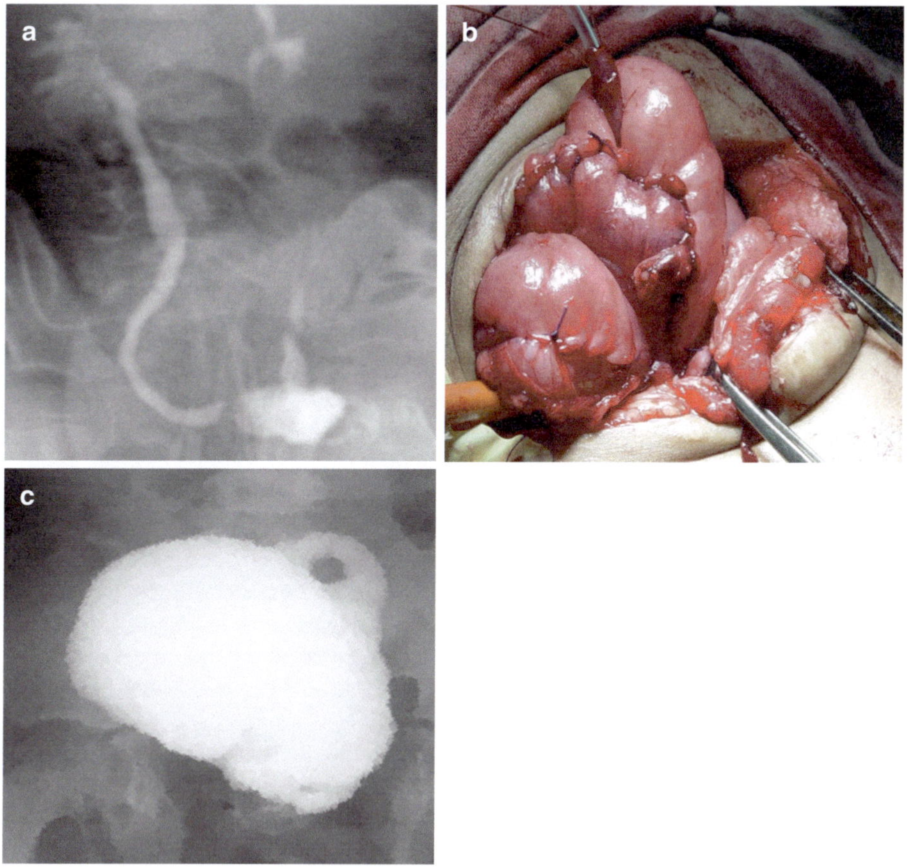

Fig. 22.11 (**a**) Pre-op cystogram—small, incontinent exstrophy bladder with bilateral VUR. (**b**) Operative picture of completed donut augmentation with "in situ" Mitrofanoff and fundoplication effect. (**c**) Post op cystogram – adequately augmented bladder showing no VUR and the circum appendicular ileal loop not allowing reflux through the appendix

adhesive intestinal obstruction was released by laparotomy, the other complications healed spontaneously. Calculi in the augmented were seen in 12, of which six were removed by open cystolithotomy and the others with small calculi are being followed up. Recurrent UTI was seen in 13, of whom three had persistent VUR (one new scar in DMSA).

Discussion

Most reports on the results of exstrophy surgery focus on urinary continence, with variable emphasis on volitional voiding, the need for CIC, the need for bladder augmentation, the benefits of a catheterizable stoma, and the protection of upper tracts.

The benefits achieved from surgical reconstruction must be maintained throughout the life of the child, and most major reconstructions fail in this regard, especially as regards reliable adult life continence and protection of the kidneys. The reconstructed exstrophy, sans BA, has or develops urodynamic abnormality, which, coupled with VUR (persistent or recurrent), takes a toll on renal function [8]. The results of bladder neck surgery and bladder capacity achieved are less than ideal. Thus a degree of dryness achieved is often lost in teenagers/adults, partly due to greater expectations beyond childhood and continuing urodynamic deterioration. In a recent American study of long-term results in exstrophy, several relevant issues came to light: Reliable continence was mainly achieved in augmented bladders with a catheterizable stoma, which, however, was achieved after many surgical procedures in the individual patient [9].

Management of exstrophy has challenges that, though applicable universally, have special relevance in a developing country. Many children have "failed exstrophy," including dehiscence or redehiscence of attempted bladder turn-in, poorly executed epispadias repair, neglected exstrophy with a small polypoid bladder, continuing incontinence after bladder turn-in, failed bladder neck surgery, and deteriorating upper tracts. Some of them with a stenotic bladder outlet and small bladder capacity with HUN with dilating VUR are of considerable concern in the long term. Meanwhile, these children are unable to attend school, the use of diapers is becoming prohibitively expensive, and their troubles are compounded by UTIs, calculi, and progressive renal failure (20% in this report). Many are hypertensive in adult life.

Repeated surgery without BA fails to bring relief to these patients, with attendant costs and hopelessness. We believe that BA, a reliable Mitrofanoff, ureteric reimplantation, and bladder neck surgery (YDL-3/4 and BCN in ¼) are reliable reconstructions in these children.

Children who come to us without any previous reconstruction are offered bladder turn-in, epispadias repair, and fasciomuscular closure with the help of a RAM flap in infancy, avoiding the first 3 months of life. The first 3 months are avoided, as thereafter the RAM becomes more robust. The bladder outlet, bladder neck, and urethra are repaired in continuity with no attempt at "tightening" of the bladder outlet. Ureteric reimplantation is not attempted at this stage, and the child is kept on prophylaxis. A few children develop a moderate amount of continence (holding on until they reach the toilet to void and not wet). They are kept on careful follow-up for UTI. Most children, however, are offered BA at around age 5 years as a more realistic and safe long-term option. Contact and social interaction with other children and families help to reassure parents, especially as regards CIC via a catheterizable stoma. Thus, these children have a two-stage reconstruction, completed by school-going age.

In older children with a neglected/dehisced bladder plate, we have incorporated BA into the open and mobilized bladder plate, achieving abdominal closure in a single stage.

The YDL bladder neck plasty, originally described for allowing dryness with continent voiding, fails to provide reliable results in this regard. Instead, there are undesirable effects on the unaugmented bladder as the procedure consumes some of the already small bladder capacity as well as inflicts undesirable urodynamic changes in the bladder that remains. This results not only in poor continence but also upper tract pathology, as shown by HUN and diminished eGFR. BA offers a reliable solution, although it necessitates to lifelong CIC. Large low-pressure storage capacity is created, providing better continence, better protection, and recovery of upper tracts. This also allows a "longer" and narrower YDL plasty, as the residual capacity of the native bladder is not a concern. The YDL allows for the greater safety of pop-off if CIC is delayed, but not for voiding via naturalis.

Exstrophy is associated with VUR, and when the bladder is urodynamically abnormal, there is a dilating VUR. Lowering bladder pressure by BA does not (unlike in augmented neurogenic or valve bladder) reliably eliminate VUR in many children. This can be a cause of repeated UTIs and renal scars. Thus, a ureteric reimplantation becomes necessary. Unlike some centers, we have not undertaken ureteric reimplantation at the time of bladder turn-in, as these bladders are often unhealthy and ureters are of fine caliber in an infant. Ureteric reimplantation has been done at the time of BA when the bladder plate improves in quality after bladder turn-in. Some were done in the colonic segment of the donut augment when the bladder was very small.

These children will need lifelong CIC, which should be easy and painless, and allow a 12 Fr catheter for draining urine and mucus. A catheterizable stoma rather than periurethral CIC is essentially preferable, generally using the appendix implanted into the bladder plate. The "in situ" appendix in the "doughnut" ileocecal augmentation with its ileal periappendiceal cuff provides a non-refluxing, well-vascularized channel without any implantation into the already small bladder. It also provides catheter drainage to the "dependent" area of the bladder–augment cavity without impinging on the sensitive trigone.

The above reconstruction shows excellent results, with dryness with 3–4 hourly CIC in 95%, resolution of VUR in 165 of 194 renal units, and resolution of persisting HUN. There was a significant improvement in eGFR ($p = 0.036$) in children with subnormal eGFR, indicating a degree of reversibility in renal damage.

The supply and cost of catheters is an important factor for an individual with lifelong CIC. We insist on a clean and dry catheter, which could be used for even 6 months. The family is supplied with a cloth catheter bag with multiple channels in which a set of catheters (feeding tube or Nelcath) is kept after cleaning with tap water. This allows the catheter to dry before the next use and is not a source of UTI [9]. Additionally, the child is encouraged to keep the catheter "in situ," with its outlet plugged, between CIC sessions during the first year or so after surgery. This makes intermittent bladder drainage easy at school and also prevents skin-level stomal stenosis. Daily bladder washouts using drinking water are insisted upon. The low incidence of calculi is possibly the outcome [10, 11] (Fig. 22.12).

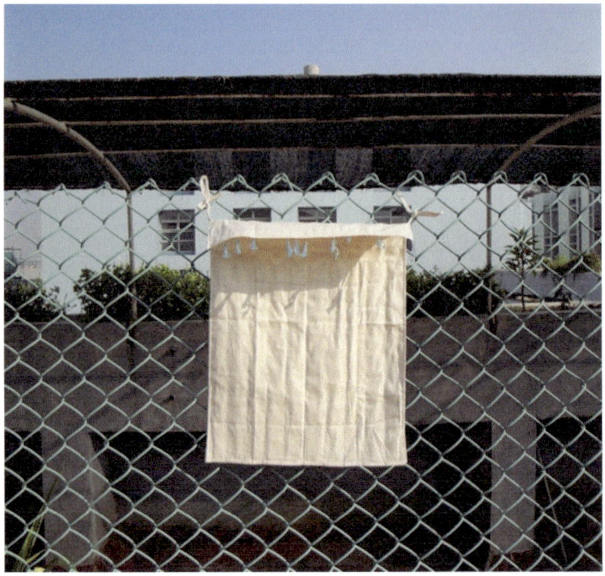

Fig. 22.12 Cloth catheter bag with catheters in place drying in the sun

Conclusion

We describe a method of treating exstrophy by an effective and safe two-step reconstruction including BA and Mitrofanoff CIC as an integral part of the reconstruction. This has yielded reliable results for more than 90% of the children treated. The chief hurdle is the crossing of the psychological barrier of accepting CIC, which is accepted either after many failed attempts at reconstruction or, preferably, by counseling from the very start, helped by contact with other reconstructed children.

References

1. James Sam C, Kurian JJ, Kishore R, Arunachalam P, Sen S. Management and outcome in dehisced exstrophy with a simplified bladder re-closure and further reconstruction. J Pediatr Urol. 2020;16(6):836.e1–8.
2. Gearhart JP, Leonard MP, Burgers JK, Jeffs RD. The Cantwell-Ransley technique for repair of epispadias. J Urol. 1992;148(3):851–4.
3. Barla RK, Sen S. Skin cover in epispadias repair by dorsal transposition of a ventral island flap: a modification of the Pippi Salle technique. Pediatr Surg Int. 2015;31(11):1099–102.
4. Sen S, Zachariah N, Chacko J, Thomas G. Buttressing the divided bladder neck by a rectus abdominis muscle flap to prevent urethral recanalisation in paediatric urinary incontinence. Pediatr Surg Int. 2003;19(1–2):124–6.
5. Sen S, Arunachalam P, Sam CJ. Non-obstructive, non-refluxing uretero-colonic anastomosis by colonic sero-muscular excision and extra mural peri-ureteric wrap – a new technique in 17 children. J Pediatr Urol. 2021;17(1):99.e1–7.
6. Babu R, Sudipta S. Augmentation in exstrophy. In: Babu R, editor. Dysfunctional and neurogenic bladder, medical and surgical management. 1st ed. Singapore: Notion Press; 2021. p. 181–92.

7. Sudipta S, Viju J. "Doughnut Augmentation"- ieocaecal segment with in-situ appendix used as a simple but effective bladder augment/substitute in very small bladders. J Pediatr Urol. 2008;4(1):S40.
8. Diamond DA, Bauer SB, Dinlenc C, Hendren WH, Peters CA, Atala A, Kelly M, Retik AB. Normal urodynamics in patients with bladder exstrophy: are they achievable? J Urol. 1999;162(3):844–5.
9. Harris KT, Villela NA, Alam R, Wu WJ, Artigas P, DiCarlo HN, Gearhart JP. The exstrophy experience: a national survey assessing urinary continence, bladder management, and oncologic outcomes in adults. J Pediatr Urol. 2023;19(2):178.e1–7.
10. Sam CJ, Jagadeesan CT, Sen S, Arunachalam P, Appalaraju B, Das PT. Urinary tract infection in pediatric patients on clean intermittent catheterization via a mitrofanoff port with reused catheters – any association with catheter sterility? J Indian Assoc Pediatr Surg. 2020;25(2):91–5.
11. Kisku S, Sen S, Karl S, Mathai J, Thomas RJ, Barla R. Bladder calculi in the augmented bladder: a follow-up study of 160 children and adolescents. J Pediatr Urol. 2015;11(2):66.e1–6.

Kidney and Bladder Exstrophy: Considerations and Caution

23

Sangeeta Hingorani

Introduction

The worldwide prevalence of chronic kidney disease (CKD) in children is 15–74.7 cases per million children [1]. The most common cause of CKD in children is congenital abnormalities of the kidney and urinary tract (CAKUT), which accounts for 29–40% of cases of CKD depending on region and database [2]. CKD is a state of irreversible damage to the kidneys with reduction of kidney function and represents a continuum of disease from mild kidney abnormalities with normal metabolic function and solute handling to end-stage kidney disease (ESKD).

Given that CAKUT, which includes obstructive uropathy, neurogenic bladder, and hypoplastic and dysplastic kidneys with or without vesicoureteric reflux, is the major cause of CKD in children, understanding the diagnosis, need for follow-up and ongoing monitoring, and prevention of progression is important for all practitioners caring for these children. This chapter will focus primarily on the exstrophy-epispadias complex, of which bladder exstrophy (BE) is the most common type, accounting for 71–83% of cases [3]. These complex malformations involve the lower abdominal wall, bladder, and pelvic floor and often necessitate multiple reconstructive surgeries and procedures. Many of the procedures are designed to obtain urinary continence, normal appearance of the genitalia, sexual function, and to preserve kidney function. Though initial thoughts were that children with exstrophy had normal kidneys, as kidney function measured by serum creatinine was normal, we have now learned that CAKUT-associated abnormalities are increased in prevalence in children with BE. Baseline abnormalities are then compounded by

S. Hingorani (✉)
University of Washington School of Medicine, Department of Pediatrics, Division of Nephrology, Seattle Children's Hospital, Seattle, WA, USA
e-mail: sangeeta.hingorani@seattlechildrens.org

A. R. Shukla, R. S. Joshi (eds.), *Bladder Exstrophy and Epispadias*, https://doi.org/10.1007/978-3-031-91238-2_23

reconstructive surgeries and obstructive complications and urinary tract infections, which can further impact an already abnormal kidney parenchyma [3].

Summary of Literature

There are few large studies of patients with BE evaluating long-term kidney function in a systematic and comprehensive way. And comparisons between studies are also difficult given varying surgical techniques used and varying modalities to evaluate kidney function (Tables 23.1 and 23.2).

In a retrospective cross-sectional study from a single-referral center in Tel Aviv of patients followed by pediatric urology from birth to the present time, investigators evaluated kidney function, including serum creatinine and urine protein to creatinine ratio; calculated an estimated glomerular filtration rate (GFR) using the Schwartz formula or 24-hour urine collection for creatinine clearance; and measured blood pressure [3]. Imaging studies included a kidney ultrasound and DMSA scan. Forty-three patients were included in this study, of whom 39 were diagnosed with BE. Kidney evaluation occurred at a median of 9 years of age (range of 1–24 years). Overall, 26 patients (60%) completed kidney evaluations. The median estimated GFR was 127.5 mL/min/1.73 m^2 with an interquartile range of 103–140/1.73 m^2; a decreased GFR was present in only 12% of patients. Elevated blood pressures were recorded in 29% of patients at follow-up, and 36% (10) of patients had albuminuria or proteinuria, and the latter were more common in patients who had a bladder augmentation. Imaging studies revealed scarring in 61% of patients evaluated, and abnormalities on ultrasound, including urinary tract dilatation, were seen in 46% of patients. The overall prevalence of any type of kidney abnormality, whether structural or functional, was seen in 32 (74%) of patients evaluated. Risk factors identified for scarring on DMSA scans were the presence of urinary tract dilatation on US and persistent infections or a history of kidney stones. None of the risk factors studied were associated with structural or functional declines or changes in kidney function [3].

Another recent study by Joshi et al. of children with BE cared for as part of a US-India Multi-Institutional Bladder Exstrophy Collaboration at a Civil Hospital in

Table 23.1 Normal glomerular filtration rate (GFR) in children and adolescents [12]

Age	Mean GFR ± SD (mL/min/1.73 m^2)
1 week (males and females)	41 ± 15
2–8 weeks (males and females)	66 ± 25
>8 weeks (males and females)	96 ± 22
2–12 years (males and females)	133 ± 27
13–21 years (males)	140 ± 30
13–21 years (females)	126 ± 22

Table 23.2 Comparison of kidney outcomes from 1979 to 2021 [4]

Authors and year of publication	Surgical technique used to repair bladder exstrophy	Sample size	Measurement of renal injury (IVP, RUS, VCUG, DMSA, eGFR)	Mean length of follow-up (Years)	Renal outcomes
Demaria et al., 1979	MSRE	22 (22 BE)	Imaging—IVP Labs—Creatinine	8.7	3/22 (14%) had renal findings on IVP 100% had normal Creatinine
Husmann et al., 1988	MSRE	68 (68 BE)	Imaging—IVP, VCUG Labs—Creatinine	12.7	8/68 (13%) had renal scarring 3/68 (4%) had renal insufficiency
Mesrobian et al., 1988	MSRE	103 (32 had BE repair, 71 diverted)	Imaging—IVP, VCUG, and RUS Labs—Creatinine	8	6/24 (25%) hydronephrosis 100% normal Creatinine
Grady and Mitchell 1999	CPRE	24 (18 BE, 6 CE)	Imaging——RUS, VCUG Labs—Creatinine (only available in 5/24 Pts)	4	98% of the renal units have no evidence of deterioration on serial RUS
Bolduc et al., 2002	MSRE	57 (49 BE, 8 CE)	Imaging—RUS, VCUG, DMSA	4.5	14/57 (24%) had renal scarring 2/57 (3.5%) renal insufficiency
Gargollo et al., 2008	CPRE	32 (32 BE)	Imaging only—RUS, DMSA, VCUG	5	9/32 (28%) had up to 4 episodes of pyelonephritis 7/32 (22%) had hydronephrosis 6 (19%) had cortical defects
Ebert et al., 2009	One stage reconstruction	17 (16 BE, 1 PE)	Imaging—RUS, DMSA Labs—eGFR	18.7	4/17 (24%) had UTIs 3/17 (18%) had unilateral smaller kidney 100% normal renal function

(continued)

Table 23.2 (continued)

Authors and year of publication	Surgical technique used to repair bladder exstrophy	Sample size	Measurement of renal injury (IVP, RUS, VCUG, DMSA, eGFR)	Mean length of follow-up (Years)	Renal outcomes
Schaeffer et al., 2012	MSRE	53 (53 BE)	Imaging—RUS Labs—eGFR	15.1	1/53 (1.8%) had CKD stage 2
Ellison et al., 2017	CPRE	30 (30 BE)	Imaging—RUS Labs—eGFR	9.7	16/30 (53%) had hydronephrosis 4/30 (13%) had CKD stage 2
Giron et al., 2017	One stage reconstruction	15 (15 BE)	Imaging—RUS, VCUG Labs—Creatinine	10.3 years	100% normal kidneys 100% normal Creatinine
Sinatti et al., 2021	Multiple techniques (Single stage and two stage repair)	48 (38 BE, 7 PE and 3 CE)	Imaging—RUS, VCUG Labs—eGFR	18 years	36/48 (75%) had recurrent UTIs 2/48 (4%) had hydronephrosis 1/48 (2%) had CKD stage 2

BE bladder exstrophy, *CE* cloacal exstrophy, *PE* penile epispadias, *MSRE* modern staged repair of exstrophy, *CPRE* complete primary repair of exstrophy

Ahmedabad, India were prospectively followed from 2010 to 2020, reported more extensively on kidney outcomes 1–10 years after BE surgery [4]. Of the 72 patients included in this study, 60 had either primary BE surgery or a redo of their BE surgery. Of these, 4 patients had an eGFR <90 mL/min/1.73 m^2, and 36 had an eGFR >120 mL/min/1.73 m^2. Twenty children had kidney scarring seen on DMSA scans. In this study, neither urinary reflux nor the presence of kidney scars was associated with a decline in eGFR after adjustment for age, sex, and duration of follow-up. Additionally, abnormal DMSA scans were not associated with microalbuminuria or urinary reflux. This population had a surprisingly low rate of urinary tract infections, precluding analysis of any associations with exposures or outcomes [4].

A study of 42 patients born with BE between 1937 and 1968, of whom 25 were contacted at a median of 50 years (range 37–69 years), found that 15 of 25 (60%) of patients had normal creatinine levels or mild CKD based on eGFR with a mean eGFR of 66 mL/min/1.73 m^2 and 3 patients were on kidney replacement therapy: (1) on hemodialysis and (2) had a kidney transplant (PMID 19136304). Childhood surgical and clinical courses were reviewed, and the ESKD was thought to be from progressive scarring of their upper tracts due to progressive hydronephrosis from bladder outlet obstruction, kidney stones, and a history of febrile urinary tract infections after closure. MRI imaging showed scarring in the kidneys of varying degrees from mild to severe in 20 of the 25 patients. Dilatation of the ureter and/or kidney pelvis was seen in 11 patients. Ten patients had recurrent kidney stones throughout their adult life [5].

Smaller, single-center studies have reported varying degrees of kidney function, from normal in all 16 study patients with BE with a mean serum creatinine of 0.85 mg/dL (0.8–1.0) after a mean follow-up of 19.4 years. Fourteen patients had normal kidney US, while only 3 had a smaller kidney and stable DMSA scan without any evidence of scarring [6]. Other studies have found that only 1 child of the 27 with normal GFR at the time of bladder neck reconstruction developed stage 2 CKD after 10 years of follow-up. Imaging studies in this cohort of patients demonstrated mild hydronephrosis (2 patients), moderate (5 patients), and severe (2 patients), with the remaining US being normal. No correlation was found between the presence or severity of hydronephrosis and eGFR [7]. In a study of 23 adult patients aged 18–57 years who had exstrophy-epispadias complex and presented to an adult urology practice, 10 of 23 were noted to have CKD stage 2 or higher, though only one patient had CKD stage 5 and 7 had hydronephrosis on US. Most patients had a history of kidney stones and pyelonephritis [8].

Nephrology Evaluation

The pediatric urologic patient may present to the nephrologist at any time during their clinical course. Ideally, those with a pre-natal diagnosis of bladder exstrophy or CAKUT will be known to nephrology, or nephrology will be involved early in their diagnosis and treatment course. Close communication between urology and nephrology is essential to provide a collaborative approach in the evaluation, prevention, and management of kidney disease. A thorough history and physical examination with a particular focus on risk factors for pre-existing kidney disease, birth weight, gestational age, family history of kidney disease, dialysis, or transplants, and a review of systems elucidating kidney and urinary symptoms (edema, dysuria, nocturia, enuresis, and hematuria) should be performed. Also, a review of the patient's urologic diagnosis, medications, past and planned surgical treatment courses, history of urinary tract infections, and kidney stones is essential to understanding risk factors for the development and progression of CKD. Additional consideration should be given to whole genome sequencing in patients with CAKUT, as approximately 25% of patients will have an identified genetic mutation [9].

Screening and ongoing monitoring of kidney outcomes in patients with bladder exstrophy

Monitoring parameter	Monitoring studies	Interval for monitoring	Care provider doing the monitoring
eGFR	Serum creatinine and cystatin C	Baseline, and then yearly	Urology or nephrology
Kidney size, growth, architecture	Kidney ultrasound	Baseline, annually through 3 years and then every 3–5 years based on kidney function or other complications; recommended during adolescence growth spurt	Urology or nephrology
Albuminuria/ proteinuria Normal albuminuria <30 mg/g creatinine Normal proteinuria <300 mg/g creatinine or <0.2	Urinalysis and spot urine albumin/ protein to creatinine ratio	Yearly	Urology or nephrology
Growth	Height and weight	Yearly and/or at each visit	Pediatrician, urology, nephrology
Blood pressure	Oscillometric BP or manual BP and ABPM when >8 years of age	At each visit, yearly	Pediatrician, urology, nephrology—24-hour ABPM study
Kidney stones	Urinalysis; urine calcium to creatinine ratio; 24-hour urine stone risk profile Ultrasound or Fast CT	If there is a suspicion of stones	Urology or nephrology
Electrolyte abnormalities	Serum levels of Na, K, Cl, HCO3, glucose, calcium, and phosphorus	Baseline, yearly if presence of CKD or failure to gain weight and grow	Pediatrician, urology, or nephrology
Prevention of kidney injury and urinary tract infections Avoidance of ibuprofen/NSAIDs and other nephrotoxic medications Good voiding and stooling habits Consider prophylactic antibiotics	Urinalyses and urine cultures when indicated VCUG and urodynamic studies	Baseline, yearly or when needed	Pediatrician, urology, nephrology
Healthy lifestyle habits	Nutrition and activity counseling	At each visit adjusted based on weight, blood pressure, albuminuria	Pediatrician at well child visits, urology and nephrology

Measuring Kidney Function

The effort to standardize the definitions of CKD has led to the Kidney Disease: Improving Global Outcomes (KDIGO) 2012 Clinical Practice Guideline (CPG) for Evaluation and Management of CKD, which includes kidney function based on GFR and the presence of urinary albumin and excretion rate [10]. There are five stages of CKD, with lower stages (e.g., stage 1) representing higher GFR. The diagnosis of CKD in pediatric patients over the age of 2 years requires fulfilling one of the following criteria: (1) eGFR of 45–59 mL/min/1.73 m^2 (Stage3a) and 30–44 mL/min/1.73 m^2 (Stage3b) for 3 months or (2) eGFR >60 mL/min/1.73 m^2 accompanied by markers of functional kidney abnormalities such as proteinuria, albuminuria, renal tubular disorders, or pathologic abnormalities, or evidence of structural damage based on imaging or history (Fig. 23.1) [11].

This classification has been widely adopted since its introduction; however, it does have significant limitations in pediatric patients. While GFR is the primary criterion used to define and stage CKD, its use is challenging in younger children. In pediatric populations, the normal level of GFR varies depending on body size, age, and gender (Table 23.1) [12]. Newer estimating equations are applicable to children as young as 1 year of age and are based on serum creatinine and cystatin C levels as well as sex, age, and height. Adult GFR normal values (estimated GFR >90 mL/min/1.73 m^2) are not applicable to children before the age of 1–2 years.

With regard to laboratory studies, a baseline evaluation of estimated glomerular filtration rate (eGFR) is standard to determine kidney function and to accurately

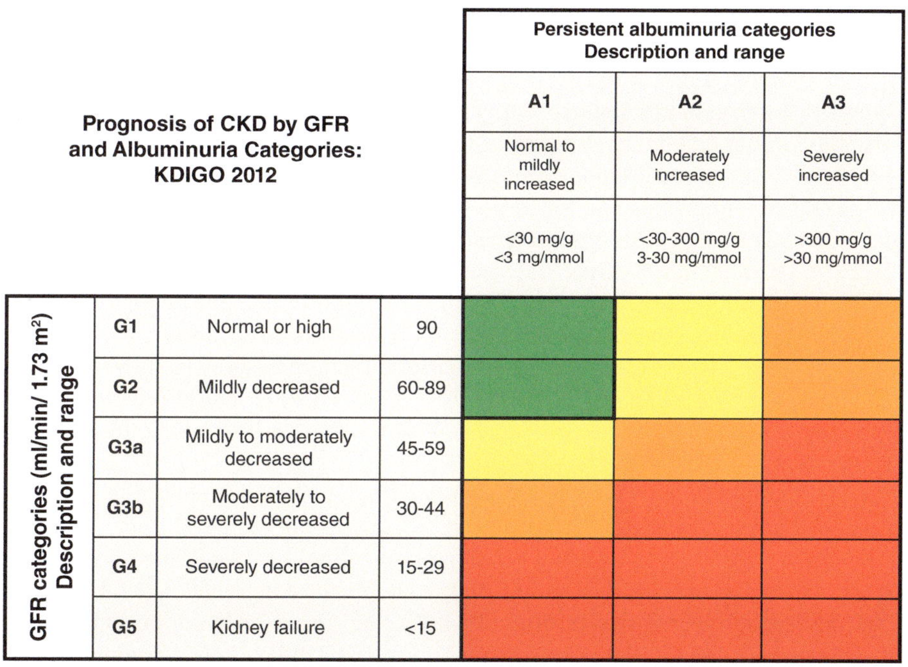

Fig. 23.1 Definition of chronic kidney disease by estimated GFR and albuminuria [12]

classify kidney injury. Alternative methods for estimating or formally measuring GFR, independent of muscle mass, have increasingly been used to either replace or supplement creatinine-eGFR. Serum cystatin C is perhaps the most feasible option for estimating GFR in such situations and is now widely available in many laboratories, either in-house or as a send-out. Cystatin C is a small protein produced by all nucleated cells and is cleared by glomerular filtration and is not significantly affected by changes in muscle mass. Cystatin C has been validated in several populations, and when used in concert with creatinine, it helps to provide a more accurate estimation of kidney function [13, 14]. Newer equations to estimate GFR in children from 1 to 25 years are currently available and are reported at multiple centers and are based on age, sex, height, serum creatinine, and serum cystatin C and are referred to as CKiDU25 equation [15]. In cases where creatinine and cystatin C give widely discrepant results, it may be necessary to consider formal measurement of GFR using nuclear medicine isotopes or iohexol [16].

Evaluation of the patient's urine, specifically focusing on the degree of proteinuria/albuminuria, can provide a baseline from which to compare subsequent studies and estimate the risk of later CKD. Similarly, attention should be paid to the serum electrolytes, especially calcium, magnesium, potassium, and phosphate, which can be markers of tubular injury. In the setting of kidney stones, urinary measurements of calcium, oxalate, uric acid, and creatinine can be informative along with a 24-hour urine collection for a stone risk profile. Increased hydration and a low-sodium diet can be helpful in the prevention and management of kidney stones prior to initiation of diuretic medications.

Evaluating Blood Pressure

Hypertension in pediatric patients with urologic abnormalities is a known complication and is common among children with CKD. In a follow-up study of 36 children with BE who underwent complete primary repair at a single institution, investigators averaged clinic visits and blood pressure readings on the same day for patients and included readings from multiple visits over time. Reimplantation, lower kidney length on US, and higher eGFR were associated with a decreased hazard of systolic or diastolic blood pressure readings >90th percentile for age and sex. No associations were found between the presence of hydronephrosis, urinary continence, pyelonephritis, and elevated systolic or diastolic blood pressures [17]. None of the patients (mean age of 8.9 years) had a systolic or diastolic blood pressure >90th percentile for age and sex, were diagnosed with hypertension, or required antihypertensive therapy.

It is important to pay close attention to the accurate measurement of blood pressure, both in the outpatient setting and when patients are admitted to the hospital. Auscultatory methods to measure blood pressure should be performed both at the onset of care and at each follow-up urology and nephrology visit. Should there be any question of hypertension or difficulty assessing suspected hypertension, the use of 24-hour ambulatory blood pressure monitoring (ABPM) is now recommended as standard of care. Recent studies in the general population demonstrated the utility of screening APBMs in diagnosing hypertension, masked hypertension (elevated ambulatory blood pressure in the presence of normal office or casual BP), white coat hypertension [elevated office or casual blood pressure in the presence of normal ambulatory BP (mean BP <95th percentile and BP load <25%)], and prehypertension [18, 19]. Another valuable data point available from a 24-hour ABPM study is nocturnal BP readings and the nocturnal dip in BP, which is defined as the percentage drop in the mean BP from wake to sleep periods. Abnormal or non-dipping is usually defined as a decline of <10%, which has been associated with development of CKD [19]. Children above the age of 7 are more likely to tolerate an ABPM study, and these are placed in pediatric nephrology clinics and interpreted by pediatric nephrologists.

Imaging Studies

Baseline radiographic studies evaluating kidney and bladder structure are often helpful in patients with concern for CKD. Renal ultrasound and more detailed examinations including DMSA scans or Lasix renograms can assess for kidney scars and differential function and perfusion and can detect urinary obstruction or hydronephrosis. CT scans may be needed in the setting of kidney stones or suspicion of kidney stones, which occur commonly in this patient population. Imaging studies such as VCUG or contrast ultrasonography can be employed when there is concern for voiding dysfunction or obstruction or in the setting of repeated urinary tract infections.

Risk Factors for Progression

The progression of CKD to ESKD results in many of the health consequences of this disease; however, the natural history and the rate of progression are both highly variable and unpredictable. Pediatric data suggests that there is a slower progression of disease in those with congenital renal disorders when compared to those with glomerular etiologies of their CKD [20]. Studies have demonstrated that the progression of CKD can be influenced by multiple factors, many of which are not modifiable (e.g., underlying renal pathology, genetics, race, age, and gender) [21]. However, some risk factors can be modified, such as obesity, hypertension, and proteinuria [22]. There is evidence in pediatric studies that hypertension and proteinuria are the most significant risk factors for CKD progression; minimizing proteinuria and maximizing blood pressure control, targeting the 50th percentile based on age, sex, and height, can slow progression of CKD [23, 24]. Treatment with either angiotensin-converting enzyme inhibitors (ACE inhibitor), or angiotensin II receptor blockers (ARBs) has been shown to be more effective for both blood pressure control and reduction in proteinuria when compared to other agents currently available [25].

It is postulated that proteinuria contributes to CKD progression due to tubular damage resulting in interstitial inflammation, fibrosis, and subsequent apoptosis of proximal tubular cells [26]. In a pediatric study of 1232 children combining the CKiD participants and children in the ESCAPE trial, investigators found that proteinuria (defined as urine protein to creatinine ratio (UPCR) on a spot sample in mg/mg) contributes to CKD progression. The median age in this combined cohort was 12 years (IQR, 8–15), and the median eGFR 47 mL/min/1.73 m^2 (IQR, 33–62). The authors reported six ordered stages with varying combinations of eGFR categories (60–89, 45–59, 30–44, and 15–29 mL/min/1.73 m^2) and UPCR categories (<0.5, 0.5–2.0, and >2.0) and calculated the risk of progression for each category. Median times to event ranged from >10 years for eGFR 45–90 mL/min/1.73 m^2 and UPCR <0.5 to <1 year in those with an eGFR 15–30 mL/min/1.73 m^2 and UPCR >2. Children with non-glomerular disease as the cause for their CKD had a slower rate of progression of their kidney disease compared to those with glomerular diseases [27].

Other risk factors for CKD progression include metabolic acidosis with a serum bicarbonate level <18 mmol/L associated with a higher risk of progression when compared to children with a serum bicarbonate level ≥22 mmol/L [2, 28].

Transplant

The goal and optimal treatment for ESKD is kidney transplant. Kidney transplant has been done successfully in children with urologic disorders, and graft survival rates at 1 and 5 years are comparable to those without urologic disorders. However, in one study of 55 patients who underwent 56 kidney transplants (only 3 had primary BE as the reason for ESKD), investigators found graft survival at 1 year was 89% and at 5 years 66%. They reported that those with a normal bladder fared better than those with an abnormal bladder at 5 years post-transplant (75% vs. 57%, respectively) and those with abnormal bladders had worse kidney function at 5 years. They also found worse kidney function in those with reflux and urinary tract infections post-transplant. High-pressure systems and residual urine volumes after voiding also contributed to the overall decline in kidney function [29]. A retrospective study from three transplant centers in France that included 14 patients with BE who had a kidney transplant at a median age of 42.8 years also found that graft survival was good, with 93% graft survival after a median follow-up of 8.2 years; graft survival out to 20 years was the same [30]. This study did not find an association between pyelonephritis and graft dysfunction. Both studies emphasize the importance of proper work-up and evaluation of bladder function and bladder pressure, evaluation for reflux, and urodynamic studies to measure post-void residual prior to kidney transplantation in this population of patients. And some advocate for prophylactic antibiotics in the first 6 months post-transplant to prevent urinary tract infections [29].

Surgical techniques have dramatically improved for children treated for BE, and the importance of close follow-up is widely recognized. However, many patients are lost to follow-up or only show up at the time of an emergency. Those patients with less complex needs and fewer surgical interventions were those most likely to be lost to follow-up [31]. However, given the risk of CKD and progression to ESKD in patients and the lack of clear risk factors, education about kidney disease and prevention is important. Close collaboration between nephrologists and urologists, along with nutritionists and social workers, is critical to maximize outcomes for these complicated patients. Careful attention to blood pressure, urine assessments for albuminuria/proteinuria, and kidney function with both serum creatinine and cystatin C is important in the long term to screen for and manage CKD. Healthy lifestyle habits, counseling, and avoidance of obesity are also important to emphasize as part of preventive care. Creation of combined urology and nephrology clinics in both the pediatric and adult specialties and transition clinics will be important to optimize management of these complex patients and allow for early recognition of kidney abnormalities and potentially early intervention and management to prevent progression and improve overall quality of life.

References

1. Warady BA, Chadha V. Chronic kidney disease in children: the global perspective. Pediatr Nephrol. 2007;22(12):1999–2009. https://doi.org/10.1007/s00467-006-0410-1.
2. Harada R, Hamasaki Y, Okuda Y, Hamada R, Ishikura K. Epidemiology of pediatric chronic kidney disease/kidney failure: learning from registries and cohort studies. Pediatr Nephrol. 2022;37(6):1215–29. https://doi.org/10.1007/s00467-021-05145-1.
3. Cleper R, Blumenthal D, Beniamini Y, Friedman S, Yosef YB, Chaim JB. Exstrophy-epispadias complex: are the kidneys and kidney function spared? Pediatr Nephrol. 2023;38(8):2711–7. https://doi.org/10.1007/s00467-023-05889-y.
4. Joshi RS, Eftekharzadeh S, Shukla AR, et al. Kidney function outcomes in patients after complete primary repair of bladder exstrophy and penopubic epispadias: results from the international bladder exstrophy consortium. J Pediatr Urol. 2023;19(1):34.e1–9. https://doi.org/10.1016/j.jpurol.2022.04.018.
5. Gobet R, Weber D, Renzulli P, Kellenberger C. Long-term follow up (37–69 years) of patients with bladder exstrophy treated with ureterosigmoidostomy: uro-nephrological outcome. J Pediatr Urol. 2009;5(3):190–6. https://doi.org/10.1016/j.jpurol.2008.11.007.
6. Ebert AK, Schott G, Bals-Pratsch M, Seifert B, Rosch WH. Long-term follow-up of male patients after reconstruction of the bladder-exstrophy-epispadias complex: psychosocial status, continence, renal and genital function. J Pediatr Urol. 2010;6(1):6–10. https://doi.org/10.1016/j.jpurol.2009.06.002.
7. Schaeffer AJ, Stec AA, Baradaran N, Gearhart JP, Mathews RI. Preservation of renal function in the modern staged repair of classic bladder exstrophy. J Pediatr Urol. 2013;9(2):169–73. https://doi.org/10.1016/j.jpurol.2012.01.014.
8. Handa N, Bowen DK, Guo J, Chu DI, Kielb SJ. Long-term kidney outcomes in exstrophy-epispadias complex: how patients present as adults. Urology. 2021;154:333–7. https://doi.org/10.1016/j.urology.2021.01.033.
9. Werfel L, Martens H, Hennies I, et al. Diagnostic yield and benefits of whole exome sequencing in CAKUT patients diagnosed in the first thousand days of life. Kidney Int Rep. 2023;8(11):2439–57. https://doi.org/10.1016/j.ekir.2023.08.008.
10. Andrassy KM. Comments on 'KDIGO 2012 clinical practice guideline for the evaluation and management of chronic kidney disease'. Kidney Int. 2013;84(3):622–3. https://doi.org/10.1038/ki.2013.243.

11. Inker LA, Astor BC, Fox CH, et al. KDOQI US commentary on the 2012 KDIGO clinical practice guideline for the evaluation and management of CKD. Am J Kidney Dis. 2014;63(5):713–35. https://doi.org/10.1053/j.ajkd.2014.01.416.
12. National Kidney F. K/DOQI clinical practice guidelines for chronic kidney disease: evaluation, classification, and stratification. Am J Kidney Dis. 2002;39(2 Suppl 1):S1–266.
13. Nehus EJ, Laskin BL, Kathman TI, Bissler JJ. Performance of cystatin C-based equations in a pediatric cohort at high risk of kidney injury. Pediatr Nephrol. 2013;28(3):453–61. https://doi.org/10.1007/s00467-012-2341-3.
14. Blufpand HN, Tromp J, Abbink FC, et al. Cystatin C more accurately detects mildly impaired renal function than creatinine in children receiving treatment for malignancy. Pediatr Blood Cancer. 2011;57(2):262–7. https://doi.org/10.1002/pbc.23119.
15. Pierce CB, Munoz A, Ng DK, Warady BA, Furth SL, Schwartz GJ. Age- and sex-dependent clinical equations to estimate glomerular filtration rates in children and young adults with chronic kidney disease. Kidney Int. 2021;99(4):948–56. https://doi.org/10.1016/j.kint.2020.10.047.
16. Ng DK, Schwartz GJ, Warady BA, Furth SL, Munoz A. Relationships of measured iohexol GFR and estimated GFR with CKD-related biomarkers in children and adolescents. Am J Kidney Dis. 2017;70(3):397–405. https://doi.org/10.1053/j.ajkd.2017.03.019.
17. Kanabolo D, Cain M, Brown M, et al. Long term renal outcome and risk of elevated blood pressure in children undergoing complete primary repair of bladder exstrophy (CPRE). J Pediatr Urol. 2023;19(4):370.e1–7. https://doi.org/10.1016/j.jpurol.2023.03.013.
18. Pao E, Gove NE, Flynn JT, Hingorani S. Ambulatory blood pressure and endothelial dysfunction in hematopoietic cell transplantation recipients. Biol Blood Marrow Transplant. 2018;24(8):1678–84. https://doi.org/10.1016/j.bbmt.2018.04.024.
19. Hermida RC, Ayala DE, Smolensky MH, Fernandez JR, Mojon A, Portaluppi F. Sleep-time blood pressure: unique sensitive prognostic marker of vascular risk and therapeutic target for prevention. Sleep Med Rev. 2017;33:17–27. https://doi.org/10.1016/j.smrv.2016.04.001.
20. Warady BA, Abraham AG, Schwartz GJ, et al. Predictors of rapid progression of glomerular and nonglomerular kidney disease in children and adolescents: the chronic kidney disease in children (CKiD) cohort. Am J Kidney Dis. 2015;65(6):878–88. https://doi.org/10.1053/j.ajkd.2015.01.008.
21. Parsa A, Kanetsky PA, Xiao R, et al. Genome-wide association of CKD progression: the chronic renal insufficiency cohort study. J Am Soc Nephrol. 2017;28(3):923–34. https://doi.org/10.1681/ASN.2015101152.
22. Fathallah-Shaykh SA, Flynn JT, Pierce CB, et al. Progression of pediatric CKD of nonglomerular origin in the CKiD cohort. Clin J Am Soc Nephrol. 2015;10(4):571–7. https://doi.org/10.2215/CJN.07480714.
23. Wong CS, Pierce CB, Cole SR, et al. Association of proteinuria with race, cause of chronic kidney disease, and glomerular filtration rate in the chronic kidney disease in children study. Clin J Am Soc Nephrol. 2009;4(4):812–9. https://doi.org/10.2215/CJN.01780408.
24. Wuhl E, Schaefer F. Therapeutic strategies to slow chronic kidney disease progression. Pediatr Nephrol. 2008;23(5):705–16. https://doi.org/10.1007/s00467-008-0789-y.
25. Dionne JM. Evidence-based guidelines for the management of hypertension in children with chronic kidney disease. Pediatr Nephrol. 2015;30(11):1919–27. https://doi.org/10.1007/s00467-015-3077-7.
26. Nolin AC, Mulhern RM, Panchenko MV, et al. Proteinuria causes dysfunctional autophagy in the proximal tubule. Am J Physiol Renal Physiol. 2016;311(6):F1271–9. https://doi.org/10.1152/ajprenal.00125.2016.
27. Furth SL, Pierce C, Hui WF, et al. Estimating time to ESRD in children with CKD. Am J Kidney Dis. 2018;71(6):783–92. https://doi.org/10.1053/j.ajkd.2017.12.011.
28. Panzarino V, Lesser J, Cassani FA. Pediatric chronic kidney disease. Adv Pediatr Infect Dis. 2022;69(1):123–32. https://doi.org/10.1016/j.yapd.2022.03.008.

29. Crowe A, Cairns HS, Wood S, Rudge CJ, Woodhouse CR, Neild GH. Renal transplantation following renal failure due to urological disorders. Nephrol Dial Transplant. 1998;13(8):2065–9. https://doi.org/10.1093/ndt/13.8.2065.
30. Marchal S, Kalfa N, Iborra F, et al. Long-term outcome of renal transplantation in patients with congenital lower urinary tract malformations: a multicenter study. Transplantation. 2020;104(1):165–71. https://doi.org/10.1097/TP.0000000000002746.
31. Haddad E, Sancaktutar AA, Palmer BW, Aston C, Kropp BP. Who, where, and why are patients lost to follow-up? A 20-year study of bladder exstrophy patients at a single institution. J Pediatr Urol. 2018;14(3):276.e1–6. https://doi.org/10.1016/j.jpurol.2017.12.022.

Role of Nursing in the Early Care of Patients with Bladder Exstrophy

24

Carolyn Fazzini, Amber Heberling, Aseem R. Shukla, and Dana A. Weiss

Introduction

Holistic care is crucial for nurses caring for patients with bladder exstrophy (BE). Nurses are central from the moment of birth, through the pre- and post-operative periods, and into ongoing follow-up. They provide initial reassurance at diagnosis, explain complex medical procedures and terms, assist with inpatient care, and help families navigate the healthcare system for necessary supplies. Additionally, they address key psychosocial concerns and often serve as the primary contact for families.

Effective communication is essential to manage the comprehensive health of children with BE. Nurses act as empathetic advisors, engage in critical assessments, and ensure efficient information flow from medical providers. They advocate for patients during transitions and disseminate BE knowledge across medical teams. In outpatient settings, nurses build lasting relationships with patients and families, using various educational methods such as verbal discussions, diagrams, and written materials, supplemented by online community access. Techniques like teach-back ensure families understand and retain the information shared.

This chapter details the extensive role of nursing throughout the early stages of a child's life with BE.

C. Fazzini (✉) · A. R. Shukla · D. A. Weiss
Children's Hospital of Philadelphia, Philadelphia, PA, USA
e-mail: fazzinic@chop.edu; ShuklaA@chop.edu; WeissD1@chop.edu

A. Heberling
Seattle Children's Hospital, Seattle, WA, USA

A. R. Shukla, R. S. Joshi (eds.), *Bladder Exstrophy and Epispadias*,
https://doi.org/10.1007/978-3-031-91238-2_24

Birth to Surgery

Inpatient (Fig. 24.1)

Nursing care for patients with BE starts at birth. The delivery team uses silk to tie the umbilical stump, avoiding abrasions that a clamp might cause on the bladder. Once the baby is stable in the NICU or nursery, nurses begin educating parents on bladder care until surgical repair is needed. They emphasize the importance of keeping the bladder covered, protected, and moist to prevent irritation, while ensuring the umbilical stalk remains dry. This can be achieved using everyday items like kitchen plastic wrap or clear adhesive bandages such as Tegaderm. Beneath the wrap, a protective moisturizer like Carasyn Hydrogel or saline should be applied. Saline can be bought or made at home with water and table salt.

- Recipe for saline—To make saline, use 4 cups (1000 mL) of distilled water or 4 cups of boiled tap water. Water should be boiled for about 20 min. When water is lukewarm, add 2 teaspoons (10 mL) of non-iodized salt. Mix until the salt is dissolved. Label the container (bottle or jar) with the date and store it in the refrigerator for up to 2 weeks.

Before hospital discharge, especially if surgical repair is delayed, nurses provide additional guidance and reassurance on general care. Beyond covering the bladder, they advise using latex-free products and discuss the high risk of fungal infections near the bladder. To prevent diaper dermatitis, fungal infections, and skin breakdown, it's important to regularly moisturize and dry the skin of the lower abdomen, buttocks, and groin. Nurses encourage parents to keep in touch with the outpatient

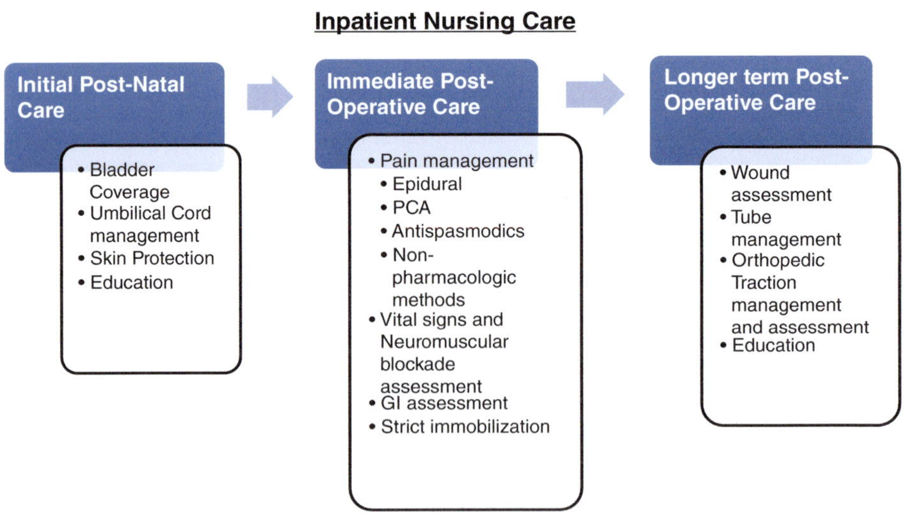

Fig. 24.1 Inpatient nursing care: Phases of care and key points to monitor and assess

clinic about any skin issues. Despite these precautions, babies can still engage in normal activities like using a regular car seat, doing tummy time, bathing, and even going to the pool or beach.

Outpatient (Fig. 24.2)

Each hospital follows specific protocols leading up to surgery with the primary goals of maintaining healthy skin and ensuring normal growth and weight gain for the patient.

Surgery Preparation and Education

Before surgery, an anemia screening is conducted by the primary care provider. Additionally, blood typing and crossmatching are completed as part of the anesthesia clearance. To guide antibiotic selection, some centers may perform a bladder plate culture 2 weeks prior to surgery. Others might conduct this culture on the day of surgery to address any early signs of fever and to inform treatment decisions. However, some centers may choose not to perform this culture at all.

General Assessment and Education

A social determinant of health screening is essential to identify families needing additional resources to ensure appropriate nutrition and general care for their child. This may necessitate a social work consultation to provide comprehensive access to

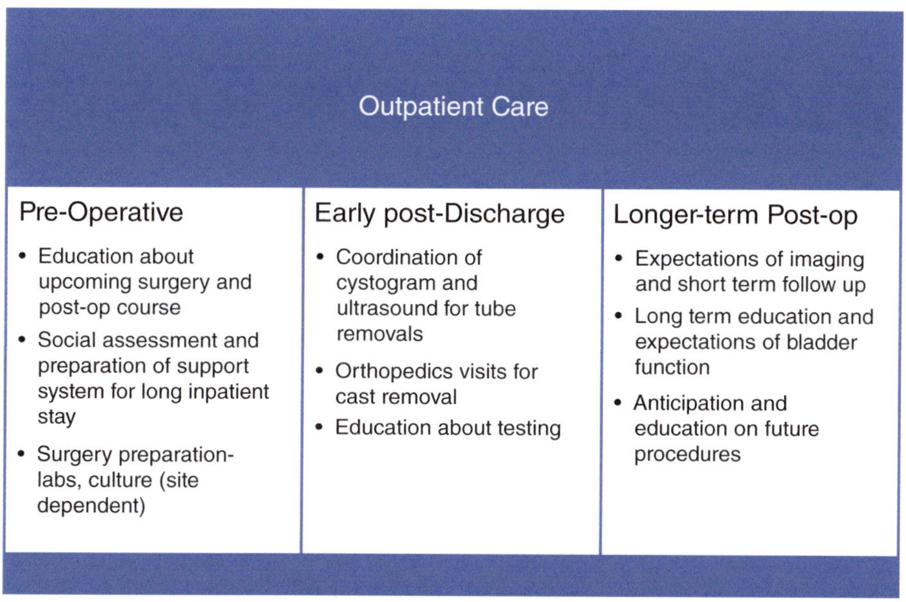

Fig. 24.2 Outpatient nursing care: phases of care and key points of assessment and education

necessary resources. Understanding how families will manage logistics for appointments, including potential issues with flights or long-distance travel, is crucial. Financial challenges related to insurance coverage or lost wages due to prolonged hospital stays and frequent appointments are common. Support such as FMLA paperwork and other resources should be provided and reassessed after surgery.

Logistics regarding the care of siblings and accommodation for parents during hospital stays must also be planned. If there are barriers in these areas, a social work consultation is recommended to thoroughly assess available resources. Essential requirements include access to running water at various temperatures, temperature-controlled environments, well-lit areas for wound care, and necessary medical equipment and medications. Considerations for travel logistics, especially when the child is in a brace or spica cast, are critical. It is important to note that the child may not fit in standard strollers or highchairs, which could be a financial burden.

Reducing anxiety involves preparing the family for what to expect. Setting realistic timelines for surgery and post-operative recovery, including time in the NICU, regular wards, and overall hospital stay, helps manage expectations and alleviate stress. Repeatedly discussing the plan for post-operative care, including immobilization, tube placement, and removal schedules, provides reassurance and helps families feel more at ease.

Providing educational handouts during preoperative visits can be very beneficial, as families often need time to learn and process information across multiple encounters. These materials should cover the basics of BE, what to expect during and after surgery, and details on post-operative care, particularly regarding the various surgical tubes and their maintenance. Information on the type of orthopedic traction—such as external fixation, SPICA cast, or other braces—which often worries families the most, should also be included.

Nurses play a crucial role in reinforcing the surgeon's explanations, detailing what will happen during the surgery. Visual aids like diagrams, images, or even dolls set up with external fixations can enhance understanding. It's important that nurses not only repeat this information but also provide written documents to complement verbal discussions.

For families unfamiliar with hospital settings, understanding inpatient procedures can be overwhelming. Nurses should explain the daily routines, including who will perform specific checks and when these will occur, helping families plan and prepare. Detailed information about inpatient logistics is also essential, such as who can stay overnight and what personal items to bring from home. This guidance helps manage expectations and reduces the stress of adapting to the hospital environment.

Post-operative Nursing Care

Inpatient (Fig. 24.1)

Post-operative inpatient nursing is crucial for successful surgery outcomes. It requires nurses skilled in the anatomy and physiology of patients recovering from

BE surgery. Nurses continuously monitor pain control, wound integrity, signs of adverse events, urine output, and infection risks. After the initial critical period, they also provide essential teaching to families about post-discharge care.

Pain Control

Most patients receive an epidural for pain management post-surgery. Nurses play a vital role in monitoring the epidural's effectiveness and potential side effects. They maintain open communication with the anesthesia and pain management teams to adjust treatment based on the patient's condition. The head of the bed (HOB) is kept elevated at 30 degrees for 24 h to reduce the risk of opioid migration. Nurses check the epidural insertion site every 8 h for any signs of infection or mechanical issues like bloody, serous, or purulent drainage or any disruption of the tube.

Regular assessments include checking vital signs every 4 h and continuous monitoring of pulse oximetry and cardiorespiratory status while the epidural is in place. Pain intensity and scores are evaluated at least every 4 h or more frequently as needed. Close monitoring for neuromuscular blockade is essential to prevent complications such as hypotension, muscle weakness, and paralysis. Early signs to watch for include tingling around the mouth or lips, tremulousness, a metallic taste, inconsolable crying in infants, or general agitation. More severe symptoms, indicating urgent medical intervention, include hypotension, seizures, ventricular dysrhythmias, and cardiac arrest.

The primary objective of post-operative pain management is to control pain effectively while gradually reducing opioid use and avoiding medications that could alter mental status. Pain assessment in children varies by age and includes self-reported pain scores, behavioral observations, and clinical indicators such as changes in heart rate, blood pressure, oxygen saturation, and respiratory patterns. Treatment may involve adjustments to the epidural, as well as administering IV and oral pain medications.

It is crucial to integrate non-pharmacologic methods, especially for infants. These include repositioning, providing consistent support from family or nursing staff, reducing environmental stimuli like lights and noise, and offering comfort items such as pacifiers, toys, or blankets. Techniques such as playing soothing music, massage, therapeutic breathing, and guided imagery can also be effective. Referrals to child life specialists can help parents understand and apply these non-medication pain relief strategies that are suitable for their child's age.

During the initial recovery phase when infants cannot be physically held, nurses instruct parents on comforting techniques. As the child's condition stabilizes, nurses also guide parents on safely holding their child, who may be in a brace or cast.

Wound and Tube Assessments

Nurses continuously monitor skin integrity, wound condition, potential urinary tract infections, and catheter care. This vigilant monitoring ensures early detection and management of complications, maintaining the overall well-being of the patient.

Wound assessment is crucial for preventing complications such as wound breakdown, which commonly occurs at the penopubic junction and may involve the bladder or urethra. In cases where a wound breakdown leads to a fistula, diverting urine flow is essential, as some small fistulas may heal spontaneously. For those that do not heal on their own, surgical intervention for closure might be necessary later. More frequently, superficial wound breakdowns occur, which do not penetrate into the urinary tract. These should be carefully monitored for infection and managed with appropriate skin care to prevent further deterioration.

Nursing care also includes monitoring IV sites for signs of phlebitis or infiltration during infusions and ensuring catheters remain patent until they can be safely removed. Epidural sites should be checked every 8 hours for any abnormal drainage.

Immobilization

During periods of immobilization, it is critical to monitor the child for potential complications arising from reduced mobility. These can include respiratory infections due to atelectasis, decreased appetite affecting nutritional intake and wound healing, and constipation. Constipation not only increases the risk of urinary tract infections but also leads to abdominal distention and straining, which can adversely affect wound healing. Effective catheter care is imperative and varies depending on the surgical approach used. Typically, children have a urethral catheter, a suprapubic catheter, and two ureteral stents, occasionally accompanied by a wound drain. These devices must be regularly checked for patency, kept clean and free from bowel contamination, and secured against accidental displacement.

GI Function and Constipation

Monitoring gastrointestinal function and nutrition is crucial for two main reasons. Adequate nutrition is vital for effective wound healing, while regular bowel movements help prevent abdominal distention and straining that could impair the healing process. During the immediate post-operative period, abdominal girth should be measured every 8 h to monitor for any signs of distention, which can indicate serious complications like abdominal compartment syndrome. This condition, characterized by abdominal pain, increased distention, shortness of breath, hypotension, and oliguria, requires urgent notification of the surgical team. If there is no significant distention, the patient's diet is typically advanced starting from the first post-operative day and gradually increased. If constipation occurs, interventions such as suppositories or enemas may be employed.

Orthopedic Care

Orthopedic management in exstrophy patients involves both urologic oversight and complex orthopedic procedures. Immediate post-operative care includes hourly neurovascular assessments for the first 24 h, then every 4 h or as needed. These assessments focus on bilateral comparisons of pulses, capillary refill, skin color, temperature, sensation, movement, and any signs of edema. Nurses must be vigilant about new-onset edema, particularly if a patient has been positioned on one side for extended periods.

For those in spica casts or undergoing external fixation with Buck's traction, routine skin assessments every 8 h are mandatory. Log rolling the patient every 2 h is recommended to prevent pressure injuries, and special attention is needed to pad the skin under braces or casts and to float heels off the bed to prevent pressure sores. The initial 5 days post-surgery are typically the most critical with restricted movement, after which the cast or brace may be opened for cleaning, and the child can be held by family.

Routine pin care for external fixation involves daily assessments and changing of dressings as needed. Pin sites should be cleaned with a solution of half water and half hydrogen peroxide, using a fresh cotton swab or gauze for each pin. Nursing care plans should ideally coordinate patient bathing and bedsheet changes with pin care routines. Any signs of infection at pin sites, such as fever, purulent drainage, or redness, must be immediately reported to the orthopedics team.

Nurses efficiently cluster various assessments during care activities, such as during the two-hourly log rolls, to simultaneously manage pain relief, check skin integrity, perform neurovascular assessments, and ensure the proper functioning of tubes and drains. This comprehensive approach helps prevent complications and ensures thorough and continuous care.

Parental Teaching

Nurses play a crucial role in educating parents about the timeline and expectations during both the inpatient stay and the subsequent outpatient post-operative course. The duration of the inpatient stay can vary, typically ranging from a week to 6 weeks, with most lasting about 2–3 weeks. Parents are educated on signs to monitor that could indicate complications, such as skin integrity issues, signs of infection, and urinary tract infections.

To ensure families can adequately care for their child at home, nurses employ teaching methods like repeat-back or teach-back. These techniques confirm that the family understands the care procedures and knows how to respond to potential complications. Parents are taught to perform regular assessments for skin health, infection prevention, and urinary tract health once the child is home.

It's also vital for families to understand the appropriate steps to take if complications arise. Nurses clarify which situations warrant a direct trip to the emergency room, which issues should lead to a call to the medical office, and how to handle non-urgent concerns. Information about who to contact for urgent matters and the appropriate hospital for emergencies, especially if they live far from the care center, is provided. During these discussions, nurses also consider social and economic factors that might affect care, offering support such as language interpretation and help navigating the healthcare system. Planning for the logistics of follow-up appointments, especially travel arrangements, is also discussed to ensure smooth post-operative management.

Outpatient (Fig. 24.2)

Once the child has been discharged, care shifts from the inpatient nurse to the outpatient nursing team. This time is critical for close communication with the family to review any concerns. Depending on the care center, patients may be discharged with one or multiple tubes in place and often are still in traction devices.

In addition, the family will be scheduled for a series of close follow-up visits with various imaging studies. The outpatient nurse can provide expectations for ultrasounds as well as for cystograms to assess bladder integrity before cycling and to assess vesicoureteral reflux. Once bladder cycling with a suprapubic tube is complete, then the child will have the tube removed, so the nursing team can provide expectations for this clinic procedure as well.

In the long term, the outpatient nursing team can keep in close contact during the initial 6–12 weeks post-operatively with ongoing education and expectations. Then, as families continue to follow up at longer and longer intervals, they will continue to support the physician in education and expectations.

Conclusion

Nursing care is essential in complementing and enhancing the treatment provided by physicians from the immediate postnatal period through long-term post-operative care. This chapter has outlined the foundational teaching and management strategies employed prior to surgery and during the critical post-operative phase. Collaborating with an experienced exstrophy nursing team not only streamlines care but also ensures a safer post-operative period and an overall enhanced experience for the patient, their family, and the entire care team.

Bibliography

Ahn JJ, Shnorhavorian M, Katz C, Goldin AB, Merguerian PA. Early versus delayed closure of bladder exstrophy: a national surgical quality improvement program pediatric analysis. J Pediatr Urol. 2018;14(1):27.e1–5. https://doi.org/10.1016/j.jpurol.2017.11.008.

Balthazar AK, Finkelstein JB, Williams V, Lee T, Lajoie D, Logvinenko T, Kim YJ, Chacko S, Borer JG, Lee RS. Enhanced recovery after surgery for an uncommon complex urological procedure: the complete primary repair of bladder exstrophy. J Urol. 2023;210(4):696–703. https://doi.org/10.1097/JU.0000000000003593.

Haffar A, Hirsch A, Morrill C, Harris TGW, Crigger C, Garcia A, Maxon V, Di Carlo HN, Monitto C, Gearhart JP, Hunsberger JB. Perioperative management of primary classic bladder exstrophy: a single institutional pathway to success. J Pediatr Urol. 2024;20(3):406.e1–7. https://doi.org/10.1016/j.jpurol.2024.01.010.

Roth E, Goetz J, Kryger J, Groth T. Postoperative immobilization and pain management after repair of bladder exstrophy. Curr Urol Rep. 2017;18(3):19. https://doi.org/10.1007/s11934-017-0667-x.

The Impact of Physical Therapy on the Bladder Exstrophy-Epispadias Complex

25

Sarah Cooper and Caroline Bergh

Introduction

Physical therapists are musculoskeletal specialists that are uniquely qualified to assist in the development of muscle strengthening and facilitating the progression of coordination of the pelvic floor musculature. This is particularly essential in the development of a functional bladder for those with exstrophy-epispadias complex as surgical repair and reconstruction typically occur in infancy or early childhood. With only about 25% expected to void per urethra without reliance on catheterization or urinary diversion, intensive physical therapy intervention could have a significant impact on continence, quality of life, and health in BEEC [7].

S. Cooper (✉) · C. Bergh
Department of Physical Therapy, Children's Hospital of Philadelphia, Philadelphia, PA, USA
e-mail: CooperS1@chop.edu; BerghC@chop.edu

A. R. Shukla, R. S. Joshi (eds.), *Bladder Exstrophy and Epispadias*, https://doi.org/10.1007/978-3-031-91238-2_25

Pelvic Floor Musculature

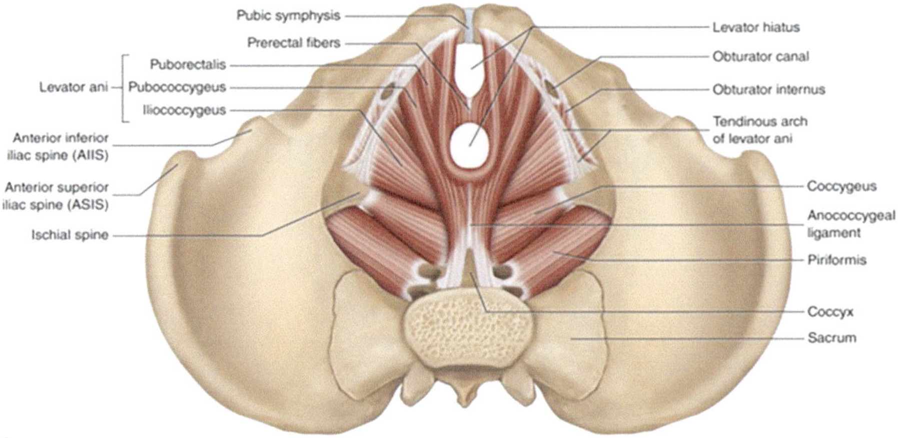

C

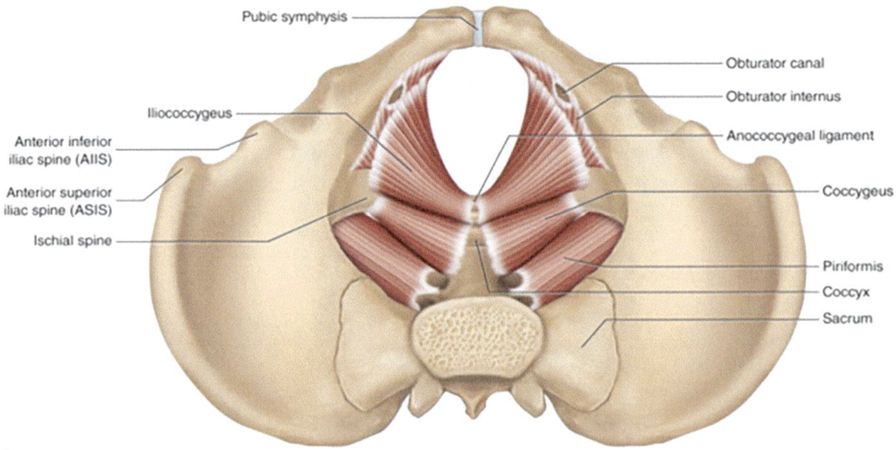

D

The pelvic floor spans from the sacrum and coccyx to extend to the pubis and ischium. Pelvic floor musculature provides support for the organs of the pelvic cavity and allows flexion of the sacrum and coccyx. These muscles also control the movement of bodily fluids through the urethra and anus. Pelvic floor muscles are under voluntary control, unlike the smooth muscles of the bladder, colon, and rectum. Pelvic floor muscles can inhibit smooth muscle involuntary contraction through voluntary muscle control. Three muscles (puborectalis, pubococcygeus, and iliococcygeus) form a major portion of the pelvic floor, collectively known as the levator ani, and serve to carry the weight of the abdominal and pelvic organs. Specifically, the puborectalis provides active control of the anorectal angle by opening the anus and the urogenital hiatus during defecation. The pubococcygeus is a sling-like muscle that provides support to the overall pelvic floor area, and the iliococcygeus supports the pelvic floor by providing a shelf for organs to rest. The coccygeus (deep) also provides support to the pelvic floor. The levator ani and coccygeus form a region of the pelvic diaphragm known as the anal triangle [12].

It is vital to remember that the muscles of the pelvic floor do not operate in isolation. Organs and muscles of the respiratory system are critical in supporting pelvic floor functionality. It is important to have postural support superiorly at the larynx and inferiorly with the pelvic floor. The diaphragm is a major pressure regulator, separating the thoracic and abdominal cavities. Additionally, the proximity of the pelvic floor muscles to the prime movers of the pelvis and lower extremities is also important to note, specifically, the piriformis and obturator internus, which both serve as external rotators of the hip. The obturator internus has a direct connection to the pelvic floor via shared fascial attachments, as strengthening of the obturator internus allows for increased overflow strengthening to the pelvic floor. Therefore, a dysfunction in the pelvic floor should be considered a dysfunction of the core.

Muscular Differences in BEEC

It is theorized that bladder exstrophy-epispadias exstrophy complex (BEEC) arises from a disturbance within the development of the mesoderm, specifically the premature rupture of the cloacal membrane, from a mechanical obstruction of mesodermal migration, or disruption of the cellular functioning resulting in abnormal development. As a result, disruption occurs to the structural alignment of the pelvis, sacrum, and SI joint. Additionally, the anatomical alignment of the pelvic floor musculature is also impacted. The levator ani muscle bulk is generally smaller, and presentation includes a flattened, twisted, externally rotated which impacts the ability to provide adequate support to the pelvic girdle as well as the organs of the genitourinary system [14].

Physical Therapy Evaluation

Dysfunctional voiding is one component of pelvic health impairments that can impact age-appropriate participation, social-emotional well-being, functional mobility, access to education, and quality of life. Timing of interventions, such as pelvic health physical therapy (PT), is critical in the development of continence in addressing pelvic health dysfunctions [6].

Pelvic floor development begins in the early months of infancy, and therefore it is important to initiate PT evaluations to determine what limitations a child has early on in their BEEC journey. Ideally, evaluations are completed preoperatively as recommendations can be made to encourage strengthening and development of the appropriate musculature prior to surgical intervention.

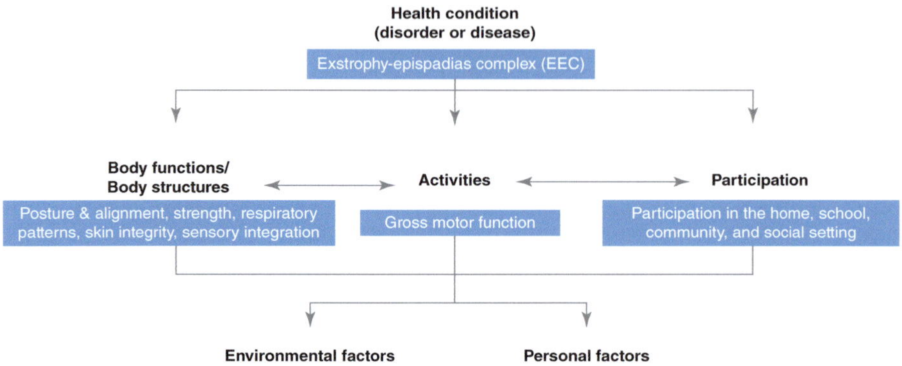

Fig. 25.1 International classification of functioning, disability, and health (ICF) model

Following surgical intervention, most children experience a period of delayed development and loss of strength. Although most children can recover to their baseline without PT intervention, it is questioned if this is lost time for continued development and strengthening. As maximum strength and function is ideal for continence, it cannot be said that this does not impact a child's potential for continence in the future. When considering timing of a PT evaluation post surgery, a PT evaluation should be completed once a child is cleared to bear weight through their lower extremities.

A child should continue to be monitored and evaluated to identify areas of need. The goals of the child and family will change as the child ages and should be reflective of the current development and function of their muscles. A child will benefit from different goals during the pre-potty training stage as compared to the post-potty training stage. As potty training will look different in a child with BEEC, it is important to identify the needs at these specific stages.

The International Classification of Functioning, Disability, and Health (ICF) can be utilized to identify the important components of a PT evaluation within the participation, activity, and impairment level. Utilizing the ICF Model (Fig. 25.1), physical therapists treat the impairments associated with health conditions, including pelvic floor dysfunctions, such as BEEC. Therapeutic goals are established to allow for the application of common principles in the treatment of bowel and bladder impairments. Goals are targeted to address pelvic floor strength and coordination while allowing for bladder capacity growth and creating optimal biomechanical alignment during voiding while also supporting increases in participation and independence in social and educational settings, quality of life, and reducing the burden of care on caregivers.

Participation

The primary goal of treatment in BEEC is to improve the quality of life for the child, which can be significantly impacted by urinary incontinence. This impact can be significant in the school, home, and social setting, including extracurricular participation such as sports and social activities, including sleepovers, vacations, and playgroups. Patient-reported outcome measures, including the cross-cultural continence-specific pediatric quality-of-life measurement tool (PinQ) and Dysfunctional Voiding Symptom Score (DVSS), can be used to qualitatively measure the effect of BE and corresponding symptoms in the home and community setting.

Activity

An extensive history of bladder and bowel habits should be obtained. Questions should include if the child is able to undress and dress independently, transfer on and off the toilet, and complete hygiene independently, if the child is currently on a voiding schedule, and if the child is currently toilet trained for bowel movements. The current posture and equipment the child is using in the bathroom, including stools, toilet inserts, and toddler toilets, should be noted. A picture can be obtained to assess the posture and positioning on the toilet. An extensive bladder log can be completed to determine the length of any dry intervals. This can include the use of pull-ups or pads and the frequency at which these are changed. It is also important to ask about the frequency and consistency of bowel movements. The Bristol stool scale and urine color chart can be used to identify any concerns with constipation or dehydration [17].

Given the differences in anatomy and muscular development in bladder exstrophy, it is important to assess overall gross motor development in this population. The Peabody Developmental Motor Scales Third Edition (PDMS-3) is a comprehensive, reliable, and valid standardized test used to measure motor skills for children under 5 years. The gross motor core subset is the culmination of three subtests: body control, body transport, and object control if the child is over the age of 12 months [5]. The Bruininks-Oseretsky Test of Motor Proficiency, Third Edition (BOT-3), is a comprehensive, reliable, and valid standardized test utilized to measure motor skills for children over the age of 5 years. The gross motor composite is the culmination of two subtests: body coordination and strength and agility [2]. Although these assessments are good indicators of overall gross motor function, they do not provide information regarding the quality of movement and the use of specific muscle groups. Therefore, additional assessments of the impairment level are necessary. A gait analysis can also be beneficial in identifying areas in need of further investigation at the impairment level. It can be common to see increased out-toeing with slower cadence and velocity [15].

Impairment

The impairment level assessment for the BEEC population can be broken down into distinct categories: posture and alignment, ROM and flexibility, strength, respiratory patterns, skin integrity, and sensory integration.

Posture and Alignment: When assessing posture and alignment, it is important to look at both static and dynamic in a variety of positions, including standing, sitting, and quadruped. Altered posture can be indicative of muscle imbalances and asymmetries resulting in movement dysfunction. It is common to see a widened base of support in all developmental positions and bilateral out-toeing. During dynamic movement, genu valgus at the knee is often seen due to weakness of the hip musculature. It is also common to see an anteriorly tilted pelvis due to weakness in the abdominals and limited flexibility in the hip flexors.

Range of Motion and Flexibility: Limited range of motion at a joint or limited flexibility of a muscle can lead to movement dysfunction and affect the efficiency of surrounding musculature. In comparison, excessive range of motion can lead to lack of stability, again resulting in movement dysfunction. The retroverted acetabulum sometimes seen in BE can result in limited internal rotation and excessive external rotation [15]. While an anterior pelvic tilt can lead to tightness in the hip flexors.

Strength: Strength assessment is imperative in identifying weakness of muscle groups that can lead to dysfunction and limited success at the participation level. It is important to assess functional strength, including both power and endurance. Formal manual muscle testing can be completed with patients of appropriate age [10]. For those younger, a functional assessment can be completed, and any lateral asymmetries should be noted. Key muscle groups to assess include the pelvic floor, hips (specifically gluteus medius and obturator internus), and abdominals (specifically transverse abdominis).

Respiratory Patterns: Breathing patterns can be indicative of the primary muscles used during respiration in various positions and during different functional movements. Given the close relationship between the respiratory muscles and pelvic floor function, it is important to assess breathing patterns to determine areas of dysfunction. The ratio of diaphragm to chest can provide an objective measure, while reports of accessory muscle use can provide more subjective information.

Skin Integrity: Scars can result in adhesions and restrictions that limit the mobility and function of tissue. The modified Vancouver scar scale (MVSS) can be used to assess the pliability, height, vascularity, and pigmentation of each scar [9]. Scars go through a well-defined period of change and maturation during 120 days following surgery; therefore, it is important to assess each scar during each evaluation [4].

Sensory Integration: Sensory awareness of both external and internal stimuli can be impacted in the BEEC population. It is important to assess the child's current level of sensation, specifically interoception. Interoception is the ability to sense internal signals that can allow us to identify a need, such as needing to void or eat. It is predicted that this signal is limited in those with BE due to the poor storing ability and capacity of the bladder.

Physical Therapy Intervention

As a child ages and advances through their BE journey, the needs and goals will continue to shift and progress. The primary focus of PT throughout the BEEC journey is on the development and function of the muscles that support continence and gross motor development. This will look different throughout each stage and will be based on the clinical findings of the evaluation. Prior to the initiation toilet training, it is recommended that a child demonstrate readiness skills for toileting. Acquisition of these readiness skills, which range from understanding toileting language to being comfortable with sitting on the toilet, typically starts between 22 and 30 months of age [13]. Achievement of "toilet trained" typically occurs between 36 and 39 months of age, with initiation of the process starting at approximately 24 months of age [11]. It is important to know that these milestones typically occur later for children with BEEC who usually train for bowel movements prior to urination. It is best to work through the developmental progression of toileting based on the child's skill level vs age to minimize frustration for the child and family.

Pre-toilet Training

Based on early development of the pelvic floor and associated musculature, timely evaluation and treatment are imperative to success. Therefore, based on the exam findings (i.e., deficits in range of motion, weakness, balance, and coordination), it may be indicated to initiate PT treatment prior to closure and immediately after, identified as the pre-toileting stage. Activities will focus on facilitating gross motor development, specifically highlighting abdominal activation and trunk rotation. Based on the evaluation, positioning to support a more neutral alignment of the hips may be recommended. The use of props such as rolled towels or blankets can be used to achieve this while still allowing for free movement of the lower extremities. It is important to highlight that positioning in prone, or tummy time, is safe and necessary for development prior to closure. It is recommended to utilize a flat, even surface and ensure no toys or objects are underneath the abdomen near the exposed bladder. Depending on the child's age and developmental stage, they may be spending a significant amount of time in supine or positioned on their back.

Postoperatively the child will likely be restricted from weight-bearing through the lower extremities and may be placed in a cast or traction. Unless otherwise instructed by the surgical team, it is still advised to encourage play in a variety of developmental positions, including supine, side-lying, sitting, and prone. This can be achieved with the assistance of a caregiver and use of blankets, towels, and pillows for positioning.

Once cleared for weight-bearing by the medical team, a PT evaluation will identify any areas of regression that occurred. The focus to treatment at this time will be to return the child to their gross motor baseline while continuing to facilitate continued progression of gross motor skills and muscle development. Once the skin has fully closed at the areas of the incisions, a daily scar massage can be initiated. This is important to stimulate blood flow and help reduce the buildup of scar tissue, which will improve mobility and function of the surrounding tissue [3].

Toilet Training

When the child is approaching the stage of toilet training, it is important to appreciate each step that is required to be utilizing the bathroom. This includes identifying the urge, mobilizing to the bathroom, undressing, transferring on the toilet, maintaining positioning on the toilet, voiding and/or defecating, hygiene, transferring off the toilet, and dressing. Each stage may require modification or assistance based on the current functional and cognitive abilities, especially at the beginning of the process. As we know, recognizing the urge to void, interoception, can be diminished or absent in a child with BE; a voiding schedule with use of caregiver or alarm reminders may be needed. Identifying the time it takes a child to get to the bathroom will help determine the need for closer bathroom accommodation at school or the use of portable toilets. Easily managed clothing such as dresses or elastic waistbands can be beneficial during the undressing process when zippers, snaps, and buttons are challenging. Adaptive equipment such as stools, toilet seat inserts, or toddler toilets can assist in obtaining the appropriate posture on the toilet. The ideal toilet posture for toileting is a squatting position with the trunk leaning forward, hips flexed greater than 90 degrees, feet supported and flat, and feet hip-width distance apart [1, 16] (Fig. 25.2). This position assists in the relaxation of the puborectalis muscle during defecation [16]. As it may be difficult to obtain a urine stream despite relaxation of the pelvic floor muscles, different techniques can be used to fully empty the bladder. When positioned ideally as described above, use diaphragmic breaths to ensure relaxation of the pelvic floor and surrounding muscles. Use of sustained exhalation can create a slight downward pressure while encouraging ongoing relaxation—utilize pinwheels, bubbles, whistles, or images to help. Bending the trunk completely over the legs or tapping the lower abdomen in the area of the bladder can trigger a contraction of the detrusor to assist with emptying. Lastly if cleared by the child's medical team, gently bearing down can also be used to assist in complete emptying of the bladder. Depending on the amount of time the child can go while being dry, it may be best to limit voiding attempts at first. For example, it is is not recommended to start a child on a voiding schedule of every 30 minutes if that is their dry interval. It is recommended to start with 2-3 voids per day and to focus on the steps of voiding rather than the volume of the void. This will assist with developing the skills required to void while minimizing frustration.

Post-toilet Training

Once a child has become more comfortable in the bathroom, they may begin to show signs of motivation to reduce or eliminate some of the modifications that are in place. The areas of focus will be determined by the child and caregiver goals as

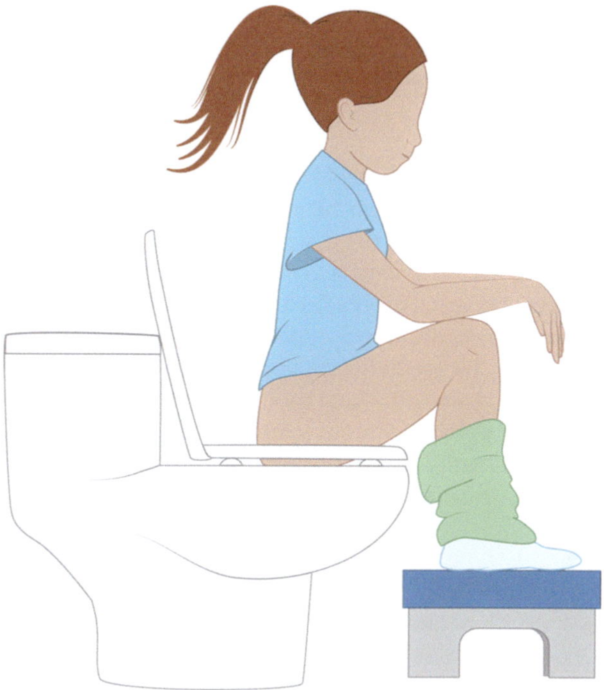

Fig. 25.2 Toilet posture

well as the areas of most potential as determined by the PT evaluation. The development of interoception can assist with identifying the urge to utilize the bathroom independently as well as the ability to identify if the pelvic floor muscles are relaxed or contracted. Recognizing what action the pelvic floor muscles are completing is an important step in both voiding and continence. Neuromuscular control of the pelvic floor is limited secondary to atypical development. Therefore, neuromuscular re-education of the pelvic floor and the surrounding musculature is needed to learn relaxation and contraction of the muscles before strengthening can be initiated. The pelvic floor muscles should be strengthened for both endurance and power. This will assist in continence as the bladder slowly fills throughout the day but also specifically during high levels of abdominal pressure, such as coughing, sneezing, laughing, and jumping. However, most importantly, the pelvic floor muscles should be trained in a variety of positions and movements to reflect the dynamic activities needed for independent mobility. As previously discussed, the pelvic floor doesn't function in isolation. Therefore, it is important to address areas of dysfunction or weakness in the surrounding muscle groups, highlighting the transverse abdominis, obturator internus, and the diaphragm.

Day Versus Night

As continence is a learned behavior, it is important to note that daytime continence is achieved prior to nighttime continence and that it is common to have intervals of being dry or close to being dry during the day while continuing to be wet overnight. With typical development, as bladder capacity increases, interoceptive awareness develops, and bladder hygiene is established, patients will have increased success with remaining dry overnight, transitioning from a brief/diaper to a pad to absorbent underwear to regular underwear. However, this progression may look different in BE due to the small bladder size and limitations in interoception and pelvic floor strength. Strategies can be implemented to assist in decreasing wetness overnight. The act of double voiding, where the child would void prior to the start of a bedtime routine, which is expected to take less than 20–60 min to complete (i.e., bath/shower, brush teeth, read, etc.,) and immediately before turning out the lights to allow for one additional opportunity to empty the bladder before sleep. Nighttime alarms can be used to wake the child at intervals throughout the night to void. Bed-wetting alarms will detect moisture and will wake the child or caregiver to initiate transition to the bathroom to complete the voiding. The social and life goals of the child and family should be considered when choosing a nighttime strategy and may change during various stages of life.

Constipation

Due to the proximity of the bladder and rectum, it is important to consider and then address regular emptying of the bowels and the impact on achieving urinary continence. Due to the limited range of control of the pelvic floor, a child may have difficulty with relaxation and elongation of the pelvic floor during evacuation. Therefore, it is important to address neuromuscular control of the pelvic floor in its entirety. Abdominal massage and regularly timed toilet sits can help alleviate constipation in addition to the postural, developmental, and neuromuscular re-education previously discussed [8]. Pharmaceuticals may be necessary to support regular bowel movements and overall urinary health and should be discussed with the medical team.

References

1. APTA. Proper toilet posture. In: Patient education; 2023. https://www.aptapelvichealth.org/info/proper-toileting-posture. Accessed 15 Aug 2023.
2. Bruininks RH, Bruininks BD. Bruininks-Oseretsky test of motor proficiency. 2nd ed. Pearson Assessments; 2005. https://www.pearsonassessments.com/store/usassessments/en/Store/Professional-Assessments/Motor-Sensory/Bruininks-Oseretsky-Test-of-Motor-Proficiency-%7C-Second-Edition/p/100000648.html. Accessed 5 Sept 2023
3. Deflorin C, Hohenauer E, Stoop R, van Daele U, Clijsen R, Taeymans J. Physical management of scar tissue: a systematic review and meta-analysis. J Altern Complement Med. 2020;26(10):854–65. https://doi.org/10.1089/acm.2020.0109.
4. Fayzullin A, Ignatieva N, Zakharkina O, Tokarev M, Mudryak D, Khristidis Y, Balyasin M, Kurkov A, Churbanov S, Dyuzheva T, Timashev P. Modeling of old scars: histopathological, biochemical and thermal analysis of the scar tissue maturation. Biology. 2021;10(2):136.

5. Folio MR, Fewell RR. Peabody developmental motor scales examiner's manual. 2nd ed. Austin: Pro-Ed; 2000.
6. Franco I, editor. Pediatric incontinence: evaluation and clinical management. 1st ed. Wiley; 2015.
7. Maruf M, Manyevitch R, Michaud J, Jayman J, Kasprenski M, Zaman MH, Benz K, Eldridge M, Trock B, Harris KT, Wu WJ. Urinary continence outcomes in classic bladder exstrophy: a long-term perspective. J Urol. 2020;203(1):200–5.
8. McClurg D, Lowe-Strong A. Does abdominal massage relieve constipation? Nurs Times. 2011;107(12):20–2.
9. Nguyen TA, Feldstein SI, Shumaker PR, Krakowski AC. A review of scar assessment scales. Semin Cutan Med Surg. 2015;34(1):28–36. https://doi.org/10.12788/j.sder.2015.0125.
10. Palmer ML, Epler M. Principles of examination techniques. In: Palmer ML, Epler M, editors. Clinical assessment procedures in physical therapy. Philadelphia: JB Lippincott; 1990. p. 8–36.
11. Pathak P, Ring JD, Delfino KR, Dynda DI, Mathews RI. Complete primary repair of bladder exstrophy: a systematic review. J Pediatr Urol. 2020;16(2):149–53. https://doi.org/10.1016/j.jpurol.2020.01.004.
12. Raizada V, Mittal RK. Pelvic floor anatomy and applied physiology. Gastroenterol Clin North Am. 2008;37(3):493–509., vii. https://doi.org/10.1016/j.gtc.2008.06.003.
13. Schum TR, Kolb TM, McAuliffe TL, Simms MD, Underhill RL, Lewis M. Sequential acquisition of toilet-training skills: a descriptive study of gender and age differences in normal children. Pediatrics. 2002;109(3):e48. https://doi.org/10.1542/peds.109.3.e48.
14. Stec AA. Embryology and bony and pelvic floor anatomy in the bladder exstrophy-epispadias complex. Semin Pediatr Surg. 2011;20(2):66–70. https://doi.org/10.1053/j.sempedsurg.2010.12.011.
15. Sutherland D, Pike L, Kaufman K, Mowery C, Kaplan G, Romanus B. Hip function and gait in patients treated for bladder exstrophy. J Pediatr Orthop. 1994;14(6):709–14. https://doi.org/10.1097/01241398-199414060-00004.
16. Tosun ÖÇ, et al. Are clinically recommended pelvic floor muscle relaxation positions really efficient for muscle relaxation? Int Urogynecol J. 2022;33(9):2391–400.
17. Yensen CP, Pendergrass JA, Smith SW, Lloveras LA, Vollmer TR. Teaching practitioners to use the bristol stool form scale. Behavior Analysis in Practice. 2025:1–1.

Psychological Implications of Bladder Exstrophy-Epispadias

26

Christina M. Rouse

Pediatric Psychology

As seen throughout this book, bladder exstrophy-epispadias complex (BEEC) is a spectrum of genitourinary conditions that affect not only the child but the entire family unit. The physical and mental struggles of living with BEEC begin in infancy with bladder reconstruction, possible surgeries and adjustments in childhood, and health and symptom maintenance throughout adulthood [1]. Therapy can be a useful tool at any stage of development, depending on the needs of the child and family. Every family is different in functioning, resiliency, severity of medical condition, and access to care; therefore, the plan for each family should be individualized. This type of work is best conducted by a psychosocial specialist that understands the nuances of BEEC, which can include clinical social workers, pediatric psychologists, child psychiatrists, and child life specialists trained in urological concerns. In addition, introducing the family to behavioral health services early in medical care (e.g., infancy or early childhood) can help with acceptance when seeking psychological services in the future [2].

Pediatric psychology is a specialty that includes emotional and behavioral support for children and adolescents with various chronic medical conditions. Pediatric psychologists are commonly embedded in pediatric hospital divisions and can be utilized in inpatient, outpatient, and multidisciplinary settings [3]. Pediatric psychologists can be involved as early as birth in the fetal or neonatal inpatient hospital units to support caregivers of children with BEEC. As the child continues to develop, the child and their caregivers can meet with a specific type of pediatric psychologist that is trained in working with children with urological concerns, often known as a "uropsychologist." If a urology team does not have a uropsychologist, a pediatric psychologist that focuses on coping with chronic health concerns is a great

C. M. Rouse (✉)
Division of Urology, Children's Hospital of Philadelphia, Philadelphia, PA, USA

A. R. Shukla, R. S. Joshi (eds.), *Bladder Exstrophy and Epispadias*, https://doi.org/10.1007/978-3-031-91238-2_26

equivalent. A uropsychologist is part of the urology medical team and engages in a wide range of therapy interventions for urological diagnoses. These include but are not limited to symptoms of depression and/or anxiety surrounding medical treatment, medication, or procedures; adherence to medical regimen; behavioral concerns inhibiting progress; and preparation for surgery or procedures [4]. These interventions are applied differently at each stage of the lifespan and will be expanded upon in this chapter.

Infancy

Since caregivers of children with BEEC are typically aware of medical anomalies prenatally, the stress and decision-making start before they meet their child. Giving birth to a child and preparing to be a caregiver is a stressful endeavor; adding a complex medical concern into the mix can create more difficulty and feelings of unease in the process. The focus of therapy during this time is on the caregivers making medical decisions for their child. Caregivers will follow the guidance of the surgeons and medical team; however, these decisions are typically complex and are easier to handle if they are processed in a nonjudgmental and safe environment. Therapy for these concerns tends to focus on validating caregiver hesitations with consenting to medical procedures, normalizing their emotional experiences, and discussing fears they have for their child as they develop [5]. Because the child is not able to voice preferences or concerns at this stage in development, caregivers may feel this burden and worry about the consequences of making choices for their child's body. Greater trust with the medical team also increases the caregivers' confidence in surgical decision-making [5], and strong communication throughout the process from the medical team improves caregiver-provider relationships [6].

In addition to medical and mental health providers, caregivers may consult with their trusted family members and/or friends and social media networks [5]. Caregivers with a mutual goal of learning about surgery and living with specific medical conditions can create groups within social media (e.g., Facebook groups) to connect with other families with similar struggles. Through this route, caregivers can learn about surgeries and procedures that are preferred, suggest providers that are knowledgeable about the condition, ask questions they may not feel comfortable asking medical providers, and understand development through childhood with the medical condition. These connections can help with the decision-making process at a young age and provide peace of mind to caregivers who are unsure of how to navigate their child's medical condition.

At this stage, some caregivers are processing the long-term struggles a child with BEEC may face throughout their development [7]. Frequent topics include how to manage peer questions as they develop through childhood, whether the child will resent the caregivers for the medical decisions that they make for them, or whether they will live a fulfilling life (e.g., sexual functioning and appearance, fertility, and ability to procreate). Caregivers typically think ahead for their child and want to remove as many obstacles as possible so the child can live a close-to-normal life.

Answering these questions as a provider is difficult, as individual differences play a role in how the child develops. Uropsychologists encourage caregivers to focus on each stage of development in smaller increments, rather than trying to solve concerns that could occur in the future. This helps reduce the level of anxiety and create a more balanced approach to the child's development.

Childhood

In this stage of development, children may undergo a series of changes and are able to verbalize more of their preferences and struggles with caregivers. Since bladder reconstruction is typically completed during infancy, the child with BEEC will be guided by their medical team to determine how to maintain continence or medical stability in childhood, which can be based on the preference of the family and severity of the medical condition. This can include a vesicostomy, voiding schedule, or catheterization if a plan is not already established. At times, these recommendations can be overwhelming, and it can be difficult to help the child adjust to frequent medical appointments, procedures, and regimens. In addition, children become more self-aware of their differences at this stage, and guidance is needed for both children and their families with navigating BEEC as they begin to attend school with peers.

Children with BEEC may notice the differences between themselves and peers during this stage of development. A concern for caregivers at this stage of development can include keeping the child's medical condition private from other peers in shared restrooms at school (e.g., hiding medical supplies such as diapers/pull-ups, and catheters) or frequent incontinence causing them to need to get changed into clean clothes [2]. Children may have access to a private restroom at either the nurse's office or another space in the school to mitigate these concerns; however, this may also cause peers to notice the differences in routine and ask personal questions about their special privileges. Another disparity they may see or learn is that their genitalia appear different from peers or siblings, as differences may be pointed out by others if they are sharing a restroom. As a result, caregivers are placed in a difficult position to explain these differences to their child and help them navigate these questions from others. Another struggle that may become more apparent is the number of medical appointments, procedures, and/or surgeries the child may need to attend during the school year. These absences are occasionally noticed by peers and questioned, which can be uncomfortable for the child. The child may also feel disappointment in missing classroom time or preferred outings (e.g., field trips) due to medical necessity.

Caregivers are encouraged to have open conversations with their child about privacy and how to handle these difficult conversations. These concerns can be discussed with their medical or mental health provider, and coping strategies can be taught in therapy to help accept their medical condition and the differences that are noticed. Uropsychologists will use role-playing and role reversal (e.g., switching roles so the child pretends to be the other person asking intrusive questions and the

Table 26.1 Examples of questions and responses regarding BEEC

Questions	Responses
"Why do you use a different bathroom?"	"I have a medical condition"
	"I don't want to talk about it"
	"I just have to do it"
	"Please respect my privacy"
"Why does your [private area] look different than mine?"	"It is none of your business"
	"I don't want to talk about it"
	"That is not an appropriate question"
	"Please stop asking that question"
"Why do you wear diapers/pull-ups?"	"I have a medical condition"
	"It is none of your business"
	"That is not an appropriate question"
	"I don't know what you are talking about"
"Why do you miss so much school?"	"I have a medical condition"
	"I just need to do it"
	"I don't talk about this with other people"
	"Please respect my answers"

caregiver/mental health provider is the child) as a strategy to help children feel prepared and confident about answering these questions [8], whether it is to deflect peer inquiries or answer with a preferred amount of information about their medical concern (see Table 26.1). This choice is left up to the child and their family, and boundaries are discussed in therapy sessions to make sure their privacy is respected. Although examples of responses are provided for different peer inquiries, these responses can also be applied to family or friends that may be asking intrusive questions. The idea is to provide a preferred amount of information and set boundaries as needed. Regardless of the reason, caregivers of the child may feel uncomfortable sharing information with extended family members or friends and can choose carefully what information they share with others.

During this stage of development, children with BEEC may have changes to their medical regimen, whether they are learning how to achieve continence, attending increased medical appointments (e.g., catheterization training, pelvic floor physical therapy), or preparing for additional procedures and/or surgeries (e.g., video urodynamics, reversal of vesicostomy, appendicovesicostomy). Children may be learning to catheterize during childhood for the first time, and both parents and children may fear pain associated with catheterization if they were not catheterized starting at birth [9]. Psychological support is helpful to assist parents with encouraging and supporting their child while also providing the child with ways to feel in control of their medical care. Exposure and response prevention is a common technique used for introducing catheterization to the child [4], including small challenges of using the catheter (e.g., touching it to the site, inserting it only a small amount, putting the catheter fully inside).

At times, children with medical conditions struggle with adherence to their medical regimen. These difficulties can be due to low motivation, limited ability to understand the importance of the regimen, or preference to be like peers that do not have medical conditions. Children at this stage may dismiss the need to engage in their regimen; as a result, caregivers struggle to find ways to persuade the child with BEEC to comply. Structured behavioral modifications can be useful, as uropsychologists encourage caregivers to use positive reinforcement and incentives as a way to help children adhere to their urological regimen [4]. If developmentally appropriate, the reason for the medical regimen can also be explored and used as a motivator (e.g., achieving continence). Different types of therapy are applied based on the presenting concerns and are typically tailored individually to each child and their family.

Adolescence

Adolescence is a time of many mental and physical changes that are challenging for any individual to experience. Adding in a complex medical condition can exacerbate this stressful time and cause tension between caregivers and the adolescent with BEEC. Each adolescent differs with the types of concerns they may experience; however, the most common struggles include symptoms of anxiety, depression, irritability, struggles with adherence to medical regimens, fear of peers' awareness about the condition, and how to handle social and/or romantic relationships. Bullying or teasing by peers can occur if others are aware of the medical condition and ostracize the individual with BEEC [10], and action should be taken by caregivers and school staff to ensure safety in the school environment. Therapy can be a useful tool during this stage of development to figure out how to ignore others, problem-solve how to preserve privacy, and maintain safety in school or extracurricular environments if they are fearful of peers targeting them verbally or physically. This topic is difficult for adolescents to discuss with caregivers, mental health providers, and school staff; therefore, a gentle approach and practicing patience about handling these concerns are helpful in allowing the adolescent to feel comfortable discussing solutions to these issues.

Even if the adolescent had not previously demonstrated emotional concerns about their medical condition (e.g., symptoms of anxiety, depression, or irritability), adolescence brings awareness to their differences from same-aged peers and a frustration with having to engage in medical care. During this stage, medical providers may be introducing difficult topics, such as long-term care, potential procedures and/or surgeries, transitioning to adult care, or increased medical care to help achieve or continue continence. Often, caregivers expect the adolescent to have the same level of urgency to maintain good medical health; however, adolescents may have different priorities that may not match the caregiver. Concerns can include a preference to focus on social relationships or situations unrelated to BEEC. Regardless of caregivers' opinions on the non-medical struggles, it is important at this stage to provide validation for these conflicting emotions to maintain a strong relationship with the child while also setting boundaries and rules for engaging in medical care.

During adolescence, individuals tend to struggle with adherence to their medical regimen, whether it be catheterization, taking medication, or following medical recommendations. This behavior can be frustrating for caregivers and medical providers when the adolescent does not see the importance of adherence to prevent further medical concerns as an adult. Therapy helps with normalizing the frustration over having a lifelong medical diagnosis and genital anomaly, reexamining future goals, and finding creative ways to make adherence easier. Adolescents may also benefit from therapy focusing on emotional concerns surrounding their diagnosis and feeling different from their peers [11]. Cognitive behavioral therapy and motivational interviewing can be useful tools in helping adolescents think more rationally and helpfully about their medical concerns while also creating goals that fit their values and continued health maintenance [2].

A sensitive topic that may be brought up in therapy with adolescents includes discomfort and embarrassment regarding sexual activity. Conversations about sex and sexuality are encouraged to start around puberty to give adolescents and caregivers more helpful expectations about future sexual functioning, which can include any surgeries (e.g., penile surgery to create a longer phallus) or concerns they may have prior to sexual activity with a partner [12]. When the adolescent is interested in romantic partners, there is a fear that the partner may not accept the look of their genitalia and/or struggles in their ability to engage in sexual activity [13]. During this stage of development, same-aged peers may not be as accepting of the differences in appearance and ability, and a sense of trust is necessary between partners to help assuage these fears. If the adolescent struggles with rejection, these concerns can be addressed in therapy or with trusted individuals (e.g., caregivers, close friends, and family). Therapy can be helpful at this stage to allow the adolescent to ask uncomfortable questions in a nonjudgmental environment, especially regarding psychological and sexual functioning. There is unfortunately no guide to handling each nuanced situation; however, validation and being present are great ways to support the adolescent with these struggles.

Adulthood

The transition from adolescence to adulthood with a medical condition is complicated and difficult for most families. The main struggle includes establishing care with a new hospital system, one that may not connect to the pediatric hospital. In addition, adult care tends to cause hesitation, ambivalence, and fear not only for individuals with BEEC but also for caregivers [14]. As a result, many individuals and families prefer to keep their care within the children's hospital for as long as possible, which can be difficult with pediatric providers who do not know the complexities of adult care. Individuals that wait to start this process further into adulthood may find themselves transitioning much later than necessary and struggling to find the care they need from the right providers.

Although a difficult topic, many pediatric providers encourage the discussion of transition early in adolescence (as early as 14 years old) to help the individual with BEEC to prepare for a successful switch to adult care to maximize quality of life and independence [15]. In this way, they can try out different adult providers while still under the care of their pediatric urologist and be more thoughtful about the process. Social workers in the pediatric hospital can also provide a plethora of information regarding the transition, and this can be done slowly over time to help with emotional distress associated with moving to adult care. In addition, there are creative ways for individuals with BEEC to have their medical information contained within a portable medical summary (PMS) to help corroborate their medical file for an easier transition to adult care [16]. This type of summary involves the pediatric providers creating a template for the individual with BEEC that will be used by adult medical providers to learn about the individual's medical and mental health history, list of specialty providers in other medical divisions, and plans for health maintenance in adulthood. A helpful addition could include individual differences that are important for trust with future providers. These improvements in medical care are still new to most medical institutions but are becoming a way of helping adolescents and young adults with medical complexity to maintain their health through adulthood.

Despite these improvements, health maintenance can be difficult at this stage of life, as adult-based hospitals tend not to initiate contact for missed appointments, reminders for routine visits, or assistance with health maintenance. Adults with BEEC that underwent major reconstructive surgery as a young child may encounter long-term complications that require follow-up with an adult urologist [17]. These complications can occur at any age, and adult urologists tend to not be as familiar with pediatric congenital conditions [18]. In addition, other specialties or disciplines may need to be included in adult care, such as orthopedics, general surgery, neurosurgery, endocrinology, nephrology, oncology, cardiology, gastroenterology, gynecology, and behavioral health [14]. As a result, finding adult care with this many subspecialties in the same hospital system with adult urologists that understand BEEC can be stressful and difficult and should be started earlier to increase success.

Although adults with BEEC are not frequently seen for therapy, there are emotional struggles that they may face as they get older. These individuals may experience anxiety surrounding body image, self-esteem, sexuality, and sexual functioning [13]. Although there is a preference for adult-based providers with a focus on medical concerns, this specialty can be hard to find in the community. Most behavioral health providers have a skill set for general emotional concerns (e.g., anxiety, depression, irritability), which may still benefit an individual with BEEC even if the provider does not specialize in medical conditions. As an adult with BEEC, sexual activity, incontinence, fertility, and genital appearance can be stressful, and health-related quality of life tends to be impaired from adolescence into adulthood [19, 20]. Even when the individual with BEEC is in good health as an adult, psychiatric concerns can still be present, including anxiety, depression, low self-esteem, poor body concept, and social withdrawal [20].

Like adolescence, struggles to find romantic partners can include fearing rejection due to the appearance or function of genitalia. Male adults tend to have more struggles with genital functioning overall [21]. Males may experience anxiety about genital appearance even when they have normal genitalia or regular erections and ejaculation [21, 22]. Female adults tend to have better outcomes with cosmetic reconstruction; however, there are still concerns with sexual satisfaction overall and anxiety about engaging in sexual activity [20]. In one study focused on outcomes of adults with BEEC, 40% of men and 50% of women were unsatisfied with sexual functioning [23]. Although not commonly seen, there are targeted programs focused on helping adolescents and young adults talk openly about sexual functioning, perception of pleasure, and having a more relational-affective approach to sexuality [13]. If groups or programs are not available, individual therapy is recommended [24]. The psychologist or therapist can focus on answering questions, openly discussing these topics, and reducing anxiety about judgment from future sexual partners.

In addition to these stressors, fertility can be a topic of discussion between partners, and this can cause strain in a romantic relationship. While individuals with BEEC are at risk for infertility, some have been successful with reproduction. Male adults may benefit from different treatment options, including assisted reproductive techniques or surgical sperm retrieval [21, 23], and there have been successful pregnancies for female adults with BEEC [25]. Pregnancy outcomes can be optimized through a successful transition from pediatric to adult urological care, understanding of BEEC and management of complications, and a planned surgical approach to delivery [26]. Despite great medical care, the risks of infertility are still high for individuals with BEEC due to reconstructive surgery affecting reproductive ability [23]. While there are other options for individuals with infertility to become parents, the emotional struggles of not being able to conceive should not be overlooked or invalidated. This is largely dependent on the individual and their values (e.g., not all individuals with BEEC may feel this way); therefore, it is best to check in with the individual with BEEC surrounding their preference about this topic.

Future Directions

Many of the psychological strategies suggested through this chapter have been gathered and learned through outpatient therapy with individuals with BEEC across development. These individuals are the greatest source of real-time information on difficult topics, and their honesty continues to provide a framework for providers and families to assist them through medical and mental health difficulties. With minimal information provided on the coping and difficulties these individuals experience, many strategies attempted may occur through trial and error. The most important strategy that a caregiver can implement is validation, whether the caregiver agrees or disagrees with the individual's perception. Through connecting with and understanding the individual with BEEC, providers and families can provide a safe, supportive environment for them throughout their lifespan.

References

1. Ebert AK, Reutter H, Ludwig M, Rösch WH. The exstrophy-epispadias complex. Orphanet J Rare Dis. 2009;4(1):1–17.
2. Haddad E, Hayes LC, Price D, Vallery CG, Somers M, Borer JG. Ensuring our exstrophy-epispadias complex patients and families thrive. Pediatr Nephrol [Internet]. 2023; https://doi.org/10.1007/s00467-023-06049-y.
3. Schast AP, Reiner WG. Pediatric psychology in genitourinary anomalies. Urol Clin N Am. 2010;37(2):299–305.
4. Rouse CM. Pediatric psychology in a urology division: unifying complex medical and mental health treatment. Curr Urol Rep. 2023;24(1):17–24.
5. Chan KH, Panoch J, Carroll A, Wiehe S, Downs S, Cain MP, et al. Parental perspectives on decision-making about hypospadias surgery. J Pediatr Urol. 2019;15(5):449.e1–8.
6. Labrie NHM, Van Veenendaal NR, Ludolph RA, Ket JCF, Van Der Schoor SRD, Van Kempen AAMW. Effects of parent-provider communication during infant hospitalization in the NICU on parents: a systematic review with meta-synthesis and narrative synthesis. Patient Educ Couns. 2021;104(7):1526–52.
7. Mednick L, Gargollo P, Oliva M, Grant R, Borer J. Stress and coping of parents of young children diagnosed with bladder exstrophy. J Urol. 2009;181(3):1312–7.
8. Abeditehrani H, Dijk C, Neyshabouri MD, Arntz A. Beneficial effects of role reversal in comparison to role-playing on negative cognitions about other's judgments for social anxiety disorder. J Behav Ther Exp Psychiatry. 2021;70:101599.
9. Selekman RE, Sanford MT, Ko LN, Allen IE, Copp HL. Does perception of catheterization limit its use in pediatric UTI? J Pediatr Urol. 2017;13(1):48.e1–6.
10. Wilson CJ, Pistrang N, Woodhouse CRJ, Christie D. The psychosocial impact of bladder exstrophy in adolescence. J Adolesc Health. 2007;41(5):504–8.
11. Taskinen S, Suominen JS, Mattila AK. Health-related quality of life and mental health in adolescents and adults operated for bladder exstrophy and epispadias. Urology. 2015;85(6):1515–9.
12. Sinatti C, Waterschoot M, Roth J, Van Laecke E, Hoebeke P, Spinoit AF. Long-term sexual outcomes in patients with exstrophy-epispadias complex. Int J Impot Res. 2021;33(2):164–9.
13. Di Grazia M, Pellizzoni S, Tonegatti LG, Rigamonti W. Psychosexual development management of bladder exstrophy epispadias in complex patients. J Pediatr Urol. 2017;13(2):199.e1–5.
14. Lambert SM. Transitional care in pediatric urology. Semin Pediatr Surg. 2015;24(2):73–8.
15. Peycelon M, Misseri R. The basics of transition in congenital lifelong urology. World J Urol. 2021;39(4):993–1001.
16. Chouteau WA, Allen SR. Implementation of a portable medical summary for adolescents and young adults with medical complexity in transition to adult health care. J Pediatr Nurs. 2019;48:35–41.
17. Wood D, Baird A, Carmignani L, De Win G, Hoebeke P, Holmdahl G, et al. Lifelong congenital urology: the challenges for patients and surgeons. Eur Urol. 2019;75(6):1001–7.
18. De Win G, De Kort L, Learner H, Noah A, Dautricourt S, Nijman R, et al. Long-term risks of childhood surgery. J Pediatr Urol [Internet]. 2023; Available from: https://www.sciencedirect.com/science/article/pii/S1477513123003029
19. Dellenmark-Blom M, Sjöström S, Abrahamsson K, Holmdahl G. Health-related quality of life among children, adolescents, and adults with bladder exstrophy–epispadias complex: a systematic review of the literature and recommendations for future research. Qual Life Res. 2019;28(6):1389–412.
20. Ebert A, Scheuering S, Schott G, Roesch WH. Psychosocial and psychosexual development in childhood and adolescence within the exstrophy-epispadias complex. J Urol. 2005;174(3):1094–8.
21. Rubenwolf P, Thomas C, Thüroff JW, Stein R. Sexual function, social integration and paternity of males with classic bladder exstrophy following urinary diversion. J Urol. 2016;195(2):465–70.

22. Tourchi A, Hoebeke P. Long-term outcome of male genital reconstruction in childhood. J Pediatr Urol. 2013;9(6, Part B):980–9.
23. Van den Eede E, Sterckx M, Vangelabbeek K, Dunford C, Noah A, Wood D, et al. An observational study on the sexual, genital and fertility outcomes in bladder exstrophy and epispadias patients. J Pediatr Urol. 2023;19(1):36.e1–7.
24. Park W, Zwink N, Rösch WH, Schmiedeke E, Stein R, Schmidt D, et al. Sexual function in adult patients with classic bladder exstrophy: a multicenter study. J Pediatr Urol. 2015;11(3):125.e1–6.
25. Bujons A, Lopategui DM, Rodríguez N, Centeno C, Caffaratti J, Villavicencio H. Quality of life in female patients with bladder exstrophy-epispadias complex: long-term follow-up. J Pediatr Urol. 2016;12(4):210.e1–6.
26. Dy GW, Willihnganz-Lawson KH, Shnorhavorian M, Delaney SS, Amies Oelschlager AM, Merguerian PA, et al. Successful pregnancy in patients with exstrophy–epispadias complex: a University of Washington experience. J Pediatr Urol. 2015;11(4):213.e1–6.

Reproductive and Sexual Health in Bladder Exstrophy

27

Raimund Stein and Margarett Shnorhavorian

Reproductive and sexual health is a priority for individuals affected by the bladder exstrophy-epispadias complex (BEEC). Bladder exstrophy is considered a difference in anatomy with long-term effects on sexual and reproductive function. BEEC, however, has not been associated with genetic or endocrine differences that would pose any further compromised fertility potential. Further, it is not associated with an increased risk of gender dysphoria. In a study of 62 adolescents and adults with BEEC, no gender dysphoria was reported [1]. This chapter will review current knowledge regarding reproductive and sexual health in women and men with BEEC and recommendations for care to optimize these outcomes.

Females

Reproductive Outcomes in Women with BEEC

Pregnancy is possible in patients with primary reconstruction or primary or secondary urinary diversion [2–5]. Grady et al. showed in their review that 1/3 of the patients do have a desire to have children [2]; however, 1/3 of the patients required fertility treatment [2, 6, 7]. In one study, only 4/19 females conceived naturally within 1 year of unprotected intercourse [7]. This indicates that there seems to be a

R. Stein (✉)
Center for Pediatric, Adolescent and Reconstructive Urology, University Medical Center Mannheim, Medical Faculty Mannheim Heidelberg University, Mannheim, Germany
e-mail: raimund.stein@umm.de

M. Shnorhavorian
University of Washington, Department of Urology, Seattle, WA, USA

Seattle Childrens Hospital, Division of Pediatric Urology, Seattle, WA, USA
e-mail: Margarett.shnorhavorian@seattlechildrens.org

A. R. Shukla, R. S. Joshi (eds.), *Bladder Exstrophy and Epispadias*, https://doi.org/10.1007/978-3-031-91238-2_27

reduction in reproductive function in females with BEEC. Urinary tract infections, upper tract dilatation, and problems with catheterization ± urinary incontinence are the main complications during pregnancy and, in most cases, are temporary [2, 5, 8]. *Delivery should be performed in a center with experience in urological malformations and urinary diversions.* Most deliveries are done through a cesarean section, which is the preferred and recommended method for delivery with a low complication rate [2, 5, 8–11].

Approximately 13% (10–52%) develop uterine prolapse before pregnancy and around 50% during or after pregnancy [2]. The incidence of prolapse does not seem to be correlated to pelvic osteotomy at the time of closure [2], but the degree of symphyseal diastasis (9.1 vs. 6.1 cm) seems to be the most significant risk factor [12].

Sexual Function in Women with BEEC

Women with bladder exstrophy (40–100%) report being sexually active, and 90% report the ability to achieve orgasm; however, one in five women with BEEC reported dyspareunia [9, 13–17]. Several studies reported that the Female Sexual Function Index (FSFI) score of women with BEEC is below normal scores, indicating that *sexual dysfunction is a significant concern* [9, 16–19].

Incontinence during sexual activities plays an important role in sexual dysfunction [19–21]. Patients with urinary diversion have the same scores compared to those with reconstruction of the bladder. In one study, the FSFI was the same in 9 sexually active females compared to a normal control group from the same place [22].

Females with BEEC report a *high rate of dissatisfaction with the appearance of their external genitalia.* A nationwide study of patient-reported outcome measures (PROMs) from the USA demonstrated that more than half of the patients are dissatisfied with the appearance of their external genitalia, and 74 out of 130 females had surgery in order to use a tampon or have penetrative intercourse [9]. Studies from large institutions also report a high rate of dissatisfaction [23, 24]. However, surgery of the female external genitalia is not without risk, as 3 out of 26 females experienced partial loss of their clitoris [24].

Future Directions: Reproductive and Sexual Outcomes in Women with BEEC

There is clearly a need for further research to better understand and improve reproductive and sexual function outcomes in women with BEEC. In a recent survey promoted online by the Association for the Bladder Exstrophy Community (A-BE-C)—an international support network for patients and families with BE—113 women with BEEC responded to the question, "What topics do you think are important to study in bladder exstrophy?" Areas identified by these women for future research included sexual function, fertility, pregnancy, risk of child with BE, mental health, UTIs, body image, transition of care into adulthood, education of the adult urologist and other providers, chronic pain, uterine prolapse, and genital reconstruction. . By far the most common response was regarding mental health and body image, followed by sexual dysfunction, together making up 33.5% of the responses [9].

Males

Reproductive Outcomes in Men with BEEC

Fertility is impaired in most men with BEEC for multiple reasons. In addition to complications of the reconstruction resulting in urethral strictures, recurrent epididymitis, injury of the vas deferens and the testicular vessels, and testicular abnormalities have been observed in BEEC patients. In one study, 50% of the patients had at least one abnormal finding during testicular ultrasound [25]. Recurrent epididymitis may explain the testicular abnormalities as well as the impaired fertility. In one study, 36% of 39 adult males had recurrent epididymitis, and this may increase the risk of an obstruction of the seminal ducts and, as a result impaired ejaculation [26]. In the rare case of a severe obstruction of the urethra after urinary diversion, a vesicostomy of the bladder remnant has been described to prevent recurrent epididymitis [27]. One study ($n = 14$) demonstrated that there was no difference in sperm concentration after reconstruction or urinary diversion [28]. Another study reported a higher paternity rate after primary compared to secondary urinary diversion (72% vs 28%), *suggesting that fertility is compromised after failure of primary reconstruction followed by several operations* [26]. There are only a few studies with small numbers of patients ($n = 4$–31) that include an evaluation of sperm concentration. In most series, patients have oligozoospermia, some have azoospermia (13–75%), and only a few have normal values (7.1–35%) [26, 28–31]; only one study demonstrated that 63% ($n = 8$) had normal values [32].

Most case series ($n = 7$–23) report that in patients with paternity, assisted reproductive techniques (e.g., insemination, intracytoplasmic sperm injection, and testicular sperm extraction) were used in 25–63% [6, 26, 28, 31, 33]. One study compared paternity rate with normal controls from the same place and found a significant reduction (22 vs. 45%; $p = 0.021$) [22]. *Due to the possible impairment in fertility, the option of cryopreservation should be considered quite early during puberty* [28].

Sexual Function in Men with BEEC

Sexual Activity and Satisfaction with the Appearance of External Genitalia

Most of the men with BBEC are sexually active (62–94%) [6, 26, 34]; *however, there is significant variability in reports of sexual function across studies in the literature*. In a study of men in Finland, men with BEEC have been significantly less sexually active compared to healthy controls (35 vs. 11%, $p = 0.008$) [22]. In another study of 25 adolescents and adults, 96% were sexually active and 78% were satisfied with their sexual health [35]. *Most men with BEEC report impaired satisfaction with sexual health,* e.g., *sexual intercourse, as well as the aesthetic aspects of the external genitalia and thus associated anxiety* [34, 36, 37]. There seems to be no difference between patients with primary reconstruction or primary urinary diversion [34]. Of note, in a small series of men with BEEC with a substitution phalloplasty, they are satisfied with their aesthetic, sexual, and psychological outcome [38].

A recent review on the health-related quality of life (HRQOL) in patients with BEEC suggested that the overall HRQOL is favorable; however, urinary incontinence and sexual dysfunction do have the greatest negative impact [21]. The lack of validated domain-specific instruments to measure the HRQOL makes it difficult to estimate the influence of sexual dysfunction on HRQOL. Some studies concluded that HRQOL and sexual functions are comparable to the normal population [31, 39]; other studies showed reduced HRQOL due to the aesthetic aspects of their genitalia [34], length of the penis and impairment of fertility [40], or lack of own children and sexual dysfunction [28]. In yet another study, there was only a trend to a lower level of HRQOL [37]. Ebert et al. reported that 5 out of 21 had psychiatric treatment [30].

Beginning in adolescence, boys with BEEC experience anxiety about their genital appearance, sexual activity, and relationships [15]. For men with BEEC, both the appearance of the external genitalia and urinary continence greatly impact sexual satisfaction [41]. Patient-reported outcomes in a nationwide study confirmed previous smaller studies, which demonstrated that between 30% and 50% of the adolescent boys and adult men with BEEC are not satisfied with the appearance of their external genitalia [32, 42]. An Italian study demonstrated that *a target program supporting adolescents with BEEC in psycho-sexual issues could significantly improve the psycho-sexual outcomes* [43].

Penile reconstructive techniques are available. The technique of primary and, in most cases, secondary reconstruction depends on the anatomy, what is available, and, last but not least the surgical experience. In a retrospective study with 129 patients using a modified Catwell-Ransley technique [44], 25 developed a fistula, 9 an urethral stricture and 12 patients a wound infection. After a follow-up of 88 months, satisfactory results could be achieved in 120/129 [45]. Even after multiple operations, satisfactory results can be achieved with the use of tissue expanders, and in some of the patients, a phalloplasty [46–48]. A systematic review (SR) related to the techniques, complications and, outcomes after substitution phalloplasty in patients with BEEC included 7 studies. The free radial forearm flap was used in 42 out of 47 patients with an overall complication rate of 15%. Urethroplasty, mainly using the "tube-within-the-tube" technique, was performed in 22 patients, with a complication rate of 54% (6 fistulas and 6 strictures). A prosthesis was implanted in 32/47 with a complication rate of 25% (6 erosions). The reported aesthetic, sexual, and psychological outcomes were satisfactory [38]. This SR confirmed an earlier review with 40 patients that even after multiple previous operations, the phalloplasty is an option with good aesthetic and functional results [49]. However, none of the studies used validated instruments to measure the outcome.

For secondary reconstruction of the urethra, the use of buccal mucosa is well established. The use of the buccal mucosa as an onlay or in a two-stage procedure has a lower complication rate compared to the reconstruction of the urethra using the buccal mucosa as a tube [50].

Erectile Function

Most men with bladder exstrophy are able to maintain an erection, however with some mild or moderate deficits. In two small studies ($n = 9/n = 21$), there was no statistical difference concerning the International Index of Erectile Function (IIEF) compared to a control group [22, 39]. A study including members of the Association for the Bladder Exstrophy Communities (A-BE-C) showed that scores on the IIEF-15 questionnaire ($n = 46$) for orgasmic function, sexual desire, and overall satisfaction were lower, but no difference in erectile function or intercourse satisfaction compared to controls. Penile Perception Scores (PPS) ($n = 54$) related to satisfaction with penile length and axis were also lower than prior published controls [41].

As most studies in the literature demonstrate some erectile dysfunction [26, 28, 34, 51, 52], therapy options using the guidelines for sexual health should be discussed. Especially the use of PDE5 inhibitors, of a vacuum erection device, and corpus cavernosum auto-injection therapy/intraurethral therapy with vasoactive substances can be used [53]. If there is no response/option at all, phalloplasty can be offered [38].

Ejaculatory Function

Ejaculation is impaired by the incomplete formation of the musculus bulbospongiosus as well as by the reconstruction of the external genitalia [52, 54]. However, most of the patients (68–100%) do report ejaculations independent of their history of primary reconstruction or primary/secondary urinary diversion [6, 15, 26, 29, 30, 32, 34, 47]. Two German studies ($n = 16$ and $n = 32$) showed that after reconstruction, antegrade ejaculation is possible in 84–94% if the colliculus seminalis is below the bladder neck [15, 30]. In one study with 25 males (20–27 years of age), 15 had a normal ejaculation and 8 had a retrograde ejaculation or no ejaculation at all [35]. In contrast to these studies, Salem and Eisa reported that 16 out of 30 had a retrograde ejaculation, 6 had no ejaculation, and 8 ejaculated with small volume [55]. If the patients were asked in more detail about the quality of their ejaculation, 4 out of 38 (10.5%) reported a normal ejaculation, 17 (45%) a weak and dribbling ejaculation, 8 antegrad and retrograde ejaculations, 1 only retrograde, and 8 no ejaculation [28]. Using the *Male Sexual Health Questionnaire short form for assessing ejaculatory dysfunction,* one study showed no significant differences in the outcome between different groups of reconstruction (overall score between 5 and 15) [47]. *If there is an impairment of ejaculation, sympathomimetic or antimuscarinic substances could be used as a temporarily option to improve collection of ejaculation fluid in those with impaired fertility* [53].

Recommendations

Due to the high prevalence of reproductive impairment and sexual dysfunction with potentially significant impacts on quality of life, we recommend that caregivers pay close attention to these potential issues, and *long-term comprehensive patient care for those affected by BEEC is strongly recommended.* This should include health professionals who are experienced in the fields of male and/or female reproductive, sexual, and behavioral health to promote and support individuals and families with BEEC.

Literature

1. Taskinen S, Suominen JS, Mattila AK. Gender identity and sex role of patients operated on for bladder exstrophy-epispadias. J Urol. 2016;196(2):531–5.
2. Grady R, Hafez AT, Mathews R, Ebert AK. Classic exstophy. In: deVries CR, Nijman R, editors. Congenital anomalies in children. 1. Montreal: Societe Internationale d'Urologie; 2013. p. 139–48.
3. Burbige KA, Hensle TW, Chambers WJ, Leb R, Jeter KF. Pregnancy and sexual function in women with bladder exstrophy. Urology. 1986;28(1):12–4.
4. Huck N, Schweizerhof S, Honeck P, Neisius A, Thuroff JW, Stein R. Pregnancy after urinary diversion at young ages-risks and outcome. Urology. 2017;104:220–4.
5. Bey E, Perrouin-Verbe B, Reiss B, Lefort M, Le Normand L, Perrouin-Verbe MA. Outcomes of pregnancy and delivery in women with continent lower urinary tract reconstruction: systematic review of the literature. Int Urogynecol J. 2021;32(7):1707–17.
6. Gobet R, Weber D, Horst M, Yamamoto S, Fischer J. Long-term followup (37 to 69 years) in patients with bladder exstrophy treated with ureterosigmoidostomy: psychosocial and psychosexual outcomes. J Urol. 2009;182(4 Suppl):1819–23.
7. Deans R, Banks F, Liao LM, Wood D, Woodhouse C, Creighton SM. Reproductive outcomes in women with classic bladder exstrophy: an observational cross-sectional study. Am J Obstet Gynecol. 2012;206(6):496 e1–e6.
8. Huck N, Schweizerhof S, Stein R, Honeck P. Pregnancy following urinary tract reconstruction using bowel segments: a review of published literature. World J Urol. 2020;38(2):335–42.
9. Canalichio KL, Ahn J, Artigas P, Amies Oelschlager AE, Rowe C, Merguerian P, et al. Patient-reported outcomes in adult females with bladder exstrophy: a study of long-term sexual, reproductive and urinary outcomes using social media. J Pediatr Urol. 2020;16(5):567 e1–e7.
10. Quiroz Y, Llorens E, Novoa R, Motta G, Llurba E, Porta O, et al. Pregnancy in pateints with exstrophy-epispadias complex: are higher rates of complications and spontaneous abortion inevitable? Urology. 2021;154:326–32.
11. Giron AM, Passerotti CC, Nguyen H, Cruz JA, Srougi M. Bladder exstrophy: reconstructed female patients achieving normal pregnancy and delivering normal babies. Int Braz J Urol. 2011;37(5):605–10.
12. Anusionwu I, Baradaran N, Trock BJ, Stec AA, Gearhart JP, Wright EJ. Is pelvic osteotomy associated with lower risk of pelvic organ prolapse in postpubertal females with classic bladder exstrophy? J Urol. 2012;188(6):2343–6.
13. Feitz WF, Van Grunsven EJ, Froeling FM, de Vries JD. Outcome analysis of the psychosexual and socioeconomical development of adult patients born with bladder exstrophy. J Urol. 1994;152(5 Pt 1):1417–9.
14. Woodhouse CR. The sexual and reproductive consequences of congenital genitourinary anomalies. J Urol. 1994;152(2 Pt 2):645–51.

15. Ebert A, Scheuering S, Schott G, Roesch WH. Psychosocial and psychosexual development in childhood and adolescence within the exstrophy-epispadias complex. J Urol. 2005;174(3):1094–8.
16. Deans R, Liao LM, Wood D, Woodhouse C, Creighton SM. Sexual function and health-related quality of life in women with classic bladder exstrophy. BJU Int. 2015;115(4):633–8.
17. Rubenwolf P, Thomas C, Thuroff JW, Stein R. Sexual function and fertility of women with classic bladder exstrophy and continent urinary diversion. J Urol. 2016;196(1):140–5.
18. Ebert AK, Lange T, Reutter H, Jenetzky E, Stein R, Boemers TM, et al. Evaluation of sexual function in females with exstrophy-epispadias-complex: a survey of the multicenter German CURE-Net. J Pediatr Urol. 2017;13(2):183 e1–e6.
19. Mathews RI, Gan M, Gearhart JP. Urogynaecological and obstetric issues in women with the exstrophy-epispadias complex. BJU Int. 2003;91(9):845–9.
20. Catti M, Paccalin C, Rudigoz RC, Mouriquand P. Quality of life for adult women born with bladder and cloacal exstrophy: a long-term follow up. J Pediatr Urol. 2006;2(1):16–22.
21. Holmdahl G, Dellenmark-Blom M, Nordenskjold A, Sjostrom S. Health-related quality of life in patients with the bladder exstrophy-epispadias complex and relationship to incontinence and sexual factors: a review of the recent literature. Eur J Pediatr Surg. 2020;30(3):251–60.
22. Suominen JS, Santtila P, Taskinen S. Sexual function in patients operated on for bladder exstrophy and epispadias. J Urol. 2015;194(1):195–9.
23. Stein R, Fisch M, Bauer H, Friedberg V, Hohenfellner R. Operative reconstruction of the external and internal genitalia in females with bladder exstrophy or incontinent epispadias. J Urol. 1995;154:1002–7.
24. Vanderbrink BA, Stock JA, Hanna MK. Aesthetic aspects of reconstructive clitoroplasty in females with bladder exstrophy-epispadias complex. J Plast Reconstr Aesthet Surg. 2010;63:2141–5.
25. Ebert AK, Kliesch S, Neissner C, Reutter H, Rosch WH. Testicular tumors in patients with exstrophy-epispadias complex. J Urol. 2012;188(4):1300–5.
26. Rubenwolf P, Thomas C, Thuroff JW, Stein R. Sexual function, social integration and paternity of males with classic bladder exstrophy following urinary diversion. J Urol. 2016;195(2):465–70.
27. Rösch W, Stein R. Epispadie und blasenekstrophie. In: Stein R, Beetz R, Thüroff J, editors. Kinderurologie in Klinik und Praxis. 3rd ed. Stuttgart: Thieme; 2011. p. 377–94.
28. Reynaud N, Courtois F, Mouriquand P, Morel-Journel N, Charvier K, Gerard M, et al. Male sexuality, fertility, and urinary continence in bladder exstrophy-epispadias complex. J Sex Med. 2018;15(3):314–23.
29. Ben-Chaim J, Jeffs RD, Reiner WG, Gearhart JP. The outcome of patients with classic bladder exstrophy in adult life. J Urol. 1996;155(4):1251–2.
30. Ebert AK, Bals-Pratsch M, Seifert B, Reutter H, Rosch WH. Genital and reproductive function in males after functional reconstruction of the exstrophy-epispadias complex--long-term results. Urology. 2008;72(3):566–9; discussion 9–70.
31. Baumgartner TS, Lue KM, Sirisreetreerux P, Metzger S, Everett RG, Reddy SS, et al. Long-term sexual health outcomes in men with classic bladder exstrophy. BJU Int. 2017;120(3):422–7.
32. Avolio L, Koo HP, Bescript AC, Snyder HM 3rd, Canning DA, Duckett JW Jr. The long-term outcome in men with exstrophy/epispadias: sexual function and social integration. J Urol. 1996;156(2 Pt 2):822–5.
33. D'Hauwers KW, Feitz WF, Kremer JA. Bladder exstrophy and male fertility: pregnancies after ICSI with ejaculated or epididymal sperm. Fertil Steril. 2008;89(2):387–9.
34. Traceviciute J, Zwink N, Jenetzky E, Reutter H, Hirsch K, Stein R, et al. Sexual function and quality of life in adult male individuals with exstrophy-epispadias complex-a survey of the German CURE-Network. Urology. 2018;112:215–21.
35. Sinatti C, Waterschoot M, Roth J, Van Laecke E, Hoebeke P, Spinoit AF. Long-term sexual outcomes in patients with exstrophy-epispadias complex. Int J Impot Res. 2021;33(2):164–9.

36. Mesrobian HG, Kelalis PP, Kramer SA. Long-term followup of cosmetic appearance and genital function in boys with exstrophy: review of 53 patients. J Urol. 1986;136(1 Pt 2):256–8.
37. Taskinen S, Suominen JS, Mattila AK. Health-related quality of life and mental health in adolescents and adults operated for bladder exstrophy and epispadias. Urology. 2015;85(6):1515–9.
38. Berrettini A, Sampogna G, Gnech M, Montanari E, Manzoni G, Di Grazia M, et al. Substitution phalloplasty in patients with bladder exstrophy-epispadias complex: a systematic review of techniques, complications and outcomes. J Sex Med. 2021;18(2):400–9.
39. Zhu X, Klijn AJ, de Kort LMO. Urological, sexual, and quality of life evaluation of adult patients with exstrophy-epispadias complex: long-term results from a dutch cohort. Urology. 2020;136:272–7.
40. da Cruz JA, de Mattos B, Srougi M, Nguyen H, Bonan R, Denes F, et al. Quality of life in young adult patients treated for bladder exstrophy. Cent Eur J Urol. 2016;69(2):221–4.
41. Rowe CK, Shnorhavorian M, Block P, Ahn J, Merguerian PA. Using social media for patient-reported outcomes: a study of genital appearance and sexual function in adult bladder exstrophy patients. J Pediatr Urol. 2018;14(4):322 e1–e6.
42. Diseth TH, Bjordal R, Schultz A, Stange M, Emblem R. Somatic function, mental health and psychosocial functioning in 22 adolescents with bladder exstrophy and epispadias. J Urol. 1998;159(5):1684–9; discussion 9–90.
43. Di Grazia M, Pellizzoni S, Tonegatti LG, Rigamonti W. Psychosexual development management of bladder exstrophy epispadias in complex patients. J Pediatr Urol. 2017;13(2):199 e1–e5.
44. Ransley PG, Duffy P, Wollin M. Bladder exstrophy and epispadias. In: Spitz L, Nixon HH, editors. Paediatric surgery. London: Butterworths; 1988. p. 620–32.
45. Baird AD, Gearhart JP, Mathews RI. Applications of the modified Cantwell-Ransley epispadias repair in the exstrophy-epispadias complex. J Pediatr Urol. 2005;1(5):331–6.
46. VanderBrink BA, Stock JA, Hanna MK. Esthetic outcomes of genitoplasty in males born with bladder exstrophy and epispadias. J Urol. 2007;178(4 Pt 2):1606–10; discussion 10.
47. Harris TGW, Khandge P, Wu WJ, Leto Barone AA, Manyevitch R, Sholklapper T, et al. Sexual health outcomes after penile reconstruction in the exstrophy-epispadias complex. J Pediatr Urol. 2022;18(6):747–55.
48. Djordjevic M, Kojovic V, Bizic M, Majstorovic M, Vukadinovic V, Korac G, et al. Epispadias repair after failed surgery in childhood. Eur J Pediatr Surg. 2013;23(1):67–71.
49. Sarikaya S, Ralph DJ. Mystery and realities of phalloplasty: a systematic review. Turk J Urol. 2017;43(3):229–36.
50. Markiewicz MR, Lukose MA, Margarone JE 3rd, Barbagli G, Miller KS, Chuang SK. The oral mucosa graft: a systematic review. J Urol. 2007;178(2):387–94.
51. Gupta AD, Goel SK, Woodhouse CR, Wood D. Examining long-term outcomes of bladder exstrophy: a 20-year follow-up. BJU Int. 2014;113(1):137–41.
52. Castagnetti M, Tocco A, Capizzi A, Rigamonti W, Artibani W. Sexual function in men born with classic bladder exstrophy: a norm related study. J Urol. 2010;183(3):1118–22.
53. Salonia A, Bettocchi C, Boeri L, Capogrosso P, Carvalho J, Cilesiz NC, et al. European Association of Urology guidelines on sexual and reproductive health-2021 update: male sexual dysfunction. Eur Urol. 2021;80(3):333–57.
54. Stein R, Stöckle M, Fisch M, Nakai H, Müller SC, Hohenfellner R. The fate of the adult exstrophy patient. J Urol. 1994;152:1413–6.
55. Salem HK, Eisa M. Long-term follow-up (18–35 years) of male patients with history of bladder exstrophy (BE) repair in childhood: erectile function and fertility potential outcome. J Sex Med. 2012;9(5):1466–72.

Gynecology in Bladder Exstrophy

28

Lissa Yu, Stephanie Cizek, and Lesley Breech

For many patients and families, a diagnosis of classic bladder exstrophy (CBE) includes questions about gynecologic anatomy, future menstruation, sexual health, and fertility. Patients and families may be hesitant to discuss these topics with providers but rank these highly among areas of concern [1]. This chapter will review common obstetric and gynecologic issues and associations with bladder exstrophy.

Gynecologic Anatomy

Genital anatomy is well-described in women with exstrophy, with split hair distribution at bilateral sides of the pubic symphysis [2]. The clitoris is typically bifid, and the vaginal opening and anus are anteriorly displaced, with a shortened perineum [3]. The vagina is typically shorter than normal and may occur at a slightly more

L. Yu (✉)
University of Washington School of Medicine, Department of Obstetrics and Gynecology, Division of Pediatric and Adolescent Gynecology, Seattle, WA, USA

Seattle Children's Hospital, Seattle, WA, USA
e-mail: lissayu@uw.edu

S. Cizek
Stanford University School of Medicine, Department of Obstetrics and Gynecology, Division of Pediatric and Adolescent Gynecology, Palo Alto, CA, USA

Lucille Packard Children's Hospital, Palo Alto, CA, USA
e-mail: scizek@stanford.edu

L. Breech
University of Cincinnati School of Medicine, Department of Obstetrics and Gynecology, Cincinnati, OH, USA

Cincinnati Children's Hospital Medical Center, Cincinnati, OH, USA
e-mail: Lesley.Breech@cchmc.org

A. R. Shukla, R. S. Joshi (eds.), *Bladder Exstrophy and Epispadias*,
https://doi.org/10.1007/978-3-031-91238-2_28

horizontal angle [2]. The cervix is generally located distally in the vagina along the anterior vaginal wall [3]. Mullerian anomalies are common, as described below. It should be emphasized with patients and families that ovarian function is generally normal.

The anatomy of the bifid clitoris in CBE should be carefully considered prior to undertaking genital reconstruction, as both functional and aesthetic outcomes affect a patient's future sexual health and body image [4]. Newer techniques such as three-dimensionally reconstructed magnetic resonance imaging (MRI) imaging have helped to further detail the bifid clitoral anatomy; specifically, for females with CBE, most of the clitoral body is anterior to the ischiopubic ramus attachment, with minimal connection to the pubic rami [5]. Understanding clitoral anatomy may guide pelvic floor dissection during surgery. If the neurovascular bundle may be compromised during reconstruction, leaving the clitoris as bifid may be a preferable option [6, 7].

There is a correlation between bladder exstrophy variants and Mullerian anomalies, particularly in patients who also have anorectal malformations such as cloacal exstrophy or other renal or midline anomalies [8, 9]. While the rate of uterovaginal abnormality in cloacal exstrophy has been estimated to be 87% [9] in a case series of 31 patients, the rate of Mullerian anomalies appears to be lower in CBE [9]. In a series of patients with CBE, six of 52 patients (12%) had Mullerian duplication with two separate uterine bodies [10]. Mullerian anomalies most commonly reported include duplication of the vagina and uterus (abnormal or incomplete fusion of Mullerian structures at the midline, resulting in a longitudinal vaginal septum and didelphys uterus), as well as vaginal agenesis [9, 11, 12].

Assessment of Gynecologic Anatomy

Evaluation of urologic and gynecologic anatomy should follow a trauma-informed model of care. Patients with CBE represent a population with high rates of invasive medical testing, surgical procedures, and medical photography, and evaluation of the urologic and gynecologic tracts, including exams limited to the external genitalia, may be emotionally traumatic for children and adolescents and have been associated with pediatric medical traumatic stress [13]. It is important to respect a patient's consent and bodily autonomy even at young ages, and (a) consider deferring examination until a patient is older if information gained will not impact the patient at their current age, or (b) if an exam is needed, consider using sedation for the exam and/or using ultrasound or MRI to gain information that would typically be obtained from an adult on pelvic exam.

Specific timepoints at which it may be best to assess anatomic structures include

- Infancy: At birth, the patient's uterus and ovaries are stimulated by maternal estrogen exposure in utero as well as the patient's own estrogen, produced during mini-puberty of infancy [14]. During the first 6 months of life, Mullerian structures may be more easily visible than later in childhood, making this an opportune time for imaging such as pelvic ultrasound, which can be done in conjunction with renal imaging. However, a full bladder may be necessary to clearly visualize underlying Mullerian structures with transabdominal ultrasound, which may not be possible in a patient with CBE. Of note, due to small size, the ovaries may not be readily seen on transabdominal pelvic ultrasound at this age, but families should be reassured that this does not indicate their absence.

- In early childhood, endogenous estrogen exposure is minimal, and thus gynecologic structures are often unable to be identified on ultrasound or MRI, even when structures are normal. In general, after infancy, the next timepoint to assess Mullerian anatomy is at puberty.
- Puberty: On average, menarche occurs 2–3 years after thelarche (breast bud development) [15]. Thus, thelarche is an excellent physical sign of estrogen stimulation of the body by the ovaries, and imaging of the Mullerian structures soon after thelarche can often clarify Mullerian anatomy and identify menstrual outflow tract obstructions early. Initial imaging can be performed with transabdominal pelvic ultrasound and can often be done at the time of routine surveillance renal and bladder ultrasounds. MRI remains the gold standard to delineate Mullerian anatomy; thus, if ultrasound is not possible or anatomy is unclear, an MRI may be performed to better evaluate. If there is evidence of menstrual outflow obstruction, this can be more closely monitored with surveillance imaging such as additional ultrasounds and/or MRI to time interventions as needed.

Finding "opportunistic" times to evaluate anatomy is possible when there is good collaboration between care teams: for example, abdominal surgery for other indications may be an opportunity for direct intraabdominal assessment of Mullerian structures. Even small Mullerian structures may be evaluated for a patent outflow tract by a saline perturbation technique, instilling saline through a small feeding tube through the fimbriated end of a fallopian tube and evaluating if the saline is expelled vaginally, essentially creating a "test menstruation" [16].

Proactive, early understanding of gynecologic anatomy is important for both patients and providers. Such knowledge can level expectations for patients and families around future reproductive capacity and risk of menstrual obstruction. Early identification of outflow tract obstructions can lead to prevention of dysmenorrhea and pelvic pain and may reduce the risk of endometriosis, which is more common in people with outflow tract obstructions [17]. Unidentified menstrual tract obstructions can present acutely due to severe pain, which may lead to surgical mismanagement and may be emotionally traumatic for young patients. It is important for providers to understand that acute presentation of menstrual obstruction is rarely a surgical emergency and that analgesics, drainage of obstructed fluid via interventional radiology guidance, and medical menstrual suppression should be used to temporize the clinical situation until anatomy can be fully clarified. Patients should be referred to a gynecologist/gynecologic surgeon with experience in managing these conditions for collaboration with urologists comfortable with the management of CBE.

Genitoplasty (surgical revision of the external genitalia) in pediatric patients is currently the center of surgical, social, and ethical debates, with many advocating for delayed genitoplasty in pediatric patients with atypical genitalia until patients themselves can give input regarding their own gender identity, sexual preferences, and surgical decision-making [18–20]. In these situations, "delayed" surgery often refers to waiting until the age of majority or at least after an age of assent, if there are no urgent medical indications for earlier genitoplasty. The timing of genitoplasty for CBE has historically been at the time of the primary repair, and some surgical techniques even start with the clitoral dissection and move toward the deeper pelvis [5]. In contrast, historical reports of "immediate" vs. "delayed" primary closure in CBE often refer to surgery within the first 48–72 hours of life vs. at 6–12 weeks of age [7]. Early timing for the primary closure and other surgical reconstructive procedures may require more immediate intervention, and as such, some reconstruction of the external genitalia may currently occur before patients can participate in the discussion. However, whenever possible, surgeons should carefully consider the alternative of delaying genitoplasty past infancy, until closer to or after puberty, both to allow optimal estrogenization of tissues to contribute to healing and to allow more patient autonomy in decision-making. Revision of external genitalia should be delayed until after puberty is complete and patients are able to provide input.

Puberty

Ovarian development and function are typically normal in patients with bladder exstrophy. Puberty is expected to occur at a physiologic age, although CBE and other complex urinary conditions have been correlated with poor growth and nutritional status, which may impact the timing of pubertal onset [21–23]. Typically, thelarche, or the presence of breast buds, is the first external clinical sign that estrogen levels are increasing in the body. In a series of 17 bladder exstrophy patients, menarche appeared to occur approximately at the same time as would be expected in the typical population, with menarche at age 10–12 in 6 (35%), 12–14 years in seven (41%) and after 14 years in four (24%) [24].

As with general recommendations for other patients, a first reproductive health visit with a gynecologist is recommended around ages 13–15 to address preventive health care and provide general guidance on reproductive health, in addition to addressing patient and family concerns [15]. A visit with a gynecologist around the time of puberty also provides an opportunity for patients to discuss menstrual management options. Some patients wish to continue with menses without suppression, which is appropriate so long as there is a patent outflow tract for menstrual egress. If desired or if medically indicated, a variety of menstrual suppression options exist, ranging from pills, patches, vaginal rings, injections, and implants, and include contraceptive and non-contraceptive options. Personal preference and medical contraindications help to direct the patient and family to the appropriate option.

Sexual Health and Function

Surgeries in childhood often involve both the abdomen and the perineum, leading to scarring, which may impact both functional and cosmetic outcomes. Primary closure in childhood may result in significant scarring at the mons and at the introitus. Surveys of patients with CBE reported patient concerns about self-image in relation to both scars and genital appearance [1]. Patients may vary in their acceptance and desire of abdominal surgical scar revision and may benefit from referral to plastic surgery or nonsurgical dermatologic intervention such as lasers or hair removal. Providers should refrain from making assumptions about gender identity, sexual orientation, sexual practices, or sexual desires/goals. Even when anatomy may not be typical in appearance, providers should not assume that a patient is unhappy with their own anatomy or desires surgical intervention. As patients progress from early childhood to adolescence, it is important to allow for a confidential dialogue with providers to provide appropriate recommendations based on sexual practices, address private concerns, and ensure that any desires for management, such as dilation or surgery, are being driven by the patient and not their parents or caregivers [25].

As patients become older, many engage in romantic and sexual relationships; female patients with bladder exstrophy often have unique needs. In a cohort of 26 Brazilian women, 10 felt BE limited their romantic relationships (38%), and 12 (46.2%) felt CBE limited sexual relationships. Sixteen (61.5%) of these patients felt scars limited social relationships, and 6 (20.1%) felt BE limited friendships [26]. A separate cohort of 13 sexually active female patients with BE described eight (47%) with problems in their sexual life. Of these, they specifically cited urinary incontinence during or immediately after intercourse (5/8), reduction or lack of clitoral sensitivity (4/8), dyspareunia due to introital stenosis (2/8), genital prolapse (2/8), abnormal vaginal position limiting sexual acts to specific positions only (2/8), and excessive vaginal dryness requiring lubrication (1/8) [24]. Six of the sexually active women described themselves as completely satisfied with intimacy and reported reaching orgasm. Most were unsatisfied with the cosmesis of the external genitalia, affecting body image and self-esteem as well as sexual function [24]. Female exstrophy patients may require additional management for sexual function, including pelvic floor physical therapy and sex therapy, and care should support patients' sexual preferences and needs. Questionnaires of adult women with exstrophy have demonstrated various levels of sexual dysfunction, including domains such as desire, arousal, lubrication, orgasm, satisfaction, and pain, as compared to normal controls while others have demonstrated no significant difference from controls, in all domains except pain [27, 28]. Some data have also examined sexual function in patients with continent diversions as compared to those without; sexual function appears to be similar in both groups [29, 30]. The more horizontal angle of the vagina in patients with exstrophy may affect positioning for intercourse; however, the impact of this on sexual health has not been studied.

Postoperative vaginal stenosis is common: in one study that included 11 postpubertal females who had undergone BE repair, 54% ($n = 6$) had vaginal stenosis, four of those patients underwent additional flap vaginoplasty, and all engaged in dilator therapy [27]. However, not every patient will desire to engage in vaginal sexual activity, and decisions regarding dilation therapy or surgical intervention for vaginal stenosis should be made together with the patient and should be individualized based on patients' input and sexual health needs. Some patients may choose to delay or completely avoid any intervention for vaginal stenosis if they are not planning vaginal sexual activity, and even obstructive vaginal stenosis can be medically managed using long-term hormonal menstrual suppression.

Vaginal procedures are best performed after puberty to improve healing with estrogenization of the vaginal tissue. Many vaginal procedures require postoperative dilation which should only be considered within the patient's individual readiness timeline. The use of menstrual suppression prior to patient readiness may be needed. Because of scarring after previous surgical procedures and/or congenital anatomic anomalies, many patients require additional surgical revision to permit any penetration. Revision may focus on introitoplasty and vaginoplasty or external genitalia reconstruction, including clitoroplasty, labiaplasty, and monsplasty [24, 31]. In a series of 91 female CBE patients (ages 12–30 years), 29 (31.8%) underwent vaginoplasty due to vaginal stenosis at a mean age of 15 years. 24 patients underwent perineal flap vaginoplasty, 3 had posterior cut-back vaginoplasties, and 2 had Y-V vaginoplasties. No patients in this series experienced restenosis [32]. Again, it is important to properly assess whether patients are willing and able to participate in postoperative dilation and defer surgical repair until the patient is motivated and able to dilate to minimize the risk of needing repeated interventions.

Pelvic Organ Prolapse

The anatomy of the pelvic floor musculature in patients with exstrophy, with absence of cardinal ligaments, limits the pelvic floor support and predisposes women to pelvic organ prolapse. Estimates of pelvic organ prolapse in women with bladder exstrophy suggest that 30–52% will experience prolapse with a mean age of 16 years [33–35]. In a series of 23 women, only 5 (29%) reported prolapse, of which 3 had mild and well-tolerated symptoms while the other two described their prolapse as a severe handicap [24]. In a single institutional review of 25 adult female patients with CBE and pelvic organ prolapse who underwent repair, 7 experienced unsuccessful initial repair and subsequent recurrence. After correction, all patients reported improvement in prolapse symptoms [36].

Risk factors for pelvic organ prolapse in all female patients include increasing parity and age. The symptoms of prolapse may be increased during pregnancy and postpartum [37]. Women with BE have additional risks such as congenital weakness of cardinal and uterosacral ligaments, pubic diastasis, and atypically flat and anterior levator ani muscles with a large levator hiatus [12, 38, 39], and some studies have suggested that CBE patient risk of prolapse is independent of parity [35]. Minimal data currently exist regarding the gynecologic outcomes of CBE patients into menopause and beyond. It is likely that evolving research will also help to clarify concerns in this patient population.

Multiple surgical techniques have been proposed to treat pelvic organ prolapse in CBE, though no one approach has been determined to be the standard of care [35]. For patients who desire future childbearing, uterine preservation procedures have been proposed, such as the Manchester-Fothergill and Elevate Posterior techniques, though little literature exists on the outcomes of these repairs after pregnancy is achieved or the pregnancy outcomes themselves [35, 40].

Many nonsurgical techniques, such as pessaries, have been suggested. Given differences in bony and soft tissue structure, many commonly used pessaries may not easily stay in place in patients with CBE. Finding the appropriate pessary may require a clinician well-versed in the many pessary options available. The role of a general gynecologist, urogynecologist, or urologist specialized in female pelvic medicine and reconstructive surgery may provide a natural transition into adulthood for the pediatric bladder exstrophy patient and allow for early discussion of multiple options available for management of pelvic organ prolapse in the context of the patient's life stage and desire for future pregnancy and/or uterine conservation.

Fertility

As more patients with CBE desire to become parents, increasing research has focused on fertility and pregnancy. Still, data remains limited. Because ovarian development is not affected, hormonal development is typical in patients with CBE, as noted above. Infertility, defined as failure to achieve pregnancy in 12 months of unprotected intercourse in women younger than 35 years or 6 months if older than 35 years, affects up to 15% of couples in the general population [41]. A series of six patients desiring pregnancy reported conception without assisted reproductive technology in 5/6 patients [42]. Another series reported 100% of women with CBE who desired pregnancy were able to achieve pregnancy spontaneously; however, this series followed only two women, one who conceived twice and the other once [43]. A British series reported 28 women with BE attempting pregnancy, of which 19 women (66%) were able to conceive, although only 4 (21%) conceived spontaneously within 1 year. Tubal infertility was noted as a contributory factor in most cases, consistent with the multiple previous surgeries and likelihood of subsequent adhesive disease that may affect fallopian tube function. Only 5 (26%) sought assisted reproductive technology, of which 4 underwent IVF and only one was successful, and 1 underwent ovulation induction. As this series was performed in the UK, they noted that the low uptake of assisted reproductive technology and success rate of IVF (25%) may not be consistent with practices of patients with tubal factor infertility in other parts of the world [10].

Contraception and Routine Gynecologic Care

Patients should be counseled that, in the absence of specific anatomic considerations that would prevent pregnancy, people with CBE can become pregnant and that contraception should be used if a patient is having penile-vaginal sex and pregnancy is not desired. Unplanned pregnancy has been reported in a patient with bladder exstrophy who thought conception could not occur due to the anomaly [44]. In addition, despite higher rates of infertility, many people with CBE who become pregnant will do so spontaneously [10, 45]. Finally, there is data that young patients with medically complex conditions, including vaginoplasty and pelvic reconstruction, seek additional guidance regarding sexual and reproductive health beyond what is typically provided in their care, and over half expressed anxiety regarding sexual relationships [30, 46]. Obstetrician/gynecologists knowledgeable about the patients' prior medical and surgical history may help facilitate these questions and concerns.

CBE patients should be counseled regarding contraception with similar frequency and considerations to patients without CBE. Considerations when choosing a form of hormonal contraception include renal dysfunction, hypertension, uterine anomalies, and degree of pelvic organ prolapse. Patients should undergo surveillance for cervical cancer per routine guidelines. Of note, cervical cancer screening in a patient with didelphys uterus will require a swab of each cervix, as cervical dysplasia may present differently, and a Pap examination and/or HPV testing of one cervix may be insufficient to identify and appropriately triage cervical cancer risk [47]. HPV vaccination should be recommended in concordance with routine recommendations. Additional routine gynecologic care, such as STI screening and evaluation of vaginal discharge, should be provided to patients by a provider who is familiar with the patients' medical and surgical history and with recommendations for gynecologic evaluation. False positive urine pregnancy testing in the setting of augmentation cystoplasty has been reported in both male and female patients; if urine testing does not support clinical findings, confirmation with serum beta-hCG levels should be sought [48].

Obstetric Considerations

Regarding the pregnancy itself, many case series have reported successful pregnancy in women with CBE. Specific concerns for CBE patients include the increased risks of pelvic organ prolapse, difficulty with bladder emptying (both via catheterizable channel and urethra), increased constipation, and risks to renal function. A series of patients with seven total pregnancies reported uterine prolapse in 7, acute pyelonephritis in 1, prolapsed ileal conduit in 1, and transient urinary incontinence in 1 [42]. In patients with chronic hypertension, additional maternal risks include pulmonary edema, myocardial infarction, preeclampsia, placental abruption, cesarean delivery, postpartum hemorrhage, and gestational diabetes, while fetal risks include increased fetal growth restriction, preterm birth, perinatal mortality, and congenital anomalies [49].

Mullerian anomalies, when present, are associated with known fertility and obstetric risks.

Having a Mullerian anomaly increases risks of preterm birth, primary cesarean delivery, fetal malpresentation, and premature rupture of membranes [50–52]. Patients with cloacal exstrophy have unique challenges, including bowel management, that may be in addition to the challenges faced by CBE patients in pregnancy [8]. A history of multiple prior abdominal surgeries for most patients with CBE of childbearing age adds additional challenge when planning for mode of delivery. Wu et al. reported a case of pregnancy in unrepaired CBE; these patients, though rare, pose even more unique perinatal management challenges [53].

A preconception visit with a maternal-fetal medicine physician is recommended for planning both for the pregnancy and medical optimization of underlying health conditions prior to conception, and use of contraception until pregnancy is desired to minimize risk of unplanned pregnancy. During pregnancy, close surveillance with a maternal-fetal medicine specialist, a urologist, and a nephrologist are helpful to optimize maternal health. Fetal development can be closely monitored via serial ultrasounds throughout the pregnancy. Antenatal consultation with an anesthesiologist may also be recommended. The availability of spinal anesthesia may be limited due to comorbidities involving the spine.

Techniques for cesarean delivery in patients with bladder reconstructions have highlighted the proximity of the uterus to the reconstructed genitourinary tract [54] (Fig. 28.1). Historically, patients with CBE were recommended to deliver via scheduled cesarean delivery at a location and time when urologic specialists were available for participation. Clemetson reviewed 65 pregnancies in 46 women from 1924

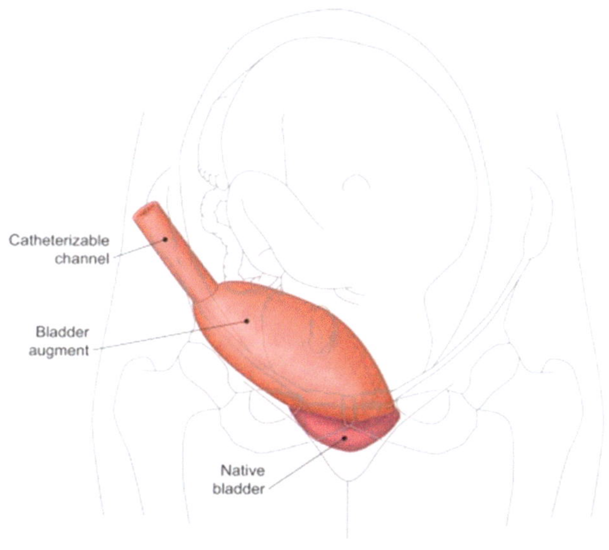

Fig. 28.1 Schematic of a pregnant patient with an augmentation cystoplasty and catheterizable channel [54]

to 1958, noting increased incidences of premature labor, malpresentation (suspected to be due to poor anterior support of the pelvic floor), obstruction, or vaginal stenosis precluding vaginal delivery. They also noted a 50% incidence of subsequent pelvic organ prolapse [55]. A series of 40 women reported that 11 patients had 14 pregnancies; those with prior urinary diversion were delivered vaginally to minimize the risk of additional surgery, while those with functional bladder closures received cesarean sections to eliminate stress on the pelvic floor or risk of injury to the bladder neck [42]. A series of 57 pregnancies in BE reported 3 sets of twins in 19 patients, with a total of 34 live births, 21 miscarriages, 1 termination, and 4 stillbirths or neonatal deaths. 42% of these patients experienced worsening prolapse symptoms, often managed by bedrest and ring pessary. All live births were delivered by cesarean, including 2 planned vaginal deliveries that resulted in cesarean section; 3 cesareans were performed earlier than scheduled due to premature labor or fetal distress [10]. Dy et al. reported a series of 12 women with 22 pregnancies, resulting in 14 live births, with 100% planned cesarean deliveries using a paramedian incision and the same surgical team. Of this group, 9 had undergone bladder augmentation, 11 required catheterization for bladder emptying, and 5 had catheterizable stomas (2 Hemi-Kock pouches, 3 Mitrofanoffs, one of which abandoned the tract due to recurrent stones). Six required urethral catheterization, and one woman voided through the urethra with an artificial urinary sphincter. Mullerian anatomy was known in nine of the 12 women, with 6 having a bicornuate uterus, one with a unicornuate uterus, and two women with typical uterine anatomy. Of the seven women with Mullerian anomaly, three had documented spontaneous abortions or termination of pregnancy, and four had live births. All patients in this group had umbilical or right lower quadrant stomas, and a vertical paramedian skin incision was used to avoid the augmented bladder and catheterizable channel, with a classical uterine incision then used for hysterotomy to avoid the reconstructed urinary tract [56] (Fig. 28.2).

Given the need for coordination and the risks of emergent cesarean delivery after a failed attempt at vaginal delivery, many centers continue to recommend a scheduled cesarean delivery. Emphasis has been placed on the importance of a surgical plan and an experienced, well-resourced team. However, Deans et al. reported the case of a singleton pregnancy delivered via emergency cesarean at 30 weeks with difficulty delivering the fetus due to adhesions from bladder reconstruction, resulting in neonatal demise despite an experienced surgical and neonatal team [10]. Additionally, cesarean delivery has its own risks, with increased risk in the CBE patient, including altered anatomy and post-surgical adhesions from prior surgeries. Vaginal delivery has been described; in one case, Duhrssen (cervical) incisions were made to facilitate a successful late preterm (36 4/7 weeks) delivery in a patient with CBE and uterine prolapse at the time of delivery, a technique that has been used on other laboring patients with uterine prolapse [57]. At present, delivery is typically

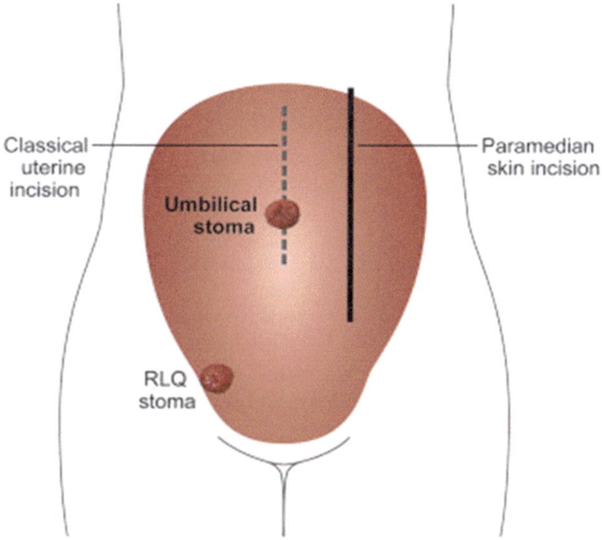

Fig. 28.2 A suggested surgical approach to Cesarean delivery. A paramedian skin incision contralateral to the catheterizable stoma is used to access the uterus, which is then entered using a classical uterine incision. Patients in this study had umbilical or right lower quadrant (RLQ) stomas [56]

recommended at early term unless an alternative indication for earlier delivery is present, ideally in a scheduled fashion with a urologist familiar with the patient's anatomy present for consultation as needed.

Delivery planning conversations, including both mode and time of delivery, should be initiated early in pregnancy and should involve shared decision-making with patients, urologists, and maternal-fetal medicine specialists. Dy et al. have argued that three components are necessary to optimize pregnancy outcomes in patients with CBE: (1) a smooth transition of care from a pediatric to adult multidisciplinary team, (2) an understanding of reconstructed urological anatomy, and (3) a planned delivery surgical approach [56]. Multidisciplinary groups have made recommendations on additional pregnancy management in the CBE patient throughout the patient's pregnancy and postpartum course, summarized here in Table 28.1. Additional studies will help to clarify recommendations for specific patient situations.

Table 28.1 Obstetric care recommendations in patients with bladder exstrophy

Preconception	1. Establish routine gynecologic care (Pap smear, menstruation management, contraception). 2. Emphasize that pregnancies should be planned. Infertility workup should be undertaken if no spontaneous conception after 6–12 months for patients <35 years of age and earlier if >35 years of age. Single embryo transfer only if in vitro fertilization is required. 3. Evaluate renal function, urinary bacterial profile, and infection history. 4. Discuss commitment to frequent surveillance schedule. 5. Discuss practical challenges of pregnancy with EEC, planned cesarean delivery at term. 6. Access information including operative notes about reconstructed anatomy, location, and path of catheterization channels.
First trimester	1. Early ultrasound confirmation of gestation, identification of multiple pregnancies, and ensuring patients are well counseled on pregnancy options. 2. Shared prenatal care between MFM and urology teams, ensuring obstetric care and delivery planning for a location with access to surgical and urologic services and comprehensive neonatal services. 3. Baseline urine specimen and culture, compare pathogen type and burden to prior positive cultures. Baseline labs to include creatinine and glomerular filtration rate. Consider renal ultrasound if not recently performed. 4. Treat positive urine cultures if new pathogens, symptomatic, and/or increased colony count compared to baseline. Asymptomatic bacteriuria is common and, in the context of a reconstructive bladder, should not be treated. Persistent urinary tract infection should prompt investigation for urological complications such as obstruction or stones. Occasionally prophylactic antibiotics may be needed.
Second/third trimester	1. Monitor for signs and symptoms of lower and upper urinary tract obstruction—image upper tracts if needed. 2. Catheterization difficulties arise due to malpositioning of conduits or channels, thus there may be a need to modify catheterization angles, positioning, change catheter size, or type. Some women may prefer to have an indwelling catheter either on free drainage or with a "flip flow tap" and may require a longer catheter if the Mitrofanoff channel becomes stretched. 3. Close observation of regular blood pressure and urinary dipstick monitoring according to standard antenatal protocols. 4. Observation of changes in bladder control; counsel patients that some incontinence may develop but is typically improved postpartum. 5. Develop a surgical approach plan, and place it in the patient's medical record.

(continued)

Table 28.1 (continued)

Delivery planning	1. Vaginal delivery may be considered based on the complexity of anatomical reconstruction and the number of past laparotomies. 2. Plan elective cesarean for 37–39 weeks with MFM, urology, and obstetrical anesthesia teams. 3. Delivery in full operating room suite with neonatal care available. 4. Regional anesthesia is provided by the obstetrical anesthesia team. 5. Consider upper paramedian/supraumbilical incision contralateral to stoma with classical uterine incision (vertical hysterotomy). 6. Consider the use of a flexible O retractor (Alexis) for circumferential retraction of abdominal contents. 7. Define the course of the ureters and their implantation into the reconstructed bladder. 8. Inflated Foley catheter balloon for defining the boundaries of the reconstructed bladder intraoperatively.
Postpartum	1. Postoperative length of stay usually 3 or 4 days. 2. Monitor for return to pre-pregnancy catheterization regimen, continence, and predisposition toward UTIs. 3. Follow-up for late complications of pregnancy including increased risk of pregnancy-related hypertensive diseases. 4. Counsel patients on future increased risk in subsequent pregnancies and iatrogenic late preterm delivery due to repeat CD following classical incision.

Adapted from Deans [10] and Dy [56]

Conclusions

The role of gynecologic care in the patient with CBE spans from infancy to adulthood. A multidisciplinary approach to the bladder exstrophy patient can optimize patient outcomes at each step of the process. Gynecologic care should be incorporated early and proactively into pediatric care for patients with CBE. Continued evaluation and management of menstruation, sexual function, fertility, pregnancy care, and pelvic organ prolapse should be included in long-term CBE follow-up.

References

1. Wilson C, Christie D, Woodhouse CR. The ambitions of adolescents born with exstrophy: a structured survey. BJU Int. 2004;94(4):607–12. https://doi.org/10.1111/j.1464-410X.2004.05010.x; discussion 612. PMID: 15329122.
2. Woodhouse CR, Hinsch R. The anatomy and reconstruction of the adult female genitalia in classical exstrophy. Br J Urol. 1997;79(4):618–22. https://doi.org/10.1046/j.1464-410x.1997.00148.x. PMID: 9126096.
3. Ebert AK, Reutter H, Ludwig M, Rösch WH. The exstrophy-epispadias complex. Orphanet J Rare Dis. 2009;4:23. https://doi.org/10.1186/1750-1172-4-23. PMID: 19878548; PMCID: PMC2777855.

4. Meyer KF, Freitas Filho LG, Martins DM, Vaccari M, Carnevale J. The exstrophy-epispadias complex: is aesthetic appearance important? BJU Int. 2004;93(7):1062–8. https://doi.org/10.1111/j.1464-410X.2004.04782.x. PMID: 15142165.
5. Benz KS, Dunn E, Solaiyappan M, Maruf M, Kasprenski M, Jayman J, Michaud JE, Facciola J, DiCarlo H, Gearhart JP. Novel observations of female genital anatomy in classic bladder exstrophy using 3-dimensional magnetic resonance imaging reconstruction. J Urol. 2018;200(4):882–9. https://doi.org/10.1016/j.juro.2018.04.071. Epub 2018 Apr 30. PMID: 29723567.
6. VanderBrink BA, Stock JA, Hanna MK. Aesthetic aspects of reconstructive clitoroplasty in females with bladder exstrophy-epispadias complex. J Plast Reconstr Aesthet Surg. 2010;63(12):2141–5. https://doi.org/10.1016/j.bjps.2010.02.005. Epub 2010 Mar 29. PMID: 20303329.
7. Promm M, Roesch WH. Recent trends in the management of bladder exstrophy: the Gordian knot has not yet been cut. Front Pediatr. 2019;7:110. https://doi.org/10.3389/fped.2019.00110. PMID: 30984727; PMCID: PMC6449419.
8. Vilanova-Sanchez A, McCracken K, Halleran DR, Wood RJ, Reck-Burneo CA, Levitt MA, Hewitt G. Obstetrical outcomes in adult patients born with complex anorectal malformations and cloacal anomalies: a literature review. J Pediatr Adolesc Gynecol. 2019;32(1):7–14. https://doi.org/10.1016/j.jpag.2018.10.002. Epub 2018 Oct 24. PMID: 30367985.
9. Suson KD, Preece J, Di Carlo HN, Baradaran N, Gearhart JP. Complexities of Müllerian anatomy in 46XX cloacal exstrophy patients. J Pediatr Adolesc Gynecol. 2016;29(5):424–8. https://doi.org/10.1016/j.jpag.2016.01.124. Epub 2016 Feb 2. PMID: 26851190.
10. Deans R, Banks F, Liao LM, Wood D, Woodhouse C, Creighton SM. Reproductive outcomes in women with classic bladder exstrophy: an observational cross-sectional study. Am J Obstet Gynecol. 2012;206(6):496.e1–6. https://doi.org/10.1016/j.ajog.2012.03.016. Epub 2012 Mar 23. PMID: 22537419.
11. Berkowitz J, Warlick C, North A, Gearhart JP. Duplicate bladder exstrophy with complete duplication of Müllerian structures. Urology. 2007;70(4):811.e15–7. https://doi.org/10.1016/j.urology.2007.07.046. PMID: 17991571.
12. Gearhart JP. The bladder exstrophy-epispadias-cloacal exstrophy complex. In: Gearhart JP, Rink RC, Mouriquand PDE, editors. Pediatric urology. Chapter 32. Philadelphia: W. B. Saunders Co; 2001. p. 511–46.
13. Hayes LC, Shepard JA, SooHoo MM, Rouse CM, Papadakis JL. Preventing pediatric medical traumatic stress in a pediatric urology outpatient setting: application of the Pediatric Psychosocial Preventative Health Model (PPPHM). J Pediatr Psychol. 2024;49(4):259–65. https://doi.org/10.1093/jpepsy/jsad064. PMID: 37738669.
14. Kuiri-Hänninen T, Sankilampi U, Dunkel L. Activation of the hypothalamic-pituitary-gonadal axis in infancy: minipuberty. Horm Res Paediatr. 2014;82(2):73–80. https://doi.org/10.1159/000362414. Epub 2014 Jul 5. PMID: 25012863.
15. American College of Obstetricians and Gynecologists' Committee on Adolescent Health Care. The initial reproductive health visit: ACOG Committee Opinion, Number 811. Obstet Gynecol. 2020;136(4):e70–80. https://doi.org/10.1097/AOG.0000000000004094. PMID: 32976378.
16. Breech L. Gynecologic concerns in patients with cloacal anomaly. Semin Pediatr Surg. 2016;25(2):90–5. https://doi.org/10.1053/j.sempedsurg.2015.11.006. Epub 2015 Nov 10. PMID: 26969232.
17. Kapczuk K, Zajączkowska W, Madziar K, Kędzia W. Endometriosis in adolescents with obstructive anomalies of the reproductive tract. J Clin Med. 2023;12(5):2007. https://doi.org/10.3390/jcm12052007. PMID: 36902794; PMCID: PMC10003989.
18. Mulkey N, Streed CG Jr, Chubak BM. A call to update standard of care for children with differences in sex development. AMA J Ethics. 2021;23(7):E550–6. https://doi.org/10.1001/amajethics.2021.550. PMID: 34351265.
19. NASPAG position statement on surgical management of DSD. J Pediatr Adolesc Gynecol. 2018;31(1):1. https://doi.org/10.1016/j.jpag.2017.12.006. PMID: 29366477.

20. Position statement on genital surgery in individuals with differences of sex development (DSD)/intersex traits. Ped Endo Soc. 2020. https://pedsendo.org/clinical-resource/position-statement-on-genital-surgery-in-individuals-with-differences-of-sex-development-dsd-intersex-traits/.
21. Gros DA, Dodson JL, Lopatin UA, Gearhart JP, Silver RI, Docimo SG. Decreased linear growth associated with intestinal bladder augmentation in children with bladder exstrophy. J Urol. 2000;164(3 Pt 2):917–20. https://doi.org/10.1097/00005392-200009020-00001. PMID: 10958756.
22. Cantürk F, Tander B, Tander B, Başoğlu T, Belet U, Aritürk E, Rizalar R, Bernay F. Bladder exstrophy: effects on bone age, bone mineral density, growth, and metabolism. Bone. 2005;36(1):69–73. https://doi.org/10.1016/j.bone.2004.07.012. Epub 2004 Dec 13. PMID: 15664004.
23. Soliman A, De Sanctis V, Elalaily R. Nutrition and pubertal development. Indian J Endocrinol Metab. 2014;18(Suppl 1):S39–47. https://doi.org/10.4103/2230-8210.145073. PMID: 25538876; PMCID: PMC4266867.
24. Catti M, Paccalin C, Rudigoz RC, Mouriquand P. Quality of life for adult women born with bladder and cloacal exstrophy: a long-term follow up. J Pediatr Urol. 2006;2(1):16–22. https://doi.org/10.1016/j.jpurol.2005.07.002. Epub 2005 Sep 6. PMID: 18947589.
25. Confidentiality in Adolescent Health Care: ACOG Committee Opinion, Number 803. Obstet Gynecol. 2020;135(4):e171–e177. https://doi.org/10.1097/AOG.0000000000003770. PMID: 32217979. https://www.acog.org/clinical/clinical-guidance/committee-opinion/articles/2020/04/confidentiality-in-adolescent-health-care.
26. Eyer de Jesus L, Dekermacher S, Pippi-Salle JL. Bladder exstrophy: we need to improve. A lot. J Pediatr Urol. 2022;18(1):38.e1–38.e11. https://doi.org/10.1016/j.jpurol.2021.11.007. Epub 2021 Nov 15. PMID: 34876380.
27. Canalichio KL, Ahn J, Artigas P, Amies Oelschlager AE, Rowe C, Merguerian P, Shnorhavorian M. Patient-reported outcomes in adult females with bladder exstrophy: a study of long-term sexual, reproductive and urinary outcomes using social media. J Pediatr Urol. 2020;16(5):567.e1–7. https://doi.org/10.1016/j.jpurol.2020.06.020. Epub 2020 Jun 21. PMID: 32698983.
28. Zhu X, Klijn AJ, de Kort LMO. Urological, sexual, and quality of life evaluation of adult patients with exstrophy-epispadias complex: long-term results from a Dutch cohort. Urology. 2020;136:272–7. https://doi.org/10.1016/j.urology.2019.10.011. Epub 2019 Nov 4. PMID: 31697953.
29. Rubenwolf P, Thomas C, Thüroff JW, Stein R. Sexual function and fertility of women with classic bladder exstrophy and continent urinary diversion. J Urol. 2016;196(1):140–5. https://doi.org/10.1016/j.juro.2015.12.099. Epub 2016 Jan 21. PMID: 26802583.
30. Ebert A, Scheuering S, Schott G, Roesch WH. Psychosocial and psychosexual development in childhood and adolescence within the exstrophy-epispadias complex. J Urol. 2005;174(3):1094–8. https://doi.org/10.1097/01.ju.0000169171.97538.ed. PMID: 16094067.
31. Harris KT, Namdarian B, Gearhart JP, Wood D. Long term outcomes in classic bladder exstrophy - The adult picture. J Pediatr Urol. 2024;20(2):157–64. https://doi.org/10.1016/j.jpurol.2023.06.028. Epub 2023 Jul 3. PMID: 37451916.
32. Cervellione RM, Phillips T, Baradaran N, Asanuma H, Mathews RI, Gearhart JP. Vaginoplasty in the female exstrophy population: outcomes and complications. J Pediatr Urol. 2010;6(6):595–9. https://doi.org/10.1016/j.jpurol.2010.01.011. Epub 2010 Mar 25. PMID: 20346733.
33. Kaufman MR. Pelvic organ prolapse and pregnancy in the female bladder exstrophy patient. Curr Urol Rep. 2018;19(3):18. https://doi.org/10.1007/s11934-018-0767-2. PMID: 29479649.
34. Mathews RI, Gan M, Gearhart JP. Urogynaecological and obstetric issues in women with the exstrophy-epispadias complex. BJU Int. 2003;91(9):845–9. https://doi.org/10.1046/j.1464-410x.2003.04244.x. PMID: 12780845.

35. Ferrer ML, Sánchez EB, Hernández LH, Linde FM, Peñalver AI, Díaz AN. The Manchester-Fothergill and the Elevate Posterior technique for the correction of a cervical elongation and large enterocele in a patient with bladder exstrophy and multiple surgeries. Int Urogynecol J. 2015;26(8):1239–42. https://doi.org/10.1007/s00192-014-2610-8. Epub 2015 Jan 13. PMID: 25578871.
36. Everett RG, Lue KM, Reddy SS, Friedlander DA, Alexander CE, Young EE, Abdelwahab M, Gandhi NM, Wright EJ, Gearhart JP. Patient-reported impact of pelvic organ prolapse on continence and sexual function in women with exstrophy-epispadias complex. Female Pelvic Med Reconstr Surg. 2017;23(6):377–81. https://doi.org/10.1097/SPV.0000000000000414. PMID: 28277470.
37. Pelvic organ prolapse: ACOG Practice Bulletin, Number 214. Obstet Gynecol. 2019;134(5):e126–42. https://doi.org/10.1097/AOG.0000000000003519. PMID: 31651832.
38. Kwong YT, Knoepp LR, Wright EJ 3rd, Chen CC. Recurrent pelvic organ prolapse in a patient with history of bladder exstrophy. Female Pelvic Med Reconstr Surg. 2012;18(1):63–5. https://doi.org/10.1097/SPV.0b013e31823bdbbe. PMID: 22453272.
39. Delancey J. Pelvic floor anatomy and pathology. In: Biomechanics of the female pelvic floor. London: Elsevier; 2016. p. 13–51. https://doi.org/10.1016/b978-0-12-803228-2.00002-7.
40. Banović V, Mikuš M, Kalafatić D, Mandić V, Orešković S. A 27-year-old patient with congenital bladder exstrophy and recurrent pelvic organ prolapse: a case report. Acta Clin Croat. 2020;59(2):373–6. https://doi.org/10.20471/acc.2020.59.02.24. PMID: 33456128; PMCID: PMC7808229.
41. Infertility workup for the women's health specialist: ACOG Committee Opinion, Number 781. Obstet Gynecol. 2019;133(6):e377–84. https://doi.org/10.1097/AOG.0000000000003271. PMID: 31135764.
42. Burbige KA, Hensle TW, Chambers WJ, Leb R, Jeter KF. Pregnancy and sexual function in women with bladder exstrophy. Urology. 1986;28(1):12–4. https://doi.org/10.1016/0090-4295(86)90172-x. PMID: 3727222.
43. Sinatti C, Waterschoot M, Roth J, Van Laecke E, Hoebeke P, Spinoit AF. Long-term sexual outcomes in patients with exstrophy-epispadias complex. Int J Impot Res. 2021;33(2):164–9. https://doi.org/10.1038/s41443-020-0248-2. Epub 2020 Mar 11. PMID: 32161399.
44. Schrey-Petersen S, Lacher M, Stepan H. Course of an unplanned and unexpected pregnancy in a 39 year-old patient with Complex bladder extrophy: a case report. J Med Case Rep. 2023;17(1):450. https://doi.org/10.1186/s13256-023-04181-9. PMID: 37898815; PMCID: PMC10613355.
45. Ebert AK, Lange T, Reutter H, Jenetzky E, Stein R, Boemers TM, Hirsch K, Rösch WH, Zwink N. Evaluation of sexual function in females with exstrophy-epispadias-complex: a survey of the multicenter German CURE-Net. J Pediatr Urol. 2017;13(2):183.e1–6. https://doi.org/10.1016/j.jpurol.2016.04.052. Epub 2016 Jul 13. PMID: 27480467.
46. Yu LX, McGowan M, Bendle K, Mullins C, Streich-Tilles T, Breech LL. Sexual and reproductive health concerns in adults with cloacal anomalies: a qualitative study. J Pediatr Surg. 2023;58(12):2300–7. https://doi.org/10.1016/j.jpedsurg.2023.08.011. Epub 2023 Aug 21. PMID: 37690871.
47. Gujral H, Bennett JA, Wright KN. Unilateral human papillomavirus infection and cervical dysplasia in a patient with two cervices. Obstet Gynecol. 2016;128(3):571–3. https://doi.org/10.1097/AOG.0000000000001511. PMID: 27500327.
48. Vasquez E, Dillon H, Hannallah A, Wang Y, Baker Z. False positive pregnancy tests in pediatric patients with augmentation enterocystoplasty. J Pediatr Urol. 2022;18(5):615.e1–615.e6. https://doi.org/10.1016/j.jpurol.2022.09.008. Epub 2022 Sep 13. PMID: 36171166.
49. American College of Obstetricians and Gynecologists' Committee on Practice Bulletins—Obstetrics. ACOG Practice Bulletin No. 203: chronic hypertension in pregnancy. Obstet Gynecol. 2019;133(1):e26–50. https://doi.org/10.1097/AOG.0000000000003020. PMID: 30575676.

50. Hua M, Odibo AO, Longman RE, Macones GA, Roehl KA, Cahill AG. Congenital uterine anomalies and adverse pregnancy outcomes. Am J Obstet Gynecol. 2011;205(6):558.e1–558.e5585. https://doi.org/10.1016/j.ajog.2011.07.022.
51. Kim MA, Kim HS, Kim YH. Reproductive, obstetric and neonatal outcomes in women with congenital uterine anomalies: a systematic review and meta-analysis. J Clin Med. 2021;10(21):4797. https://doi.org/10.3390/jcm10214797.
52. Panagiotopoulos M, Tseke P, Michala L. Obstetric complications in women with congenital uterine anomalies according to the 2013 European Society of Human Reproduction and Embryology and the European Society for Gynaecological Endoscopy classification: a systematic review and meta-analysis. Obstet Gynecol. 2022;139(1):138–48. https://doi.org/10.1097/AOG.0000000000004627.
53. Wu S, Sun J, Lv H, Zhang Y, Shang H, Zhang H, Belinson JL. Pregnancy in a woman with untreated bladder exstrophy: a case report. Case Rep Womens Health. 2018;17:11–3. https://doi.org/10.1016/j.crwh.2018.02.002. PMID: 29594008; PMCID: PMC5869060.
54. Roth JD, Casey JT, Whittam BM, Szymanski KM, Kaefer M, Rink RC, Schubert FP, Cain MP, Misseri R. Complications and outcomes of pregnancy and cesarean delivery in women with neuropathic bladder and lower urinary tract reconstruction. Urology. 2018;114:236–43. https://doi.org/10.1016/j.urology.2017.11.052. Epub 2018 Jan 3. PMID: 29305940.
55. Clemetson CA. Ectopia vesicae and split pelvis; an account of pregnancy in a woman with treated ectopia vesicae and split pelvis, including a review of the literature. J Obstet Gynaecol Br Emp. 1958;65(6):973–81. https://doi.org/10.1111/j.1471-0528.1958.tb08591.x. PMID: 13621295.
56. Dy GW, Willihnganz-Lawson KH, Shnorhavorian M, Delaney SS, Amies Oelschlager AM, Merguerian PA, Grady R, Miller JL, Cheng EY. Successful pregnancy in patients with exstrophy-epispadias complex: a University of Washington experience. J Pediatr Urol. 2015;11(4):213.e1–6. https://doi.org/10.1016/j.jpurol.2015.04.019. Epub 2015 May 27. PMID: 26092092.
57. Lachica R, Chan Y, Uquillas KR, Lee RH. Vaginal delivery after Dührssen incisions in a patient with bladder exstrophy and uterine prolapse. Obstet Gynecol. 2017;129(4):689–92. https://doi.org/10.1097/AOG.0000000000001938. PMID: 28277359.

Advocacy for the Exstrophy Community: Empowering and Encouraging the Patient and Family

29

Pamela Artigas and Emily Haddad

Introduction

The bladder-exstrophy-epispadias complex (BEEC) is a group of rare congenital diagnoses that present a multitude of medical and psychosocial challenges to the individual and their family. This condition is seen worldwide with a frequency of 2.2 cases in 100,000 in the most prevalent form of the condition, bladder exstrophy [1]. Individuals living with epispadias, bladder exstrophy, and cloacal exstrophy are at risk for being isolated and managing their medical and social challenges without support. Like all chronic conditions, living with BEEC without proper support can lead to mental distress, anxiety, depression, and other mental health conditions [2–7]. Due to this condition being rare, often hidden, and invisible, these individuals and their families may face stigma and shame as a result. To mitigate these risks, stakeholders (affected individuals and their families, the medical community specializing in these conditions, and the advocacy community) have prioritized several avenues of support. These advocacy efforts include support groups (local and international), educational platforms, summer camps, family-oriented events, international partnerships and workshops, interventions for school success and access, and advocacy for vulnerable individuals around the world to access suitable care [8].

The authors have no financial or non-financial interests to disclose.

P. Artigas (✉) · E. Haddad
Association for the Bladder Exstrophy Community (A-BE-C), Vero Beach, FL, USA
e-mail: pamela.artigas@bladderexstrophy.com

A. R. Shukla, R. S. Joshi (eds.), *Bladder Exstrophy and Epispadias*,
https://doi.org/10.1007/978-3-031-91238-2_29

Patient Advocacy

Given the challenges posed to the chronically ill and the most vulnerable, patient advocacy has become understood as the act of supporting and promoting the rights and safety of a patient or a patient group [9]. Advocacy can be informal and be a service delivered by a family, friend, or representatives from an organization. Patient advocacy organizations provide a sense of community as well as education, resources, and support. In a more formal sense, a patient advocate, nurse, or social worker may be assigned by an institution to advocate on behalf of a patient and their family. The concept of advocacy is contingent on the need and vulnerability of a person to have social support in their time of medical decision-making, medical intervention, and illness. For those with BEEC, physicians, nurses, social workers, family members, friends, and other community groups may serve as advocates for the individual through their lifespan. The goal of advocacy is to respect the integrity of the individual with BEEC and to empower and equip the individual with self-advocacy skills (including collaboration with allies) to manage their health and well-being with optimal independence and self-efficacy.

The Association for the Bladder Exstrophy Community (A-BE-C) is the only non-profit dedicated exclusively to advocating for those with BEEC around the world, established in 1998. The A-BE-C, now based in Florida, USA, in partnership with medical professionals, patient advocates, and patient families, addresses health inequities, advocating for the patient and family within the healthcare system. Additionally, the A-BE-C provides avenues for education, emotional coping, and peer support. These interventions are ultimately to promote self-advocacy and patient dignity. The A-BE-C is committed to ensuring that all affected by exstrophy can, in the words of the organization, "realize their greatest life purpose and potential" [10] (Fig. 29.1).

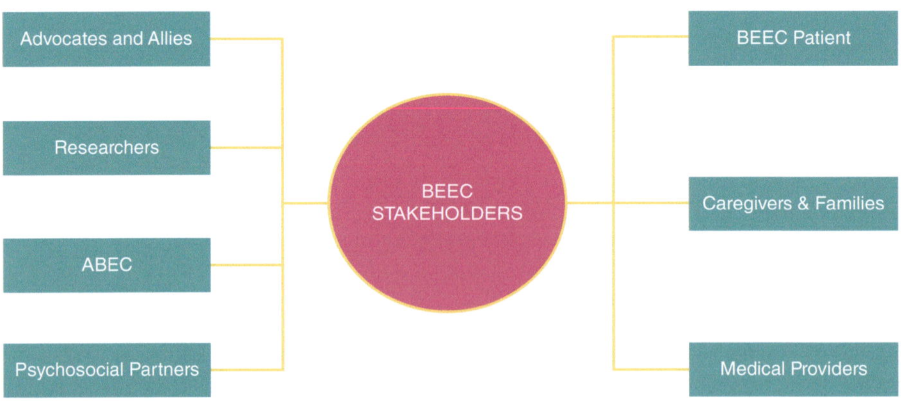

Fig. 29.1 Stakeholders engaged in advocacy for BEEC

Advocacy Needs Along the Lifespan

Upon diagnosis, education and access to care are critical. Some families in middle-income or high-income countries may receive a prenatal diagnosis, but many parents around the world first learn of BEEC soon after delivery and without any indication during pregnancy. The family is then catapulted into a world of complex, lifelong health conditions where accessing the best care can be a challenge. Importantly, the cultural beliefs about disability and difference in the community to which the child is born have major implications on acceptance and stigmatization. In communities where there is limited health literacy and limited resources, parents of children with BEEC may be encouraged to abandon their child and not welcome the child into the community. This challenge has massive implications for the adjustment of the parents of a child with BEEC. Parent and child bonding may also be interrupted by extended hospitalization, unplanned surgeries, and the shock and trauma of the diagnosis. Parents may feel powerless and overwhelmed while also coping with the reality that BEEC is a chronic and lifelong condition. Caregivers are required to evolve from novices to experts on BEEC while advocating for the child in their community and the medical setting [11].

Preparing for the developmental milestone of accessing education/school can trigger more challenges. Many children with BEEC will enter school incontinent, which is a significant concern for families. Communication with the child's teachers and school is critical to ensure the child's rights and accommodations are addressed and respected. Confidentiality and independence become more vital as teens engage in more intimate settings (athletic changing rooms, unsupervised social activities), which may require changing in front of peers. The initiation of romantic relationships and investment in peer relations during this time period have the potential to lead to episodes that may impact the individual's self-image and mental health.

Transitioning to adulthood has its own set of challenges for the individual with BEEC and their family. The importance of access to education throughout childhood becomes apparent as the adult seeks employment and is motivated for increased independence. Young adults will now be responsible for their care and must understand their childhood health history, how to access care, and avenues for self-advocacy. Furthermore, many adults consider sexual health issues such as intimacy, intercourse, and procreation, which may be challenged by the implications of their BEEC diagnosis [12, 13]. Now that those with BEEC are living longer, clinicians must educate older adults on special needs considerations to maintain a healthy quality of life.

Advocacy Interventions for the BEEC Community

Advocating for the BEEC community includes protecting, supporting, and promoting their rights to health, education, and justice. There are many tools or interventions that can be utilized, but they must be tailored to each individual and their family. This patient-centered approach is vital to respect the individual with BEEC

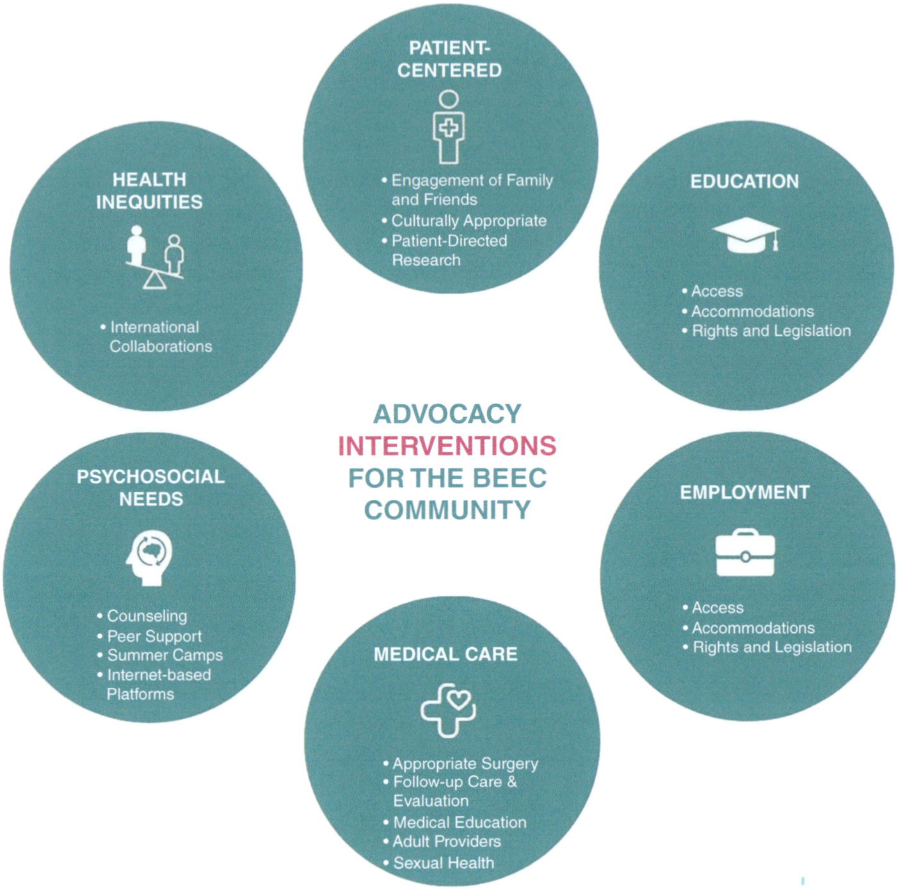

Fig. 29.2 Advocacy interventions for the BEEC community

and their culture, patient-family values, access to care and resources, and individual uniqueness. Peer support, local support groups, summer camps for children, and annual conferences are several interventions that may enhance quality of life, increase health literacy, and reduce isolation for the affected person and their family. These are psychosocial tools that may be in addition to or supplement other more individualized approaches such as behavioral health counseling.

Educational advocacy through legislation/public policy and advocating for specific individuals' accommodations in their school setting is imperative for this population's academic success. International surgical workshops and collaborations for BEEC address global health inequities by raising awareness and enhancing access to optimal interdisciplinary care (Fig. 29.2).

Image 29.1 Teen panel at Annual A-BE-C conference

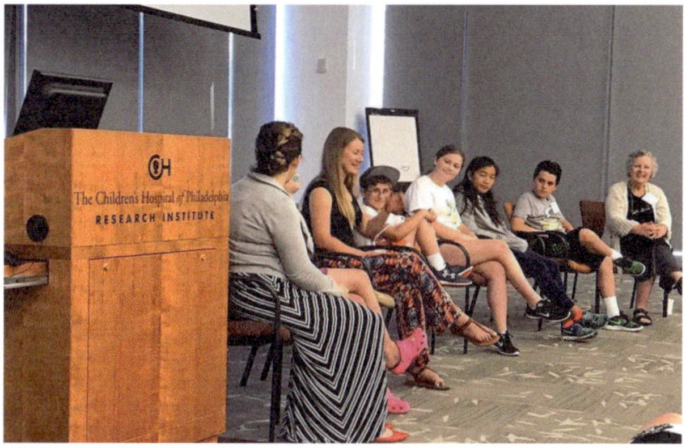

Peer Support

It is understood that individuals with chronic illnesses benefit from being introduced to one another to create a sense of community and reduce feelings of isolation [14]. Mentorship and peer-to-peer consultation may enhance the individual's self-determination, self-directed advocacy, and motivation to seek medical care and pursue their academic, career, and social goals. These peer support options are available locally, nationally, and internationally within the BEEC community. The use of internet-based communication has undoubtedly increased access and networking. There are many informal social media support groups that are age and disease specific and directed to BEEC patients and families. A-BE-C directed events and annual conferences, hospital-oriented groups, and summer camps provide opportunities for those with BEEC and their families to meet one another (Image 29.1).

Local Support Groups

Hospital institutions have begun prioritizing peer support and patient-family advisory committees to extrapolate the strength and benefit of the community itself as a valuable partner. These formal support groups and activities allow families to share their knowledge and experience, and provide emotional support around various challenges faced (medical decision-making, coping with major surgeries, disclosure, navigating the school setting, etc.) [15]. Furthermore, local support groups are also created by the patients and families themselves as separate entities that act as informal support networks. Parent-parent, parent-affected adult, and teen-affected adult are a few variations of beneficial support arrangements that can have lasting effects on a family's experience navigating the management of BEEC. These support networks exist in many countries throughout the world (see Fig. 29.3) and are

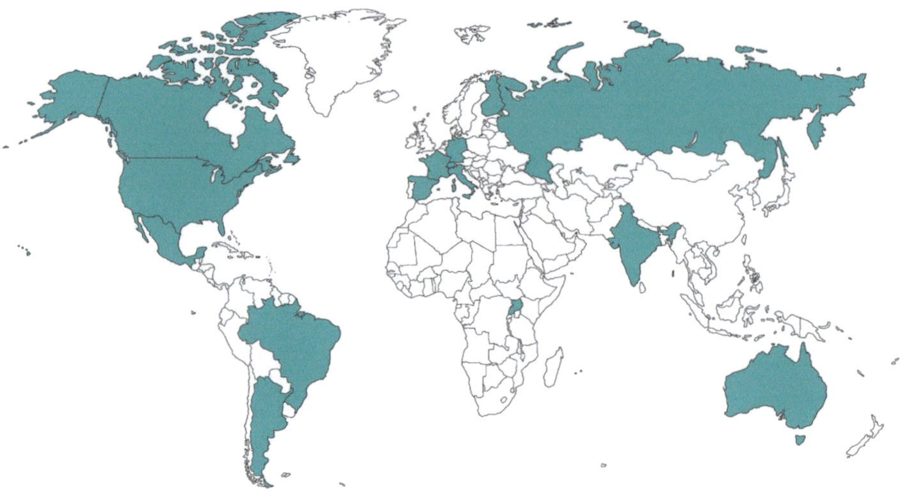

Fig. 29.3 Map of support groups for BEEC

primarily web-based. However, often these groups have in-person meetings when possible. The majority of these groups are also integrated into the A-BE-C global network, and communication is transferred back and forth to share ideas, activities, care opportunities, and emotional support.

Summer Camps for Youth

The opportunity to meet others with BEEC and similar conditions may alter a child's perspective and ease a caregiver's anxiety and fears. The ability to see an adult or older teen with BEEC thriving in their psychological health, academics, career, intimate relationships, athletics/sports, etc. is a major benefit of peer support. This support can be accessed via summer camps like Youth Rally (www.youthrally.org) and Ostomy Canada Youth Camp (www.ostomycanada.ca), which are available to pre-teens and teens regardless of financial status, citizenship, etc. [16, 17]. Counselors with similar conditions provide guidance, support, encouragement, mentorship, and an adult example of resilience and determination. In turn, the motivation to become a counselor and explore altruism in adulthood for the younger generation may motivate the younger, struggling, and insecure child with BEEC to improve their independence and social skills. The community-oriented aspect of these camps encourages compassion, unity, and togetherness, thus reducing isolation and loneliness. The therapeutic aspect of summer camp can be easily promoted by medical teams and advocates for the BEEC community. Local summer camps, teen retreats, or day camp opportunities for chronic illnesses in general or provided by your urology team/hospital also provide opportunities for community, peer support, and informal education.

A-BE-C Initiatives and Opportunities

Collaborating with a team of dedicated parents and patients, international exstrophy experts, and dedicated pediatric and adult urologists, the A-BE-C supports all those affected by BEEC. A-BE-C provides parents, caregivers, and persons living with bladder exstrophy tools and resources to help manage their condition throughout their lifetime by providing awareness, education, advocacy, and ongoing support to help navigate the medical and psychosocial issues.

Centers of Excellence

The diagnosis of bladder exstrophy, cloacal exstrophy, and epispadias can be isolating and overwhelming for caregivers. The ability to find specialized care quickly and easily is important for these rare conditions. Many primary care physicians, gynecologists, and obstetricians have never heard of the BEEC diagnoses. Awareness and education can help bridge the gap between provider and patient, removing barriers of isolation and fear. A-BE-C, after consultations with leading BEEC experts volunteering on the organization's advisory committee, established a Centers of Excellence program in 2018 to identify comprehensive care centers dedicated to BEEC. BEEC programs based at children's hospitals throughout the world apply to be considered a Center of Excellence and are required to meet criteria exemplifying their experience, commitment, and interdisciplinary programming. A peer review selection process ensues where the BEEC Advisory Committee reviews and selects applications for designation.The availability of designated Centers of Excellence, which are shared on the organization's webpage, then supports caregivers of children born with BEEC in finding accurate information and expert treatment [10].

Medical Advisory Council

Families have support and guidance from many of the world's experts in the treatment and management of BEEC through A-BE-C's dedicated medical advisory council, which includes surgeons, nurses, and psychosocial specialists. These specialists collaborate with A-BE-C to promote education about living with BEEC through workshops, educational webinars, and patient and physician panels. These medical advisory council members collaborate with A-BE-C to create free online resources such as downloadable handouts, videos, and books related to BEEC [10].

US-Based Initiatives: Policy and Legislation

A-BE-C is 1 of 30 patient and physician advocacy organizations that work to advance awareness and education about bladder health through the Urology Care Foundation Bladder Health Alliance [18]. Recognizing that millions of Americans suffer from a variety of bladder health conditions such as BEEC, the alliance secured House and Senate resolutions supporting the designation of November as "National Bladder Health Month" in the United States. Resolution 604 recognizes that those affected by bladder conditions have a significant impact on their health and quality of the life, which could lead to depression, social isolation, and loss of self-esteem, and supports the critically underfunded need for medical and behavioral research to better understand and treat bladder conditions [19].

Annual Conferences

For one weekend every summer (month of June or July), A-BE-C, in partnership with Center of Excellence designees, joins families and healthcare providers to offer an opportunity to share experiences, knowledge, and support around BEEC. Each year's conference strives to unite families to build community and provide the latest medical information. As the conference is held in North America, most attendees come from all over the United States and Canada. However, as the A-BE-C community is global, all of those affected by BEEC around the globe are welcome and encouraged to attend. These conferences allow for a special opportunity for individuals with BEEC to share their stories and meet specialized medical professionals who can guide them on their exstrophy journey (Image 29.2).

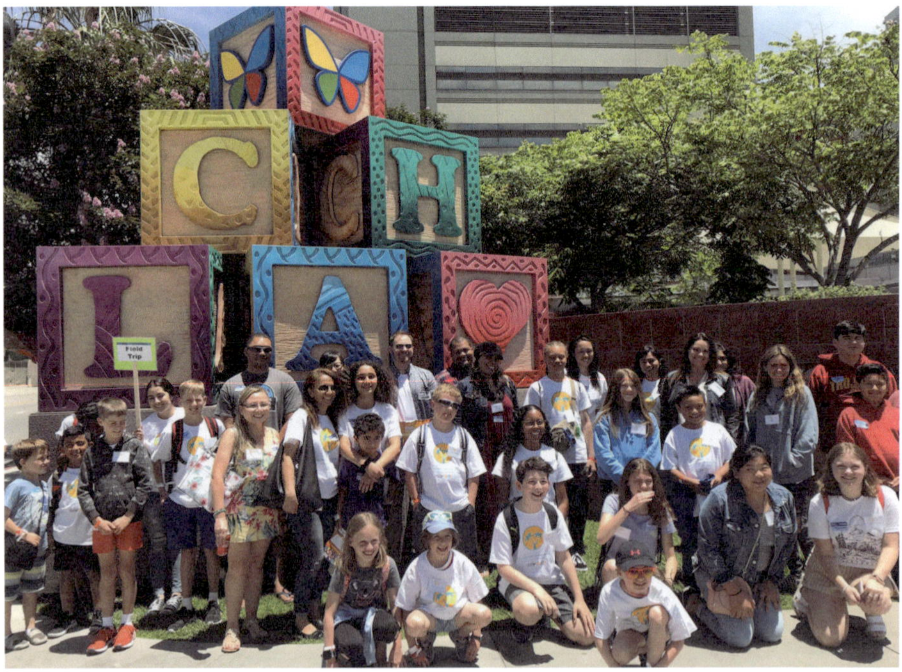

Image 29.2 Annual A-BE-C conference

Global Health Inequities

Pediatric urology is still in its early infancy as an independent specialty in many areas of the world. The need for fellowship-trained pediatric urologists working exclusively for children is paradoxically most acute where the need is the greatest. This deficit has resulted in a volume of children worldwide in urgent need of complex surgical reconstruction that would lead to quantifiable improvements in health, productivity, reduced healthcare expenditure, and quality of life. Providing points of access to quality healthcare from centers that are demographically large but deficient in pediatric surgical expertise remains a massive unmet need. To complicate matters, very few surgeons worldwide are qualified to treat children with BEEC. As a result, these children are often abandoned, left untreated, or multiple attempted repairs are unsuccessful.

Global Health Initiatives

A-BE-C volunteers, global partners, and its medical advisory council members facilitate care and consultation to reduce gaps in global health inequities and enhance outcomes. The A-BE-C prioritizes the following global health initiatives to address these challenges (Fig. 29.4).

The US-India Bladder Exstrophy Collaborative commenced in 2009 as a consortium bringing together leading US and Canada-based children's hospitals partnering with one of the largest public hospitals in Asia—the Civil Hospital-Ahmedabad that serves as the tertiary safety-net hospital for a state with a population of 60 million [20]. [This collaboration is detailed elsewhere in this compendium.] Patients from the region with BEEC receive the full spectrum of care with international and Indian surgeons during this workshop and are provided education, peer support, and

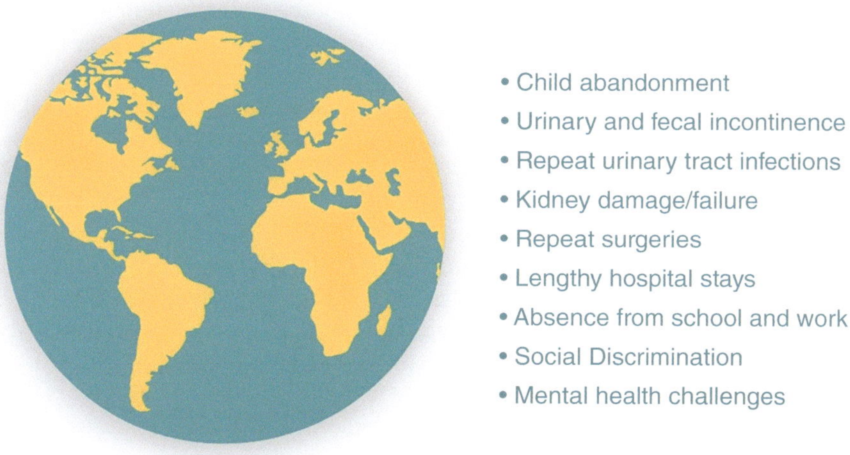
• Child abandonment
• Urinary and fecal incontinence
• Repeat urinary tract infections
• Kidney damage/failure
• Repeat surgeries
• Lengthy hospital stays
• Absence from school and work
• Social Discrimination
• Mental health challenges

Fig. 29.4 Priorities of global health initiatives

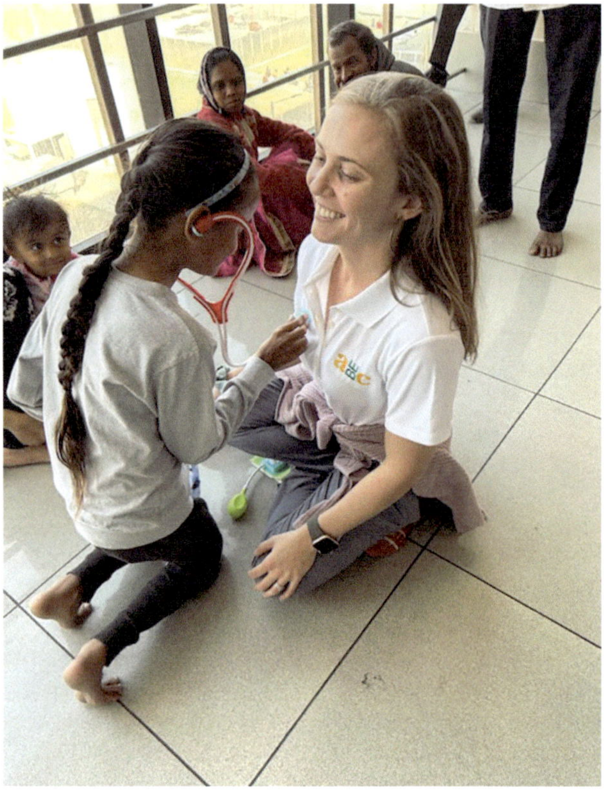

Image 29.3 Affected adult/social worker provides medical play at India workshop

advocacy interventions in addition to their surgical or medical interventions (Image 29.3). The A-BE-C partners with the Collaboration to facilitate travel for some children with BEEC and their responsible surgeons from many parts of South Asia, Central Asia, and Africa to travel to India during the Collaboration date to receive care while providing crucial training to the accompanying surgeons. A-BE-C also has an initiative in the sub-Saharan country of Uganda, which prioritizes care for children and adults in that region while cross-training surgeons, nurses, social workers, and patient advocates. In addition to life-changing surgical interventions, the organization's role is to facilitate peer support sessions covering topics such as coping with differences, negotiating peer and family situations, managing discrimination and bullying, and school advocacy. A-BE-C volunteers provide medical play with the children (see Image 29.4) to ease the families' fears and utilize teaching dolls to enhance their health literacy and improve coping and self-efficacy.

The (A-BE-C) network chain attempts to create a lifeline for families and children with BEEC worldwide. A portion of the organization's fundraising efforts are dedicated to transporting individuals, their families, and their local doctors to travel to International Centers of Excellence for treatment and training, respectively. As many children with BEEC are abandoned by their parents and experience

Image 29.4 Bunji, a teaching doll with A-BE-C volunteers

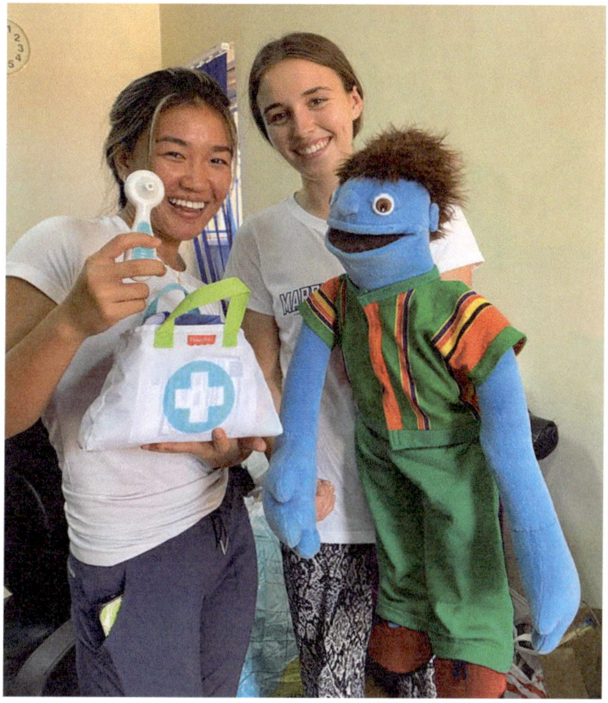

discrimination and bullying from their peers due to ignorance of BEEC, the A-BE-C provides education and psychosocial interventions to empower families to advocate for the rights of their children.

Advocacy Considerations

Adult Care for BEEC

In the past, many patients with classic bladder exstrophy, the most common presentation of the exstrophy-epispadias complex, had poor surgical outcomes. Previous generations (depending on severity, which varies per person) had lower survival rates and poorer quality of life due to limited surgical knowledge, surgical success, uncertain longevity of reparative procedures and consequences, and less technology. The primary focus was on pediatrics (infants, young children, adolescents, and their parents), treated in the pediatric urology setting due to the onset of condition severity at birth. However, the thriving and growing "adults with exstrophy" population in the United States and worldwide has needs that differ significantly from the pediatric population.

Adult urologists familiar with this population's complex surgical procedures and their complications are essential for adulthood, as urinary and reproductive function remains a lifelong struggle. Additionally, adult providers may need more familiarity with issues specific to this population, such as reconstructive surgeries and their complications. The increasing patient workload of adult urology providers due to an aging American population is another competitor to the transition of some of the more complicated urologic conditions. Adults with exstrophy are often turned away for care from adult urologists and have nowhere to go for treatment. The A-BE-C is contacted in these situations where the adult needs assistance advocating for themselves and navigating the system to identify care. Appropriate transitional arrangements to adult care must be made to ensure this is achieved. A-BE-C's *Center of Excellence* transition models support early introduction to the adult provider. This can be accomplished in a joint clinic where adult and pediatric providers are present [21].

Patient-Directed Research

Centers of Excellence use the A-BE-C network to recruit study participants. The A-BE-C helps promote patient-centered studies in these collaborative efforts [22]. Social media is, in turn, used to improve patient outcomes and empower those with BEEC to be actively involved in the progression of care. Most BEEC research to date is focused on surgical outcomes and clinician-derived research priorities. There are few patient-reported studies or patient-generated or patient-directed research on the adult exstrophy community's needs from their healthcare providers. In 2018, the A-BE-C began a new initiative to better meet the needs of a growing adult population with bladder exstrophy. The organization contacted their young adult and adult population with a survey and individual interviews to understand what adults with exstrophy need from their providers. Comprehensive care of young adult and adult patients fell into seven (6) major categories: teens and puberty, maintenance of childhood revisions and diversions, adulthood health maintenance, men's and women's health, psychosocial concerns, and effective self-advocacy as an adult [21].

Patient Advisory Councils

A-BE-C's patient advocacy strategy is grounded in a patient-centered perspective that improves independence, empowerment, and healthcare accessibility for BEEC patients. This multi-level approach provides patients and families with the support, education, tools, mentorship, and peer-to-peer connection to improve their quality of life. To better address this aim, the A-BE-C has several new patient advocacy initiatives, including establishing a Patient Advisory Council in 2023. The first step to enhancing patient advocacy strategy is learning the needs of BEEC patients and understanding the specific issues and challenges they face. A thorough needs assessment and ongoing consultation and collaboration are meant to improve the self-advocacy skills of those affected by BEEC while simultaneously improving clinical care standards based on the prioritized needs defined by those affected by BEEC.

Conclusion

Due to medical advancements and improved social awareness regarding difference and disability, individuals with BEEC are living longer with improved quality of life. The importance of early intervention, proper surgical management, and prioritizing a positive relationship with a medical team is paramount. Lifelong follow-up regarding continence, voiding efficiency, kidney health, sexual health, psychosocial needs, and other urological complications is mandatory. Thus, the focus on advocacy interventions along the lifespan, such as peer support, may effectively enhance self-advocacy later in life. Positive long-term outcomes can be achieved for the BEEC population when adequate support is provided, adequate access to care/education/employment is granted, and the individual with BEEC is provided respect and dignity as a primary team member capable of self-advocacy.

References

1. Jayachandran D, Bythell M, Platt MW, Rankin J. Register based study of bladder exstrophy-epispadias complex: prevalence, associated anomalies, prenatal diagnosis and survival. J Urol. 2011;186:2056–60.
2. Apple RW. Children and adolescents coping with chronic illness and disability. Int J Child Adolesc Health. 2017;10:495–508.
3. Deans R, Liao L, Wood D, Woodhouse C, Creighton SM. Sexual function and health-related quality of life in women with classic bladder exstrophy. BJU Int. 2015;115:633–8. https://doi.org/10.1111/bju.12811.
4. Dellenmark-Blom M, Sjöström S, Abrahamsson K, Holmdahl G. Health-related quality of life among children, adolescents, and adults with bladder exstrophy-epispadias complex: a systematic review of the literature and recommendations for future research. Qual Life Res. 2019;28:1389–412. https://doi.org/10.1007/s11136-019-02119-7.
5. Baird AD. Exstrophy in the adolescent and young adult population. Semin Pediatr Surg. 2011;20:109–12. https://doi.org/10.1053/j.sempedsurg.2010.12.006.
6. Pennison MC, Mednick L, Rosoklija I, Grant R, Price D, Huang L, Ziniel S, Borer JG. Health related quality of life in patients with bladder exstrophy: a call for targeted interventions. J Urol. 2014;191:1553–7. https://doi.org/10.1016/j.juro.2013.09.089.
7. Holmdahl G, Dellenmark-Blom M, Nordenskjöld A, Sjöström S. Health-related quality of life in patients with the bladder exstrophy-epispadias complex and relationship to incontinence and sexual factors: a review of the recent literature. Eur J Pediatr Surg. 2020;30:251–60. https://doi.org/10.1055/s-0040-1713178.
8. Haddad E, Hayes L, Price D, Vallery C, Somers M, Borer J. Ensuring our exstrophy-epispadias patients and families thrive: multidisciplinary and integrated psychosocial services. J Pediatr Nephrol. 2023;
9. Selanders L, Crane PC. The voice of florence nightingale on advocacy. Online J Issue Nurs. 2012;17:1.
10. Association for the Bladder Exstrophy Community (A-BE-C). 2022. www.bladderexstrophy.com. Accessed 1 Nov 2023.
11. Murrey M, Kratz L. Chapter 1: Introduction. In: Living with bladder exstrophy: a book for families. Wake Forest: Association for the Bladder Exstrophy Community; 1996.
12. Anderson DL, Murray CD, Hurrell R. Experiences of intimacy among people with bladder exstrophy. Qual Health Res. 2013;23:1600–12. https://doi.org/10.1177/1049732313509409.

13. Lee C, Reutter HM, Grässer MF, Fisch M, Noeker M. Gender-associated differences in the psychosocial and developmental outcome in patients affected with the bladder exstrophy-epispadias complex. BJU Int. 2006;97:349–53. https://doi.org/10.1111/j.1464-410x.2005.05910.x.
14. Kaufman N. Peer-to-peer support helps people improve their chronic condition therapy outcomes. Canary Health Chronic Disease Programs; 2022. https://www.canaryhealth.com/peer-to-peer-support-imporves-chronic-condition-therapy-neal-author/. Accessed 9 Jan 2023
15. Price D, Grant R, Anderson L. I don't believe everyone here has bladder exstrophy: one hospital's experience with support group services. Dialogues Pediatr Urol. 2016;37:5–6.
16. Youth Rally Sumner Camp. 2023. www.youthrally.org. Accessed 1 Nov 2023.
17. Ostomy Canada Society. Ostomy Camp Canada. 2023. www.ostomycanada.ca. Accessed 1 Nov 2023.
18. Urology Care Foundation. (2023). www.urologyhealth.org. Accessed 1 November 2023.
19. Senate Resolution 604. National Bladder Month; 2016. https://www.govinfo.gov. Accessed 1 Nov 2023.
20. Joshi RS, Shrivastava D, Grady R, Kundu A, Ramji J, Reddy PP, Pippi-Salle JL, Frazier JR, Canning DA, Shukla AR. A model for sustained collaboration to address the unmet global burden of bladder exstrophy-epispadias complex and penopubic epispadias: the international bladder exstrophy consortium. JAMA Surg. 2018;153:618–24. https://doi.org/10.1001/jamasurg.2018.0067.
21. Artigas P. What adults need. AUA News 27.5. 2022:19.
22. Rowe CK, et al. Using social media for patient-reported outcomes: a study of genital appearance and sexual function in adult bladder exstrophy patients. J Pediatr Urol. 2018;14(4):322.e1–6.

Index

A. R. Shukla, R. S. Joshi (eds.), *Bladder Exstrophy and Epispadias*, https://doi.org/10.1007/978-3-031-91238-2

D

P

MIX
Papier aus verantwortungsvollen Quellen
Paper from responsible sources
FSC® C105338

If you have any concerns about our products,
you can contact us on
ProductSafety@springernature.com

In case Publisher is established outside the EU,
the EU authorized representative is:
Springer Nature Customer Service Center GmbH
Europaplatz 3, 69115 Heidelberg, Germany

Printed by Libri Plureos GmbH
in Hamburg, Germany